BIOLOGY OF THE
UTERUS
Second Edition

BIOLOGY OF THE UTERUS

UTERUS

Second Edition

Edited by

RALPH M. WYNN, M.D.

Professor, Departments of Obstetrics & Gynecology
and Anatomy & Cell Biology
Wayne State University School of Medicine
Detroit, Michigan

and

WILLIAM P. JOLLIE, Ph.D.

Professor and Chairman, Department of Anatomy
Medical College of Virginia
Virginia Commonwealth University
Richmond, Virginia

PLENUM MEDICAL BOOK COMPANY
NEW YORK AND LONDON

Library of Congress Cataloging in Publication Data

Biology of the uterus / edited by Ralph M. Wynn and William P. Jollie. — 2nd ed.
     p.   cm.
   Includes bibliographies and index.
   ISBN 0-306-43057-6
   1. Uterus. I. Wynn, Ralph M. II. Jollie, William P.
   [DNLM: 1. Uterus — anatomy & histology. 2. Uterus — physiology. WP 400 B615]
QP265.B543   1989
599′.016 — dc19
DNLM/DLC   89-3540
for Library of Congress   CIP

The previous edition of this work was published by Plenum Press in
1977 under the title *Biology of the Uterus*. That volume, in turn,
was a revision of *Cellular Biology of the Uterus,* published by
Appleton-Century-Crofts in 1967.

© 1989, 1977, 1967 Plenum Publishing Corporation
233 Spring Street, New York, N.Y. 10013

Plenum Medical Book Company is an imprint of Plenum Publishing Corporation

Printed in the United States of America

Contributors

L. L. Anderson
Department of Animal Science
Iowa State University
Ames, Iowa 50011

John D. Aplin
Departments of Obstetrics and
Gynaecology, Biochemistry, and
Molecular Biology
University of Manchester
Manchester M13 0JK, England

Christine Bergeron
Departments of Pathology and
Obstetrics and Gynecology
McGill University and
The Sir Mortimer B. Davis Jewish
General Hospital
Montreal, Quebec H3T 1E2,
Canada

W. C. Cole
Division of Cardiovascular Sciences
St. Boniface Research Institute
Department of Physiology
University of Manitoba
Winnipeg, Manitoba R2H 2AG,
Canada

Allen C. Enders
Department of Human Anatomy
University of California School of
Medicine
Davis, California 95616

Alex Ferenczy
Departments of Pathology and
Obstetrics and Gynecology
McGill University and
The Sir Mortimer B. Davis Jewish
General Hospital
Montreal, Quebec H3T 1E2,
Canada

R. E. Garfield
Departments of Neurosciences and
Obstetrics and Gynecology
McMaster University, Health
Sciences
Hamilton, Ontario L8N 3Z5,
Canada

Randall L. Given
Department of Anatomy and
Neurosciences
University of Texas Medical
Branch
Galveston, Texas 77550

Frank C. Greiss, Jr.
Department of Obstetrics and
Gynecology
Bowman Gray School of Medicine
of Wake Forest University
Winston-Salem, North Carolina
27103

CONTRIBUTORS

Gabor Huszar
Department of Obstetrics and
Gynecology
Yale University School of Medicine
New Haven, Connecticut 06510

C. Y. Kao
Department of Pharmacology
State University of New York
Downstate Medical Center
Brooklyn, New York 11203

Wendell W. Leavitt
Departments of Biochemistry and
Obstetrics and Gynecology
Texas Tech University Health
Sciences Center
Lubbock, Texas 79430

Harland W. Mossman
Department of Anatomy
University of Wisconsin-Madison
Madison, Wisconsin 53706

A. I. Musah
Department of Animal Science
Iowa State University
Ames, Iowa 50011

Ronan O'Rahilly
Carnegie Laboratories of
Embryology
California Primate Research Center
Davis, California 95616

Helen A. Padykula
Department of Cell Biology
University of Massachusetts
Medical School
Worcester, Massachusetts 01655

Earl L. Parr
Department of Anatomy
School of Medicine
Southern Illinois University
Carbondale, Illinois 62901

Margaret B. Parr
Department of Anatomy
School of Medicine
Southern Illinois University
Carbondale, Illinois 62901

Elizabeth M. Ramsey
Department of Embryology
Carnegie Institution of Washington
Baltimore, Maryland 21210

James C. Rose
Departments of Physiology and
Obstetrics and Gynecology
Bowman Gray School of Medicine
of Wake Forest University
Winston-Salem, North Carolina
27103

Melvyn S. Soloff
Department of Biochemistry
Medical College of Ohio
Toledo, Ohio 43699

Michael P. Walsh
Department of Medical
Biochemistry
University of Calgary
Calgary, Alberta T2N 4N1, Canada

Ralph M. Wynn
Departments of Obstetrics and
Gynecology and Anatomy and
Cell Biology
Wayne State University School of
Medicine
Detroit, Michigan 48201

Preface

Almost a quarter of a century has elapsed since *Cellular Biology of the Uterus,* the predecessor of the present volume, was planned. During that period, especially in the decade since the publication of the last edition of *Biology of the Uterus,* new information in the field has been so voluminous as to require major revisions of most of the chapters, the addition of several new chapters, and the collaboration of a second editor to facilitate the selection of appropriate experts as authors. As in prior editions, a balance has been struck between classical biology and modern biochemistry and biophysics. The inclusion of basic histological and embryological information provides a necessary, though often lacking, background for the protein chemist and molecular biologist and a bridge between the cell biologist and clinician. Thus, major practical problems in human reproduction, such as the genesis of endometrial carcinoma and the cause of the initiation of labor, may be approached on a firm scientific footing.

The current edition deals primarily with the biology of the uterus itself (comparative and human) rather than placentation or pregnancy and thus is a synthesis of data derived from many techniques, both conventional and modern. As it is clearly beyond the competence of any one scientist to prepare such a text on the basis of personal knowledge and experience, the aid of 22 distinguished scientists was enlisted. All of these authors, acknowledged experts in their respective fields, agreed to extensive revisions of their chapters in the previous edition or preparation of entirely new contributions.

A scholarly history of uterine biology has been retained to illustrate the evolution of studies from superstition to speculation to science. The chapters on comparative anatomy and embryology of the human genitourinary tract have been revised by their original authors. It is noteworthy that Dr. Mossman's chapter was prepared on the occasion of that distinguished scientist's 90th birthday. An extensively revised chapter on vascular anatomy and a new chapter on vascular physiology of the uterus, emphasizing the nonpregnant condition, precede the final 12 chapters, which stress cell biology. Comparative embryology of the müllerian derivatives provides the basis for predicting and analyzing the cellular response of the uterus to hormones. The chapters on vascular anatomy and physiology illustrate the dominant role of blood vessels in critical uterine functions such as menstruation and pregnancy, the effects on uterine blood flow of hormones, oxygenation, vasoactive amines, and prostaglandins, and the changes in uterine arteries as they relate to preeclampsia and retardation of intrauterine growth.

Two entirely new complementary chapters on biochemistry and cell biology of the endometrium bridge the gap between morphology and biochemistry and illustrate the crucial role of receptors in endocrine regulation of uterine activity. The cytoskeletal proteins, the biochemistry of the cellular surface, the extracellular matrix, and the secretory components of the endometrium are discussed as they relate to implantation and associated phenomena. The interrelations of the actions of steroid and peptide hormones, receptor status, synthesis of nucleic acids and proteins, and regulation of gene expression are detailed in one of the new pivotal chapters of this edition. The chapter on delayed implantation has been revised and extended to include a discussion of the uterus during early implantation, with detailed data derived from studies of marsupials and several orders of eutherian mammals. Delayed implantation strikingly illustrates the mediation of the developmental rate of one organism (the unimplanted blastocyst) by the internal environment (the uterus) of another. A new chapter on the implantation reaction discusses experimental techniques and hormonal sensitization of the endometrium for implantation. Contributions of electron microscopy to the understanding of several fundamental problems in reproductive biology are well documented. In particular, the role of prostaglandins in the initiation of decidualization and the importance of apoptosis as the mode of cellular death in uterine epithelium are discussed. A short but stimulating chapter on the role of stem cells in the regeneration of the primate uterus presents work currently in progress in the author's laboratory.

The chapter on the human endometrium, which encompasses histology and scanning and transmission electron microscopy, has been expanded to include a detailed discussion of the endometrial vascular changes in normal and hypertensive pregnancies. The information derived from transmission electron microscopy deals with basic problems, such as the origin and significance of the nucleolar channel system and the functions of the decidua, and clinical applications, such as the morphological effects of contraceptives and the cause of menstruation. The morphological correlates of preeclampsia and other abnormal gestational states are illustrated. The chapter on pathology of the endometrium advances the thesis that hyperplasia and neoplasia may have fundamentally different causes in this tissue.

Two of the three chapters dealing with biochemistry, electrophysiology, and ultrastructure of the myometrium are entirely new. The need for collaboration between the electron microscopist and the biochemist in elucidating the contractile mechanism of the myometrium is amply demonstrated. Although much more is known about skeletal muscle than about smooth muscle, the major data concerning the provision of energy and the proteins of the contractile mechanisms of mammalian myometrium are presented. The organelles of smooth muscle are discussed in detail, with particular emphasis placed on the role of gap junctions in myometrial contractility. The chapter on electrophysiology of the myometrium focuses on patterns of ionic distribution and resting potential and their modifications by hormonal and gestational influences. Current experiments dealing with single-cell myometrial preparations are discussed authoritatively in appropriate detail.

The last two chapters, the second of which is entirely new, discuss the uterine regulation of ovarian function and the endocrine control of parturition. Effects of hysterectomy on ovarian function and luteolytic action of the uterus are analyzed. The effects of ovarian and adrenal steroids, prostaglandins, and oxytocin on uterine activity in several species, including man, are discussed. Although the emphasis of the volume as a whole is not on pregnancy, the final chapter is obviously relevant to experimental biologists, endocrinologists, and obstetricians.

Even though each of the chapters is a self-contained unit, which provides a critical review and a comprehensive list of references for the graduate student, the intended interdisciplinary orientation is best achieved by reading the chapters in the order in which they appear. The volume is designed to serve as an introduction for the academic clinician to the scientific foundations of reproductive biology, as a suggestion to the basic scientist of significant applications of uterine biology, and as a bridge between morphologists and pathologists on the one hand and biochemists and physiologists on the other. If new or enhanced interdisciplinary collaboration is stimulated by this volume, the efforts of the authors and the editors will be rewarded.

Detroit, Michigan   Ralph M. Wynn
Richmond, Virginia   William P. Jollie

Contents

4 Vascular Anatomy 57

ELIZABETH M. RAMSEY

5 Vascular Physiology of the Nonpregnant Uterus 69

FRANK C. GREISS, JR., AND JAMES C. ROSE

6 Cellular Biochemistry of the Endometrium 89

JOHN D. APLIN

7   Cell Biology of the Endometrium   131

WENDELL W. LEAVITT

8   The Endometrium of Delayed and Early Implantation   175

RANDALL L. GIVEN AND ALLEN C. ENDERS

9 The Implantation Reaction   233

MARGARET B. PARR AND EARL L. PARR

13 Biochemistry of the Myometrium and Cervix 355

GABOR HUSZAR AND MICHAEL P. WALSH

14 Electrophysiological Properties of Uterine Smooth Muscle 403

C. Y. KAO

15 Ultrastructure of the Myometrium 455

W. C. COLE AND R. E. GARFIELD

16 Uterine Control of Ovarian Function 505

L. L. ANDERSON AND A. I. MUSAH

17   Endocrine Control of Parturition   559

MELVYN S. SOLOFF

Index   609

History

ELIZABETH M. RAMSEY

Our present knowledge of uterine structure and function has been achieved, slowly and laboriously, over the course of many centuries. Only bit by bit have facts emerged through the obscuring mists of superstition, tradition, and speculation.

Since the human uterus, at least in its gross anatomy, is not a particularly complicated organ, one may wonder why anyone who had once held a uterus in his hand and perhaps made a simple sagittal section through it would have failed to grasp its pattern. That of course is the crux of the matter. The early physicians did not hold the uterus in their hands; many never even set eyes on one. Religion and law both forbade dissection of human bodies until surprisingly recent times, and all concepts of reproductive tract anatomy were based on findings in animals. Since most of the animals observed had duplex or bicornuate uteri, extrapolation to the human produced many erroneous and bizarre theories.

1. Greece

In tracing the development of medical concepts, it is customary to begin with the Golden Age of Greece. This is an appropriate starting place for consideration of the history of the uterus, too. What then is to be found on this subject in the Hippocratic Corpus, which embodies the thought of the great Father of Medicine and his contemporaries in the fourth century B.C.? At that time, the uterus was believed to consist of a number of cavities exhibiting angulations and horns, its lining studded with "tentacles" or "suckers." Tubes and ovaries were not identified or even mentioned. On the other hand, external portions of the reproductive tract that were accessible to inspection, the perineum, the vagina, the cervical os, and the labia, were carefully noted and described in terms still recognizable.

The extensive studies of Aristotle fell within the same period. We tend to think of Aristotle as a philosopher rather than a scientist, but in classical times learned men were versed

ELIZABETH M. RAMSEY ● Department of Embryology, Carnegie Institution of Washington, Baltimore, Maryland 21210.

in all fields of knowledge, and Aristotle was the greatest biologist of his era. His studies dealt exclusively with animals, and he frankly stated that he knew nothing of the reproductive tract of man. His concept of the uterus as bicornuate was arrived at by analogy with the animals he had studied, and so too was his concept of ''cotyledons'' within the uterus, similar to those of cattle (cf. the Hippocratic ''tentacles''). Unfortunately, Aristotle's drawings of the reproductive organs have been lost, for we may be sure that they would tell us a great deal about his ideas. An example of his careful and perceptive work survives in a sketch of a dogfish embryo attached to the maternal brood pouch. In it, incidentally, we can see a striking similarity to the condition of the mammalian embryo *in utero*. Aristotle's research in an indirectly related field, that of the development of the chick embryo, should be mentioned because it laid the basis for embryological investigation for centuries to come. Subsequently, as other types of embryos became available for study, investigators used the classic chick terminology to describe them, often causing confusion, some of which persists to our day.

2. Alexandria

When the torch of intellectual eminence passed from Greece to Alexandria in Egypt around the beginning of the Christian era, many Greek physicians journeyed to that great center. Here, for a time, dissection of human bodies was permitted, specifically those of executed criminals. The trio consisting of Herophilus of Chalcedon and Rufus and Soranus, both of Ephesus,

Table 1. Chronology

Century	Practitioner	Birth and death (active)	Place of birth; training; activity
B.C.			
Fourth	Hippocrates	460–377	Greece
	Aristotle	384–322	Greece
	Herophilus of Chalcedon	(300)	Greece; Alexandria; Rome
A.D.			
First	Rufus of Ephesus	(98–117)	Greece; Alexandria; Rome
Second	Soranus of Ephesus	(110)	Greece; Alexandria; Rome
	Galen	130–?200	Pergamon; Asia Minor; Alexandria; Rome
Ninth to 12th	School of Salerno		
14th	Mondino dei Luzzi	1275–?	Italy
15th	Leonardo da Vinci	1452–1519	Italy
	Berengario da Carpi	?1480–1550	Italy
16th	Vesalius	1514–1564	Brussels; Louvain and Paris; Padua
	Colombo da Cremona	1516–1559	Italy
	Eustachio	1520–1574	Italy
	Fallopio da Modena	1523–1562	Italy
17th	William Harvey	1578–1657	England; Cambridge and Padua; London
	Marcello Malpighi	1628–1694	Italy
	Regnier de Graaf	1641–1673	Holland
18th	Caspar Friedrich Wolff	1733–1794	Germany
	John and William Hunter	(1774)	England
19th	Johannes Peter Müller	1801–1858	Germany
20th	Hitschmann and Adler	(1908)	Germany
	Robert Schroeder	(1930)	Germany

characterizes this era (Table 1). The first two continued the tradition of a bicornuate uterus but identified uterine tubes as separate entities. Herophilus thought that the tubes entered the urinary bladder, but Rufus corrected this misconception. Both identified the ovary but were unaware of its function. Rufus modified earlier opinions of the shape of the uterus by describing it as similar to a "cupping vessel," and he differentiated a fundus with two cornua from the cervix, and both from the vagina.

Soranus, who was especially cognizant and appreciative of his indebtedness to earlier workers and in his own turn profoundly influenced his successors until well into the 16th century, reminds us how knowledge and understanding were slowly growing as each successive investigator "stood upon the shoulders" of his predecessors. Soranus' *Gynecology* was one of the great works of the early Christian centuries (available to us in a fine translation by Owsei Temkin of the Johns Hopkins Department of Medical History). Although it deals chiefly with the clinical matters of Soranus' primary interest, it does incorporate the findings of his anatomic studies. The work is not illustrated, but a drawing in a ninth-century manuscript depicts the uterus as Soranus conceived it (Fig. 1). Shaped like a cupping vessel, as Rufus said, it has recognizable parts with modern names. Internally, Soranus described "two folds" in the fundus of nulliparae that disappear when the uterine cavity becomes "rounded and stretched" in pregnancy. Despite many progressive opinions, Soranus entertained some curious misconceptions. Thus, he considered the cervix of girls before puberty to have a spongy consistency similar to the lungs and agreed with Herophilus that the tubes enter the urinary bladder (perhaps a confusion with the round ligaments?). He supported Aristotle's idea of

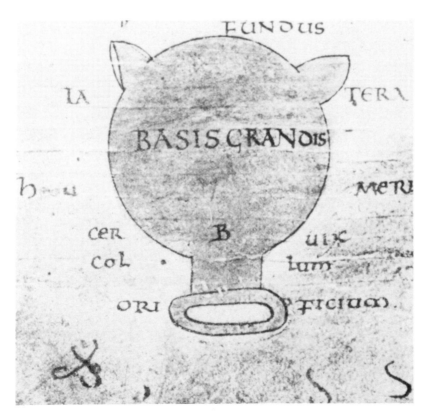

Figure 1. Earliest known representation of the anatomy of the uterus. It embodies Soranus' conception of the organ and appears in a Muscio text of the ninth century. From Weindler (1908). Courtesy of the National Library of Medicine, Bethesda, MD.

cotyledons, regarding the nipplelike projections as provisions for intrauterine suckling to accustom the fetus to a function in which he would need to be proficient at birth. Soranus advanced the understanding of the function of the ovary to some degree but called the organ a female testis. His successors copied him in this idea down to the 17th century. The *Gynecology* is particularly distinguished by its tone of dispassionate objectivity. Soranus fought against superstition and espoused rationalism; he assailed many inherited and contemporary opinions but without rancor; his clinical histories were refreshingly clear in an age of verbosity and circumlocution. Indeed, they often sound more like the 19th than the second century A.D.

3. Rome

Following the decline of Alexandria as an intellectual center in the first century of the Christian era, Rome became the lodestone for physicians as well as for other men of learning. The life and work of Galen may be regarded as spanning the period of this shift and as, in many ways, forming Rome's finest and most typical product.

Galen did not have Soranus' special interest in gynecology, but his treatises included observations on all aspects of the human body and its normal and pathological function, so that the reproductive tract received a share of his attention. As far as the uterus is concerned, he adopted the opinions of two of his predecessors: Rufus' belief that the tubes are connected with the uterus rather than the urinary bladder, and Aristotle's belief that the endometrial surface is cotyledonary. But to each he made additions of his own: to Rufus' that the tubes have large, patent lumina through which the ova are conducted to the uterine cavity, and to Aristotle's that the vessels supplying menstrual blood open into the crypts of the cotyledons. The animal background of his work led to the opinion that the uterus is multilocular—this although the monkey was one of the animal species he investigated.

The great name of Galen was perhaps too great, for slavish adherence to his opinions stultified progress for more than 1000 years after his death. "According to Galen" or "as Galen said" provided the final word on all aspects of medical science and clinical practice throughout the Middle Ages.

During the period of the Roman Empire, gynecology was an important facet of medical practice, but the invention of surgical instruments and the elaboration of operative techniques were of greater interest than the investigation of morphology and physiology. This preoccupation with practicalities was characteristic of the mode of Roman thought and was paralleled by the fact that organization of the hospital system was Rome's greatest contribution to medicine in general.

When Rome in its turn declined, there developed an active and considerable body of Byzantine medicine in Constantinople. However, it was neither original nor creative but was grounded in the study of ancient documents. In gynecology the major name we remember is that of Oribasius, who dealt almost exlusively with clinical practice, as did his colleagues.

4. The "Dark Ages"

Throughout Europe the millennium following Galen's death, properly designated the Middle Ages, fully merits its more usual title, the "Dark Ages." The eager enthusiasm, the creative curiosity, the humanism of Greece and Alexandria were gone, replaced by dusty scholasticism and blind dependence on "the authorities." These attitudes were not confined to scientists, of course. In the broad field of philosophy, which covered a multitude of disciplines, "according to Aristotle" was as decisive an answer to all inquiries as "according to Galen" was in medicine. The writings of earlier scientists were copied, revised, interpreted, quoted (and often misquoted) in thousands of volumes. The practice of medicine, guided by inherited dicta, was of greater interest than investigation of its anatomic and physiological bases.

The influence of Arabic medicine, reaching Europe at this time via Spain, gave added impetus to scholasticism and traditionalism. Scientific medicine was little advanced by the infusion, and gynecological knowledge hardly at all.

In one spot the old spark was kept alive during the dark centuries. At Salerno in Sicily, inquiring spirits congregated, and some advances were made—few, however, in the field of human reproduction. For the most part, even here, the era witnessed elaboration of inherited theories and opinions, particularly the theory of the multicompartmented uterus. The old magic number seven was the most favored one, and particularly approved was the fanciful idea that male embryos develop in the three right-hand cells, females in the left three, and hermaphrodites in the middle one (Fig. 2). The reams of recorded debates on this doctrine are reminiscent, in their heat and involved reasoning, of the discussions that engrossed theologians at the time as to how many angels could dance on the head of a pin! Another popular anatomic belief was that the female reproductive tract is the mirror image of the male: the vagina, a penis turned inside out; the uterus, analogous to the scrotum; and so forth.

None of these theories, of course, was ancestral to present-day knowledge. They are cited only as illustrating the numerous blind alleys along the tortuous path by which that knowledge has been achieved.

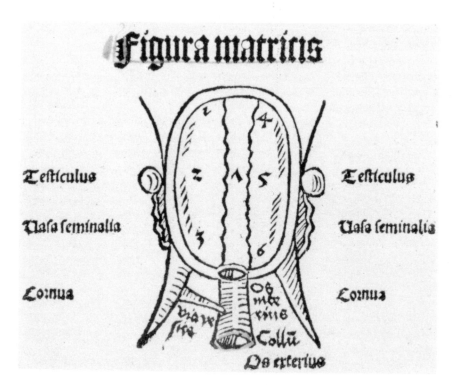

Figure 2. A drawing illustrating the doctrine of the seven-chambered uterus. From Hundt (1501). Courtesy of the National Library of Medicine, Bethesda, MD.

5. *Renaissance*

Although the fall of Constantinople in 1453 is usually accepted as the beginning of the renaissance in Europe, with entry of fresh intellectual air and scientific curiosity, there was, of course, no sharp cutoff date for the Middle Ages. There had been numerous evidences of the "Medical Awakening" long before that specific date. The first founding of universities in the 13th century and their subsequent growth and spread throughout Europe were in no small measure responsible. Most of the universities established medical faculties, and teachers and students proliferated. Slowly, dependence on the ancient authorities waned, particularly as study of the human body commenced. For the latter, the year 1315 may be considered a landmark date, for in that year at the University of Bologna, Mondino dei Luzzi performed the first authorized public dissection of a human body for scientific purposes in modern times.

The burgeoning spirit of the Renaissance in the graphic arts was secondarily reflected in anatomic investigation, an effect both helpful and delightful to us in our present consideration. As never before, medical texts were now illustrated, often by skilled and famous artists. A full series of plates might be assembled describing, without a single word of text, the development of knowledge of the reproductive tract in these centuries. Typical examples in Figs. 3–9 show the feeling for artistic representation as well as for the scientific concepts that the writers wished to show.

Thus, in Mondino's drawing (Fig. 3) we see a uterus with cervix and vagina much as we know it. Tubes and ovaries are not shown, but we do see the lower ends of the vessels thought to convey menstrual blood to the mammary glands, there to be converted into milk in pregnancy. Mondino still believed that the interior of the uterus was divided into compartments, but he introduced the then radically new idea that the organ is fixed and does not migrate in the abdominal cavity, as was previously maintained.

Chronologically, Leonardo da Vinci comes next, and in his famous sketches are reflected the current ideas of his day as well as his own. In the drawing in Fig. 4, ovaries, tubes, and ligaments are depicted. In Fig. 5, the full extent of the uterus-to-breast vessels is clearly shown. The uterus appears to be lobular, though not actually divided, and from the beautiful drawing in Fig. 6 it can be confidently deduced that Leonardo considered the cavity of the pregnant uterus to be single. The very modern appearance of the uterus in this drawing may be compared with that of Rymsdyk's drawing for Hunter (Fig. 11) made nearly 300 years later.

Almost contemporary with Leonardo was Berengario da Carpi, one of whose drawings is reproduced in Fig. 7. Here and in his text Berengario is unequivocal in statement of his belief that the uterus has a single chamber. "Es purum mendacium dicere . . ."—it is a pure lie—to say that the uterus has seven cavities. This statement is reiterated by his equally dogmatic contemporary, Nicola Massa, who expressed it "Decepti sunt etiam . . ."—deceived are they also—who believe that the uterus contains several cells; indeed there is only one. Long years of argument about this matter would thus seem to be definitively terminated, but some years later Dryander published a charmingly naive drawing (Fig. 8) in which a dimple at the fundus of the uterus denotes the presence of a septum dividing the cavity. Old ideas die hard!

With Vesalius we reach one of the high points of Renaissance anatomy. He was born in Brussels, educated at Louvain and Paris, and eventually settled in Padua, and his career demonstrates both the commanding position of Italy at this time and the internationalism of science. The latter feature is reinforced by the record of students flocking to Vesalius' lectures and demonstrations from every country in Europe, including Britain, Poland, and Russia. In 4 years at Padua, on the basis of personally conducted anatomic studies, Vesalius prepared his epoch-making work, *De humani corporis fabrica*. Nothing in anatomic science has been the same since that publication, any more than cosmology has been the same since publication of Copernicus' *De revolutionibus orbium coelstium*. Interestingly, both treatises appeared in the same fateful year, 1543.

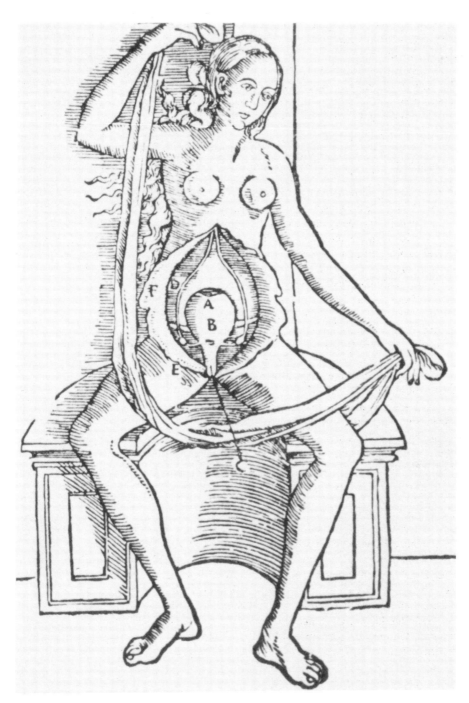

Figure 3. Female genital tract according to Mondino as illustrated in a 1541 German translation of his work. Note indentation at fundus of uterus, indicating compartmentalization. From Mondino dei Luzzi, per J. Dryandrum (1541). Courtesy of the National Library of Medicine, Bethesda, MD.

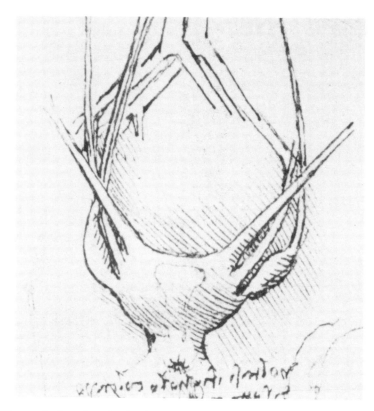

Figure 4. Uterus and adnexa in a drawing by Leonardo da Vinci. From the *Quaderni d'Anatomia* (1513). Courtesy of the National Library of Medicine, Bethesda, MD.

We know that Vesalius dissected the female cadaver; the frontispiece of the *Fabrica* shows him presiding over such a dissection. He was clear about the size and shape of the uterus and about its single cavity, though he agreed with Galen that a septum partly divides it. He corrected opinion as to the shape and course of the adnexa and identified the muscular and decidual layers of the uterine wall. The terms "uterus" and "pelvis" were first used in his treatise, though he still called the ovaries the female testicles (Fig. 9).

Three distinguished pupils of Vesalius carried on the progress that he initiated. Colombo da Cremona described and named the labia and vagina and was the first to record a case of congenital absence of both uterus and vagina. Eustachio studied the vasculature of the whole body, and one illustration in his *Atlas* includes an admirable drawing of the blood vessels of the pelvis (Fig. 10). Fallopio da Modena made the definitive description of the uterine tubes, which we know by his name, though he disclaimed priority, remembering Herophilus' and Rufus' description some 1800 years earlier. Fallopio gave the "aqueous humor of the ovary" its modern name "corpus luteum" and described the hymen and clitoris correctly and noted that it is the integrity of the uterine ligaments that prevents uterine prolapse.

6. Seventeenth to Early Twentieth Centuries

By the end of the 16th century the conditions outlined at the beginning of this brief history had been fulfilled in all essentials. Men had held the human uterus in their hands, had made

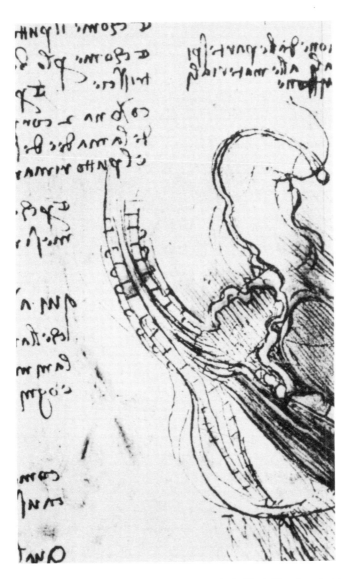

Figure 5. Organs of the female genital tract as drawn by Leonardo da Vinci. The uterus is lobular though not subdivided. The "milk vein" is clearly shown. From the *Quaderni d'Anatomia* (1513). Courtesy of the National Library of Medicine, Bethesda, MD.

sagittal and many other sorts of sections through it, and were clear about its gross morphology. Major attention was turned to other components of the reproductive tract. To consider such important contributions as de Graaff's well-known work on the ovary or Harvey's revolutionary concept, *omne ex ovo* (all life comes from the egg), would carry us too far afield. The placenta, however, is closely enough allied to the uterus to justify a word about the work of John and William Hunter, who settled old problems about its nature and blazed new trails in the understanding of the mechanism whereby it acts as a nutritive and excretory pathway for maternal–fetal exchange. In particular, they scotched the old idea that maternal and fetal vessels are anastomosed end to end in the placenta, rendering the two bloodstreams continuous. They showed conclusively that there is maternal blood in the intervillous space and demonstrated the "curling arteries" of the endometrium (Figs. 11 and 12).

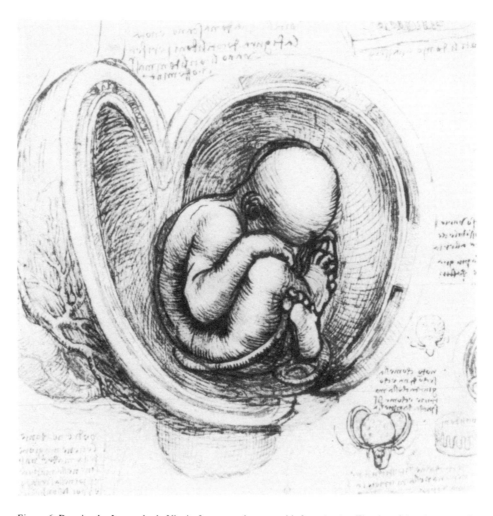

Figure 6. Drawing by Leonardo da Vinci of an opened uterus with fetus *in situ.* The rim of the placenta and a coil of the umbilical cord are seen. From the *Quaderni d'Anatomia* (1513). Courtesy of the National Library of Medicine, Bethesda, MD.

During the same period, study of the embryology and histology of the reproductive tract gained momentum, made possible by the development of a practical microscope and techniques of tissue fixation and staining. The prolonged influence of Aristotle's studies of avian embryology has been mentioned, but with, at first, relatively crude, simple lenses, direct observation of mammalian embryos got under way. The perfected compound microscope came in the 18th century. The primary goal of the early embryological studies was to resolve the conflict between the theories of preformation (''a fully formed embryo exists in the ovary'') and epigenesis (''there is a gradual building up of parts''). Our present knowledge that the latter is in fact the case recognizes the work, among a great many others, of such men as Malpighi, a successor to Mondino in the chair of medicine at Bologna; Wolff, whose name is familiar as the eponym of the mesonephros and mesonephric ducts; and Müller, whose name stands in similar relation to the paramesonephric ducts and therefore in closest possible relation to the uterus itself.

The story of reproductive tract histology was built up rapidly in comparison with the long history of gross anatomy from the time of Hippocrates to, say, Vesalius. The 19th and early

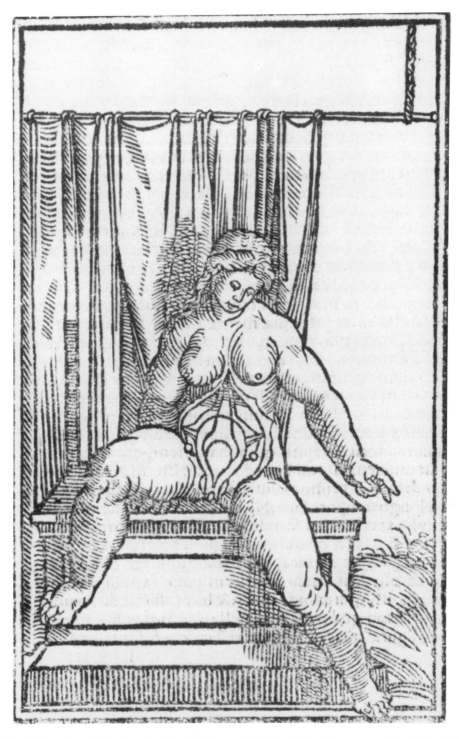

Figure 7. Female genital tract as illustrated by Berengario da Carpi. Note clear representation of the single cavity in the uterus. From Berengario (1521). Courtesy of the National Library of Medicine, Bethesda, MD.

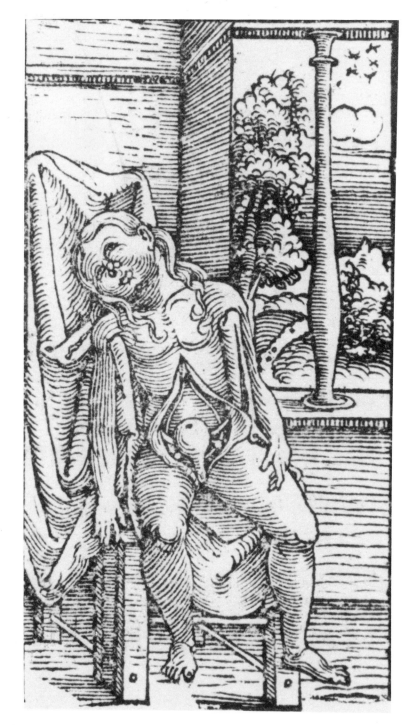

Figure 8. Female genital tract shown by Dryander. The ''dimple'' at the fundus of the uterus denotes the presence of a septum dividing the cavity. From Dryander (1547). Courtesy of the National Library of Medicine, Bethesda, MD.

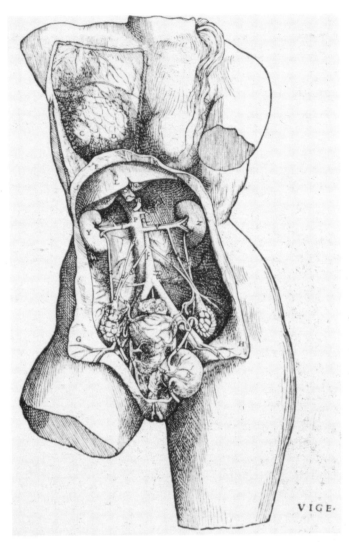

Figure 9. Vesalius' illustration of the female genital tract. From Vesalius (1543). Courtesy of the National Library of Medicine, Bethesda, MD.

20th centuries in particular saw very rapid growth of knowledge in this field. No development was more dramatic and far reaching than Hitschmann and Adler's demonstration of the hormone-controlled cyclic activity of the endometrium, which Robert Schroeder subsequently systematized into diagnostic stages. It is hard to realize that well under 100 years ago all the histological appearances characteristic of those stages were lumped together as pathological conditions under the term ''chronic endometritis.''

7. *Contemporary*

It is of course impossible to evaluate contemporary work in the same way as work of the distant past, especially at the present time, when workers are vastly more numerous in laboratories throughout the world and are employing a wide variety of techniques of study.

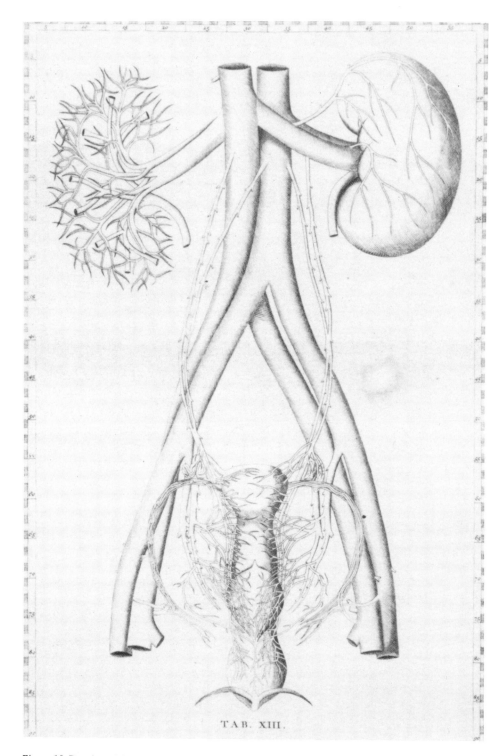

TAB. XIII.

Figure 10. Drawing of the renal and reproductive tract circulations by Pini for Eustachio. Published 1761 by Albini. Courtesy of the National Library of Medicine, Bethesda, MD.

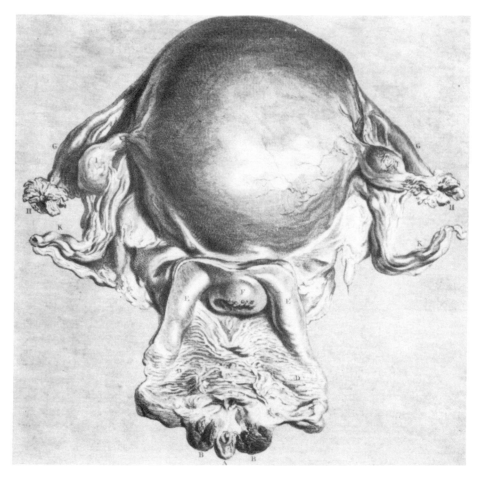

Figure 11. William Hunter's preparation of a uterus in the fifth month of pregnancy. Drawing by Rymsdyk. From Hunter (1774). Courtesy of the National Library of Medicine, Bethesda, MD.

Only time and the work of investigators in the future can determine what of today's work is worthy to stand beside the great discoveries of the past. Who are our Galens, Vesaliuses, Harveys, and Hunters?

But it is both possible and useful to identify the major trends of thought and methods of study that preoccupy contemporary researchers.

In looking back over the history of the uterus and reproductive tract, it is strikingly apparent that each burst of investigative activity has followed the development of new experimental tools and methodologies. This is also abundantly true of the present field in the decades since World War II. Greatly improved techniques, for example, electron microscopy, histochemistry, and more recently molecular biology, have permitted ever-deeper penetration into the structure of the cell and its constituent parts down to the ultimate ramifications of DNA. The radiological techniques of ultrasound and magnetic resonance scanning are permitting *in vivo* recognition of the character and activity of reproductive structures in varying physiological states. Immunocytochemistry is revealing secretory activity of structures previously regarded as inert. Even the early revelations achieved to date in these fields indicate that a whole new era has dawned. "Things will never be the same again," we say once more.

Current work focuses heavily on the role of the uterus in pregnancy. As a corollary, the fetus and placenta are drawn into a great number of studies as integral portions of the

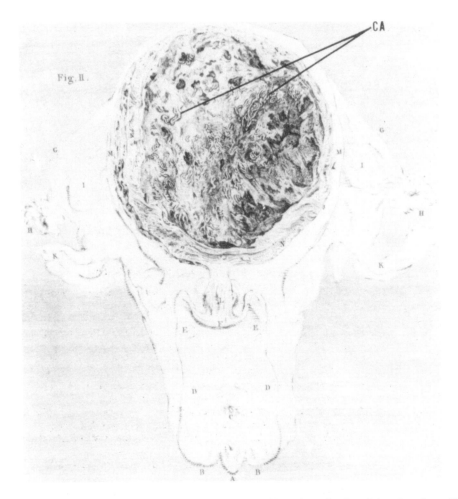

Figure 12. William Hunter's demonstration of curling arteries of the endometrium in an injected specimen. CA, curling arteries. Drawing by Rymsdyk. From Hunter (1774). Courtesy of the National Library of Medicine, Bethesda, MD.

reproductive tract. Additionally, more than ever before, the relation of the reproductive tract to the pathogenesis of diseases of pregnancy is under investigation—in particular the role of the uterine vasculature, maternal and fetal, in such cases as fetal immaturity (infants small for gestational age), preeclampsia–eclampsia, etc.—while the embryology of the tract and its occasional malfunction are regarded as responsible for many congenital anomalies and genetic diseases. Practical utilization of much of this information is already incorporated into the fields of prenatal and perinatal practice. The dissection of the human uterus would not have seemed more radical to medieval anatomists than would intrauterine surgery as practiced today to our predecessors of less than a century ago!

It is profitable to remember that history is a continuum. It is on the foundations laid by the anatomic, embryological, and histological greats of past centuries that our present—and future—understanding of the structure and functions of the reproductive tract is built. Indeed, everything presented in the following chapters of this book is part of the continuing history of the uterus.

8. References

I. Standard texts on the history of medicine. These works supply background and basic information about individuals.

Castiglioni, A., 1958, *A History of Medicine,* tr. and ed. by E. B. Krumbhaar, 2nd ed., Knopf, New York.

Garrison, F. H., 1961, *An Introduction to the History of Medicine,* 4th ed., Saunders, Philadelphia.

Mettler, C. C., and Mettler, F. A., 1947, *History of Medicine: A Correlative Text Arranged according to Subjects,* Blakiston, Toronto.

Singer, C., and Underwood, E. A., 1962, *A Short History of Medicine,* 2nd ed., Clarendon Press, Oxford.

II. Histories of the reproductive tract.

Barbour, A. H. F., 1887–1888, Early contributions of anatomy to obstetrics, *Trans. Edinburgh Obstet. Soc.* **13:**127–154.

Peillon, G., 1891, *Étude Historique sur les Organes Génitaux de la Femme,* O. Berthier, Paris.

Ricci, J. V., 1943, *The Genealogy of Gynecology,* Blakiston, Philadelphia.

III. Works dealing in greater depth with specific individuals, discoveries, and theories.

Albini, B. S., 1791, *Explicatio Tabularum Bartholomaei Eustachii,* Joannes and Hermannus Verbeek, Leyden.

Berengario, J., 1521, *Carpi Commentaria cum Amplissimis Additionibus super Anatomia Mundini,* Impressum per Hieronymum de Benedictis, Bononiae.

Corner, G. W., 1963, Exploring the placental maze. The development of our knowledge of the relationship between the bloodstream of mother and infant *in utero, Am. J. Obstet. Gynecol.* **86:**408–418.

da Vinci, L., 1513, *Quaderni d'Anatomia. III. Organi della Generazione-Embrione,* Dodici Fogli della Royal Library di Windsor, Casa Editrice Jacob Dyburad, Christiana.

Dryander, J., 1547, *Arzenei Spiegel gemeyner Inhalt derselbigen, wes bede einem Leib unnd Wundtartzt, in der Theoric, Practic und Chirurgei zusteht,* Christian Egenolph, Franckfurt am Meyn.

Hitschmann, F., and Adler, L., 1908, Der Bau der Uterusschleimhaut des geschlechtsreifen Weibes mit besonderer Berücksichtigung der Menstruation, *Monatsschr, Geburtshilfe Gynaekol.* **27:**1–82.

Hundt, M., 1501, *Antropologium de Hominis Dignitate,* Baccalarium Wolfgangum Monacenem, Liptzick.

Hunter, W., 1774, *The Gravid Uterus,* Birmingham.

Hunter, W., 1794, *An Anatomical Description of the Human Gravid Uterus, and Its Contents,* J. Johnson, London.

Kudlien, F., 1965, The seven cells of the uterus: The doctrine and its roots, *Bull. Hist. Med.* **39:**415–423.

Massa, N., 1559, *Anatomiae liber introductoris,* Venet.

Mondino dei Luzzi, 1541, *Anatomia Mundini,* per Joannem Dryandrum, In officina Christiani Egenolph, Marburg.

Ramsey, E. M., 1971, Maternal and foetal circulation of the placenta, *Ir. J. Med. Sci.* **140:**151–168.

Schroeder, R., 1930, Weibliche Genitalorgane, *Handb. Mikrosk. Anat.* **7:**329–566.

Soranus, 1956, *Gynecology,* tr. by O. Temkin, Johns Hopkins Press, Baltimore.

Vesalius, A., 1543, *De Humani Corporis Fabrica,* Basilae (facsimile, Brussels, 1964).

Weindler, F., 1908, *Geschichte der Gynäkologisch-anatomischen Abbildung,* Zahn and Jaensch, Dresden.

Comparative Anatomy

HARLAND W. MOSSMAN

In this brief consideration of some of the comparative aspects of the mammalian uterus, it is important to keep in mind that this organ develops from a pair of completely mesodermal tubes called, variously, müllerian, paramesonephric, or female ducts (see *Nomina Anatomica,* 5th ed., 1983). The whole female internal genital system of eutherian (''placental'') mammals, with the probable exception of the vagina, is basically double—two ovaries, two oviducts, and two uteri. The vagina is completely paired in monotremes and marsupials and has been reported to be partially divided by a longitudinal septum in one genus of bat (*Hipposideros*) (Karim, 1973), in the plains viscacha (*Lagostomus*) (Weir, 1971), and in the immature of some baleen whales (*Mysticeti*) (Ohsumi, 1969); otherwise, it is single in Eutheria. In most mammals, the vagina is joined by the urethra. Together they open into a common tube, the definitive urogenital sinus or vaginal vestibule, which connects both to the surface. Often this vestibule is nearly as long as the vagina proper. However, in woman it is represented by only the shallow space between the two labia minora.

The female ducts arise as grooves in the mesothelial lining of the peritoneal cavity, lateral to but closely alongside the mesonephric ducts about midway on the ventral surface of the mesonephroi, hence just lateral to the developing gonads. The caudal ends of the paired grooves differentiate into a pair of tubes that grow caudally in a retroperitoneal position until beyond the caudal poles of the mesonephroi (Fig. 1). Here they curve medialward until they meet at the midline, where they again turn and grow caudalward. In the human embryo they reach the urogenital sinus at about the ninth week, that is, in the early fetal stage.

Examination of embryos around this period reveals that the gubernacula, the fibro-muscular cords extending from the caudal poles of the gonads and mesonephroi to the internal inguinal rings, cross the female ducts somewhere along their medially directed portions (Fig. 1). Regardless of the eutherian species, this point of crossing marks the uterotubal junction. That portion of the female duct lateral and cephalic to the crossing becomes the oviduct, and the medial and caudal portions become the uterus plus whatever contribution the female ducts may give to the vagina (Cunha, 1975). The gubernacular fold cephalic to the crossing becomes

HARLAND W. MOSSMAN ● Department of Anatomy, University of Wisconsin-Madison, Madison, Wisconsin 53706.

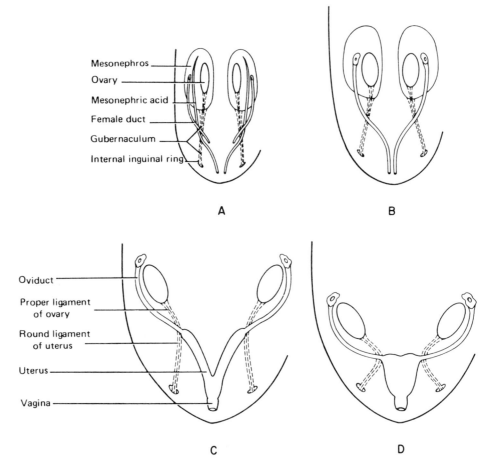

Mesonephros

Ovary

Mesonephric acid

Female duct

Gubernaculum

Internal inguinal ring

A

B

Oviduct

Proper ligament
of ovary

Round ligament
of uterus

Uterus

Vagina

C

D

Figure 1. Diagrams of ventral views of developing eutherian female internal genital systems. The vagina and urinary organs, except the mesonephroi, are not shown. A: Early fetal stage. B: Later fetal stage. C: Definitive stage in the case of a long bicornuate uterus with minimal caudal migration of the ovaries. D: Definitive stage in the case of a simplex uterus with maximal caudal migration of the ovaries.

the proper ligament of the ovary, and that caudal to the crossing becomes the round ligament of the uterus. These two ligaments may be difficult to distinguish in adults of some species. However, the proper ligament of the ovary can almost always be seen, and it always attaches at the uterotubal junction. The round ligament of the uterus usually can be found attaching at the same area but on the opposite side of the uterotubal junction. Yet in some species, especially the ruminants, the round ligament of the uterus often can be traced from the internal inguinal ring only to about the center of the broad ligament, where it fans out and cannot be followed to its original connection with the proper ovarian ligament. The fact that these ligaments always attach, at least during development, to the uterotubal junction, regardless of the type of adult uterus (duplex, bicornuate, or simplex), is evidence that the simplex uterus is developed by fusion of the entire paired uterine portions of the female ducts and is not derived just from their originally fused portion as seen in an early fetus. Also, the complexity of the arrangement of the musculature of the human uterus, and presumably that of other simplex uteri, is explainable on this basis (Goerttler, 1930).

Clinicians know that partial or complete duplication of the uterus is common among anomalies of the tract in women, and this is probably the result of failure of the female ducts to fuse in the normal manner. Another well-known abnormality is ectopic endometrium (endometriosis). This is sometimes explained as implantation of endometrium derived from menstrual detritus refluxed through the oviducts. When one realizes that, unlike the intestine, the whole uterus—mucosa, musculature, and serosa—is of mesodermal origin, one wonders whether ectopic endometrium may not possibly develop *in situ* as the result of the abnormal presence of factors comparable to those that induce the differentiation of endometrium in its normal location. Certainly from what is known of differentiation potential and induction mechanisms during embryonic development, this is perhaps the most logical explanation of ectopic endometrium.

Discussion of the comparative anatomy of the uterus is hindered by lack of data on many mammalian genera and the unreliability of many of the data in the literature. Authors have frequently described uteri as bicornuate without mentioning whether or not they have examined the lumen carefully to be sure that there is a common endometrium-lined corpus and a single cervical canal connecting to the vagina. Then, too, in many eutherians, especially the smaller ones, it is necessary to study microscopic sections of the cervical area to ascertain where true endometrium of the gestational portion of the uterus meets the cervical mucosa. Even with microscopic examination, identification of the true cervical region and canal can be difficult because, as the literature shows, in many mammals, especially the smaller ones, the epithelium of the canal is essentially like that of the vagina, and its glands, if any are present, are often similar to those of the true or gestational endometrium. Colburn *et al.* (1967) found such histological conditions in the squirrel monkey (*Saimiri*), where the cervical region is, however, easily recognized by its gross appearance. In fact, most of the commonly studied mammals have cervices easily identified grossly and microscopically because they are in general similar to that of woman. However, the limited literature on less-well-known and wild eutherians indicates that the more familiar histological and gross features are frequently absent (Graham, 1973), so that one must judge the extent of the true cervical region by a combination of features, including the nature and amount of muscle and connective tissues as compared with the vagina and gestational uterus, and sometimes by relatively minor variations of the mucosa from that of the rest of the uterus and the vagina. No wonder then that one finds statements that the cervix is absent or that the vagina is absent in certain species, even when some microscopic study has been done. Perhaps these statements are true, but it seems best not to accept such allegations until thorough developmental and histological studies have been made on the species under consideration. The amount of variation alleged to occur in the histological appearance of cervical mucosae is surprising, because the endometrium proper in all eutherian and marsupial mammals is basically very similar in type of gland and in the presence of both ciliated and nonciliated surface epithelial cells (Arnold and Shorey, 1985).

Fortunately, the junction between the oviduct and uterus is usually quite abrupt and therefore obvious. Yet in thick-walled simplex uteri such as the human, an appreciable part of the oviduct is actually enclosed by the myometrium but can be easily identified by its typical oviductal mucosa. In one species of bat having a simplex uterus, implantation of the blastocyst normally takes place in what at first appears to be the intramural portion of the oviduct. However, the mucosa of the area proves to be much like that of the uterine corpus; hence, the region no doubt represents a rudimentary cornu enclosed in the thick wall of the well-developed corpus (Fig. 2K) (Rasweiler, 1974).

We have, then, a basic concept of the uterus of Eutheria with which we shall proceed. Simply stated, it is that the uterus consists of two different portions, either of which may be double or parially or completely united. They are (1) the gestational portion, lined by the specialized serous-type mucosa (endometrium), which is highly embryonic (i.e., capable of further differentiation during the estrous cycle and especially during pregnancy), and (2) the cervix, lined by a mucosa often but by no means always containing either compound mucous

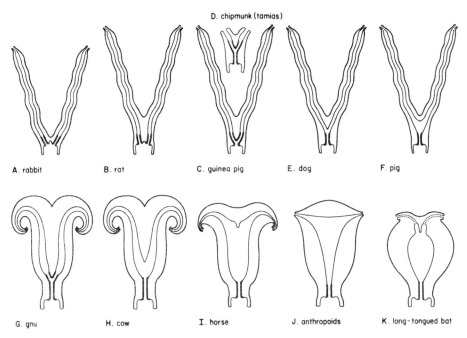

Figure 2. Diagrams of ideal frontal sections of uterine types found among Eutheria, with one known example of each type. The drawings cut the oviducts off near the uterotubal junctions and the vaginas just caudal to the cervices. Heaviest lines, cervical mucosa; thinnest lines, endometrium; dashed lines, oviduct epithelium. A–D show long duplex, of which A is the most primitive. B has caudal ends fused externally, thus resembling externally the corpus uteri of a bicornuate type. C and D have V-shaped and Y-shaped cervical canals, respectively. E and F are long bicornuate types. E has a very short corpus that rarely permits a single fetus to extend from one cornu to the other. The corpus of F permits a fetus with its placenta in one cornu to extend into the other. G is a medium-length duplex type with a Y-shaped cervical canal. H is a medium-length bicornuate type that permits fetal membranes, but usually not the fetus, to extend into the opposite cornu. I is a short bicornuate uterus with a very short septum that is almost obliterated late in pregnancy, thus permitting the membranes and sometimes the fetus to extend into both cornua. J and K are simplex uteri. In J, the cornua are represented by only the lateral angles of the lumen and surrounding tissue. In K, the cornua appear as short tubular pits with surrounding tissue continuous with the intramural portion of the oviducts; the blastocyst attaches in one of these pits. K is modified from Rasweiler (1974).

glands or a mucous epithelium and so structured with connective tissue and smooth muscle that it acts as a sphincter for the gestational period. With only a few dubious exceptions, all eutherian uteri are composed of these two portions.

I also consider the following interesting questions and hope to throw some light on them. Why have various groups of mammals evolved so many modifications of the simple primitive paired tubular uteri? Why has the trend been toward a completely fused simplex types? Are uterine types correlated with such things as litter size, degree of maturity at birth, placental structure, body build, and size of the adult female? Do these comparative data give us any significant insight into uterine structure and function in women?

1. Types of Uteri

Three classic types of mammalian uteri are usually described. (1) The duplex type has two separate tubes often joined externally at their cervical ends but always opening independently into two cervical canals. These canals usually open separately into the vagina but in some species may join within the cervical region (Fig. 2C,D,G) and then communicate with the vagina by a single ostium. (2) The bicornuate type has two tubes (cornua) joined externally beginning at their cervical ends for from about 5% to about 50% of their length and always joined internally at their cervical ends to form the body (corpus), which opens by a single cervical canal into the vagina. (3) The simplex type has a single unpaired corpus externally, usually with very small rudiments of the lumina of the cornua internally. Communication with the vagina is by a single cervical canal.

An additional term, "bipartite," has been used, but unfortunately sometimes for the long bicornuate types and sometimes for the medium to short bicornuate ones. Because of this confusion, the term should be dropped. Duplex uteri have often been called bicornuate simply because their cervical ends were joined externally and perhaps were assumed to be joined internally as well. Figure 2 illustrates, names, and gives examples of the three basic types and some of the intermediates.

2. Distribution and Probable Evolution of Uterine Types

Table 1 lists the types of uteri found in the major groups of Eutheria. Two, sometimes three, distinctly different types are found in four of the groups—Megachiroptera, Microchiroptera, Rodentia, and Artiodactyla. These are categories with numerous genera and are thus more likely to show a wide range of anatomic characters. Insectivora and Carnivora are also multigeneric but at present are known to have only one uterine type each; however, this may change when more genera have been examined. The finding of duplex uteri in two artiodactyl genera, *Hippotragus* (sable antelope) (Fig. 3) and *Connochaetes* (blue wildebeest), was a surprise to the author, since all the domestic and the few wild genera of this group that had been studied up to this time had had bicornuate uteri. All of the other orders have only one distinct type each, but this is to be expected since most of them contain only a few living genera.

Gestationally functional uteri probably evolved from a portion of each egg-transporting tube of primitive egg-laying mammals and were hence of the long, tubular, completely separate duplex type well known in marsupials. With the evolution of the unpaired vagina typical of eutherians, it became possible for the two uteri to fuse, first externally and finally internally, to have a single corpus and cervical canal. Once fusion occurred, it could logically continue from the long bicornuate condition through the medium to the short bicornuate and finally to the simplex type. Like most concepts of the pattern of evolution of soft parts, this is conjectural, but it has much support from both developmental and comparative anatomic evidence.

Biologists long ago discarded the so-called law of recapitulation, that ontogeny obligatorily repeats phylogeny; yet the fact of the matter is that, although there are numerous exceptions, the developmental history of an organ or system usually does in a broad general way repeat its phylogeny. The development of a simplex uterus from two female ducts certainly repeats the essential steps proposed for its evolution from the primitive paired-tube condition.

The dual nature of the female genital tract in monotremes and marsupials and the occurrence of the duplex and long bicornuate types in some of the more primitive eutherians, together with the incidence of the short bicornuate and simplex types chiefly in the most specialized eutherians, point to an evolutionary trend from duplex to simplex uterus. The presence of two or more distinct uterine types in the same order or suborder, and of the duplex type in several widely unrelated orders, suggests that the more primitive duplex and long bicornuate uterine types probably persisted until several mammalian orders became well

Table 1. Types of Uteri, Usual Litter Size Range, and Number of Recent Genera in the Major Groups of Eutheria[a]

Basic type	Long cornua — No corpus, duplex (rabbit)	Long cornua — Small corpus, bicornuate (pig)	Medium cornua — No corpus, duplex (gnu)	Medium cornua — Small corpus, bicornuate (sheep)	Short cornua, large corpus, bicornuate (horse)	Corpus only, simplex (human)	Litter size range	Number of living genera (Simpson, 1945)
Insectivora (hedgehogs, tenrecs, shrews, moles)		I		I			1–25	68
Dermoptera (flying "lemurs")	II						1	1
Megachiroptera (fruit bats)	II	I					1	21
Microchiroptera (all other bats)			II	I		I	1–3	94
Prosimii (lemurs, lorises, galagos, tarsiers)				I			1–3	22
Anthropoidea (monkeys, apes, man)						I	1–2	36
Edentates (Am. anteaters, sloths, armadillos)						I	1(4–12)P	14
Pholidota (pangolins)				I			1	1

Order				Litter size	n
Lagomorpha (rabbits, pikas)	II			1–6	10
Rodentia (rodents)	II	Y	I	1–10	337
Cetacea (whales, porpoise)			I	1	35
Carnivora (dogs, weasels, seals)		I	I	1–8	113
Tubulidentata (aardvarks)	II			1	1
Proboscidea (elephants)			I	1	2
Hyracoidea (hyraxes, dassies)		I	I	1–4	3
Sirenia (dugongs, manatees)			I	1	2
Perissodactyla (horses, tapirs, rhinos)			I	1	6
Artiodactyla[b] (cloven-hoofed mammals)		Y	I	1–2[c]	85

[a] The primary categories in this table are based on length or absence of uterine cornua because general uterine function and litter size seem to correlate more with this characteristic than with type of cervix. The table is a summary of observations by the author and data from a survey of the literature, the authors of which are too numerous to cite here. The range of litter size for each group is a combination of that of the genera within the group. For instance, since some insectivores bear only one young and others an average of 25, the range is 1–25. Asdell (1965) was the source of most of the data on litter size. I, Single cervical canal; II, paired cervical canals; Y, V- or Y-shaped cervical canal; (4–12)P, species having polyembryony.

[b] Camelidae cornua are very short, and the corpus is very large like that of horses (Ghazi, 1981).

[c] The Chinese water deer, Hydropotes, and the domestic Finnish Landrace sheep are said to bear litters of 4–6.

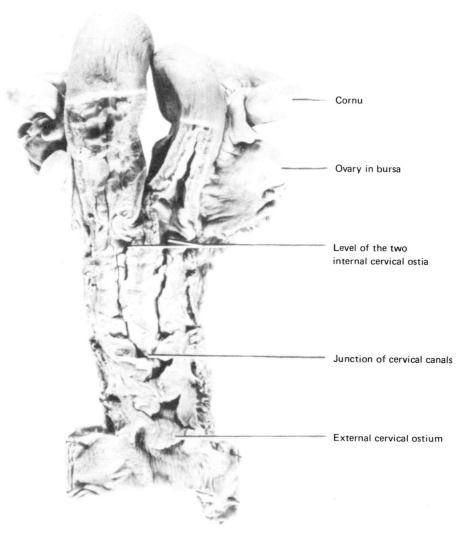

Cornu

Ovary in bursa

Level of the two
internal cervical ostia

Junction of cervical canals

External cervical ostium

Figure 3. Uterus of a sable antelope (*Hippotragus niger*). The dorsal half of the cervix and the caudal end of each cornu have been cut away to show the Y-shaped cervical canal.

differentiated from one another. If this is true, then further evolution to the medium and short bicornuate and simplex conditions probably occurred more recently and also independently in several orders. This could account for the simplex uteri of such widely unrelated groups as the anthropoids, armadillos, and bats.

Asymmetry in size of uterine cornua occurs in a few genera of each of three widely unrelated orders—Chiroptera (bats), Rodentia, and Artiodactyla (cloven-hoofed animals) (Wimsatt, 1975, 1979). In many of these, the right cornu is noticeably the larger, even in fetal and juvenile females. In one bat and five genera of ruminants, the right cornu is almost always significantly larger, although the right and left ovaries appear to be equally active in ovulation. In four other genera of bats and in one rodent, only the right ovary ovulates. In one other bat genus and another ruminant, the left ovary is more active, but the embryos almost always implant in the right cornu. These examples could represent a trend toward a type of simplex uterus. However, it is an asymmetric pattern, and all known simplex uteri are clearly symmetrical; hence, it is unlikely that they evolved in this manner.

27

COMPARATIVE
ANATOMY

3. Correlations of Uterine Types with Other Biological Features

Any attempt to correlate uterine type with reproductive or other characteristics of a species is somewhat risky because of the scattered nature of the data. Of the approximately 850 genera of eutherians (Simpson, 1945), some data as to uterine type are available on about 160, but at least a third of the data are more or less unreliable. Authors have called uteri bicornuate without making clear whether they have checked the actual nature of the cervices, either grossly or microscopically.

However, a few correlations seen undeniable. For instance, transuterine migration of blastocysts is common in species with bicornuate uteri but obviously cannot occur in those with duplex uteri: an egg or blastocyst certainly never passes through the cervix into the other uterus. Nor is there any likelihood that it would pass down one arm of a Y-shaped cervical canal and then back up the other arm into the opposite uterus. There is simply no hint of any physiological mechanism that could accomplish such a feat. The position of the implanted blastocyst, right, left, or otherwise in a simplex uterus, is apparently unrelated to which oviduct delivered it. The bat, *Glossophaga,* described by Rasweiler (1974), is apparently an exception, but here the blastocyst implants in the lumen of a rudimentary cornu from which it soon expands to occupy the corpus.

Certainly long tubular uteri are ideally adapted to gestate large litters of relatively small fetuses, whereas medium and short bicornuate and simplex types appear best for only one or two relatively large fetuses. By and large, the data substantiate this, even though there are many species with long tubular uteri that bear only one or two large young. Examples of the latter range over several orders: certain elephant shrews of the Insectivora; the African rock hares (*Pronolagus*) of the Lagomorpha; several rodents, including the spring haas (*Pedetes*) and the North American porcupine (*Erethizon*); and several carnivores, including the panda (*Ailurus*), sea otter (*Enhydra*), and apparently all seals, sea lions, and the walrus (*Pinnipedia*). These cases seem best interpreted as trends toward one or two young per pregnancy that have occurred independently in several different orders, and that may well have been the factor resulting in the parallel evolution in several groups toward a short bicornuate or simplex uterus. In fact, the uteri of the porcupine and sea otter have relatively shorter cornua than are common in their respective orders. However, the lumen of the porcupine nonpregnant uterus is coiled, thus making it much longer than the externally relatively short cornu containing it.

One of the most consistent correlations is that of the medium and short bicornuate and simplex uteri with species bearing only one or two relatively large and precocious newborn. This is especially characteristic of the hoofed mammals (Perissodactyla and Artiodactyla), primates, and edentates. The lone exceptions among the hoofed mammals are a breed of sheep, the Finnish Landrace, which normally bears an average of 3.4 young at each parturition (Bradford *et al.,* 1971), and the Chinese water deer, *Hydropotes,* which is said to bear five to seven young per pregnancy (Walker, 1964). However, no description of its uterus is known to me. The other exceptions are among the armadillos, in which a few species have apparently solved the problem of accommodating large litters to simplex uteri by "inventing" polyembryony, by which one fertilized ovum results in four to eight identical siblings. It is probable that simplex uteri were characteristic of this group long before polyembryony evolved in it. In fact, four of the six recognized living genera of armadillos bear only one or two young, which may be of the same or opposite sex and therefore probably derived from two individual eggs. Development of four or more symmetrically arranged embryos from a single blastocyst seems an ideal way to assure equally shared space in an essentially ovoid uterine lumen. If this concept is valid, then one would expect human monozygous multiple pregnancies to result in a lower ratio of nongenetic anomalies and defects such as those caused by crowding and inadequate blood supply than do dizygous and polyzygous multiple pregnancies. However, such a hypothesis may be hard to substantiate because of the many difficulties in obtaining unbiased data on human pregnancies, especially on twinning.

Multiple-litter fetuses in long tubular uteri are delivered in serial order from the most caudal to the most cephalic. It would be almost impossible for a more cephalic fetus to be forced past a more caudal one without dislodging it. Also, fetuses from such uteri are normally born enclosed in intact or nearly intact fetal membranes. Since the whole conceptus, membranes with placenta and fetus, is extruded at the same time, the fetuses must be quickly released from their membranes to prevent suffocation. Release is accomplished either by the clawing action of the newborn or by the mother or both. The umbilical cords of such young are much too short to allow them to be born through the ruptured membranes and still to maintain a functional cord attachment to an undetached placenta as is normal in most double and single births of mammals such as anthropoids, man, and ruminants.

The disposal of conceptuses that die before term is also somewhat different in tubular uteri from that in the shorter horned or simplex types. In the latter, spontaneous abortion is the rule, although occasionally the fetus is retained and either "mummified" or "skeletonized." In longer tubular uteri, retention and resorption *in situ* are almost universal except in very late pregnancy. Even if the whole litter dies, mass abortion is not common. This is true even when there is only one conceptus, as in the American porcupine. Abortion late in pregnancy sometimes occurred in our porcupine colony, but much more often resorbing conceptuses were found of exactly the same type as those seen in multiple pregnancies in other rodents and in rabbits. Although I know of no literature on the subject, it is my experience that resorption is much less frequent in insectivores and carnivores than it is in lagomorphs and rodents.

Ipsilateral uterine horn influence on the ovary, especially relating to persistence of the corpora lutea, has recently been of considerable interest to reproductive physiologists (Ginther, 1974). There is no indication that such an effect occurs in species with simplex uteri, but it has been demonstrated in those with duplex and bicornuate uteri (Fischer, 1967). There is a remote possibility that placentation limited to one side of a simplex uterus might produce such an effect, but so far there seems to be no evidence for this.

Different uterine types could have evolved in correlation with differences in body build, which in turn is certainly correlated with habitat and behavioral patterns, but there is little to indicate that this happened. Simplex uteri occur in some of the most active groups, the anthropoids and bats, as well as in some of the most sluggish, the anteaters and sloths. Medium-length bicornuate uteri are found in species given to violent activity such as the ruminants, but also in cetaceans, in which the buoyancy of their aquatic environment and the smoothness of their movements would seem to minimize traumatic effects to which ruminants are subject. Indirectly the form of the uterus may be related to some extent to numbers of litters per year and length of gestation. With the rare exceptions of Finnish Landrace sheep (Bradford *et al.*, 1971) and Chinese water deer (Walker, 1964), all eutherians with gestational periods of several months, excluding those with delayed implantation, bear only one or two relatively precocious young at a time, whereas those with very short gestational periods invariably have large litters of small altricial newborn.

One of the more enigmatic situations is found in bats. Here the young at term are unusually heavy compared with the weight of the mother and in many cases are even carried about for an appreciable period after birth. Bat uteri tend to be short-horned or simplex, as one would expect with precocious young, but why have these flying mammals not evolved low-weight young that could be left in shelters and fed by mothers unencumbered during their foraging flights? About all one can say is that the situation attests to the remarkably efficient flying ability of bats.

The strictly anthropoid type of fetal membranes—i.e., hemochorial villous placenta, rudimentary yolk sac, and rudimentary or absent allantoic vesicle—occurs only in species having simplex uteri. Every other type of fetal membrane system and placenta is found at least occasionally in species having either the long or medium-long tubular uteri. Since both the simplex uterus and the anthropoid type of fetal membrane system probably represent the most recent evolutionary step of each, it is not surprising that they should be found together. However, it is unwarranted to assume that their evolution has been in any degree causally linked. Some simplex uteri bear labyrinthine endotheliochorial placentae (sloths, anteaters, and some bats). None has diffuse or cotyledonary placentae or the large allantoic vesicles that accompany these. Therefore, one can conclude only that among recent mammals the anthropoid type of fetal membrane system is limited to species having simplex uteri, whereas some occurrences of all other types of fetal membrane systems are known in either the long or medium-long tubular uteri, both duplex and bicornuate. In other words, there is no clear evidence of any evolutionary adaptive relationships between gross uterine type and the nature of the fetal membranes.

4. Miscellaneous Aspects of the Comparative Morphology of the Uterus

Comparative aspects of a number of uterine features should be mentioned but cannot be discussed in detail in this chapter.

Considerable information on the histology of the endometrium of many mammals scattered among most of the orders is found chiefly in literature pertaining to estrous cycles or to nidation and placentation. Usually the cyclic and gestational changes are more conspicuous in the endometrium proper than in the cervical mucosa. Also, in most cases the endometrium is characterized by tubular glands of a serous type. Pardo and Larkin (1982) showed that one reason for cyclic changes in the endometrial glands of guinea pigs is their production of relaxin during pregnancy. (For an excellent electron microscopic study and interpretation of the uterine glands of swine during pregnancy, see Sinowatz and Friess, 1983.) In very small species, such as mice and shrews, glands are usually scarce, and the surface epithelium seems to be an adequate secretory substitute for them. A few, such as the elephant shrews (Macroscelididae), have definite "implantation sites," which differ from the remainder of the endometrium in various ways (Horst and Gillman, 1942; Horst, 1950).

All ruminants examined, except the Camelidae (camels, llamas, alpacas, guanacos, and vicunas), have specialized aglandular endometrial caruncles to which the chorioallantoic cotyledons attach to form the placentomes. Pigmentation (melanocytic) has long been known in the maternal caruncles and even in the intercaruncular endometrium of some parous sheep from early pregnancy into the postpartum period (Grant, 1933). Rowell *et al.* (1987) found that heavily pigmented caruncles are apparently normal in pregnant and parous muskoxen (*Ovibos moschatus*). They also discussed early pregnancy and the pathology of the uterus of this species. Wooding *et al.* (1982) in ultrastructural studies found melanocytes in sheep endometrium during the early attachment of the blastocyst. Camels have no uterine caruncles, and their placentas are diffuse like those of pigs and hippopotamuses. Also, a camel's uterus has very short coruna and a relatively large corpus (Ghazi, 1981). In fact, endometrial histology is so closely correlated with nidation and placentation that it scarcely makes sense to discuss it except in relation to these processes, and, again, this is beyond the purpose of this chapter.

A start on the comparative histology of the cervix has been made by Hafez and his colleagues. Those interested should consult Hafez (1973a,b), Hafez and Jaszczak (1972), and Graham (1973). Also, *The Biology of the Cervix* (Blandau and Moghissi, 1973) contains surveys of numerous fields of research on the nature of the cervix and its secretions.

It is known that the chemical and physical nature of cervical secretions in humans and in several laboratory and domestic mammals changes with changes in the reproductive status of the female. The secretions are adapted to allow relatively free passage of spermatozoa during estrus but are comparatively obstructive at other times. Although little is known about the structure or function of the cervix in many orders of mammals, there seems to be little question that its musculature and fibrous tissue in all mammals is designed to retain the contents of the uterus during pregnancy. In addition to the many possible chemical and physical functions of cervical mucus demonstrated or suggested by modern studies, it seems to me that its continuous production and movement toward the vagina during pregnancy must be an effective barrier to invasion of the uterus by microorganisms. Its slow outward flow probably equals or exceeds the rate at which bacteria and other infectious organisms can penetrate it from the vagina. It seems almost certain that a similar protection is at work in all viviparous mammals, but it is not known how it is accomplished in those believed to lack cervical glands.

In my experience, all mammals have functional anastomoses between branches of the ovarian artery and branches of the uterine artery of the same side. These are so large that ligation of the uterine or the ovarian artery does not deprive either organ of an adequate blood supply. In fact, the human simplex uterus is reputed to have enough cross anastomoses on its wall and between its muscle layers to allow ligation of both the ovarian and the uterine arteries on one side without serious consequences, at least to the uterus. Excellent illustrations and descriptions of the blood supply of the female internal genitals of several domestic and laboratory mammals are given by Del Campo and Ginther (1972, 1973), Ginther (1974), and Ginther et al. (1974). They studied vascular injections primarily to find a pathway that might explain the well-known direct unilateral influence of a uterine horn on the ovary of the same side. Ghazi (1981) described and illustrated clearly the blood supply of the internal genitals of camels.

Moffat (1959) demonstrated sphincteric structures at the origin of each segmental branch of the rat uterine artery. It is unknown how these may function and whether similar mechanisms occur in other mammals. However, Wragg (1959), during perfusion of rats' uteri with their own blood under near-normal pressure and temperature, noted brief periods of reverse flow in the segmentals from the uterus toward the main uterine artery. Presumably the reversal was caused by intrauterine contraction of muscle in such a pattern and sequence that arterial blood was forced backward out of the capillaries and small arteries. This phenomenon occurred rather commonly, but no physiological explanation could be found for it. Such a mechanism could force blood that had been widely distributed in the uterus into arterial anastomoses with the ovarian arterial supply and might be the pathway for the local unilateral effect of the uterus on the ovary. Obviously this is merely a possibility founded on very little evidence, and much more investigation must be done to indicate its validity or nonvalidity as an explanation for the ''local effect'' enigma. (See Kardon et al., 1982, for a scanning electron microscopic study of the intraarterial cushions. Also see Liebgott, 1984, for possible vascular effects of contraction of the mesometrial portion of the longitudinal uterine musculature.)

In man and the few other mammals that have been studied, the lymph vessels draining a visceral organ almost parallel the arteries supplying the organ. This was shown clearly in the sheep and goat by Staples et al. (1982). Although too few species have been studied in this respect to make a comparison significant, it is reasonable to expect that the lymphatics of the viscera of all mammals conform to this basic pattern.

The innervation of the human uterus is described in all the major anatomic textbooks, and the few studies on the gross anatomy of the innervation in common domestic and laboratory mammals show no essential differences. Peters et al. (1987) identified the individual sensory nerves supplying each portion of the female reproductive tract of the laboratory rat and presented an excellent diagram of their distribution. This diagram should be helpful in the use of this easily available animal for the study of sensory nerve function and control of pain arising in the reproductive organs. However, for a complete understanding of the innervation of such organs, electron microscopic, histochemical, cytochemical, and physiological studies are necessary. Although these aspects are beyond the purpose of this chapter, an ultrastructural study by Buchanan and Garfield (1984) on the little brown bat (*Myotis lucifugus*) is well worth our attention as an excellent piece of research in itself and for their suggestion of a very useful animal for such investigations. The myometrium of this bat is heavily innervated. The great uterine size change during a pregnancy cycle requires remarkable anatomic and physiological adjustments of its nervous system. These changes are extreme in bats because the weight of their usually single fetus at term is often a third of that of its nonpregnant mother.

With the exception of the vagina, the female internal genital organs of mammals are suspended by mesenteries. The early fetal ovary is attached to the ventromedial surface of the mesonephros by the mesovarium. An embryonic broad ligament attaches the cephalic portion of the female (müllerian) duct of the early fetus to the ventral or ventrolateral surface of the mesonephros as long as the latter persists and the remainder of the duct to the dorsal or dorsolateral abdominal and pelvic walls. The gubernaculum crosses the female duct and traverses the broad ligament, dividing it into a more cephalic portion, the mesosalpinx, and a more caudal portion, the mesometrium. During the gradual caudal migration of the fetal ovary, the mesonephros degenerates, increasing the length and looseness of both the mesosalpinx and the mesovarium and thus usually allowing them to unite at their bases and to have a common attachment to the dorsal body wall. Because of this union, the mesovarium of the adult is sometimes considered part of the broad ligament, although it was originally a completely separate structure (*Nomina Anatomica,* 1966).

Obviously the type of uterus and the degree of caudal migration of the ovary and uterus toward or into the pelvis have much to do with the nature of the broad ligament of the adult. For instance, the ovary, oviduct, and uterus of rabbits remain near their embryonic location; hence, the rabbit's mesosalpinx and mesometrium are extensive in the cephalocaudal direction. Rats, on the contrary, have marked migration of the ovary and oviduct toward the uterus, the ovary being almost against the tubal end of the uterus and the oviduct tightly convoluted beside the ovary; thus, the extent of the mesosalpinx, particularly at its tubal edge, is apparently much reduced.

The relationship of the uterine musculature to the broad ligament seems to vary greatly among mammalian groups, but apparently no comprehensive comparative study of this has ever been made. Frequently, as in the porcupine, *Erethizon,* the longitudinal layer from each side of the uterus extends out onto the mesometrium to form a very conspicuous band about as wide as the diameter of the nonpregnant cornu. In other species, the mesometrial musculature is an irregular network, heaviest among the major blood vessels and the round ligament.

Hibernating mammals, such as the ground squirrels, marmots, hedgehogs, and tenrecs, use the broad ligament (and incidentally the mesovarium and mesorchium also) as major fat storage depots. However, a narrow but sharply limited band adjacent to the cornu and oviduct remains fat-free. It is a striking sight in a well-fattened hibernator to see the fat-laden portion of the broad ligament end abruptly in a thick, almost squared edge along the center of which is attached the delicate transparent uterine portion suspending a very narrow, almost threadlike anestrous uterus. Certainly in such mammals there are definitely delimited fields of potential steatoblasts, fields in which these cells are inconspicuous during most of the gestation and lactation periods.

In certain myomorph rodents, a group of glandular cells occurs in the myometrium in the area of attachment of the mesometrium. These cells have been studied intensively in the mouse and rat. Their morphology is closely correlated with the reproductive cycle, and, although they are thought to be endocrine secretors, this supposition has been difficult to verify. Even their origin is uncertain but probably lies in stromalike cells of the area. Bulmer *et al.* (1987) reviewed evidence of their origin and differentiation. For other recent literature, consult Pardo and Larkin (1982), Stewart (1985), and Tarachand (1986).

5. Summary and Conclusions

The eutherian internal genital system is basically paired except for the vagina.

Three primary types of uteri are recognized: duplex, bicornuate, and simplex; but there are significant intermediate types.

The more specialized medium and short bicornuate and simplex types apparently have evolved independently in several mammalian orders.

Uterine type is in some cases clearly correlated with other features of reproductive biology of the species: transuterine migration of blastocysts almost certainly cannot occur in duplex uteri; except for cases of polyembryony, large litters occur only in the longer tubular duplex or bicornuate uteri, not in the medium and short bicornuate or simplex types.

Polyembryony is probably a recently evolved mechanism to adapt a species with a simplex uterus to simultaneous gestation of multiple young.

Fetuses from long tubular uteri have short umbilical cords and are normally born with their membranes relatively intact; those from medium and short bicornuate and simplex uteri are typically large and precocious and are born through ruptured membranes, leaving the placenta and its umbilical cord still attached and functional until the newborn begins to breathe air.

Dead fetuses in long tubular uteri are usually resorbed *in situ;* only those in late gestation are aborted. Those of medium- and short-horned and simplex types are more commonly aborted.

Anything comparable to the important ipsilateral influence of the uterine horn and conceptus on the ovary is unknown in species with simplex uteri.

There is little evidence of a correlation between uterine type and body build or activity of the female.

As far as is known, all eutherians with several months of active gestation have large precocious newborn and medium to short bicornuate or simplex uteri, whereas those with very short gestational periods usually have large litters of small altricial newborn and long tubular uteri.

Microscopic study of the cervical region is necessary, especially in smaller species, to ascertain whether a given uterus is duplex or bicornuate.

Differences between mammalian groups in uterine mucosal histology are often great, especially with respect to changes during estrous and pregnancy cycles.

Free anastomoses of uterine blood vessels with those of the ovaries appear to be universal among mammals.

Man and the few other mammals investigated have closely similar uterine lymph drainage and innervation.

The human uterus, although no doubt evolved from a long duplex type, is in its present form ill-adapted to the gestation of more than one fetus.

The comparative anatomy and embryology of an organ or organ system can give a useful background and understanding of its biology.

ACKNOWLEDGMENTS. Much of the information presented was gathered during preparation of a monograph on vertebrate fetal membranes (Mossman, 1987).

6. References

Arnold, R., and Shorey, C. D., 1985, Structure of the uterine luminal epithelium of the brush-tailed possum (*Trichosurus vulpecula*), *J. Reprod. Fertil.* **74:**565–573.

Asdell, S. A., 1965, *Patterns of Mammalian Reproduction,* 2nd ed., Constable, London.

Blandau, R. J., and Moghissi, K., 1973, *The Biology of the Cervix,* University of Chicago Press, Chicago.

Bradford, J. E., Quirk, J. F., and Hart, R., 1971, Natural and induced ovulation rate of Finnish Landrace and other breeds of sheep, *Anim. Prod.* **13**:627–635.

Buchanan, G. D., and Garfield, R. E., 1984, Myometrial ultrastructure and innervation in *Myotis lucifugus,* the little brown bat, *Anat. Rec.* **210**:463–475.

Bulmer, D., Peel, S., and Stewart, I., 1987, Review. The metrial gland, *Cell Differ.* **20**:77–86.

Colburn, G. L., Walker, J. B., and Lang, C. M., 1967, Observations on the cervix uteri of the squirrel monkey, *J. Morphol.* **122**:81–88.

Cunha, G. R., 1975, The dual origin of the vaginal epithelium, *Am. J. Anat.* **143**:387–392.

Del Campo, C. H., and Ginther, O. J., 1972, Vascular anatomy of the uterus and ovaries and the unilateral luteolytic effect of the uterus: Guinea pigs, rats, hamsters, and rabbits, *Am. J. Vet. Res.* **33**:2561–2578.

Del Campo, C. H., and Ginther, O. J., 1973, Vascular anatomy of the uterus and ovaries and the unilateral luteolytic effect of the uterus: Horses, sheep, and swine, *Am. J. Vet. Res.* **34**:305–316.

Fischer, T. V., 1967, Local uterine regulation of the corpus luteum, *Am. J. Anat.* **121**:425–442.

Ghazi, R., 1981, Angioarchitectural studies of the utero-ovarian component in the camel (*Camelus dromedarius*), *J. Reprod. Fertil.* **61**:43–46.

Ginther, O. J., 1974, Internal regulation of physiological processes through local venoarterial pathways: A review, *J. Anim. Sci.* **39**:550–564.

Ginther, O. J., Dierschke, D. J., Walsh, S. W., and Del Campo, C. H., 1974, Anatomy of arteries and veins of uterus and ovaries in rhesus monkeys, *Biol. Reprod.* **11**:205–219.

Goerttler, K., 1930, Die Architektur der Muskelwand des menschlichen Uterus und ihre funktionelle Bedeutung, *Morphol. Jahrb.* **65**:45–128.

Graham, C. E., 1973, Functional microanatomy of the primate uterine cervix, in: *Handbook of Physiology,* Sect. 7: *Endocrinology,* Vol. II, *Female Reproductive System,* Part 2 (R. O. Greep and E. B. Astwood, eds.), pp. 1–24, Williams & Wilkins, Baltimore.

Grant, R., 1933, The pigmentation of the uterine mucosa in the ewe, *Vet. J.* **89**:271–274.

Hafez, E. S. E., 1973a, The comparative anatomy of the mammalian cervix, in: *The Biology of the Cervix* (R. J. Blandau and K. Moghissi, eds.), pp. 23–56, University of Chicago Press, Chicago.

Hafez, E. S. E., 1973b, Anatomy and physiology of the mammalian uterotubal junction, in: *Handbook of Physiology,* Sect. 7: *Endocrinology,* Vol. II, *Female Reproductive System,* Part 2 (R. O. Greep and E. B. Astwood, eds.), pp. 87–95, Williams & Wilkins, Baltimore.

Hafez, E. S. E., and Jaszczak, S., 1972, Comparative anatomy and histology of the cervix uteri in non-human primates, *Primates* **13**:297–314.

Horst, C. J., van der, 1942, Some observations on the structure of the genital tract of *Elephantulus, J. Morphol.* **70**:403–429.

Horst, C. J., van der, 1950, The placentation of *Elephantulus, Trans. R. Soc. S. Afr.* **32**:435–629.

Horst, C. J. van der, and Gillman, J., 1942, Pre-implantation phenomena in the uterus of *Elephantulus, S. Afr. J. Med. Sci.* **7**:47–71.

Kardon, R. H., Farley, D. B., Heidger, P. M., Jr., and Van Orden, D. E., 1982, Intra-arterial cushions of the rat uterine artery: A scanning electron microscope evaluation utilizing vascular casts, *Anat. Rec.* **203**:19–29.

Karim, K. B., 1973, Occurrence of a bicornuate vagina in the Indian leaf-nosed bat, *Hipposideros fulvus fulvus* (Gray), *Curr. Sci.* **42**:62–63.

Liebgott, B., 1984, Mesometrial smooth muscle in the mouse: Its control of uterine blood flow, *Anat. Rec.* **208**:365–374.

Moffat, D. B., 1959, An intra-arterial regulating mechanism in the uterine artery of the rat, *Anat. Rec.* **134**:107–124.

Mossman, H. W., 1987, *Vertebrate Fetal Membranes,* Rutgers University Press, New Brunswick, NJ.

Nomina Anatomica, 1966, 3rd ed., Excerpta Medica, New York.

Nomina Anatomica, 1983, 5th ed., Williams & Wilkins, Baltimore and London.

Ohsumi, S., 1969, Occurrence and rupture of vaginal band in the fin, sei, and blue whales, *Sci. Rep. Whale Res. Inst. (Tokyo)* **21**:85–94.

Pardo, R. J., and Larkin, L. H., 1982, Localization of relaxin in endometrial gland cells of pregnant, lactating and ovariectomized hormone-treated guinea pigs, *Am. J. Anat.* **164**:79–90.

Peters, L. C., Kristal, M. B., and Komisaruk, B. R., 1987, Sensory innervation of the external and internal genitalia of the female rat, *Brain Res.* **408**:199–204.

Rasweiler, J. J., IV, 1974, Reproduction in the long-tongued bat, *Glossophaga soricina.* II. Implantation and early embryonic development, *Am. J. Anat.* **139**:1–35.

Rowell, J., Betteridge, G. C. B., and Fenwick, J. C., 1987, Anatomy of the reproductive tract of the female muskox (*Ovibos moschatus*), *J. Reprod. Fertil.* **80**:431–444.

Simpson, G. G., 1945, The principles of classification and a classification of mammals, *Bull. Am. Mus. Nat. Hist.* **85**:1–350.

Sinowatz, F., and Friess, A. E., 1983, Uterine glands of the pig during pregnancy: An ultrastructural and cytochemical study, *Anat. Embryol.* **166**:121–134.

Staples, L. D., Fleet, I. R., and Heap, R. B., 1982, Anatomy of the utero-ovarian lymphatic network and the composition of afferent lymph in relation to the establishment of pregnancy in the sheep and goat, *J. Reprod. Fertil.* **64**:409–420.

Stewart, I., 1985, Immunoglobulin G in the decidua basalis and metrial gland of the pregnant mouse uterus, *J. Reprod. Immunol.* **7**:275–278.

Tarachand, U., 1986, Metrial gland: Structure, origin, differentiation, and role in pregnancy, *Biol. Res. Pregnancy Perinatol.* **7**:34–36.

Walker, E. P., 1964, *Mammals of the World,* Johns Hopkins University Press, Baltimore.

Weir, B. J., 1971, The reproductive organs of the female plans viscacha, *Lagostomus maximus, J. Reprod. Fertil.* **25**:365–373.

Wimsatt, W. A., 1975, Some comparative aspects of implantation, *Biol. Reprod.* **12**:1–40.

Wimsatt, W. A., 1979, Reproductive asymmetry and unilateral pregnancy in Chiroptera, *J. Reprod. Fertil.* **56**:345–357.

Wooding, F. B. P., Staples, L. D., and Peacock, M. A., 1982, Studies of trophoblast papillae on the sheep conceptus at implantation, *Am. J. Anat.* **134**:507–516.

Wragg, L. E., 1959, Growth and regression of uterine vessels in the rat, *Anat. Rec.* **133**:637–654.

7. Bibliography

Asdell, S. A., 1965, *Patterns of Mammalian Reproduction,* 2nd ed., Constable, London.

Kimball, F. A., ed., 1980, *The Endometrium,* S. P. Medical and Scientific Books, New York, London.

Mossman, H. W., 1987, *Vertebrate Fetal Membranes,* Rutgers University Press, New Brunswick, NJ.

3

Prenatal Human Development

RONAN O'RAHILLY

The prenatal development of the human uterus is presented here primarily from the viewpoint of morphology. It should be needless to stress that other considerations—from the fields of biochemistry and endocrinology, for example—are also necessary for a proper understanding of uterine development. Moreover, a developmental account of the uterus necessitates that attention be given to the urinary system, because "the urinary and reproductive organs . . . form an inseparable whole in the adult organism" (Felix, 1912) as they do also in the embryo and fetus.

The determination of the precise sequence and timing of developmental events necessitates the use of a staging system. The first 8 postovulatory weeks of human development (i.e., those following the ovulation and fertilization that resulted in pregnancy) have been subdivided into 23 Carnegie stages (O'Rahilly and Müller, 1987), formerly termed "horizons" by Streeter. The stages, which are mostly 2 days apart, are based on morphological criteria such as the appearance of the eyes and the limb buds. The detailed use of the staging system has been described in a number of different regions, such as the reproductive system (O'Rahilly, 1983). Greatest length is the most useful measurement (O'Rahilly and Müller, 1984), but it should be emphasized that such expressions as "at the 18-mm stage" should be replaced by "at 18 mm" because the single and variable criterion of embryonic length is not in itself sufficient to establish a stage. Unfortunately, at the present time a satisfactory staging system for the fetal period (i.e., 8 weeks to birth) is not available.

1. Urinary Preliminaries

"The concept of the pronephros does not apply to the human embryo" (Torrey, 1954), but the mesonephros is closely associated with the development of the reproductive pathway, particularly in the male. Hence, a consideration of the urinary system is necessary.

RONAN O'RAHILLY • Carnegie Laboratories of Embryology, California Primate Research Center, Davis, California 95616.

The hindgut appears at 20 days (stage 9). As described in detail elsewhere (O'Rahilly and Muecke, 1972), the intermediate mesoderm becomes visible at about 22 days (stage 10) and provides the nephrogenic cord. The ridge occupied by the developing mesonephros was described in about 1765 by the eminent embryologist of Berlin, Kaspar Friedrich Wolff, whose name has frequently been associated with mesonephric structures. At 24 days (stage 11), the mesonephric duct develops as a solid rod *in situ* from the nephrogenic cord or perhaps from ectodermal buds lateral to the somites.

At the same time, the nephrogenic tissue develops into nephric vesicles, which are connected by tubules to the mesonephric duct (Fig. 1). By 26 days (stage 12), the duct acquires a lumen. Although the mesonephric duct at first ends blindly, it soon becomes attached to the terminal part of the hindgut, which is henceforth known as the cloaca. (The cloaca maxima in Rome was the main sewer that led into the Tiber.) At about 28 days (stage 13), as the ureteric bud is about to form or has even appeared, the mesonephric ducts may already open into the cloaca. Within a few days, the urorectal septum (the origin of which is disputed) appears to "descend" and divide the cloaca into the primary urogenital sinus and the rectum. By the seventh week, urinary pressure is believed to cause rupture of the cloacal membrane, thereby allowing the urogenital sinus to communicate with the exterior, i.e., with the amniotic cavity.

In summary, two features directly relevant to the establishment of the female reproductive pathway, namely, the urogenital sinus and the two mesonephric ducts, have appeared by 6 weeks.

The mesonephric ducts persist to a variable degree in the female. Koff (1933) found them intact at 56 mm but interrupted at 63 mm. Their openings were occluded by 75 mm, and, in a 77-mm fetus, only the rostral portions in the broad ligaments remained. The caudal parts are said usually to "lose their connections with the urogenital sinus and either disappear completely or migrate cranially . . . and disappear at a later stage" (Koff, 1933). Others have

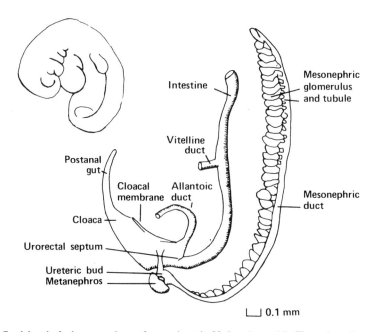

Figure 1. Caudal end of a human embryo of approximately 32 days (stage 14). The embryo (inset drawing) is 5.7 mm in length and possesses 38 pairs of somites. In this left lateral view, the mesonephric duct can be seen to enter the cloaca. Near the junction, the ureteric bud extends into the metanephros. The urorectal septum will shortly appear to "descend" and divide the cloaca into the primary urogenital sinus and the rectum. The paramesonephric duct will appear in less than a week. Based on Shikinami (1926).

denied the existence of a rostral migration, however, and it has been claimed that the caudal ends of the mesonephric ducts are quite durable structures (Witschi, 1970).

Various mesonephric remains may be found in postnatal life. For example, the caudal portions of the mesonephric ducts may persist lateral to the uterus and vagina, where the unnecessary and historically unjustified name "Gärtner's ducts" has been employed. When a mesonephric duct persists in the fetal cervix, it may present an ampulla, which sends branches into the substance of the cervix (Meyer, 1909). In addition, cranial to the ampulla, the mesonephric duct possesses a muscular coat that may persist even after degeneration of the epithelium (Huffman, 1948). Mesonephric remnants may appear in the adult cervix as either tubules or cysts, and the latter may give rise to adenomatous proliferations or to adenocarcinoma.

Mesonephric structures also may be seen in the broad ligament and have given rise to a ridiculous system of eponyms (Gardner *et al.*, 1948). The epoophoron, which includes mesonephric tubules and a portion of the mesonephric duct, was found to be present constantly (Duthie, 1925), although no evidence of secretory activity was observed on electron microscopy (Beltermann, 1965). As seen with the light microscope, the mesonephric duct is situated closely external to the musculature of the uterine tube. It is usually moderately convoluted, possesses its own muscular investment, and is lined by a nonciliated low cuboidal epithelium. The mesonephric tubules are generally more highly convoluted, may display their own musculature, and are lined by ciliated and nonciliated low columnar or cuboidal epithelium.

Additional structures that may be found in the broad ligament include the paroophoron and rete tubules. Not all the structures in this area, however, are necessarily mesonephric in origin.

2. The Paramesonephric Ducts

The paramesonephric duct was first noted in 1825 by the eminent physiologist of Koblenz, Johannes Müller. In accordance with one of the principles of the *Nomina Anatomica*, however, eponymous terms should be avoided whenever possible.

The paramesonephric ducts arise as variable invaginations in the mesonephros during the sixth week (stage 16; Faulconer, 1951). The invagination (Figs. 2 and 3) involves a precise area of the coelornic epithelium at the level of the third thoracic somite (Felix, 1912), and it occurs in both sexes. The site of the infolding later becomes the abdominal ostium of the uterine tube, and scattered irregularities of the margin form the beginnings of the future fimbriae. Accessory tubes, which end blindly, may be found in female embryos, and one of them may persist as the appendix vesiculosa (Monroe and Spector, 1962).

The site of origin of the paramesonephric duct differs from the rest of the mesonephric ridge by virtue of the taller cells of its epithelium. The mesonephric duct lies close to this portion of the epithelium (hence the appropriate name "paramesonephric duct"), but it is clearly separated from it throughout (Gruenwald, 1941). It has been shown in the chick embryo that the mesonephric duct induces the "paramesonephric plaque," as the epithelial area may be termed (Didier, 1973b).

As each paramesonephric duct grows caudally through the mesenchyme, the adjacent mesonephric duct acts as a guide for it, as has been shown experimentally in the chick embryo (Gruenwald, 1941, 1942). The caudal growth of the paramesonephric duct takes place probably by multiplication of its own cells, at least in the chick embryo (Didier, 1968). Three main segments (Fig. 4) may be distinguished rostrocaudally (Gruenwald, 1941): (1) a portion separated from the mesonephric duct by mesenchyme, (2) a portion separated by basement membrane only, and (3) a portion fused with the mesonephric duct without the intervention of a basement membrane. Thus, the growing caudal tip of the paramesonephric duct lies within

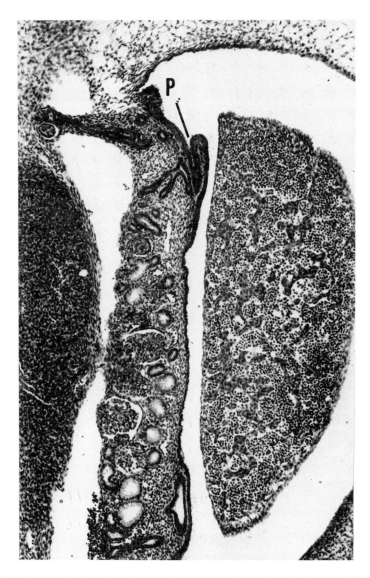

Figure 2. Photomicrograph of coronal section through an embryo of approximately 41 days and 11 mm in length (stage 17). The mesonephros is cut longitudinally and the coelom, containing a portion of the liver, appears to its right. Mesonephric glomeruli and tubules are visible, as is a small portion of the mesonephric duct. Adjacent to the last, a funnel-shaped depression, the paramesonephric duct (P), can be seen to communicate with the coelom. Section selected by Koff (1933).

the basement membrane of the mesonephric duct, and it is possible that the mesonephric duct contributes cells to the paramesonephric canal (Frutiger, 1969). The sheath of connective tissue surrounding the paramesonephric duct develops *in situ* from a strip of differentiated mesothelium (Didier, 1973a,b). It has been claimed that a portion of the mesenchyme is derived from the cells of the paramesonephric duct itself (Gruenwald, 1959). It has also been claimed that the mesenchyme surrounding the paramesonephric ducts shows differentiation from its earliest appearance in female (18.5 mm) but not in male (16 mm) embryos (Candreviotis, 1967).

It is believed that ''hormone-dependent development of the urogenital tract occurs via an

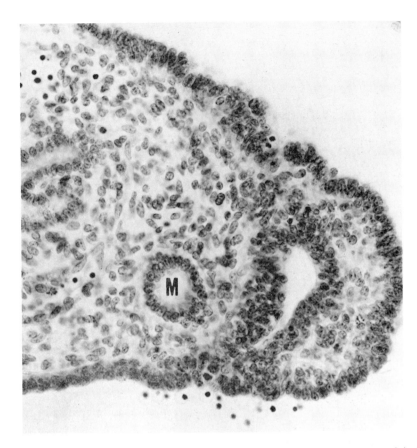

Figure 3. Photomicrograph showing transverse section of the mesonephric (M) and paramesonephric ducts at approximately 41 days (stage 17) in a 14.2-mm human embryo. The site of the paramesonephric invagination can be seen on the surface of the mesonephros. From Faulconer (1951).

interaction between epithelium and stroma in which the stroma plays a decisive role in mediating the unique morphological response of epithelium to sex hormones by inducing specific patterns of epithelial morphogenesis'' (Cunha, 1976).

Abnormally arrested growth of a mesonephric duct is accompanied by absence of the accompanying paramesonephric duct at corresponding levels. Furthermore, because of the absence of the mesonephric duct, the ureteric bud fails to develop, and hence unilateral renal agenesis is a frequent accompaniment of uterus unicornis and an associated defective uterine tube.

The rate of elongation of the paramesonephric duct is so precisely regulated that "it provides us with an additional definable character for determining the level of development of any given specimen falling within this general period" (Streeter, 1948). The length of the paramesonephric duct can be correlated closely with the level of development of other parts of the embryo, such as the number of semicircular ducts present in the ear (Fig. 5). Thus, from the status of paramesonephric development, "one can arrive at the degree of development of an organ as remote and comparatively unrelated as the inner ear" (Streeter, 1948).

Asymmetric development of the urogenital system is characteristic of certain vertebrates. In most birds, for example, the right ovary is smaller and shows a tendency toward testicular differentiation, and the right oviduct ceases to develop. Indeed, from its first appearance, the left paramesonephric duct of the chick embryo is longer than that on the right. In the human,

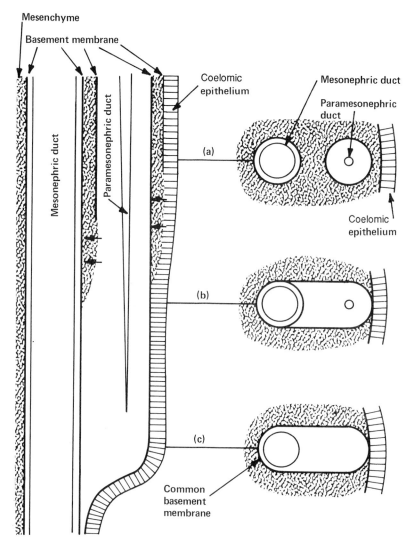

Figure 4. Diagram of longitudinal and transverse sections through the developing mesonephric and para-mesonephric ducts. Rostrally, at level (a), the two ducts are separated by mesenchyme, and each has its own basement membrane. At level (b), the two ducts are no longer separated by mesenchyme but by basement membrane only. Caudally, at level (c), the two ducts are enclosed in a common basement membrane. The small arrows indicate cellular contributions from the coelomic epithelium to the paramesonephric duct and from the paramesonephric duct to the surrounding mesenchyme. Based on Gruenwald (1959).

some isolated references to asymmetric urogenital development may be found, such as a smaller right mesonephros. The length of the left uterine tube during fetal life is generally from 1 to 3 mm less than that of the right (Hunter, 1930). A systematic study of asymmetry in human urogenital development, however, does not seem to have been published.

The mesonephric duct, as seen from "in front," develops two gentle curves that enable vertical, horizontal, and vertical portions to be distinguished successively in its course (Fig. 6). As the paramesonephric duct extends caudally, it adopts a similar arrangement so that, during the eighth week, three parts can be detected: rostral vertical, middle transverse, and caudal vertical. Both the mesonephric and the paramesonephric ducts are enclosed in urogenital folds of peritoneum that later give rise to the broad ligaments.

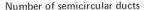

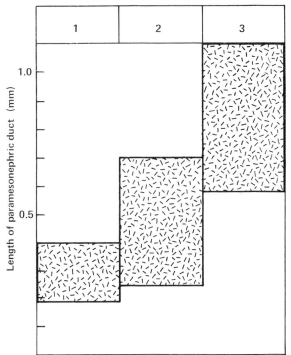

Figure 5. Graph to show the close relationship between the length of the paramesonephric duct and the number of semicircular ducts in the internal ear at approximately 44 days (stage 18). The paramesonephric duct attains a length of 0.5 mm only in those embryos that possess two semicircular ducts, and a length of 1 mm only in those that display all three semicircular ducts.

At 7 weeks, the paramesonephric ducts have generally not yet reached the urogenital sinus (Fig. 6), although a ventral projection of the dorsal sinusal wall is found between the openings of the mesonephric ducts (Vilas, 1934). This has been given the unsatisfactory name "müllerian tubercle," but it will be referred to here as the "sinusal tubercle." The usual description that the solid tips of the fused paramesonephric ducts "push forward the epithelium of the posterior wall of the urogenital sinus" to form the tubercle (Koff, 1933) does not appear to be correct. The projection first formed (the primary tubercle) is believed to subside and soon be replaced by the definitive tubercle, that is, a connective tissue proliferation that represents the future urethrovaginal septum (Frutiger, 1969). The primary and secondary tubercles are not formed by the pressure of the paramesonephric ducts, because those canals have not yet reached the urogenital sinus. The sinusal tubercle is perhaps best regarded as "a site at which three types of epithelium meet and very likely mingle" (Glenister, 1962): sinusal, mesonephric, and paramesonephric.

As soon as the paramesonephric ducts "come into close contact with each other they begin to fuse even before their tips reach the urogenital sinus" (Koff, 1933). The fusion (Fig. 6) takes place initially by means of the external walls; then the cavities come together, being separated by merely a median septum. Finally, the septum becomes resorbed, and the cavities become single. Remnants of the septum between the right and left ducts may be found either rostrally or caudally. By the end of the embryonic period proper (8 weeks), ductal fusion has resulted in the formation of the "genital canal" (Matějka, 1959) or so-called uterovaginal canal. Luminal fusion is evident by stage 23 in both male and female embryos (Fig. 6).

In the event that the paramesonephric ducts do not progress sufficiently caudally, a uterus may not be formed (uterine aplasia). In other instances, uterine nodules may be found (Rokitansky–Küster–Hauser syndrome). Unilateral aplasia results when one paramesonephric duct fails to develop adequately (unicornuate uterus). In some cases, a uterine nodule may appear on the defective side (pseudounicornuate uterus). The paramesonephric ducts may

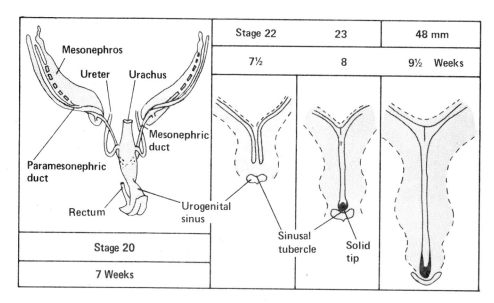

Figure 6. Scheme to show the fusion of the paramesonephric ducts. At 7 weeks (stage 20), the ducts are separated widely from each other. Their paramesonephric position, i.e., the way in which they accompany the mesonephric ducts, is well shown. The rostral vertical and middle transverse portions of each duct have formed, and the caudal vertical part develops within a few days (stage 22). The ducts then become apposed (stage 22) and fused (stage 23). In addition, the sinusal tubercle has appeared and has become related to the solid tip of the fused paramesonephric ducts. Early in the fetal period, a remnant of the median septum can still be seen rostrally. The external contour of the developing uterus is shown by interrupted lines. Based on Hunter (1930) and Koff (1933).

retain their duality externally as well as internally, resulting in two hemiuteri, which may be bicornuate and bicervical or bicornuate and unicervical. All of these anomalies arise during the embryonic period proper, i.e., the first 8 postovulatory weeks. Unfortunately most of the classifications proposed for uterine and vaginal anomalies are either exceedingly complicated or oversimplified (Monie and Sigurdson, 1950; Zanetti *et al.*, 1978; Buttram, 1983).

In addition to the mesonephric remains already described in the broad ligament, tubules believed to be of paramesonephric origin have been reported, and accessory uterine tubes have been recorded. Cysts have been noted, and the appendix vesiculosa may perhaps be considered as a hydropic accessory uterine tube.

Primary paramesonephric epithelium consists of the cellular lining of the unfused and fused portions of the paramesonephric ducts (Lauchlan, 1972). Included are tubal, endometrial, probably endocervical, and possibly ectocervical epithelium, the prostatic utricle (at least in part), and the appendix testis. Secondary paramesonephric epithelium consists of cells similar to those lining the derivatives of the paramesonephric ducts but located external to the original ductal epithelium. The superficial (so-called germinal) epithelium of the ovary is the chief source of the secondary cells, but a far wider potential distribution has been recorded. That the epithelium is a very unusual tissue has long been appreciated (Gruenwald, 1942). Its abnormal differentiation (peritoneal metaplasia) has frequently been invoked to account for at least some cases of endometriosis. Other theories, however, are not lacking, such as the detachment of islands from the paramesonephric ducts. It would appear that "no uniform pathogenesis of dystopic endometriosis can be given" (Sanfilippo and Niedobitek, 1965).

The development of the paramesonephric ducts in the male fetus has been described in detail by Glenister (1962). The caudal, fused portion of the ducts becomes joined to the urogenital sinus by a solid utricular cord. The cord then lengthens and becomes separated from the sinus by bilaterial outgrowths of sinusal epithelium, which give rise to a single sinu-utricular cord. The caudal paramesonephric remnant becomes confined within the developing prostate and merges with the sinu-utricular cord. The composite rudiment then acquires a lumen and becomes greatly dilated. Postnatally the utricle is highly variable but, in some instances, is markedly glandular. In brief, "the prostatic utricle has a composite origin, its cranial portion being formed from the paramesonephric ducts and the caudal end from the mixed epithelium covering the colliculus seminalis" (i.e., the sinusal tubercle). It would seem, therefore, that the prostatic utricle corresponds developmentally to the uterus and perhaps to the vagina; hence the old term "utriculus masculinus," which was given to it by Weber in 1836, although the structure was probably first recognized by Morgagni in 1762. Variations in the position of the male vagina, or vaginalike diverticulum, have been recorded (Bowdler *et al.*, 1971).

The appendix testis, present in 92% of adult males, is believed to be formed by the cranial end of the paramesonephric duct (Rolnick *et al.*, 1968). Frequently it contains tubular remnants of that duct and is covered by an abundant and folded layer of paramesonephric epithelium that resembles closely that of the fimbriated end of the uterine tube (Sundarasivarao, 1953). The appendix epididymidis is generally, although not universally, held to be mesonephric in origin.

The relevant events of the embryonic period proper are summarized in Table 1. Bilaterally situated paramesonephric ducts have grown caudally and fused together in both male (Fig. 7) and female embryos. In the latter, the future uterus is thereby establish (Fig. 8).

Table 1. Early Development of Reproductive Pathway

Stage	Pairs of somites	Embryonic length (mm)	Age (days)	Features
9	1–3	1.5–2.5	20	Hindgut appears
10	4–12	2–3.5	22	Intermediate mesoderm is recognizable
11	13–20	2.5–4.5	24	Mesonephric ducts develop
12	21–29	3–5	26	Mesonephric ducts become attached to cloaca
13	30–?	4–6	28	Ducts may open into cloaca
14		5–7	32	Gonadal ridges appear
15		7–9	33	Urogenital sinus is distinguishable
16		8–11	37	
17		11–14	41	Paramesonephric ducts develop
18		13–17	44	
19		16–18	48	
20		18–22	51	Paramesonephric ducts are separated widely
21		22–24	52	
22		23–28	54	Sinusal tubercle has appeared; para-mesonephric ducts are apposed
23		27–31	56	Paramesonephric ducts have fused together, and their solid tip is attached to urogenital sinus

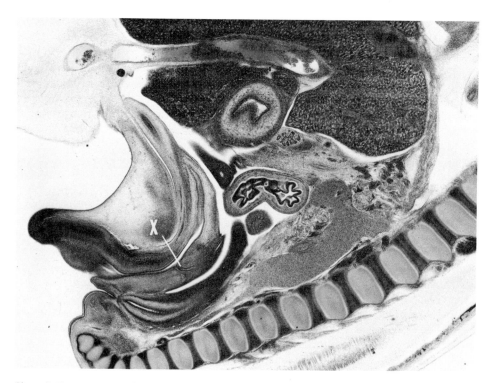

Figure 7. Photomicrograph of a sagittal section through the caudal end of a male embryo of the eighth week (stage 22), 27.5 mm in length. The section is almost in the median plane. From before backward, the genital tubercle, urogenital sinus, urorectal septum, rectum, and cartilaginous vertebral centra can be identified. The point where the fusing paramesonephric ducts reach the urogenital sinus is marked X.

3. *The Vaginal Controversy*

The development of the vagina has been discussed in detail elsewhere (O'Rahilly, 1977).

Most writers have described some type of bilateral proliferation that unites with the solid paramesonephric tip and takes part in the formation of the vagina. Although some authors had considered these to be of mesonephric or paramesonephric origin, Koff (1933) maintained that the sinuvaginal bulbs were bilateral epithelial evaginations from the dorsal wall of the urogenital sinus. They were said to appear in the region of the sinusal tubercle, which thereby became obliterated at 63 mm. The bulbs became largely solidified by 77 mm through proliferation of their lining epithelium and then fused with the solid paramesonephric tip. Bulmer (1957) referred to them as dorsolateral projections of the sinusal cells at 65 mm and also described a third and median proliferation of the dorsal wall of the sinus, as noted previously by Vilas (1934). These three initial elements were said to fuse at 94 mm to form a single sinusal upgrowth. Wells (1959) concluded that the sinuvaginal bulbs "are not discrete evaginations of the urogenital sinus" but "merely regions of junction of two kinds of epithelium," namely, that of the paramesonephric ducts and that of the urogenital sinus. (See also Chapter 2 of this volume.)

Witschi (1970) emphasized that the "old misconceptions" of previous authors were based on the assumption that the vagina grows rostrally, whereas actually, he maintained, it grows caudally.

The vaginal canal becomes occluded by a cellular mass termed the "vaginal plate" (Fig.

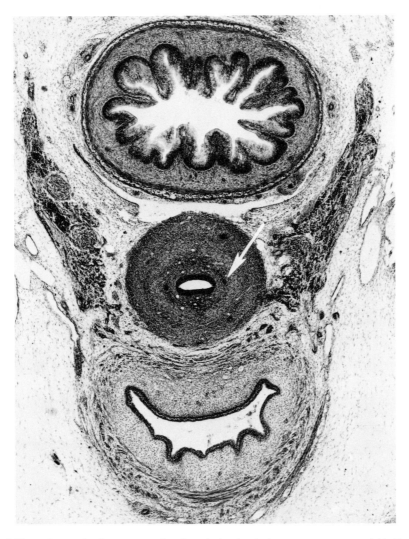

Figure 8. Photomicrograph of a cross section through the developing rectum, uterus, and bladder at 11 postovulatory weeks (69 mm). The thick wall of the uterus is evident. The mesonephric duct is present immediately lateral (arrow) to the uterine lumen (cf. Koff, 1933, Plate 1, Fig. G). The rectouterine pouch is visible behind the uterus.

9), which is generally said to be, at least initially, of paramesonephric and sinusal (or sinuvaginal) origin (Koff, 1933; Bulmer, 1957). Histochemical studies seem to be more in accord with a mesonephric origin (Forsberg, 1963, 1965). Witschi (1970) described a vaginal bud formed from the solid paramesonephric tip together with lateral wings of mesonephric duct blastema (Fig. 9). The vaginal plate is first seen distinctly at about 60–75 mm, and its formation is complete at about 140 mm. Finally, when the cells of the plate desquamate, the vaginal lumen is formed (Fig. 10).

The formation of the vaginal plate is followed immediately by extensive growth caudally, so that at 105 mm the vaginal rudiment approaches the vestibule (Witschi, 1970). It has been assumed in the past that the tissue added, either to line or to replace the vaginal segment, was pushed rostrally from the caudal end of the vaginal rudiment. Witschi (1970), however,

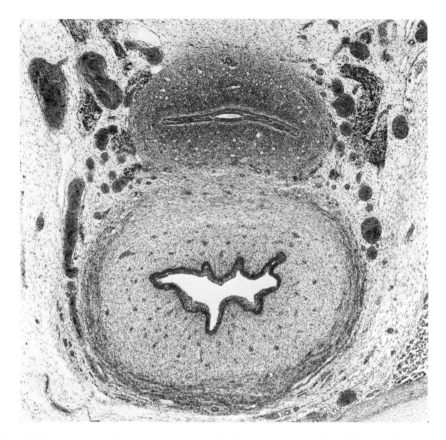

Figure 9. Photomicrograph of a cross section through the developing cervix uteri and bladder at 13 postovulatory weeks (100.5 mm). According to Koff (1933; see his Plate 2, Fig. C), the section shows the original lumen and the vaginal plate. According to Witschi (1970), however, the fins on each side of the lumen consist of "irregularly arranged cells of mesonephric duct blastema."

stressed that "the lower end of the vagina is sliding down along the urethra to its separate opening" into the vestibule.

The development in the mouse has recently been reinvestigated (Bok and Drews, 1983; Mauch *et al.,* 1985). The paramesonephric ducts fuse with the caudal parts of the mesonephric ducts, so that the latter are incorporated into the vaginal plate. The sinuvaginal bulbs are the caudal parts of the mesonephric ducts. The vagina develops by downgrowth of mesonephric and paramesonephric ducts along sinusal ridges. After regression of the mesonephric ducts and the sinusal ridges, the definitive vagina of the mouse is formed by the paramesonephric ducts. Forsberg (1978), however, continues to stress "the uniqueness of human vaginal development" and denies either a purely paramesonephric origin or a dual origin (Koff's paramesonephric and sinusal epithelia or Witschi's paramesonephric and mesonephric epithelia) in the human, although he accepts a dual origin in the mouse.

The uterovaginal canal at 75 mm presents a rostral dilatation, which represents the cavity of the body, and also a dilatation in the cervix, which "marks the region where the lateral fornices of the vagina develop" (Koff, 1933). The transition between pseudostratified columnar and stratified squamous epithelium at "17 weeks" has been assumed to represent the cervicovaginal junction (Davies and Kusama, 1962).

Cavitation in the vaginal plate can be observed at 151 mm (Fig. 10), and by 162 mm (Fig. 11) the vaginal lumen is complete except at its cranial end, where the fornices are still solid

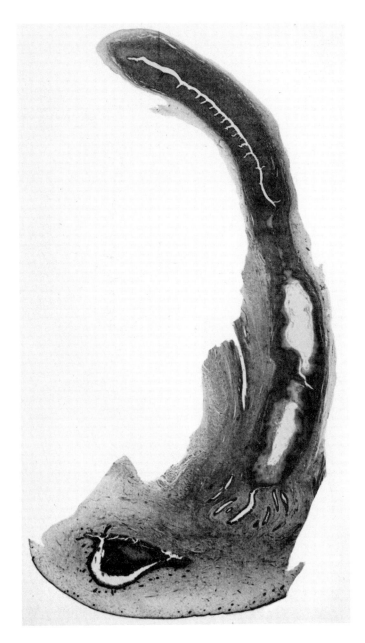

Figure 10. Sagittal section through the uterus and vagina at 17 postovulatory weeks (151 mm). The corpus is small and its lumen is relatively narrow, whereas glands are evident in the cervix. The posterior fornix appears higher in position than the anterior. The vaginal plate is still solid in its upper part. Degeneration of the central cells of the lower part of the plate indicates early formation of the vaginal lumen. A portion of the urethra can be seen in longitudinal section in front of the lower part of the vagina. From Hunter (1930, Plate 3, Fig. 15), courtesy of the Carnegie Institution of Washington. Compare Koff (1933, Plate 3, Fig. G).

(Koff, 1933). The fornices become hollow at approximately 170 mm. By about 180 mm, the genital canal has access to the exterior (Bulmer, 1957).

Although it is agreed that at least the body of the uterus is derived from the fused paramesonephric ducts, the development of the vagina has long been and still remains controversial. In brief, it is admitted that the epithelium of the vagina is derived from one or more of

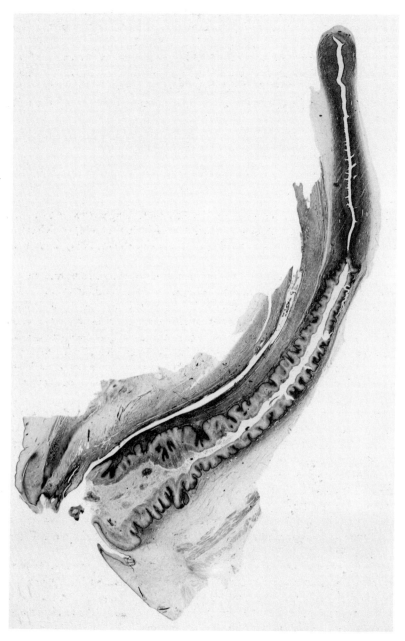

Figure 11. Median section through the uterus and vagina at about $17\frac{1}{2}$ postovulatory weeks (162 mm). The corpus is small, and glands are more evident in the cervix. The fornices are still solid, but elsewhere the vaginal plate has become completely hollowed. The vaginal lumen communicates with the urogenital sinus through the hymeneal opening. The hymeneal membrane and the fossa (navicularis) vestibuli vaginae can be detected posteriorly. The posterior part of the hymen is lined internally by vaginal epithelium and externally by sinusal epithelium. The urethra can be seen in longitudinal section in front of the vagina. Compare Koff (1933, Plate 3, Fig. H).

the following sources: the mesonephric ducts, the paramesonephric ducts, or the urogenital sinus. Thus, the origin of the vaginal epithelium has been claimed to be (1) mesonephric ("wholly a derivative from sinus or Wolffian epithelium; it is difficult to establish which," Forsberg, 1973); (2) mesonephric and paramesonephric (the epithelium of the vagina "is contributed in almost equal measures by oviduct and mesonephric duct proliferations," Witschi, 1970); (3) paramesonephric (Walz, 1958); (4) paramesonephric and sinusal ("l'origine . . . est double, müllérienne et sinusale," Agogué, 1965; Forsberg, 1973; Cunha, 1975, in the mouse); or (5) sinusal (Politzer, 1955; "the sinus upgrowth . . . forms the whole of its epithelial lining," Bulmer, 1957; Matějka, 1959; Fluhmann, 1960; Ulfelder and Robboy, 1976).

4. The Fetal Uterus

The fetal period has not been staged, and the most useful single criterion of developmental progress is the greatest length of the fetus (exclusive of the lower limbs), which corresponds approximately to the sitting height postnatally (O'Rahilly and Müller, 1984). Body weight and foot length are also of value.

Apart from possible differences in the differentiation of paramesonephric mesenchyme during the embryonic period (Candreviotis, 1967), no noticeable difference in the form and degree of development of the urogenital duct system in the male and the female is found until the ninth week, 35 mm (Glenister, 1962). Sexual differentiation of the reproductive pathway begins early in the fetal period and is attributed to the influence of gonadal hormones. The fetal testis is believed to produce not only a masculinizing hormone but also a paramesonephric inhibitor (Jost, 1972). Consequently, the mesonephric ducts become dominant in the male fetus, whereas the paramesonephric ducts are allowed to pursue their development in the female. The heterologous ducts in each sex regress for the most part.

Presumably once the paramesonephric ducts come into apposition and begin to undergo fusion, one may speak of a uterus in the female fetus. Hunter (1930) used the term "uterus" at 36 mm, and Koff (1933) at 37 mm. The rostral limit of the organ is at first V-shaped, being formed by the approximation of the free portions of the paramesonephric ducts, which may now be termed uterine tubes (Fig. 6).

Hunter (1930) found a distinct constriction between the cervix and body as early as 36 mm. At 43 mm, he noted that the body of the organ appears to be slightly twisted, "a constant feature" that "persists throughout fetal life." Furthermore, the cervix is characterized by a fusiform thickening of the surrounding mesenchyme, which, although present at 48 mm (Fig. 6), becomes marked by 75 mm.

In some instances, the internal median septum between the fusing paramesonephric ducts may persist in whole (uterus septus) or in part (uterus subseptus). Such anomalies would be expected to arise between 8 and 10 postovulatory weeks (30–50 mm). In some cases (communicating uteri), an opening between the demicavities may be found at the level of the isthmus.

Early in the fetal period (48 mm), the sinusal tubercle in the female attains its maximal development and then declines and disappears (Koff, 1933). The fusion of the paramesonephric ducts to form the genital canal is complete at 56 mm (Koff, 1933), and by that time the septum between the fused ducts has generally disappeared entirely. The canal grows in length by further fusion of the paired paramesonephric ducts rostrally, by interstitial growth and cellular multiplication, and by continued caudal growth of the solid tip of the canal.

The cervix is generally believed to be of paramesonephric origin (Koff, 1933; Forsberg, 1965; Witschi, 1970), but it has been claimed that its mucous membrane is derived from the urogenital sinus (Fluhmann, 1960), so that the precise limits of the paramesonephric and sinusal contributions to the cervix remain uncertain (Davies and Kusama, 1962). The cervical glands appear at 100–120 mm (Koff, 1933; Eida, 1961). The position of the future ostium uteri is indicated at 112 mm by differentiation of the mesoderm surrounding the stratified polygonal epithelium of the caudal part of the genital canal (Bulmer, 1957). The vaginal rudiment reaches the level of the greater vestibular glands at 130 mm and makes contact with the vestibule, at which time the vaginal downgrowth equals the uterine rudiment in length (Witschi, 1970). At about this time the maternal and fetal organisms become flooded with increasingly high concentrations of estrogenic steroids, and organ responsiveness begins in the fetal vagina (Witschi, 1970). No indication of hormonal stimulation, however, is noted in the body of the organ (Witschi, 1970).

At 130 mm, "the cervix is not sharply separated from the corpus, but at least two-thirds of the entire uterus [is] set off by a narrow isthmus against the short, bulbous corpus" (Witschi, 1970). The isthmus and the *museau de tanche* have been identified during the "5th month" of fetal life (Bouton and Maillet, 1971). A constriction between the body and cervix, however, has been recorded as early as at 36 mm (Hunter, 1930).

Some stratification at 130 mm presages the differentiation of the mucosa, muscularis, and serosa (Witschi, 1970). By 139 mm, the uterine body is a single, rounded swelling, although a shallow notch remains at the point of junction of the right and left paramesonephric ducts. More of the free portion of the ducts continues to be taken into the body of the organ, so that the round ligaments, which were originally attached laterally, become anchored to the ventrolateral angles of the body (Hunter, 1930). By 139 mm (Hunter, 1930), and perhaps even as early as 37 mm (according to an illustration in Koff, 1933), the body, cervix, and vagina are concave ventrally (Fig. 11) in relation to the abdominal viscera, especially the well-developed urinary bladder.

The glands of the corpus begin as outpouchings of the simple columnar epithelium at 151 mm (Koff, 1933). The solid epithelial primordia of the anterior and posterior fornices of the vagina can be seen (Fig. 11), and they may perhaps be detected even as early as at 130 mm (Matějka, 1959). Furthermore, "it is noteworthy that the anterior fornix is lower than the posterior fornix developmentally and not due to the cervicovaginal angulation as is commonly taught" (Koff, 1933). The anlagen of the palmate folds of the cervix are present at 160 mm (Hunter, 1930).

Although estrogen sensitivity has spread over the entire length of the vagina by 162 mm, "the epithelium of the endocervix is only slightly stimulated. It has changed from cuboidal to cylindrical cells, and mucoid development starts in the grooves of the many narrow folds" (Witschi, 1970).

In Carnegie fetuses of 142 and 151 mm, areas suggestive of future adenosis in the vagina have been seen (A. T. Hertig, personal communication, 1976). The association between postpubertal vaginal adenosis and maternal treatment with diethylstilbestrol (DES) is the subject of numerous publications (Edelman, 1986).

5. *The Second Half of Prenatal Life*

Smooth muscle cells are found in the wall of the uterus immediately before the middle of prenatal life (Hunter, 1930; Valdés-Dapena, 1957; Song, 1964; Witschi, 1970). According to Hunter, the differentiation begins in the periphery, and the site of its greatest activity is at first in the area of the cervix. In another investigation, however, smooth muscle was observed to be well differentiated in the corpus at 180 mm, although it was absent from the wall of the cervix (Davies and Kusama, 1962). It has been estimated that muscular tissue in the uterus during fetal life is approximately 35–47% of the organ (Clarke, 1911).

It has been claimed that, at 185 mm, not only the vagina and its fornices but also the cervical canal is lined by stratified squamous epithelium, so that the squamocolumnar junction is situated very high; i.e., entropion is present (Eida, 1961). In another study, however, the squamocolumnar junction has been found some distance external to the ostium, "so that the so-called 'congenital ectropion' already existed" (Davies and Kusama, 1962). Moreover, the ectropion was present "from 22 weeks to term when estrogenic effects were maximal and again at 22 months after birth when estrogenic effects were absent" (Davies and Kusama, 1962). These differing views may perhaps be attributed at least in part to individual variation.

A well-marked fundus is visible by 227 mm, and "the change in the form of the upper limit of the uterus from a V-shaped notch to a convex curve . . . is due to the general thickening of its walls, brought about by the growth and development of muscle tissue" (Hunter, 1930). The fundus projects well above the uterotubal junction and is distinctly bent ventrally. The corpus becomes anteverted upon the cervix (341 mm), and the cervix is somewhat, although not definitively, anteflexed upon the vagina (Hunter, 1930). The body of the uterus now presents its adult form, although not its adult position, and the peritoneal relations resemble closely those found in adult life.

The endometrial alterations in the fetal uterus are said to resemble successively the cyclic changes in the adult mucosa (Song, 1964). In the newborn, the endometrium generally resembles, but does not duplicate, either the proliferative or the secretory mucosa of the adult. In rare instances it resembles progestational endometrium, and decidual transformation as well as appearances analogous to menstrual changes (and attributed to estrogen withdrawal) may be encountered.

The endometrium at birth presents a low columnar or cuboidal epithelium (Fluhmann, 1960). The cervical epithelium during the last trimester reacts by proliferation and conversion to a mucinous epithelium, attributed either to estrogen alone or to a combination of estrogen and progesterone (Davies and Kusama, 1962). In the newborn, the cervical epithelium "appears typical of a stratified or pseudostratified columnar epithelium" and contains migrating leukocytes (Davies and Kusama, 1962). The basal cells are clear, and the superficial, columnar cells are mucinous and periodic acid-Schiff positive. The vaginal epithelium is stratified squamous and shows intense estrogenic stimulation.

Histochemical studies indicate that the development of the cervix precedes that of the corpus during fetal life (Szamborski and Laskowska, 1968). The junction between the cervical

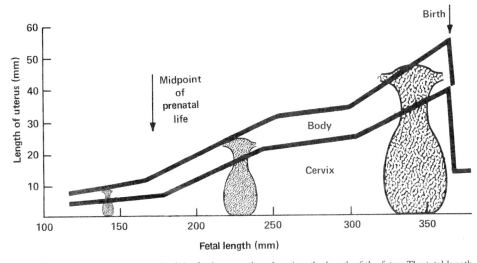

Figure 12. Graph showing the length of the fetal uterus plotted against the length of the fetus. The total length and also that of the cervix are indicated. The gradients of both before the midpoint of prenatal life are resumed after birth. During the second half of prenatal life, however, the growth of the cervix is augmented temporarily under hormonal influence. From the data of Hunter (1930).

Table 2.   The Development of the Uterus during the Fetal Period[a]

Fetal length (mm)	Approximate age (postovulatory weeks)	Features
36	9	Uterus is distinguishable as an organ
36–43		Constriction occurs between body and cervix
48–75	10	Thickened mesenchyme indicates cervix
56	10½	Median septum has usually disappeared
60–75	11	Vaginal plate becomes distinct and fuses with solid para-mesonephric tip
62–130		Vaginal rudiment grows caudally
63		Mesonephric ducts begin to disappear in female
100–120	15	Cervical glands appear
112		Position of future ostium is visible
130	17	Isthmus is readily distinguishable; layers of uterus begin to be defined
135		Cervix is about 5 mm in length
151	19	Glands of body appear; solid fornices are evident
162–180	20	Smooth muscle cells are distinguishable
170		Fornices become hollow
180	21	Canalization of vagina is complete
190	22	Cervix is about 10 mm in length
215–295	24	Body is about 10 mm in length
227	25	Fundus is well marked
240	26	Cervix is about 20 mm in length
305	34	Cervix is about 25 mm in length
341	40	Anteversion is noted, and an indication of anteflexion

[a]Modified slightly from O'Rahilly (1973).

and vaginal epithelia is very variable at term. In some areas the vaginal epithelium extends up to the edge of the ostium, whereas in others "congenital ectropion" is observed. No evidence is found for an actual migration of the vaginal epithelium with displacement of the cervical epithelium or *vice versa* (Davies and Kusama, 1962). The site and pattern of the squamo-columnar junction vary considerably in postnatal life. The predominant pattern in childhood is one of entropion (Hamperl and Kaufmann, 1959).

Late in fetal life (at about 240 mm), the uterus undergoes an increased linear growth in relation to most bodily dimensions (Scammon, 1926). Immediately after birth, however, the length and weight of the organ diminish sharply until it assumes basically the dimensions that it would have attained had its early fetal growth rate remained unchanged (Fig. 12). The secondary prenatal growth increment is attributed chiefly to a hormone (probably placental in origin), which, being lost at birth, allows the uterus to decline to its level of typical growth. The sudden postnatal reduction in length is associated mainly with the cervix rather than with the body of the uterus (Hunter, 1930). In a more recent study, the growth of the isthmus has been plotted separately, although unfortunately fetal lengths are not included (Bouton and Maillet, 1971). Measurements of the lower uterine segment during pregnancy have been made by ultrasonic scanning (Morrison, 1972). However, measurement of the isthmus is difficult even in the adult (Danforth, 1947). Additional measurements of prenatal weight have been published (Morii, 1958).

The development of the uterus during the fetal period is summarized in Table 2. Representative photomicrographs are reproduced in Figs. 8 to 11.

ACKNOWLEDGMENT. This work was aided by research grant No. HD-16702, Institute of Child Health and Human Development, National Institutes of Health.

Agogué, M., 1965, Dualité embryologique du vagin humain et origine histologique de sa muqueuse. *Gynécol. Obstét.* **64**:407–414.

Beltermann, R., 1965, Elektronenmikroskopische Untersuchungen am Epoophoron des Menschen, *Arch. Gynaekol.* **200**:275–284.

Bok, G., and Drews, U., 1983, The role of the wolffian ducts in the formation of the sinus vagina: An organ culture study, *J. Embryol. Exp. Morphol.* **73**:275–295.

Bouton, C., and Maillet, M., 1971, Contribution à l'étude de l'organogénèse utérine chez le foetus humain, *C. R. Assoc. Anat.* **56**:261–275.

Bowdler, J. D., Dey, D. L., and Smith, P. G., 1971, Embryological implications of the male vagina, *J. Anat.* **110**:510.

Bulmer, D., 1957, The development of the human vagina, *J. Anat.* **91**:490–509.

Buttram, V. C., 1983, Müllerian anomalies and their management, *Fertil. Steril.* **40**:159–163.

Candreviotis, N., 1967, Die spezifische Differenzierung des Mesenchym in den Anlagen der Genitalorgane des Menschen, insbesondere des Müllerschen Ganges bei der Frau und ihre Beziehung zur Histogenese der Endometriose, gegrundet auf embryologisch-histologische Untersuchungen, *Zentralbl. Gynaekol.* **89**:369–382.

Clarke, H. R., 1911, A contribution to the origin of uterine muscle in relation to blood-vessels, *J. Obstet. Gynaecol. Br. Emp.* **20**:85–104.

Cunha, G. R., 1975, The dual origin of vaginal epithelium, *Am. J. Anat.* **143**:387–392.

Cunha, G. R., 1976, Epithelial–stromal interactions in development of the urogenital tract, *Int. Rev. Cytol.* **47**:137–194.

Danforth, D. N., 1947, The fibrous nature of the human cervix, and its relation to the isthmic segment in gravid and nongravid uteri, *Am. J. Obstet. Gynecol.* **53**:541–560.

Davies, J., and Kusama, H., 1962, Developmental aspects of the human cervix, *Ann. N.Y. Acad. Sci.* **97**:534–550.

Didier, E., 1968, Données expérimentales sur la formation du canal de Müller chez l'embryon d'oiseau, *Ann. Embryol. Morphog.* **1**:341–350.

Didier, E., 1973a, Recherches sur la morphogénèse du canal de Müller chez les oiseaux. I. Étude descriptive, *W. Roux Arch. Entwickl. Mech. Org.* **172**:271–286.

Didier, E., 1973b, Recherches sur la morphogénèse du canal de Müller chez les oiseaux. II. Ètude expérimentale, *W. Roux Arch. Entwickl. Mech. Org.* **172**:287–302.

Duthie, G. M., 1925, An investigation of the occurrence, distribution and histological structure of the embryonic remains in the human broad ligament, *J. Anat.* **59**:410–431.

Edelman, D. A., 1986, *DES/Diethylstilbestrol. New Perspectives,* MTP, Lancaster.

Eida, T., 1961, Entwicklungsgeschichtliche Studien über der Verschiebung der Epithelgrenze an der Portio vaginalis cervicis, *Yokohama Med. Bull. Suppl.* **12**:54–63.

Faulconer, R. J., 1951, Observations on the origin of the Müllerian groove in human embryos, *Contrib. Embryol. Carnegie Inst.* **34**:159–164.

Felix, W., 1912, The development of the urinogenital organs, in: *Manual of Human Embryology,* Vol. 2 (F. Keibel and F. P. Mall, eds.), pp. 752–979, J. B. Lippincott, Philadelphia.

Fluhmann, C. F., 1960, The developmental anatomy of the cervix uteri, *Obstet. Gynecol.* **15**:62–69.

Forsberg, J.-G., 1963, *Derivation and Differentiation of the Vaginal Epithelium,* Institute of Anatomy, Lund.

Forsberg, J.-G., 1965, Origin of vaginal epithelium, *Obstet. Gynecol.* **25**:787–791.

Forsberg, J.-G., 1973, Cervicovaginal epithelium: Its origin and development, *Am. J. Obstet. Gynecol.* **115**:1025–1043.

Forsberg, J.-G., 1978, Development of the human vaginal epithelium, in: *The Human Vagina* (E. S. E. Hafez and T. N. Evans, eds.), pp. 3–19, North-Holland, Amsterdam.

Frutiger, P., 1969, Zur Frühentwicklung der Ductus paramesonephrici und des Müllerschen Hügels beim Menschen, *Acta Anat.* **72**:233–245.

Gardner, G. H., Greene, R. R., and Peckham, B. M., 1948, Normal and cystic structures of the broad ligament, *Am. J. Obstet. Gynecol.* **55**:917–939.

Glenister, T. W., 1962, The development of the utricle and of the so-called "middle" or "median" lobe of the human prostate, *J. Anat.* **96**:443–455.

Gruenwald, P., 1941, The relation of the growing müllerian duct to the wolffian duct and its importance for the genesis of malformations, *Anat. Rec.* **81**:1–19.

Gruenwald, P., 1942, Primary asymmetry of the growing müllerian ducts in the chick embryo, *J. Morphol.* **71**:299–305.

Gruenwald, P., 1959, Growth and development of the uterus: The relationship of epithelium to mesenchyme, *Ann. N.Y. Acad. Sci.* **75**:436–440.

Hamperl, H., and Kaufmann, C., 1959, The cervix uteri at different ages, *Obstet. Gynecol.* **14**:621–631.

Huffman, J. W., 1948, Mesonephric remnants in the cervix, *Am. J. Obstet. Gynecol.* **56**:23–40.

Hunter, R. H., 1930, Observations on the development of the human female genital tract, *Contrib. Embryol. Carnegie Inst.* **22**:91–108.

Jost, A., 1972, A new look at the mechanisms controlling sex differentiation in mammals, *Johns Hopkins Med. J.* **130**:38–53.

Koff, A. K., 1933, Development of the vagina in the human fetus, *Contrib. Embryol. Carnegie Inst.* **24**:59–90.

Lauchlan, S. C., 1972, The secondary Müllerian system, *Obstet. Gynecol. Surv.* **27**:133–146.

Matějka, M., 1959, Die Morphogenese der menschlichen Vagina und ihre Gesetzmässigkeiten, *Anat. Anz.* **106**:20–37.

Mauch, R. B., Thiedemann, K.-U., and Drews, U., 1985, The vagina is formed by downgrowth of Wolffian and Müllerian ducts, *Anat. Embryol.* **172**:75–87.

Meyer, R., 1909, Zur Kenntnis des Gartnerschen (oder Wolffschen) Ganges besonders in der Vagina und dem Hymen des Menschen, *Arch. mikroskop. Anat.* **73**:751–792.

Monie, I. W., and Sigurdson, L. A., 1950, A proposed classification for uterine and vaginal anomalies, *Am. J. Obstet. Gynecol.* **59**:696–698.

Monroe, C. W., and Spector, B., 1962, The epithelium of the hydatid of Morgagni in the human adult female, *Anat. Rec.* **142**:189–193.

Morii, T., 1958, Statistical studies on the weights of female internal genital organs of human fetus, *Shikoku Acta Med.* **13**:212–230.

Morrison, J., 1972, The development of the lower uterine segment, *Aust. N.Z. J. Obstet. Gynaecol.* **12**:182–185.

O'Rahilly, R., 1973, The embryology and anatomy of the uterus, in: *The Uterus* (H. J. Norris, A. T. Hertig, and M. R. Abell, eds.), pp. 17–39, Williams & Wilkins, Baltimore.

O'Rahilly, R., 1977, The development of the vagina in the human, *Birth Defects* **13**:123–136.

O'Rahilly, R., 1983, The timing and sequence of events in the development of the human reproductive system during the embryonic period proper, *Anat. Embryol.* **166**:247–261.

O'Rahilly, R., and Muecke, E. C., 1972, The timing and sequence of events in the development of the human urinary system during the embryonic period proper, *Z. Anat. Entwicklungsgesch.* **138**:99–109.

O'Rahilly, R., and Müller, F., 1984, Embryonic length and cerebral landmarks in staged human embryos, *Anat. Rec.* **209**:265–271.

O'Rahilly, R., and Müller, F., 1987, *Developmental Stages in Human Embryos*, Publication 637, Carnegie Institution of Washington, Washington, D.C.

Politzer, G., 1955, Zur normalen und abnormen Entwicklung der menschlichen Scheide, *Anat. Anz.* **102**:271–278.

Sanfilippo, S., and Niedobitek, F., 1965, Zur Pathogenese einer Endometriose im Bereich des Lumbalmarkes bei Spina bifida, *Arch. Gynaekol.* **200**:452–462.

Scammon, R. E., 1926, The prenatal growth and natal involution of the human uterus. *Proc. Soc. Exp. Biol. Med.* **23**:687–690.

Shikinami, J., 1926, Detailed form of the Wolffian body in human embryos of the first eight weeks, *Contrib. Embryol. Carnegie Inst.* **18**:49–61.

Song, J., 1964, *The Human Uterus: Morphogenesis and Embryological Basis for Cancer,* Charles C. Thomas, Springfield, IL.

Streeter, G. L., 1948, Developmental horizons in human embryos. Description of age groups XV, XVI, XVII, and XVIII, being the third issue of a survey of the Carnegie Collection, *Contrib. Embryol. Carnegie Inst.* **32**:133–203.

Sundarasivarao, D., 1953, The Müllerian vestiges and benign epithelial tumours of the epididymis, *J. Pathol. Bacteriol.* **66**:417–432.

Szamborski, J., and Laskowska, H., 1968, Some observations on the developmental histology of the human foetal uterus, *Biol. Neonat.* **13**:298–314.

Torrey, T. W., 1954, The early development of the human nephros, *Contrib. Embryol. Carnegie Inst.* **35**:175–197.

Ulfelder, H., and Robboy, S. J., 1976, The embryologic development of the human vagina, *Am. J. Obstet. Gynecol.* **126**:769–776.

Valdés-Dapena, M. A., 1957, *An Atlas of Fetal and Neonatal Histology,* J. B. Lippincott, Philadelphia.

Vilas, E., 1934, Zur Entwicklung der menschlichen Scheide, *Anat. Anz.* **79**:150–151.

Walz, W., 1958, Über die Genese der sogenannten indirekten Metaplasie im Bereich des Müllerschen-Gang-Systems, *Z. Geburtshilfe Gynaekol.* **151**:1–21.

Wells, L. J., 1959, Embryology and anatomy of the vagina, *Ann. N.Y. Acad. Sci.* **83:**80–88.

Witschi, E., 1970, Development and differentiation of the uterus, in: *Prenatal Life* (H. C. Mack, ed.), pp. 11–35, Wayne State University Press, Detroit.

Zanetti, E., Ferrari, L. R., and Rossi, G., 1978, Classification and radiographic features of uterine malformations, *Br. J. Radiol.* **51:**161–170.

4

Vascular Anatomy

ELIZABETH M. RAMSEY

Most of the blood vessels of the body maintain a high degree of stability once they are fully formed. Changes associated with advancing years creep on slowly, almost imperceptibly, and only dramatic episodes of disease or trauma call forth the vessels' inherent capacity for regeneration. The blood vessels of the uterus, however, and particularly those of the endometrium, form an exception to this generalization. In them, stability gives place to a high degree of variability. The variability is of two sorts, for the regularly recurring interruptions of vascular pattern associated with the menstrual cycle are themselves interrupted at irregular intervals by the vascular upheavals occasioned by pregnancy. The efficiency with which the vessels adapt to this demanding schedule forms the dividing line between normal function and pathology. The factors that produce vascular variability also control the cyclic changes in the parenchymatous tissues of the endometrium, in large part secondarily via the blood vessels. The latter may therefore with justice be regarded as dynamic determinants of endometrial activity and as such merit a detailed consideration of their anatomy and physiology.

In the first edition of this book the gross and microscopic anatomy of the blood vessels of the uterus and the stages of their transformation into the uteroplacental vasculature were presented in some detail. The reader is referred to that volume and to Boyd and Hamilton (1970) and Ramsey and Donner (1980) for full descriptions. Only a brief review is given here to serve as the basis for consideration of current studies.

Uterine and uteroplacental vasculature and circulation are so similar in all primate species examined to date that any one of them may be regarded as essentially representative of all. In experimental studies the rhesus monkey has been extensively employed. Some of the illustrations presented here record observations made in that species. Where pertinent differences occur, they are noted.

ELIZABETH M. RAMSEY • Department of Embryology, Carnegie Institution of Washington, Baltimore, Maryland 21210.

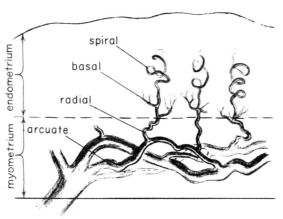

Figure 1. Schematic representation of uterine arteries. After Okkels and Engle (1938).

1. Basic Aspects of Architecture and Physiology of Uterine Arteries

1.1. Nonpregnant

Figure 1 shows that the major arterial blood supply to the uterus is derived from the uterine arteries. This is augmented by small, variable increments from the ovarian arteries. The spiral arteries, which constitute prolongations of the radials, project into the endometrium, terminating in a capillary plexus that reaches to the subepithelial zone. These arteries respond to hormonal stimuli throughout the menstrual cycle. Their coiling is progressively accentuated, and they continue ever further into the endometrium, as shown in Fig. 2a,b. This growth is under the influence of estrogen supplied by the growing ovarian follicle. Intermittent constriction of the arteries at the myometrial–endometrial junction, as seen in Fig. 2c, occurs throughout the cycle. Following ovulation, if no implantation occurs, the arteries regress. When follicular support of the endometrium wanes, with regression of the follicle, the arterial constrictions create ischemia, which in turn occasions the necrosis and hemorrhage of menstruation. The basal arteries, which are small, stubby branches of the radial arteries, do not respond to hormonal stimuli and remain unaltered throughout the cycle.

Uterine veins are long, vertical vessels roughly paralleling the course of the glands. Localized dilatations, "lakes," occur at the points of intersection of connecting veins. The lakes fluctuate in size and apparently serve as reservoirs to cushion changes in blood volume and rate of flow. Uterine veins, assisted by ovarian veins, effect drainage from the uterus. The participation of ovarian veins is greater in monkeys than in humans.

Histologically the radial arteries are characterized by stout elastic membranes separating the endothelium and the media, with scattered elastic fibrils intermingled with muscle cells in the media and irregular elastic membranes in the adventitia. The spiral arterial continuations of the radials gradually lose their elastic membranes as they pass through the endometrium, although a loose fibrillar network persists as far as the subepithelial region. The basal arteries contain almost no elastic tissue but have abundant muscle with particularly large individual cells that contain more cytoplasm and larger nuclei than do the muscle cells of other uterine arteries.

1.2. Pregnant

When pregnancy occurs, the spiral arteries do not regress, but the changes that have occurred in them are continued and augmented by the action of the corpus luteum of pregnan-

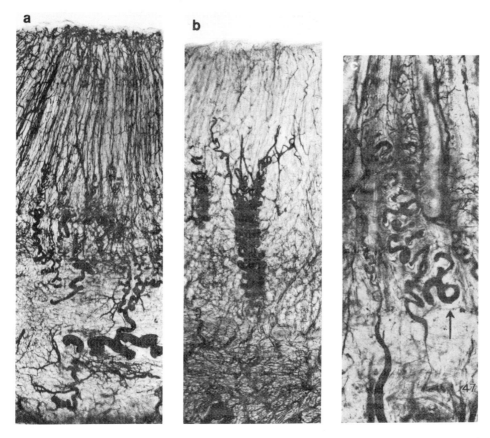

Figure 2. (a) Cross section of the uterine wall of a rhesus monkey on day 12 of the menstrual cycle. Several spiral arteries show minimal coiling in the lower third of the endometrium. The straight distal ends reach almost to the surface epithelium. (b) The endometrium and inner layer of the myometrium in another monkey on day 17 of the menstrual cycle. The abundant coiling of a spiral artery is seen in the middle third of the endometrium. The straight distal ends reach three-fourths of the way to the surface epithelium. (c) The myometrial–endometrial junction (arrow) in a third monkey on the 11th day of the cycle. The deeper portion of the spiral artery and the immediately adjacent portion of the radial artery show marked constriction. All specimens injected with India ink. All from Bartelmez (1957).

cy. The vessels continue to grow even after the trophoblastic invasion has effected communication between the arteries and the intervillous space, at which time the designation "uteroplacental arteries" becomes appropriate. Indeed, this growth of the arteries continues until the end of the first trimester, with resultant coiling and back-and-forth looping of the vessels to enable them to accommodate themselves to the constantly shrinking endometrial diameter. At midterm, when enlargement of the uterus by growth of its parts is replaced by enlargement by stretching, the coils are paid out, more completely so in the monkey than in man. Concomitantly with growth and coiling, the terminal portion of the artery undergoes progressive dilatation in all primate species studied. The mechanism by which the dilatation is effected is described later in this chapter. Figure 3 illustrates these developments.

Uterine veins react passively to pregnancy. The pressure of the growing conceptus obliterates many of them, and the remaining ones become distended by the increasing volume of blood from the intervillous space that they must handle. Orifices of exit from the intervillous space persist in all regions of the placental base. There is no "marginal sinus" or any

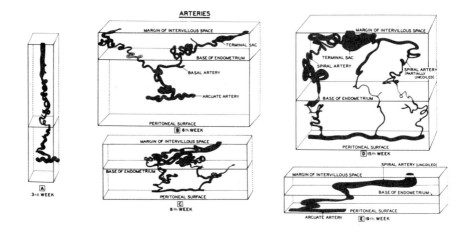

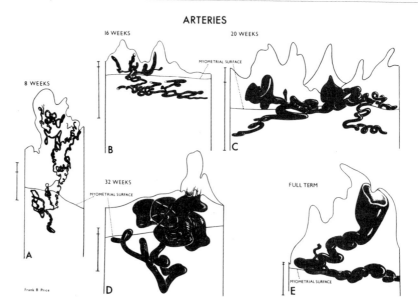

Figure 3. Diagrammatic representations of the course and configuration of the uteroplacental arteries in the rhesus monkey (top) and man (bottom) at comparable stages of gestation. From Harris and Ramsey (1966). The qualitative similarity between rhesus and man is apparent. The quantitative differences are largely occasioned by the thicker muscularis and the almost total disappearance of the decidua basalis in man versus other nonhuman primates.

predilection for drainage from the margin of the placenta. However, large veins do drain that area, and there is usually a major wreath of veins within the epiplacental angle.

Circulation of blood through the placenta is accomplished by the head of pressure of maternal systemic blood, which forces maternal blood in characteristic "spurts" deep into the intervillous space before lateral dispersion occurs. Thus, the villi in the area supplied by individual spiral arteries are bathed by the oxygen- and nutrient-carrying afferent streams, and metabolic transfer occurs across the walls of the terminal villi. The maternal blood rendered venous by this exchange is forced out of the intervillous space through orifices in the placental base by further inflowing blood. Pressure differentials are small but adequate for this mechanism (Fig. 4).

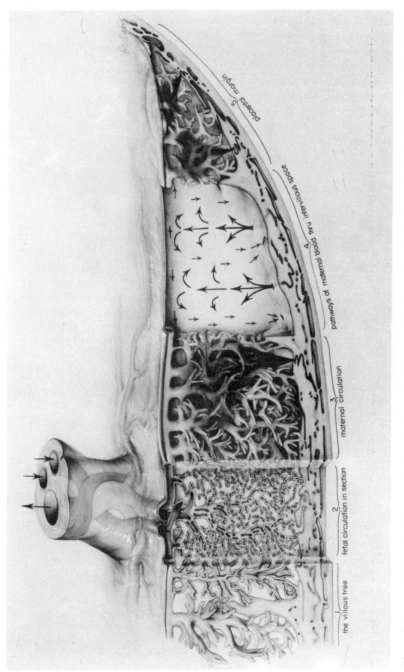

Figure 4. A composite drawing of the primate placenta showing its stricture and circulation. Drawing by Ranice W. Crosby, *Carnegie Year Book*, 1961–1962.

2.   Interaction of Trophoblast and Decidua

The interaction between fetal trophoblast and maternal decidua has long aroused interest, in particular the effects exerted by the trophoblast on the maternal blood vessels. Boyd and Hamilton (1956) and Hamilton and Boyd (1960) summarized the early studies to which they themselves contributed extensively.

At their earliest contact with the trophoblast, at implantation, the endometrial capillaries resist erosion. The trophoblast flows around them and engulfs them. During the first week, however, capillary walls are penetrated by trophoblast, and maternal blood seeps into lacunae, forerunners of the intervillous space, which are then forming in the trophoblastic shell. As the trophoblast penetrates the endometrium more deeply, it reaches the spiral arteries proper and "taps" them. Arterial blood then enters the intervillous space under higher pressure, thus forming the earliest stage of placental circulation.

Subsequent developments have been intensively studied in recent years by the international team of Brosens, Robertson, Dixon, and Pijnenborg, leading to formulation of the widely recognized "physiological concept" described in the following paragraphs (Brosens *et al.,* 1967, 1977; Pijnenborg *et al.,* 1980, 1981, 1986).

By the eighth week trophoblast has entered the arterial lumina at the orifices of entry in the placental base (Fig. 5a). Clumps of trophoblastic cells may temporarily plug one or another orifice. It should be noted that certain investigators are of the opinion, based on ultrasound studies and chorionic villus sampling, that there is complete obstruction of all the uteroplacental arteries so that there is no entry of blood into the intervillous space before 12 weeks (Hustin *et al.,* 1988). Retrograde extension of trophoblast within arterial channels occurs as a "drip" along the endothelial lining. The process reaches the myometrial–endometrial junction by the end of the 12th to 13th week in the human. The penetration is a little deeper in humans than in other primates; in fact, the process continues into the myometrial portion of the arteries. This deep localization is considered by some to represent a new wave of trophoblastic invasion.

In the second phase of trophoblastic action, trophoblast enters the arterial wall itself and replaces the fixed tissues of the media, which do not regenerate (Fig. 5b). The endoarterial trophoblast is embedded in a matrix of fibrin. By elimination of the elastic tissue and muscle of its wall, the contractile capacity of the artery is destroyed, and the pressure of the blood in the

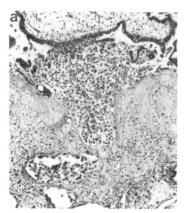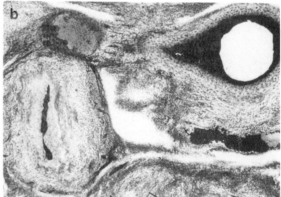

Figure 5. (a) A photomicrograph showing trophoblast in a human uteroplacental artery. Trophoblast fills the arterial lumen and "drips" into proximal coils of the artery, seen in cross section. From Ramsey *et al.* (1976). (b) A photomicrograph showing coils of two spiral arteries underlying the placenta in a rhesus monkey on the 102nd day of pregnancy. The coil on the right shows replacement of the vessel wall by trophoblast. In the vessel on the left the wall is replaced by fibrosis. India ink injection. Carnegie specimen C-679, section B125.

lumen distends it. It is in this way that the dilatation of the terminal portion of the uteroplacental arteries as shown in Fig. 3 is effected, i.e., by trophoblastic action on the walls of the arteries.

In the final third of pregnancy the majority of the trophoblast disappears from the arterial wall and is replaced by fibrous connective tissue containing very few residual isolated trophoblastic cells (Fig. 5b). In the human being, although in no other primate studied, isolated trophoblastic cells, often called "wandering cells" or "giant cells," are found throughout the decidua and often deeper in the myometrium. These are large pleomorphic cells, sometimes clumped. Nuclei vary in size and shape and usually are single (Fig. 6). They have been variously identified as syncytiotrophoblast or cytotrophoblast. The prevalent opinion at present is that they are specialized forms of cytotrophoblast. It may be postulated that these cells, attacking the arteries from without, may augment the action of the intraarterial cells, thus causing greater and more persistent terminal sac formation in the human (Fig. 3) than in the placenta of other primates. Differing opinions expressed by investigators of this point leave the matter open for future settlement (Harris and Ramsey, 1966; Ramsey et al., 1976; Pijnenborg et al., 1980). The arterial changes occur only in arteries in communication with the intervillous space. No comparable changes occur in the veins.

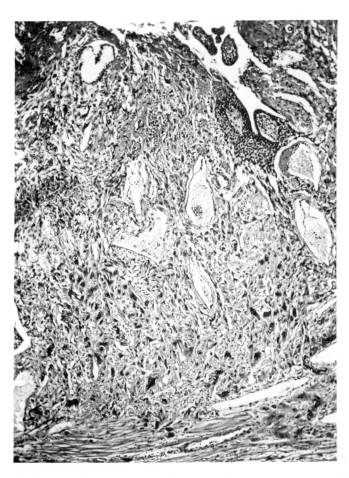

Figure 6. Trophoblastic giant cells are seen invading the uterine wall in a human pregnancy of the 17th week. Villous attachment above with a few layers of muscle at the bottom of the photomicrograph. University of Virginia specimen U18-2.

Originally regarded as pathological phenomena, such arterial changes are now recognized as normal (Sheppard and Bonnar, 1974), indeed as essential, for they establish a mechanism for control of volume, speed, and pressure of inflow of maternal blood into the intervillous space. When these physiological changes are lacking, pathological changes may develop in the course of pregnancy, and the fetus may be adversely affected.

The intermittent constrictions of spiral arterial stems seen in the basalis in the menstrual cycle continue into pregnancy (Martin *et al.*, 1964), when they lead to intermittent flow into the intervillous space (Figs. 7 and 8). The action is independent from one arterial stem to another and has no connection with the generalized contractions of the myometrium (Braxton Hicks contractions). The intrinsic constrictions last approximately 12 sec and doubtless permit mixing of blood in the intervillous space (Ramsey *et al.*, 1979).

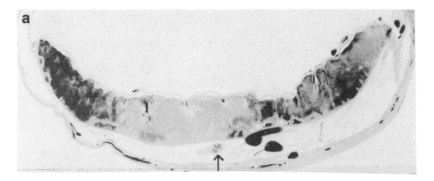

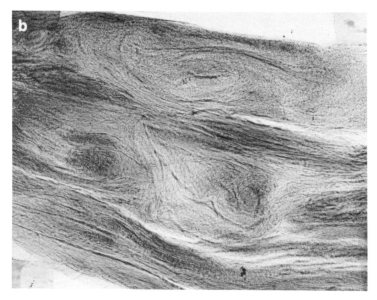

Figure 7. (a) Cross section of the uterine wall of a monkey 123 days pregnant. Placenta *in situ*. Note central anemic area in the placenta. A patent cross section of the spiral artery supplying the area is at arrow. The vessel is bloodless. (b) The same specimen 5 mm deeper in the block. The artery supplying the anemic area is seen crossing the myometrial–endometrial junction. Its complete occlusion, apparently by vasospasm, explains the bloodlessness of the area of placenta it supplies. From Ramsey (1959).

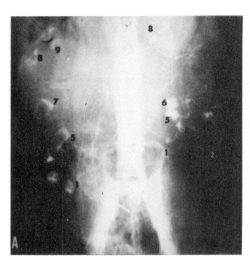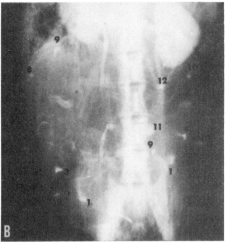

Figure 8. Photographs of radiograms of a rhesus monkey 125 days pregnant labeled to show that different spiral arterioles are patent in two successive contraction cycles. Recalling that the rhesus placenta is bidiscoid, note in comparing the two radiograms that in B entries 4–7 in the right placenta and 6–8 in the left are not seen, but two new entries, 9–8, appear in the left placenta. From Ramsey *et al.* (1963).

3. Contemporary Studies

The close temporal relationship between bursts of scientific activity and discovery and the development of new tools and techniques has frequently been noted. Such a relationship often comes about when an impasse has been reached and further progress with existing technology is impossible. Such an event occurred in the first part of the present century, when classical techniques of sectioning, staining, preparation of three-dimensional models, and conventional radiology approached the horizons of usefulness. Currently a great variety of new techniques have raised the curtain on whole new realms and given rise to vast new concepts: transmission and scanning electron microscopy, cytochemistry, immunohistochemistry, ultrasound, and magnetic resonance imaging, to list but a few (Al-Timimi and Fox, 1986).

Two new points of view also characterize study of the uterus at the present time. The first is preoccupation with the pregnant state. This shift in interest may have come about in part because the fundamentals of nonpregnant structure and function had been reasonably well established and also because a large part of research in reproduction is now carried out by obstetricians in clinical institutions with special interest focused in this direction. The second, closely related interest is in the role played by uterine vasculature and circulation in the pathogenesis of disorders of pregnancy.

Of course not all of the refined new techniques have been employed in studying uterine blood vessels, which are the focal point of interest in this chapter, but use of various pertinent ones has supplied important information.

If the sequential development of knowledge of the structure of uterine blood vessels is reviewed, it is seen that the classical concept of vascular wall as composed of connective tissue, muscle, and elastic tissue was automatically applied to uterine vasculature in the first instance. It was Hitschmann and Adler's (1908) identification of cyclic changes in the endometrium that provided the first inkling that the uterine vessels are "different."

Brosens *et al.* (1967), in their formulation of the "physiological concept" previously described, elucidated an important aspect of this difference, requiring the addition of the trophoblast and fibrinoid as new components of arterial walls that replace muscle and elastic tissue.

Simultaneously histochemists were showing that the placenta is important in the maintenance of hormonal balance in the maternal–placental–fetal unit and that the placenta itself actually produces hormones. The first peptides to be identified were hCG and hPL, and these were followed by many others (Al-Timimi and Fox, 1986). Immunohistochemistry and immunofluorescence then were used to show that by use of antisera specifically developed for the purpose, it is possible to identify individual hormones in various locations. For uterine vessels these techniques have permitted demonstration of specific types of trophoblast in the walls and elsewhere in the reproductive tract. These include the characteristic ''intermediate type'' between cytotrophoblast and syncytiotrophoblast and several subtypes of cytotrophoblast (Bulmer and Johnson, 1985; Gaspard et al., 1980; Kurman et al., 1984; Gosseye and Fox, 1984; Nelson et al., 1986; Wynn, 1972). Although the syncytiotrophoblast, rather than the villous cytotrophoblast, has generally been considered to be the hormonally active form of trophoblast, the specialized transitional and intermediate forms of trophoblast now are considered to be hormonally active as well (Wynn, 1972; Kurman et al., 1984).

Another altered component of the spiral arteries that have been invaded by trophoblast is the basement membrane. By studying the immunofluorescence of such arteries after treatment with appropriate antisera, Wells et al. (1984) demonstrated that antigens characteristic of endovascular trophoblast, specifically AA3, are present in the areas of trophoblastic invasion. Since the invading trophoblast lacks AA3 in its interstitial form, it was suggested that it creates its own basement membrane once it has entered the artery. Aplin and Campbell (1985), in their study of cytotrophoblast of the chorion laeve, found the trophoblast there similarly active in formation of matrix.

From consideration of the still highly incomplete body of information about normal uterine vessels, investigators have postulated that in certain pathological conditions such as intrauterine growth retardation and preeclampsia–eclampsia, failure of the ''physiological changes'' to occur may be basic to the development of the clinical syndromes. If the normal replacement of muscle and elastic tissue in the myometrial segments of the spiral arteries does not occur, the vessels may not distend and thus be unable to accommodate the volume and flow of maternal blood required by the developing fetus (Brosens, 1988; Brosens et al., 1972, 1977; Jones, 1980; Teasdale, 1987). Sheppard and Bonnar (1976; 1980) also studied the failure of physiological changes and the formation of atherosis in the vessels and concluded that these features are not specifically related to preeclampsia. Further discussion of this subject is found in Wynn's Chapter 11 in this volume.

These examples of current trends in research reinforce the statement made in the introduction to this chapter that the uterine blood vessels may be regarded as ''dynamic determinants'' of endometrial activity. Now it is clear that the vessels are in fact determinants of activity in all phases of the reproductive cycle and in the pathogenesis of some major disorders of pregnancy.

4. References

Al-Timimi, A., and Fox, H., 1986, Immunohistochemical localization of follicle-stimulating hormone, luteinizing hormone, growth hormone, adrenocorticotrophic hormone and prolactin in the human placenta, *Placenta* **7**:163–172.

Aplin, J. D., and Campbell, S., 1985, An immunofluorescence study of extracellular matrix associated with cytotrophoblast of the chorion laeve, *Placenta* **6**:469–480.

Bartelmez, G. W., 1957, The form and the functions of the uterine blood vessels in the rhesus monkey, *Carnegie Contrib. Embryol.* **36**:153–182.

Boyd, J. D., and Hamilton, W. J., 1956, Cells in the spiral arteries of the pregnant uterus, *J. Anat. (Lond.)* **90:**595.

Boyd, J. D., and Hamilton, W. J., 1970, *The Human Placenta,* Heffer, Cambridge.

Brosens, I., 1988, Morphology of the utero-placental vessels at term, *Troph. Res.* **3:**61–68.

Brosens, I., Robertson, W. B., and Dixon, H. G., 1967, The physiological response of the vessels of the placental bed to normal pregnancy, *J. Pathol. Bacteriol.* **93:**569–579.

Brosens, I. A., Robertson, W. B., and Dixon, H. G., 1972, The role of the spiral arteries in the pathogenesis of preeclampsia, *Obstet. Gynecol. Ann.* **1:**177–191.

Brosens, I., Dixon, H. G., and Robertson, W. B., 1977, Fetal growth retardation and the vasculature of the placental bed, *Br. J. Obstet. Gynaecol.* **84:**656–664.

Bulmer, J. N., and Johnson, P. M., 1985, Antigen expression by trophoblast populations in the human placenta and their possible immunobiological relevance, *Placenta* **6:**127–140.

Gaspard, U. J., Huston, J., Reuter, A. M., Lambotte, R., and Franchimont, P., 1980, Immunofluorescent localization of placental lactogen, chorionic gonadotrophin and its alpha and beta subunits in organ cultures of human placenta, *Placenta* **1:**135–144.

Gosseye, S., and Fox, H., 1984, An immunohistological comparison of the secretory capacity of villous and extravillous trophoblast in the human placenta, *Placenta* **5:**329–348.

Hamilton, W. J., and Boyd, J. D., 1960, Development of the human placenta in the first three months of gestation, *J. Anat.* **94:**297–328.

Harris, J. W. S., and Ramsey, E. M., 1966, Morphology of human uteroplacental vasculature, *Carnegie Contrib. Embryol.* **38:**43–58.

Hitschmann, F., and Adler, L., 1908, Der Bau der Uterusschleimhaut des geschlechtsreifein Weibes mit besonderer Berücksichtigung der Menstruation, *Monatsschr. Geburtshilfe Gynaekol.* **27:**1–82.

Hustin, J., Schaaps, J.-P., and Lambotte, J., 1988, Anatomical studies of the utero-placental vascularization in the first trimester of pregnancy, *Troph. Res.* **3:**49–60.

Jones, C. J. P., and Fox, H., 1980, An ultrastructural and ultrahistochemical study of the human placenta in maternal pre-eclampsia, *Placenta* **1:**61–76.

Kurman, R. J., Main, C. S., and Chen, H.-C., 1984, Intermediate trophoblast: A distinctive form of trophoblast with specific morphological, biochemical and functional features, *Placenta* **5:**349–369.

Martin, C. B., Jr., McGaughey, H. S., Jr., Kaiser, I. H., Donner, M. W., and Ramsey, E. M., 1964, Intermittent functioning of the uteroplacental arteries, *Am. J. Obstet. Gynecol.* **90:**819–823.

Nelson, D. M., Meister, R. K., Ortman-Nabi, J., Sparks, S., and Stevens, V. C., 1986, Differentiation and secretory activities of cultured human placental cytotrophoblast, *Placenta* **7:**1–16.

Okkels, H., and Engle, E. T., 1938, Studies on the finer structure of the uterine blood vessels of the macacus monkey, *Acta Pathol. Microbiol. Scand.* **15:**150–168.

Pijnenborg, R., Dixon, G., Robertson, W. B., and Brosens, I., 1980, Trophoblastic invasion of human decidua from 8 to 18 weeks of pregnancy, *Placenta* **1:**3–20.

Pijnenborg, R., Robertson, W. B., Brosens, I., and Dixon, G., 1981, Trophoblast invasion and the establishment of haemochorial placentation in man and laboratory animals, *Placenta* **2:**71–91.

Pijnenborg, R., Robertson, W. B., and Brosens, I., 1986, Morphological aspects of placental ontogeny and phylogeny, *Placenta* **6:**155–162.

Ramsey, E. M., 1959, Vascular anatomy of the utero-placental and foetal circulation in: *Oxygen Supply to the Human Foetus* (J. Walker and A. C. Turnbull, eds.), pp. 67–79, Blackwell, Oxford.

Ramsey, E. M., and Donner, M. W., 1980, *Placental Vasculature and Circulation,* Georg Thieme, Stuttgart.

Ramsey. E. M., Corner, G. W., Jr., and Donner, M. W., 1963, Serial and cineradiographic visualization of maternal circulation in the primate (hemochorial) placenta, *Am. J. Obstet. Gynecol.* **86:**213–225.

Ramsey, E. M., Houston, M. L., and Harris, J. W. S., 1976, Interactions of the trophoblast and maternal tissues in three closely related primate species, *Am. J. Obstet. Gynecol.* **124:**647–652.

Ramsey, E. M., Chez, R. A., and Doppman, J. L., 1979, Radioangiographic measurements of the internal diameters of the uteroplacental arteries in rhesus monkeys, *Am. J. Obstet. Gynecol.* **135:**247–251.

Sheppard, B. L., and Bonnar, J., 1974, The ultrastructure of the arterial supply of the human placenta in early and late pregnancy, *J. Obstet. Gynaecol. Br. Commonw.* **81:**497–511.

Sheppard, B. L., and Bonnar, J., 1976, Ultrastructure of arterial walls with extreme intrauterine growth retardation, *Br. J. Obstet. Gynaecol.* **83:**948.

Sheppard, B. L., and Bonnar, J., 1980, Ultrastructural abnormalities of placental villi in placentae from pregnancies complicated by intrauterine fetal growth retardation: Their relationship to decidual spiral artery lesions, *Placenta* **1:**145–156.

Teasdale, F., 1987, Histomorphometry of the human placenta in pre-eclampsia associated with severe intrauterine growth retardation, *Placenta* **8:**119–128.

Wells, M., Hsi, B.-L., Yeh, C.-J. G., and Faulk, W. P., 1984, Spiral (uteroplacental) arteries of the human placental bed show the presence of amniotic basement membrane antigens, *Am. J. Obstet. Gynecol.* **150:**973–977.

Wynn, R. M., 1972, Cytotrophoblastic specializations: An ultrastructural study of the human placenta, *Am. J. Obstet. Gynecol.* **114:**339–355.

Vascular Physiology of the Nonpregnant Uterus

FRANK C. GREISS, JR., and JAMES C. ROSE

One would expect that a proper appreciation of uterine vascular responses during pregnancy would be dependent on an understanding of those basic factors that control blood flow to the nonpregnant uterus. This is the logical approach, but that is not how it happened. Prior to 1950, observations of both nonpregnant and pregnant uterine vascular changes consisted of descriptive morphology (Ramsey, 1949) and descriptive physiology. The latter was limited by the primitive technologies then available. In his classic studies, Markee (1932) described cyclic changes in endometrium transplanted into the eyes of rabbits. These correlated with the ovarian cycle. He also described the marked vasodilatation that followed estrogen stimulation. Similarly, MacLeod and Reynolds (1938) observed the "red hyperemia" that occurred in nonpregnant uteri after estrogen injection. Few other vascular responses were reported in nonpregnant animals.

When the technologies developed during World War II were applied to more precise quantitative measurements of uterine vascular responses, primary attention was directed to the gravid uterus. Perhaps this was because the new technologies were still too primitive to measure the very low uterine blood flow rates present in the nonpregnant state. Alternately, it is possible that the logical investigative approach was bypassed as the new clinician–researchers of the post-World War II era aimed to obtain basic knowledge that could be applied clinically as soon as possible. For whatever reasons, experiments were initially performed on gravid animals, and these observations, influenced by the quantitatively pervasive responses of the placental circulation, obscured reactivities of the nonplacental circulation.

It has only been during the last two decades that attention has focused on the nonpregnant uterine vasculature. Such experiments have been facilitated by the development of the chronic animal model unimpeded by the stresses of anesthesia and acute operative procedures. The

FRANK C. GREISS, JR. ● Department of Obstetrics and Gynecology, Bowman Gray School of Medicine of Wake Forest University, Winston-Salem, North Carolina 27103. JAMES C. ROSE ● Departments of Physiology and Obstetrics and Gynecology, Bowman Gray School of Medicine of Wake Forest University, Winston-Salem, North Carolina 27103.

results obtained in nonpregnant animals have caused a complete rethinking of concepts derived from experiments in pregnant animals and have focused investigative efforts on more fundamental mechanisms.

It is the purpose of this chapter to review our current knowledge of the vascular responses of the nonpregnant uterus, to describe the responses of those portions of the uterine vasculature not supplying the placenta during the pregnancy, and to emphasize pertinent areas for future investigation. We have elected to omit any discussion of morphological observations, directing our attention instead to physiological responses. The majority of the material to be presented has been obtained from lower animals, primarily the sheep. However, where tested, the general responses of the primate uterine vasculatures seem similar to those of lower animals.

1. Fundamental Characteristics of the Uterine Vasculature

1.1. The Pressure–Flow Relationship

Relatively few observations of this basic relationship have been reported. In acute experiments in nonpregnant ewes pretreated with estradiol and progesterone injections, Greiss and Anderson (1974) described a curvilinear line with convexity to the flow axis consistent with an autoregulated vasculature (Fig. 1). Since the reported data were normalized, the slope of the relationship was not defined, but the control uterine blood flow (UBF) values suggest significant resting vascular tonus in these circumstances. Such a relationship is not unexpected in a predominantly muscular organ and is thought to reflect vasodilatory responses to accumulating metabolites during reductions in perfusion pressure. This interpretation is supported by the observations that total ischemia evokes significant reactive hyperemia and that injections of sodium cyanide or the breathing of 10% oxygen evokes significant vasodilatation (Greiss, 1971; Greiss et al., 1972).

1.2. Autonomic Influences

1.2.1. Adrenergic Stimulation

During pregnancy, sympathetic nerve stimulation significantly increases uterine vascular resistance in in vivo experiments in the ewe (Greiss and Gobble, 1967). In vitro, stimulation of

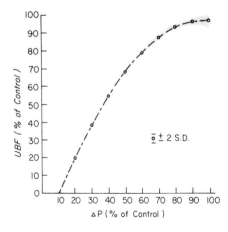

Figure 1. Pressure–flow relationship in nonpregnant ovine uterus. Curvilinearity to the uterine blood flow (UBF) axis indicates an autoregulatory vascular bed. From Greiss and Anderson (1974).

the periarterial sympathetic nerves of perfused segments of uterine arteries from nonpregnant animals causes vasoconstriction (α_1-adrenergic receptors) (Ford *et al.,* 1984). Since norepinephrine (NE) evokes vasoconstriction in nonpregnant ewes, it can be inferred that sympathetic nerve stimulation *in vivo* would cause similar effects.

The actions of NE, epinephrine, and isoproterenol have been studied extensively in ewes (Greiss, 1971, 1972, 1978; Naden and Rosenfeld, 1985b; Magness and Rosenfeld, 1986). Both NE and epinephrine cause marked uterine vasoconstriction proportionately greater (sixfold) than that induced in the systemic vascular bed as a whole. The NE-induced vasoconstriction is similar in the myometrial, endometrial, and caruncular blood vessels and is totally blocked by phenoxybenzamine at the 10 mg/kg level (Fig. 2). With epinephrine, total blockade occurs at the 3 mg/kg level, and vasodilatation occurs at the 10 mg/kg phenoxybenzamine level. This is blocked by propranolol (Fig. 3). The peripherally acting sympathomimetic drug phenylephrine causes vasoconstriction similar to that of NE. Since vasoconstriction has been demonstrated in pregnant ewes with other sympathomimetic agents (Greiss and Van Wilkes, 1964), it is probable that similar effects occur in the nonpregnant uterine vascular bed.

Isoproterenol, 10 μg, injected into the descending aorta causes a 40% decrease in uterine vascular resistance. This effect is also blocked by propranolol.

These observations indicate that both α_1- and β-adrenergic receptors are present in the vasculatures of the nonpregnant uterine vascular beds and respond classically to appropriate stimuli.

1.2.2. Cholinergic Stimulation

The effects of cholinergic drug and parasympathetic nerve stimulation on the uterine vasculatures are controversial. Perhaps this is related to the fact that whereas ACh-containing nerve terminals have been demonstrated in the uterine vascular walls of dogs, pigs, and man, no similar vasodilator nerve plexuses have been found in cats, rabbits, cows, or sheep (Bell, 1972). Shabanah *et al.* (1964) reported the effects of pelvic parasympathetic nerve stimulation and denervation on the uteri of nonpregnant and pregnant dogs. Although they reported

Figure 2. Semilogarithmic plot of uterine vascular conductance (1/resistance) responses to intraarterial norepinephrine at progressive levels of α-adrenergic blockade, illustrating responses during pregnancy, in nonpregnant ewes, and in one pregnant ewe with placental cotyledons confined to the uterine horn contralateral to the monitored uterine artery. The changes from prephenoxybenzamine (POBZ) responses in nonpregnant ewes were significantly different from those during pregnancy at the 0.1 to 1.0 mg/kg of POBZ levels, indicating a more rapid muting of the vasoconstrictor response at term pregnancy, when the placental vascular reactivity is dominant. Responses in the pregnant ewe without an ipsilateral placenta parallel those of nonpregnant ewes. From Greiss (1972).

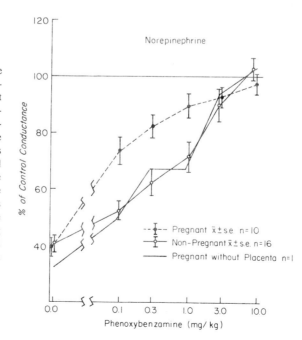

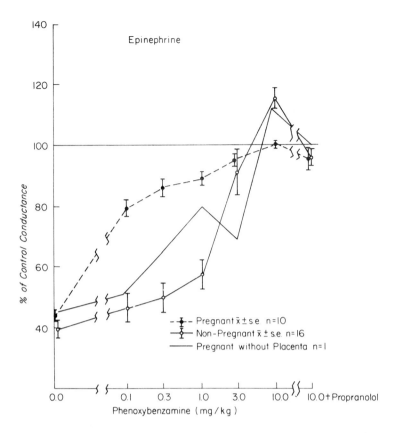

Figure 3. Semilogarithmic plot of uterine vascular conductance (1/resistance) responses to intraarterial epinephrine at progressive levels of α-adrenergic blockade and after β-adrenergic blockade, illustrating responses during pregnancy, in nonpregnant ewes, and in one pregnant ewe with placental cotyledons confined to the uterine horn contralateral to the monitored uterine artery. The changes from pre-POBZ responses in nonpregnant ewes were significantly different from those during pregnancy at the 0.1 to 1.0 mg/kg of POBZ levels, indicating a more rapid muting of the vasoconstrictor response at term pregnancy. At the 10.0 mg/kg level, vasodilatation that was blocked by propranolol occurred in the nonpregnant bed. Responses in the pregnant ewe without an ipsilateral placenta parallel those of nonpregnant ewes, including epinephrine reversal and its ablation by propranolol. From Greiss (1972).

significant effects on myometrial activity and fetal survival, UBF was not measured, so their observations are only inferential. Van Orden *et al.* (1983) observed in nonpregnant rats that neither parasympathetic decentralization nor excision of the paracervical ganglion of Frankenhauser affected estrogen-induced uterine hyperemia. However, ganglionectomy alone reduced the number of rats exhibiting normal vaginal cycles.

Greiss *et al.* (1967a) reported that electrical stimulation of sacral nerve roots two, three, and four in nonpregnant ewes at levels sufficient to evoke bladder and bowel contractions had no effect on the uterine vasculature or on myometrial activity. Similarly, transection of the sacral nerve roots evoked no immediate uterine responses. In contrast, ACh administered into the descending aorta evokes significant uterine vasodilatation (up to a 75% reduction in uterine vascular resistance) and transient uterine contractions at higher dose levels (Greiss *et al.*, 1967b).

More recently, Garris *et al.* (1986) reported that the sequential administration of ACh followed by NE induced an increase in UBF in oophorectomized estrogen-treated guinea pigs. In addition, methacholine increased the affinity of the α-adrenergic receptors for NE. These effects did not occur in oophorectomized or progesterone-treated oophorectomized guinea pigs, and the vasodilatation was blocked by phentolamine. Although these results were purported to show a cholinergic modulation of α-adrenergic receptor affinity and activity on the proper steroid hormone background, α-adrenergic stimulation has never been thought to cause vasodilatation, and another mechanism may be operable.

These observations shed minimal light on the significance of either acute or long-term tonic cholinergic stimulation on the uterine circulation. Clearly this is an area that merits further investigation.

1.3. Effects of Myometrial Contractions

Myometrial contractions decrease UBF by extrinsically narrowing blood vessels passing through the myometrium, thus increasing vascular resistance. The UBF varies inversely with the intensity and duration of uterine contractions and with the level of intercontraction tonus (Fig. 4). Increasing the frequency of contractions decreases UBF by decreasing the duration of intercontraction relaxation. Following a uterine contraction, UBF transiently rebounds above control levels, reflecting reative hyperemia. During pregnancy, the domiant placental circulation masks this myometrial response.

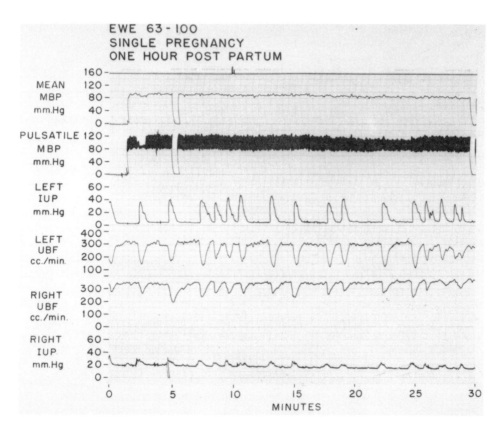

Figure 4. Postpartum recording illustrating uterine blood flow–myometrial contraction relationships. Note the inverse relationship. More intense myometrial contractions in the left uterine horn caused more marked decreases in left uterine blood flow as compared with the right uterine horn. From Greiss (1965).

1.4. Endocrine Regulation

1.4.1. Estrogens

The classic studies of Markee (1932) were first quantified in 1970. Huckabee *et al.* (1970) administered intravenous estrone to conscious previously instrumented ewes and observed a 33–600% increase in UBF after 110 min. The magnitude of the changes was inversely related to control UBF levels. Employing oophorectomized ewes chronically prepared with electromagnetic flow transducers around the uterine artery, Greiss and Anderson (1970) reported up to a 30 fold increase in UBF 1 to 2 days after the daily intramuscular administration of estradiol-17β (E_2) in sesame oil, 2.0 μg/kg. Subsequently, Killam *et al.* (1973) determined in more detail the time course and magnitude of the estrogen-induced UBF response, which has now become classic (Fig. 5). Approximately 30 min after an injection of E_2, UBF begins to rise, reaching peak levels between 90 and 120 min after injection. Such peaks are followed by a return to base line over the next 8 to 24 hr. In further studies, Still and Greiss (1976) and Greiss *et al.* (1986) showed that UBF falls off to 50% of peak levels 4 to 6 hr after injection, thereafter gradually decreasing to control levels after 24 hr. The E_2-induced vasodilatation occurs equally in the vascular beds of the myometrium, endometrium, and uterine caruncles (Rosenfeld *et al.*, 1973; Anderson and Hackshaw, 1974). Dose–response studies show that the maximum UBF evoked by E_2 occurs at the 1.0 μg/kg intravenous level, the 0.5 μg/kg level when injected into the descending aorta, and the 0.02 μg/kg level when given directly into the uterine artery. When given locally into one uterine artery or into the cavity of one uterine horn, E_2 has a unilateral effect (Killam *et al.*, 1973; Greiss and Miller, 1971).

Various estrogens have been shown to simulate the characteristic UBF response with a rank order of potency of E_2-17β > estriol > diethylstilbestrol > E_2-17α > estrone > estetrol (Resnick *et al.*, 1974; Levine *et al.*, 1984). Catechol estrogens evoke the same response, the order of potency relative to E_2 being E_2-17β > estrone > 2-OH E_2 > 2-OH estrone (Rosenfeld and Jackson, 1982). The doses of 2-OH E_2 and 2-OH estrone necessary to obtain a response comparable to that seen with E_2 are 62 and 500 times greater, respectively. *Cis-* and *trans*-clomiphene citrate also stimulate the maximum E_2 response at dose levels 20 and 1000 times greater, respectively (Still and Greiss, 1976).

Investigators have been confounded by many peculiarities of the estrogen response. For example, except after daily intramuscular injections of E_2, the sustained elevation of UBF observed at the time of ovine estrus has not been duplicated (F. C. Greiss, Jr., unpublished observations). In addition, when E_2 is infused constantly over 24 hr at 1.0 μg/kg per min, the UBF response is no different from that following a single bolus infusion (Still and Greiss, 1976). Both of these observations point to the possibility that estrogen receptor depletion and subsequent replenishment may determine the dynamics of the UBF response. For example, when repetitive intravenous boluses of 1.0 μg/kg E_2 are given at intervals varying from 1 to 24 hr, the maximum UBF response cannot be evoked repetitively with dose intervals less than every 12 to 18 hr (Greiss *et al.*, 1986). In addition, uterine cytosol receptors (R_c) are depleted to a nadir of 25% of control 2 hr after E_2 injection, then recover and approach control levels after 12 hr (Fig. 6). Perhaps the maximum single E_2 dose is pharmacological and at lower doses, more R_c would be available to permit a sustained UBF elevation. Similarly, with a constant E_2 infusion, R_c may be sustained at low levels, with depletion matching replenishment, thus blocking any further E_2 effect.

1.4.2. Progesterone

Progesterone injections alone given to conscious oophorectomized ewes have no effect on UBF. When UBF is stable on daily intramuscular injections of E_2, supplemental intramuscular progesterone in oil, 1.0 mg/kg, causes a 25% decrease in UBF (Greiss and Anderson, 1970)

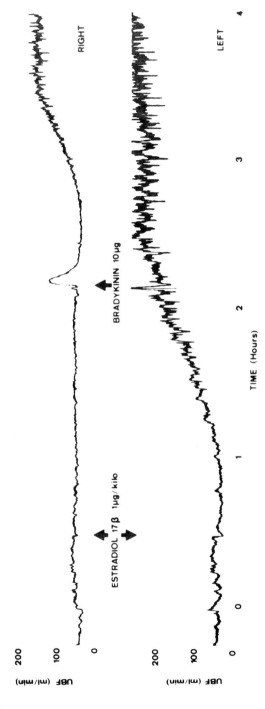

Figure 5. Bilateral UBF responses to intravenous estradiol administration in the control horn (left) and in the test horn (right) with local cycloheximide preinfusion. In the control horn, UBF began to increase 30 min after the estradiol injection, reaching maximal levels after 2 hr. Cycloheximide was infused constantly into the right uterine artery from time 0 to time 2 hr 25 min. Note that the right UBF response to estradiol was blocked until the cycloheximide infusion was stopped. From Killam *et al.* (1973).

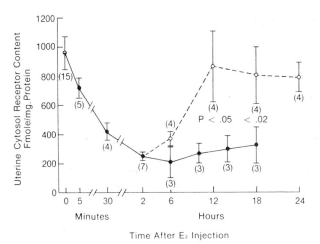

Figure 6. Uterine cytosol estrogen receptor content (mean ± SEM) after intravenous 1 μg/kg estradiol injection in continuously anesthetized (●) and previously conscious (○) ewes. Numbers in parentheses indicate number of observations. Note that in conscious ewes, receptor content approximated control levels after 12 hr. From Greiss *et al.* (1986).

(Fig. 7). Similarly, either pretreatment with daily intramuscular progesterone or progesterone injected directly into the uterine artery causes a 20–25% decrease in the UBF response to intraarterial E$_2$ (Resnik *et al.,* 1977). Such responses may be explained by the fact that progesterone depletes the quantity of R$_c$ (Clark *et al.,* 1977). When, during the concomitant administration of estrogen and progesterone, progesterone is withdrawn, UBF increases within 3 to 4 days from stable levels to approximate those levels seen following initial E$_2$ injections (Greiss and Anderson, 1970) (Fig. 7). This response could also be explained by changes in R$_c$ levels.

Distribution of UBF can be altered by ovarian steroids. During combined estrogen and progesterone injections, the fraction of UBF supplying the uterine caruncles approximates 30%, 1.5 times that observed during E$_2$ injections alone (Anderson *et al.,* 1977).

These observations of the effects of ovarian steroids on the uterine vasculature are intended to serve as a basis for subsequent discussion of their physiological significance (see Sections 3 and 4).

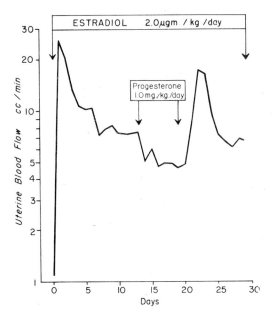

Figure 7. Effect of progesterone on ovine UBF during daily estradiol administration. With estradiol alone, UBF stabilized at low levels compared with the initial flow peak. Added progesterone decreased UBF moderately, whereas progesterone withdrawal induced a marked rise similar to the initial estradiol response. From Greiss and Anderson (1970).

2.1. Temporal Changes

Uterine blood flow varies regularly during the estrous cycles of ewes (Greiss and Anderson, 1969), cows (Ford *et al.*, 1979), and sows (Ford and Christenson, 1979), with abrupt increases occurring at or just preceding estrus, followed by reduced flows during the luteal phase of the estrous cycle. Figure 8 depicts unilateral UBF in conscious ewes throughout the estrous cycle, and Fig. 9 examines more closely the UBF changes during the days immediately preceding and during behavioral estrus. The UBF spikes preceding the prolonged UBF rise at estrus are thought to reflect intermittent spurts of E_2 secretion from maturing follicles, although this hypothesis has not been documented. The prolonged UBF rise begins 24 hr before behavioral estrus and falls off rapidly during estrus to relatively low levels at the time of ovulation, which occurs at the end of the estrus. The UBF rise follows the increased estrogen secretion that precedes the LH spike necessary to trigger ovulation and appears to be an

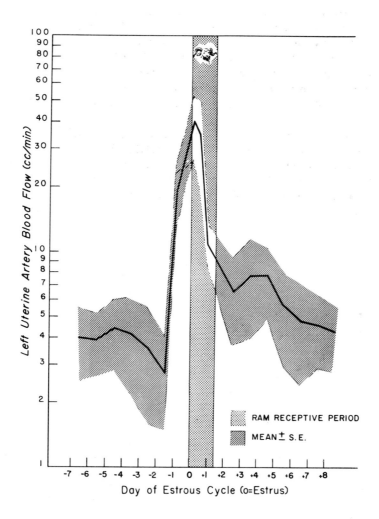

Figure 8. Semilogarithmic graph of mean uterine blood flow observations during the ovine estrous cycle. Note the prolonged rise in UBF prior to clinical estrus (ram receptive period). From Greiss and Anderson (1969).

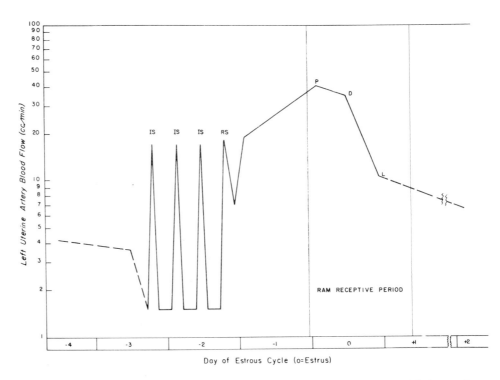

Figure 9. Semilogarithmic graph of composite uterine blood flow changes surrounding clinical estrus determined from the mean of 15 estrous cycles. Note that the onset of ram receptivity (overt estrus) approximates the peak level of UBF (P) and is preceded by isolated transient spikes (IS) 2 to 3 days preceding the prolonged UBF rise. From Greiss and Anderson (1969).

obligatory response, since UBF patterns following a conceptional estrus are not different from those following a nonconceptional estrus for the next 12 to 14 days.

2.2. *Hormonal and Other Correlates*

The rhythmic changes in UBF during the estrous cycle in each species appear to be temporally associated with the daily estrogen : progesterone ratios observed in systemic blood (Fig. 10) (Ford, 1982). The higher the estrogen : progesterone ratio, the greater is the quantity of blood flowing through the uterine vascular beds, and vice versa. We have already seen that progesterone mutes the vasodilatory response to estrogen. Although this could be caused by a progesterone-induced decrease in R_c, an indirect vasoconstrictive effect of progesterone is a possibility. A substantial body of evidence has accumulated to support the premise that ovarian steroids may influence the vasoconstrictive function of uterine periarterial adrenergic nerves with subsequent alterations in UBF. For example, estrogens reduce NE levels in uterine periarterial nerves of rats coincident with an increase in UBF (McKercher *et al.*, 1973). In oophorectomized E_2-primed ewes, the doses of NE necessary to reduce UBF to 20% of control are markedly higher than those needed to produce similar effects in intact or estrogen- and progesterone-primed ewes (Barton *et al.*, 1974). Ford *et al.*, (1977a,b) have shown that arteries from E_2-dominated ewes exhibit reduced contractility to periarterial nerve stimulation or exogenous NE stimulation. In a more recent report, Ford *et al.* (1984) demonstrated greater arterial contractility to nerve stimulation and greater α-adrenergic receptor binding in uterine arteries from gilts in the late luteal phase of the estrous cycle than in arteries from the day of

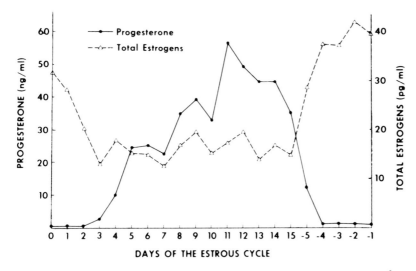

Figure 10. Concentrations of progesterone and total estrogens (estrone plus estradiol-17β) in blood collected from the vena cava of 18 nonpregnant gilts throughout an estrous cycle. Day 0 equals first day of estrus. From Ford (1982).

estrus. Finally, Ford and Reynolds (1981) observed that an increase in UBF of oophorectomized cows in response to an intraarterial injection of 1 μg E_2 could be mimicked by an intraarterial injection of the same dose of phentolamine. In direct contrast to this observation, Naden and Rosenfeld (1985a) reported that phentolamine had no detectable effect on UBF or on the UBF response to E_2 when both were given together to oophorectomized E_2-stimulated ewes. In part these opposing observations might be explained by the fact that although 1 μg of E_2 was injected in both experiments, the relative doses applied were probably much different when one considers the differences in the size and basal UBF of the uteri of the two species.

Progesterone appears to augment the responsiveness of vascular smooth muscle to catecholamines. In aortic strips, Kalsner (1969) observed that progesterone increased E_2-induced smooth muscle contractility by inhibiting the action of catechol-O-methyltransferase, thus reducing the rate of catecholamine degradation.

Although some of the evidence for adrenergic mediation of the effects of ovarian steroids is controversial at present, the evidence derived in many species makes this a promising area for continued exploration.

3. Mediators of Estrogen-Induced Vasodilatation

Obviously, a discussion of the mediators of estrogen-induced uterine vasodilatation overlaps any discussion of hormonal and other modulators of UBF patterns during the ovarian cycle. However, the principal experimental approaches used to date have taken two different tacks. The first has been to identify agents that reproduce the maximal E_2 response. Then the potential role of such agents as E_2 mediators has been tested by evaluating the effects of pretreatment with antagonists of such agents on the E_2 response. The second approach has been to explore at a cellular level receptor and metabolic changes following E_2 stimulation, usually on the background of physiological steroid hormone levels. Although the first approach has been relatively unrewarding, a review of the agents tested and their effects seems appropriate.

The effect of prostaglandins (PG) injected into the uterine artery has been studied extensively in the oophorectomized ewe. Prostaglandin E_1, PGD_2, and PGI_2 cause marked vasodilatation approximating the maximal E_2-induced effect (Still and Greiss, 1978; Resnik and Brink, 1978, 1980; Clark et al., 1981a). Prostaglandin A_1, PGA_2, and PGE_2 cause lesser but significant vasodilatation. Although Clark et al. (1975) initially reported that meclofenamate blocked or muted the E_2-induced rise in UBF in two sheep, in a later report, pretreatment with indomethacin did not alter the response (Clark et al., 1980a). Parisi et al. (1984) reported that the leukotriene receptor antagonist FPL55712 augmented the E_2-induced UBF response in rabbits. This observation raises the possibility that leukotrienes per se might inhibit or block the E_2 response. Resnik and Brink (1978) reported that $PGF_{2\alpha}$ caused vasoconstriction and concomitant myometrial contractions in the ewe.

A number of related observations may be pertinent. There is increasing evidence that adrenergic neuronal activity and vascular tone are modulated by prostaglandins. Hedqvist (1970) has shown that PGE inhibits the release of NE at nerve terminals, and Kadowitz et al. (1972) reported that $PGF_{2\alpha}$ facilitates the release of neuronal NE. Wilhelmsson et al. (1981) reported that PGE_2 and $PGF_{2\alpha}$ increase the tonus of human uterine arteries strips in vitro. Conversely, PGI_2 relaxed spontaneously active and PG- and NE-stimulated strips but did not relax nerve-stimulated strips. In view of the observations of Ford et al. (1977a,b) with $PGF_{2\alpha}$ and periarterial nerve stimulation of estrogen- or progesterone-dominated blood vessels, it appears that prostaglandins may evoke variable vascular response depending on the neuronal content of NE.

H_1 and H_2 histamine receptors have been demonstrated in the ovine uterine arteries (Resnik et al., 1976; Clark et al., 1980b). Clark et al. (1984) observed that base-line UBF was not changed by individual or combined H_1 or H_2 receptor antagonists. They further demonstrated that the vasodilatation evoked by histamine was primarily the function of the H_1 receptor agonist. With respect to the E_2-induced UBF response, Marshall and Senior (1986) reported that in the rat, either H_1 receptor blockade or combined H_1 and H_2 receptor blockade had no effect. H_2 receptor blockade alone, however, caused an early but transient muting of the E_2 response.

Clark et al. (1980c) demonstrated the presence of serotonin receptors in ovine uterine arteries. Serotonin injected into the uterine artery caused a vasoconstriction of approximately 10% of that induced by NE. The effect was attenuated by the serotonin antagonist methylsergide.

Several miscellaneous substances also have been shown to induce uterine vasodilatation similar to that following E_2. In the ewe, they include bradykinin, adenosine, ATP, ADP, AMP, and glucosamine (Still and Greiss, 1978; Greiss and Wagner, 1983; Resnik et al., 1976; Clark et al., 1981b). Vasoactive intestinal polypeptide increases myometrial blood flow in the rabbit (Ottesen and Fahrenkrug, 1981; Bardrum et al., 1986), goat (Carter et al., 1981), and ewe (Clark et al., 1981b).

The early observation that UBF does not begin to increase until 30 min after exposure to estrogen combined with the finding that the protein synthesis inhibitor cycloheximide blocks the UBF response strongly suggests that a secondary mediator(s) is ultimately responsible for the increase in UBF. Therefore, a number of investigative efforts have focused on an analysis of the classic uterine response to estrogen stimulation: an early period of fluid accumulation (water imbibition) and later uterine growth. The hypothesis that estrogen-stimulated UBF and the water imbibition are correlative physiological events is supported by the facts that they share a similar temporal relationship in response to E_2 stimulation, that they have the same quantitative response to various estrogens, and that they are both suppressed by inhibitors of protein synthesis (Hisaw, 1959). Therefore, the two responses may be mediated similarly.

In vivo, both catechol estrogens and E_2 induce vasodilatation (Rosenfeld and Jackson, 1982). In vitro, however, only catechol estrogens relax the uterine artery (Stice et al., 1985). Although pretreatment with cycloheximide blocks the effects of E_2 on UBF, it has no effect on responses to catechol estrogens (Ford *et al.*, 1986). Puromycin blocks water imbibition as well as early synthesis of protein but has no effect on later protein synthesis (Whelly and Barker, 1974; Mueller *et al.*, 1960). In contrast, actinomycin D has no effect on vasodilatation or on early peptide synthesis, but it blocks later RNA synthesis (Resnik *et al.*, 1975; Whelly and Barker, 1974; Penny *et al.*, 1981). These observations have led to the concept of two systems controlling the estrogen response: an early protein-synthesis-dependent response causing vasodilatation and water imbibition and a later uterine growth response dependent on the transcription of new RNA. A number of further observations support the premise that estrogens are converted to catechol estrogens, which mediate the early cytoplasmic response. Estradiol is converted by aromatic hydroxylation to 2- and 4-OH estradiol. Such conversion seems to be a necessary step to evoke the E_2 response that is cycloheximide sensitive (Ford *et al.*, 1986). In rats, uterine peroxidase converts E_2 to 4-OH E_2, and after estrogen stimulation, peroxidase and uterine blood volume increase (Van Orden *et al.*, 1987). The observations that cycloheximide and dexamethasone block or mute the estrogen-induced UBF response and that both block the influx of peroxidase-laden eosinophils into cells are consistent with the catechol estrogen mediation theory.

One further observation may be pertinent. Farley *et al.*, (1986) have demonstrated that the estrogen-receptor-blocking drug nafoxidine blocks uterine vasodilatation induced by either E_2 or 4-OH E_2 in rats *in vivo*. *In vitro*, only 4-OH E_2 causes vasodilatation, which is associated with a decrease in Ca^{2+} uptake. However, pretreatment with nafoxidine followed by 4-OH E_2 not only blocks vasodilatation but is associated with a marked increase in Ca^{2+} uptake. It is possible that nafoxidine may block a catechol estrogen receptor that regulates Ca^{2+} uptake.

4. Responses of the Nonplacental Uterine Vasculature during Pregnancy

The early observations of uterine vascular responses during late pregnancy include a summation of the responses of the nonplacental and placental vasculatures. Since the placental bed receives more than 75% of total UBF during late pregnancy in most species, observed responses reflected primarily those of the placental circulation, and, unfortunately, these were generalized to the entire uterus. In fact, the concept of differentially responsive vascular beds was barely mentioned. All of the early investigators fell into this trap. Perhaps one of the earliest dilemmas resulting from such observations was presented by the pressure–flow relationship (Greiss, 1966). The senior author of this chapter remembers more than one evening reviewing the data with Dr. Harold D. Green, a noted cardiovascular physiologist at Wake Forest University. Neither of us could explain the straight-line pressure–flow relationship that was compatible only with a rigid tube model. Subsequently, the answer became obvious when the differential vascular response studies permitted by the use of nuclide-labeled microspheres were performed. Investigators realized that responses of two different vascular beds (placental and nonplacental) were combining to give often erroneously interpreted results.

A priori, one would not anticipate that vascular responses of the nonpregnant uterus would change significantly during pregnancy. Instead, one would anticipate that those blood vessels supplying the placenta would be so modified as to dilate progressively and shunt blood to the placenta and that the blood vessels supplying nonplacental tissues would retain their prepregnant responsivities. In general, this is exactly what occurs, modified perhaps by the progressive reduction in the number and intensity of uterine adrenergic nerves that has been reported by numerous investigators (Thorbert, 1979; Zuspan *et al.*, 1981). However, even these changes are more prominent in areas of the uterus supplying the placenta.

Prior to definitive placentation in the ewe, the pressure–flow relationship of blood vessels supplying the caruncles and noncaruncular tissues retain their prepregnant autoregulatory

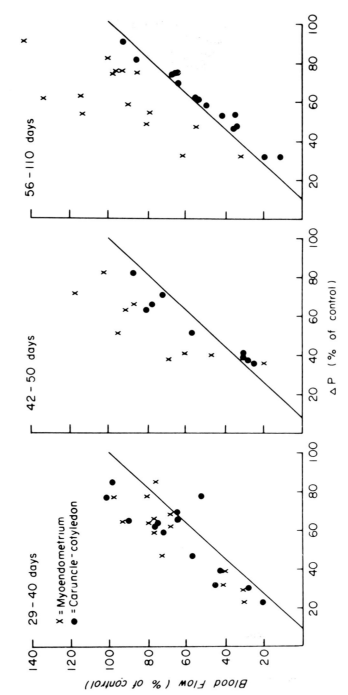

Figure 11. Comparison of caruncle–cotyledon and myoendometrial pressure–flow responses at progressive phases of ovine placentation shown with respect to a linear relationship. Before the onset of definitive placentation (40 days), responses were similar to nonpregnant ones (autoregulatory). Following definitive placentation (60 days), placental responses (caruncle–cotyledon) subtended the linear line (passive reactivity), while myoendometrial (nonplacental) responses remained autoregulatory. From Greiss *et al.* (1976).

curves (Fig. 11) (Greiss *et al.*, 1976). As definitive placentation occurs and the caruncular blood vessels progressively dilate, the pressure–flow curve of the placental circulation becomes a passive one with curvilinearity to the pressure axis. Meanwhile, the pressure–flow curve of the nonplacental circulation maintains its prepregnant autoregulatory relationship. It was the composite of these two responses that explained the originally described straight-line relationship.

Fortuitously, comparisons have been made of vasoactive responses observed during ovine pregnancy in both horns or the uterus in the rare circumstance that all of the placental blood supply was derived from one uterine horn. In the non-placenta-supplying horn, both vasodilator and vasoconstrictor stimuli closely simulated responses of the nonpregnant uterine vasculatures (Greiss, 1971, 1972) (Figs. 2, 3, and 12). Similarly, using microsphere technology, Novy *et al.* (1975) demonstrated in pregnant rhesus monkeys that myometrial blood flow was minimally reduced during uterine contractions, whereas during the subsequent relaxation phase myometrial blood flow almost doubled (reactive hyperemia), the same responses observed prior to pregnancy.

At present, it seems clear that the questions to be answered during pregnancy relate primarily to the processes that induce and maintain the placental vasculature. This position does not negate continued investigation of those factors controlling the nonplacental circulation during pregnancy. Rather it emphasizes the fact that until we better understand the nonpregnant uterine circulation, investigative efforts during pregnancy will be compromised.

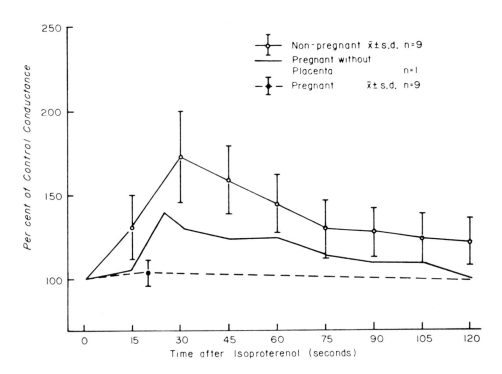

Figure 12. Comparison of uterine vascular conductance (1/resistance) responses to isoproterenol in nonpregnant and pregnant ovine vascular beds and in a uterine horn during pregnancy with placentation confined to the contralateral horn. Note the similarity of the gravid non-placenta-containing uterine vasculature with the nonpregnant one. From Greiss (1971).

During the 40 years since World War II, our understanding of both the nonpregnant and pregnant uterine vasculatures has increased appreciably. However, it appears, except in directed situations, that the progress in gross descriptive physiology permitted by many of our new technologies has reached if not passed its zenith. Further progress will not occur until we direct our investigations to the cellular and molecular levels. Moreover, it seems to us that too much attention has been directed to a maximal pharmacological response (E_2) rather than to the UBF response as it occurs physiologically. For example, mean maximum UBF levels observed during ovine estrus average about 40 ml/min, only one-third of those seen during the maximal E_2 response. It appears not only that much lower endogenous E_2 levels occur naturally, probably with more subtle effects on estrogen receptors, but that the cause(s) of these lesser increases in UBF may only be apparent within physiological ranges. Therefore, it appears that future investigations must focus attention on the background of normal fluctuations of ovarian steroids, for the investigations reviewed in this chapter increasingly suggest a subtle interaction among many endogenous systems and the normal ovarian cycle.

Finally, it must be remembered that *in vitro* experiments on isolated segments of the uterine artery reflect responses of a major supply vessel rather than those of the arterioles, which classically control vascular resistance. At present, technological limitations preclude similar experiments on these resistance vessels so that we must hope, rightly or wrongly, that the responses of these two segments of the vascular tree are similar.

> "For the soul is dead that slumbers,
> and things are not what they seem."
> Longfellow, *Song of Life*

6. *References*

Anderson, S. G., and Hackshaw, B. T., 1974, The effect of estrogen on uterine blood flow and its distribution in nonpregnant ewes, *Am. J. Obstet. Gynecol.* **119**:589–595.

Anderson, S. G., Hackshaw, B. T., Still, J. G., and Greiss, F. C., Jr., 1977, Uterine blood flow and its distribution after chronic estrogen and progesterone administration, *Am. J. Obstet. Gynecol.* **127**:138–142.

Bardrum, B., Ottesen, B., and Fahrenkrug, J., 1986, Peptides PHI and VIP: Comparison between vascular and nonvascular smooth muscle effect in rabbit uterus, *Am. J. Physiol.* **251**:E48–E51.

Barton, M. D., Killam, A. P., and Meschia, G., 1974, Response of ovine uterine blood flow to epinephrine and norepinephrine, *Proc. Soc. Exp. Biol. Med.* **145**:996–1003.

Bell, C., 1972, Autonomic nervous control of reproduction: Circulatory and other factors, *Pharmacol. Rev.* **24**:657–736.

Carter, A. M., Einer-Jensen, N., Fahrenkrug, J., and Ottesen, B., 1981, Increased myometrial blood flow evoked by vasoactive intestinal polypeptide in the nonpregnant goat, *J. Physiol. (Lond.)* **310**:471–480.

Clark, J. H., Hsueh, A. J. W., and Peck, E. J., Jr., 1977, Regulation of estrogen receptor replenishment by progesterone, *Ann. N.Y. Acad. Sci.* **286**:161–179.

Clark, K. E., Van Orden, D. E., Meldrum, D. R., Brody, M. J., and Brinkman, C. R. III, 1975, Effect of prostaglandin synthetase inhibitor meclofenamate on estrogen-induced increases in uterine blood flow in sheep, *Prostaglandins* **5**:25–29.

Clark, K. E., Stys, S. J., Austin, J. E., and Golter, M., 1980a, Prostaglandins: Mediator of estrogen-induced increases in uterine blood flow, *Proc. Soc. Gynecol. Invest.* **27**:126.

Clark, K. E., Stys, S. J., and Mills, E. G., 1980b, Histamine and serotonin: Effects on uterine blood flow, *Proc. Soc. Gynecol. Invest.* **27**:56.

Clark, K. E., Mills, E. G., Otte, T. E., and Stys, S. J., 1980c, Effect of serotonin on uterine blood flow in pregnant and nonpregnant sheep, *Life Sci.* **27**:2655–2661.

Clark, K. E., Austin, J. E., and Stys, S. J., 1981a, Effect of bisenoic prostaglandins on the uterine vasculature of the nonpregnant sheep, *Prostaglandins* **22**:333–348.

Clark, K. E., Mills, E. G., Stys, S. J., and Seeds, A. E., 1981b, Effects of vasoactive polypeptides on the uterine vasculature, *Am. J. Obstet. Gynecol.* **139**:182–188.

Clark, K. E., Mills, E. G., and Harrington, D. J., 1984, Effect of histamine receptor agonists and antagonists on the uterine vasculature, *Proc. Soc. Exp. Biol. Med.* **175**:476–482.

Farley, D. B., Ford, S. P., MacIndoe, J. H., and Van Orden, D. E., 1986, Effect of nafoxidine on uterine vasculature *in vivo* and *in vitro*, *Proc. Soc. Gynecol. Invest.* **33**:158.

Ford, S. P., 1982, Control of uterine and ovarian blood flow throughout the estrous cycle and pregnancy of ewes, sows, and cows, *J. Anim. Sci.* **55**(Suppl. 2):32–42.

Ford, S. P., and Christenson, R. K., 1979. Blood flow to uteri of sows during estrous cycle and early pregnancy: Local effect of the conceptus on the uterine blood supply, *Biol. Reprod.* **21**:617–624.

Ford, S. P., and Reynolds, L. P., 1981, Interaction of estradiol-17β and adrenergic antagonists in controlling uterine arterial flow of cows, *J. Anim. Sci.* **53**(Suppl. 1):317.

Ford, S. P., Weber, L. J., and Stormshak, F., 1977a, Response of ovine uterine arteries to nerve stimulation after perfusions of prostaglandin $F_{2\alpha}$, norepinephrine or neurotransmitter antagonists, *Endocrinology* **101**:659–665.

Ford, S. P., Weber, L. J., and Stormshak, F., 1977b, Role of estradiol-17β and progesterone in regulating constriction of ovine uterine arteries, *Biol. Reprod.* **17**:480–488.

Ford, S. P., Chenault, J. R., and Echternkamp, S. E., 1979, Uterine blood flow of cows during the oestrous cycle and early pregnancy: Effect of conceptus on the uterine blood supply, *J. Reprod. Fertil.* **56**:53–62.

Ford, S. P., Reynolds, L. P., Farley, D. B., Bhatnagar, R. K., and Van Orden, D. E., 1984, Interaction of ovarian steroids and periarterial α_1-adrenergic receptors in altering uterine blood flow during the estrous cycle of gilts, *Am. J. Obstet. Gynecol.* **150**:480–484.

Ford, S. P., Van Orden, D. E., and Farley, D. B., 1986, Effect of cycloheximide on (catechol) estrogen uterine hyperemia, *Proc. Soc. Gynecol. Invest.* **33**:224.

Garris, D. R., McConnaughey, M. M., and Dar, M. S., 1986, Estrogen modulation of uterine adrenergic-cholinergic interaction: Effects on vasoactivity and adrenergic receptors in the guinea pig, *J. Pharmacol. Exp. Ther.* **239**:270–278.

Greiss, F. C., Jr., 1965, Effect of labor on uterine blood flow: Observations on gravid ewes, *Am. J. Obstet. Gynecol.* **93**:917–923.

Greiss, F. C., Jr., 1966, Pressure–flow relationship in the gravid uterine vascular bed, *Am. J. Obstet. Gynecol.* **96**:41–47.

Greiss, F. C., Jr., 1971, Differential reactivity of the myoendometrial and placental vasculatures: Vasodilatation, *Am. J. Obstet. Gynecol.* **111**:611–625.

Greiss, F. C., Jr., 1972, Differential reactivity of the myoendometrial and placental vasculatures: Adrenergic responses, *Am. J. Obstet. Gynecol.* **112**:20–30.

Greiss, F. C., Jr., 1978, Reactivities of the nongravid uterine vasculatures: Effects of norepinephrine, *Am. J. Obstet. Gynecol.* **131**:778–779.

Greiss, F. C., Jr., and Anderson, S. G., 1969, Uterine vascular changes during the ovarian cycle, *Am. J. Obstet. Gynecol.*: 103–629–640.

Greiss, F. C., Jr., and Anderson, S. G., 1970, Effect of ovarian hormones on the uterine vascular bed, *Am. J. Obstet. Gynecol.* **107**:829–836.

Greiss, F. C., Jr., and Anderson, S. G., 1974, Pressure-flow relationship in the nonpregnant uterine vascular bed, *Am. J. Obstet. Gynecol.*:118–763–772.

Greiss, F. C., Jr., and Gobble, F. L., Jr., 1967, Effect of sympathetic nerve stimulation on the uterine vascular bed, *Am. J. Obstet. Gynecol.* **97**:962–967.

Greiss, F. C., Jr., and Miller, H., 1971, Unilateral control of uterine blood flow in the ewe, *Am. J. Obstet. Gynecol.* **111**:299–301.

Greiss, F. C., Jr., and Van Wilkes, D., 1964, Effects of sympathomimetic drugs and angiotensin on the uterine vascular bed, *Obstet. Gynecol.* **23**:925–930.

Greiss, F. C., Jr., and Wagner, W. D., 1983, Glycosaminoglycans: Their distribution and potential vasoactive action in the nonpregnant and pregnant ovine uterus, *Am. J. Obstet. Gynecol.* **145**:1041–1048.

Greiss, F. C., Jr., Gobble, F. L., Jr., Anderson, S. G., and McGuirt, W. F., 1967a, Effect of parasympathetic nerve stimulation on the uterine vascular bed, *Am. J. Obstet. Gynecol.* **99**:1067–1072.

Greiss, F. C., Jr., Gobble, F. L., Jr., Anderson, S. G., and McGuirt, W. F., 1967b, Effect of acetylcholine on the uterine vascular bed, *Am. J. Obstet. Gynecol.* **99**:1073–1077.

Greiss, F. C., Jr., Anderson, S. G., and King, L. C., 1972, Uterine vascular bed: Effectives of acute hypoxia, *Am. J. Obstet. Gynecol.* **113**:1057–1064.

Greiss, F. C., Jr., Anderson, S. G., and Still, J. G., 1976, Uterine pressure–flow relationships during early gestation, *Am. J. Obstet. Gynecol.* **126**:799–808.

Greiss, F. C., Jr., Rose, J. C., Kute, T. E., Kelly, R. T., and Winkler, L. S., 1986, Temporal and receptor correlates of the estrogen response in sheep, *Am. J. Obstet. Gynecol.* **154**:831–836.

Hedqvist, P., 1970, Control by prostaglandin E_2 of sympathetic neurotransmission in the spleen, *Life Sci.* **9**:269–278.

Hisaw, F. L., Jr., 1959, Comparative effectiveness of estrogens in fluid imbibition and growth of the rat uterus, *Endocrinology* **64**:276–289.

Huckabee, W. E., Crenshaw, C., Curet, L. B., Mann, L., and Barron, D. H., 1970, The effect of exogenous oestrogen on the blood flow and oxygen consumption of the uterus of the nonpregnant ewe, *Q. J. Exp. Physiol.* **55**:16–24.

Kadowitz, P. J., Sweet, C. S., and Brody, M. J., 1972, Enhancement of sympathetic neurotransmission by prostaglandin $F_{2\alpha}$ in the cutaneous vascular bed of the dog, *Eur. J. Pharmacol.* **18**:189–194.

Kalsner, S., 1969, Steroid potentiation of responses to sympathomimetic amines in aortic strips, *Br. J. Pharmacol.* **36**:582–593.

Killam, A. P., Rosenfeld, C. R., Battaglia, F. C., Makowski, E. L., and Meschia, G., 1973, Effect of estrogens on the uterine blood flow of oophorectomized ewes, *Am. J. Obstet. Gynecol.* **115**:1045–1057.

Levine, M. G., Miodornik, M., and Clark, K. E., 1984, Uterine vascular effects of estetrol in nonpregnant ewes, *Am. J. Obstet. Gynecol.* **148**:735–738.

MacLeod, J., and Reynolds, S. R. M., 1938, Vascular, metabolic and motility relationships in the uterus after administration of oestrin, *Proc. Soc. Exp. Biol. Med.* **37**:666–676.

Magness, R. R., and Rosenfeld, C. R., 1986, Systemic and uterine responses to α-adrenergic stimulation in pregnant and nonpregnant ewes, *Am. J. Obstet. Gynecol.* **155**:897–904.

Markee, J. E., 1932, An analysis of the rhythmic vascular changes in the uterus of the rabbit, *Am. J. Physiol.* **100**:374–382.

Marshall, K., and Senior, J., 1986, The effect of mepyramine and ranitidine on the oestrogen and anti-oestrogen stimulated rat uterus, *Br. J. Pharmacol.* **89**:251–256.

McKercher, T. C., Van Orden, L. S. III, Bhatnagar, R. K., and Burke, J. P., 1973, Estrogen-induced biogenic amine reduction in rat uterus, *J. Pharmacol. Exp. Ther.* **185**:514–522.

Mueller, G. C., Gorski, J., and Aizawa, Y., 1960, The role of protein synthesis in early estrogen action, *Proc. Natl. Acad. Sci. U.S.A.* **47**:164–169.

Naden, R. P., and Rosenfeld, C. R., 1985a, Role of α-receptors in estrogen-induced vasodilation in nonpregnant sheep, *Am. J. Physiol.* **248**:H339–H344.

Naden, R. P., and Rosenfeld, C. R., 1985b, Systemic and uterine responsiveness to angiotensin II and norepinephrine in estrogen-treated nonpregnant sheep, *Am. J. Physiol.* **153**:417–425.

Novy, M. J., Thomas, C. L., and Lees, M. H., 1975, Uterine contractility and regional blood flow responses to oxytocin and prostaglandin E_2 in pregnant rhesus monkeys, *Am. J. Obstet. Gynecol.* **122**:419–433.

Ottesen, B., and Fahrenkrug, J., 1981, Effect of vasoactive intestinal polypeptide (VIP) upon myometrial blood flow in nonpregnant rabbit, *Acta Physiol. Scand.* **112**:195–201.

Parisi, V. M., Rankin, J. H. G., Phernetton, T. M., and Makowski, E. L., 1984, The effect of a leukotriene receptor antagonist, FPL 55712, on estrogen-induced uterine hyperemia in the nonpregnant rabbit, *Am. J. Obstet. Gynecol.* **148**:365–369.

Penney, L. L., Frederick, F. J., and Parker, G. W., 1981, 17β-Estradiol stimulation of uterine blood flow in oophorectomized rabbits with complete inhibition of uterine ribonucleic acid synthesis, *Endocrinology* **109**:1672–1676.

Ramsey, E. M., 1949, The vascular pattern of the endometrium of the pregnant rhesus monkey *Macaca mulatta*, *Carnegie Contrib. Embryol.* **33**:113–147.

Resnik, R., and Brink, G. W., 1978, Effects of prostaglandins E_1, E_2, $F_{2\alpha}$ on uterine blood flow in nonpregnant sheep, *Am. J. Physiol.* **234**:H557–561.

Resnik, R., and Brink, G. W., 1980, Uterine vascular response to prostacyclin in nonpregnant sheep, *Am. J. Obstet. Gynecol.* **137**:267–270.

Resnik, R., Killam, A. P., Battaglia, F. C., Makowski, E. L., and Meschia, G., 1974, The stimulation of uterine blood flow by various estrogens, *Endocrinology* **94**:1192–1196.

Resnik, R., Battaglia, F. C., Makowski, E. L., and Meschia, G., 1975, The effect of actinomycin-D on estrogen-induced uterine blood flow, *Am. J. Obstet. Gynecol.* **122**:273–277.

Resnik, R., Killam, A. P., Barton, M. D., Battaglia, F. C., Makowski, E. L., and Meschia, G., 1976, The effect of various compounds on the uterine vascular bed, *Am. J. Obstet. Gynecol.* **125**:201–206.

Resnik, R., Brink, G. W., and Plumer, M. H., 1977, The effect of progesterone on estrogen-induced uterine blood flow, *Am. J. Obstet. Gynecol.* **128**:251–254.

Rosenfeld, C. R., and Jackson, G. M., 1982, Induction and inhibition of uterine vasodilatation by catechol estrogen in oophorectomized, nonpregnant ewes, *Endocrinology* **110:**1333–1339.

Rosenfeld, C. R., Killam, A. P., Battaglia, F. C., Makowski, E. L., and Meschia, G., 1973, Effect of estradiol-17β on the magnitude and distribution of uterine blood flow in nonpregnant oophorectomized ewes, *Pediatr. Res.* **7:**139–148.

Shabanah, E. H., Toth, A., and Maughan, G. B., 1964, The role of the autonomic nervous system in uterine contractility and blood flow. II. The role of the parasympathetic neurohormone acetylcholine in uterine motility and blood flow, *Am. J. Obstet. Gynecol.* **89:**860–880.

Stice, S. L., Van Orden, D. E., and Ford, S. P., 1985, Role of estrogen and catechol estrogen in reducing arterial tone and ^{45}Ca uptake, *Proc. Soc. Gynecol. Invest.* **32:**112.

Still, J. G., and Greiss, F. C., Jr., 1976, Effect of *cis-* and *trans-*clomiphene on the uterine blood flow of oophorectomized ewes, *Gynecol. Invest.* **7:**187–200.

Still, J. G., and Greiss, F. C., Jr., 1978, The effect of prostaglandins and other vasoactive substances on uterine blood flow and myometrial activity, *Am. J. Obstet. Gynecol.* **130:**1–8.

Thorbert, G., 1979, Regional changes in structure and function of adrenergic nerves in guinea pig uterus during pregnancy, *Acta Obstet. Gynecol. Scand. [Suppl.]* **79:**5–32.

Van Orden, D. E., Farley, D. B., and Clancey, C. J., 1983, Effect of parasympathetic decentralization and paracervical ganglion excision on reproductive function in the rat, *Biol. Reprod.* **28:**910–916.

Van Orden, D. E., Matthew, T. S., Farley, D. B., and Markham, A. L., 1987, Catechol estrogen synthesis and uterine vasodilatation: Role of uterine peroxidase, *Proc. Soc. Gynecol. Invest.* **34:**240.

Whelly, S. M., and Barker, K. L., 1974, Early effect of estradiol on the peptide elongation rate by uterine ribosomes, *Biochemistry* **13:**341–346.

Wilhelmsson, L., Lindblom, B., Wikland, M., and Wiqvist, N., 1981, Effects of prostaglandins on the isolated uterine artery of nonpregnant women, *Prostaglandins* **22:**223–233.

Zuspan, F. P., O'Shaughnessy, R., Vinsel, J., and Zuspan, M., 1981, Adrenergic innervation of the uterine vasculature in human term pregnancy, *Am. J. Obstet. Gynecol.* **139:**678–680.

6

Cellular Biochemistry of the Endometrium

JOHN D. APLIN

Morphological alterations in endometrium during the reproductive cycle are increasingly well documented. A new era has now begun in which the molecular processes that underlie these structural changes will be elucidated. Ultimately, in the foreseeable future, the molecular interactions responsible for implantation and placentation will be understood, with undoubted benefits in the clinic. Progress will depend on a combination of biochemical, molecular biological, cell biological, and morphological approaches. This chapter summarizes current information on endometrial composition with emphasis on hormone-regulated alterations in endogenous glycoproteins, proteins, and proteoglycans that may be required for successful reproduction. The main focus of attention is on the human, but results of some animal studies are also included since they may facilitate the establishment of hypotheses for testing, insofar as ethics permit, in the human. New insights into function may be gained when a prominent constituent of one species is absent or modified in another. Emphasis is placed on structural components many of which represent the end products of metabolic processes that are controlled hormonally. The underlying endocrine and metabolic processes themselves are not considered. At the time of writing, few uninterrupted lines of connection can be drawn between morphology and biochemisry, so one function of this chapter is to draw attention to areas of research in which, with recent methodological advances, progress can now be expected.

After a discussion of methodology, the chapter is organized into sections along compartmental lines, dividing the tissue into intracellular, cell surface, and extracellular domains, the last of which is further subdivided into the extracellular matrix and soluble secretions. Information is not yet sufficiently complete to justify subdividing the various endometrial cell types; indeed, the development of new molecular markers is required to facilitate the characterization of the cell populations of the endometrium and their function in the reproductive cycle.

JOHN D. APLIN ● Departments of Obstetrics and Gynaecology, Biochemistry, and Molecular Biology, University of Manchester, Manchester M13 0JK, England.

1. Methodological Comments

Molecular studies of endometrium have been impeded by the lack of a cell culture system that retains the hormonally induced proliferation and differentiation occurring *in vivo*. Methods are now available for separating epithelial and stromal elements and for subfractionating the latter into fibroblastic and bone-marrow-derived populations (Kirk and Irwin, 1980; Siegfried *et al.*, 1984; Lindenberg *et al.*, 1984; Aplin and Seif, 1985; Daya *et al.*, 1985; Kirk and Alvarez, 1986; Lala *et al.*, 1986; Oksenberg *et al.*, 1986; Wewer *et al.*, 1986; Campbell *et al.*, 1988). However, the phenotype of both epithelial and stromal cells is unstable in culture; although they retain estrogen receptors, neither cell type shows a proliferative response to estrogen (or progesterone) when cultured in isolation (Kirk and Irwin, 1980; Kleinman *et al.*, 1983; Heimann *et al.*, 1985; Cooke *et al.*, 1986).

Epithelial cells cease to express some cell surface components characteristic of the differentiated state (unpublished observations), and their secretory phenotype is altered (Campbell *et al.*, 1988), although outgrowth from explants may provide a useful model for reepithelialization after menstruation (Kirk *et al.*, 1978). For modeling early implantation, however, it is clear that careful attention will have to be paid to epithelial polarity. This model will necessitate the use of confluent cultures in which tight junctions are established (Glasser, 1985; S. R. Glasser, personal communication). Stromal cells in monolayer culture acquire some features of decidual differentiation (Vladimirsky *et al.*, 1977; Sananes *et al.*, 1978; Wewer *et al.*, 1986). Changes in either cell type may result in part from the use of inappropriate culture media, and the future use of a chemically defined medium should lead to improved results (Cooke *et al.*, 1986). However, it has also been demonstrated that, as in other epithelial systems, the differentiated state of endometrial epithelium is dependent on interaction with the underlying stroma. Thus, normal morphology and estrogen responsiveness can be restored to mouse endometrial epithelial cells after an initial period (7–10 days) in pure cell culture by recombining the epithelium with homologous stroma (Cooke *et al.*, 1986, 1987).

It is probable that for full functional differentiation, epithelial and stromal cells are required to be maintained in a correct spatial relationship within an extracellular matrix of precisely defined composition (Bissell *et al.*, 1982). In organ culture, where these relationships are preserved, essentially normal progesterone-induced differentiation can be observed after estrogen priming (Daly *et al.*, 1983). Thus, molecular studies to date, particularly of endometrial secretions, have relied in general on short-term (24–48 hr) organ or explant cultures in which cellular viability and the differentiated state are preserved. Under these conditions, soluble secretory products can be collected from the supernatant medium for analysis. Radiolabeled metabolic precursors can be added, and, given specific antibody probes, labeled macromolecular products can be immunoprecipitated from the medium to demonstrate that the product is endogenous. This methodology, although particularly useful for detecting minor components and studying biosynthesis, does not allow identification of the cell type within which biosynthesis occurs. Hence, there is the need for studies of pure (ideally, cloned) cell populations *in vitro*.

Antibodies may also be used for immunohistochemical analysis of the tissue or culture; this method provides invaluable information on spatial distribution and is especially powerful in studies of extracellular matrix and cytoskeleton, where products are immobilized in polymeric structures near the site of production. However, it can be both qualitatively and quantitatively misleading, especially in studies of soluble secretory products, which may diffuse interstitially to binding sites in adjacent or distant tissue locations. Hybridization autoradiography with labeled nucleotide probes will be more widely used in the future as the amino acid sequences of endometrial polypeptides become available. This technique will allow the spatial distribution of the corresponding mRNAs and the cell type of origin to be defined.

Another approach to the analysis of more abundant tissue polypeptides is to examine mRNA via complementary DNA libraries. These can be made using tissue exposed to different hormonal regimens, thus allowing hormone-induced or hormone-repressed products to be identified and cloned. The method has been applied successfully in rabbits, leading to the isolation of a progesterone-induced mRNA encoding a protein of calculated molecular weight 40,800 (Misrahi *et al.*, 1987). The mRNA is also found in rabbit liver, ovary, and fallopian tubes and cross-hybridizes with an mRNA found in human secretory-phase endometrium. This powerful approach will undoubtedly lead to the isolation and characterization of more endometrial products.

2. Intracellular Constituents

Many of the secretory components discussed in Section 5 and the circulating hormones and plasma proteins found in the uterus can be detected within uterine cells either because they are produced there or following endocytotic uptake (Parr and Parr, 1986). This section, however, concentrates on components the lifespan and function of which are exclusively intracellular. Three types of species are discussed: cytoskeletal components because of their importance in tissue structure; oncogene products because of their involvement in growth regulation; and components the expression of which is hormonally regulated. This approach may help provide compositional correlates of morphological development even in the absence of complete functional descriptions of the molecules that are detected.

2.1. Cytoskeletal Proteins

Actin and tubulin, the major globular protein subunits of microfilaments and microtubules, are present in all cells. However, surprisingly little information is yet available about their organization and functions in endometrium. Campbell *et al.*, (1988) have shown by immunofluorescence that freshly isolated tissue fragments consisting of glandular epithelial cells exhibit a characteristic peripheral cytoplasmic accumulation of microfilaments within each cell (Fig. 1). This arrangement may well be important in the stability of cell–cell contacts and the integrity of the epithelial sheet. Outgrowths from these aggregates have also been studied in short-term (1- to 3-day) culture (Campbell *et al.*, 1988), a procedure that provides a model for reepithelialization in the early proliferative phase. The cells migrate across the culture substratum in a cooperative manner in which the integrity of the epithelial sheet is maintained, the cells at and immediately behind the free edges of the islands becoming increasingly well spread. This behavior is typical of epithelial cells *in vitro* (DiPasquale, 1975). During the development of the outgrowths, significant alterations in the organization of the actin cytoskeleton occur (Fig. 1). The cells develop prominent stress fibers, and, with the loss of the peripheral accumulation in individual cells of the aggregates, filament bundles become evident running circumferentially and radially near the free edges of islands and outgrowths. These connect contiguous structures in adjacent members of the colony via cell–cell (adherens) junctions.

Microtubules in these cultures exhibit two characteristic forms of organization (Fig. 2): a typical, partly radial, distribution occupying all or most of the cytoplasm and forming a basketlike structure around the nucleus and an association with apical cilia. The relationship between these two microtubular systems and the components involved in integration of the basal body of the cilium into the cytoskeletal system are presently unknown. The tubulin content of rat uterus has been reported to increase during progesterone-induced differentiation (Guest *et al.*, 1986).

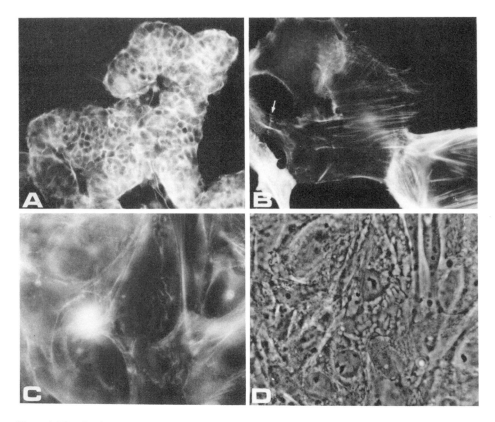

Figure 1. Visualization of actin in human endometrial epithelial cell cultures using rhodamine–phalloidin. A: Explant showing peripheral accumulation of actin in the cytoplasm consistent with an involvement in adherens-type junctions (×710). These can be seen in well-spread cells in an outgrowth (B; arrow). Stress fibers are prominent in sparser (B) and denser (C) outgrowths. D: Phase contrast of field in C. Micrographs by S. Campbell. B, C, and D ×1840.

The intermediate filament proteins show patterns of cell-type-specific expression that give information on developmental lineage and will, in due course, provide insight into cell function. Franke and co-workers have made an extensive survey of cytokeratin intermediate filament proteins and their patterns of expression in epithelial cells (Moll *et al.,* 1982). Of the more than 20 keratin polypeptides found in human epithelia, four are coexpressed in endometrial epithelial cells: these are keratins 7, 8, 18, and 19 (Moll *et al.,* 1983) (Fig. 3; Table 1). The same pattern of expression is seen in the simple epithelia of oviduct and endocervix as well as in endometrial adenocarcinoma, and it appears to persist in endometrial gland cells in the decidua of pregnancy (Khong *et al.,* 1986). The distribution of cytoplasmic keratin in endometrial epithelial cells is shown in Fig. 3 and is consistent with the existence of keratin-associated junctional structures such as desmosomes (Wynn, 1977) at the lateral intercellular boundaries that are maintained in the well-spread sheet outgrowths.

Decidualizing stromal cells exhibit interesting alterations in intermediate filament level and composition consistent with the idea that the acquisition of differentiated functions requires a specific program of intermediate filament gene expression (Table 1). In rats, vimentin increases in proportion to total decidual cell protein, whereas desmin expression increases more rapidly, from trace amounts in endometrial stroma to a level approximately equal to that of vimentin (Glasser and Julian, 1986). The appearance of desmin is correlated with mor-

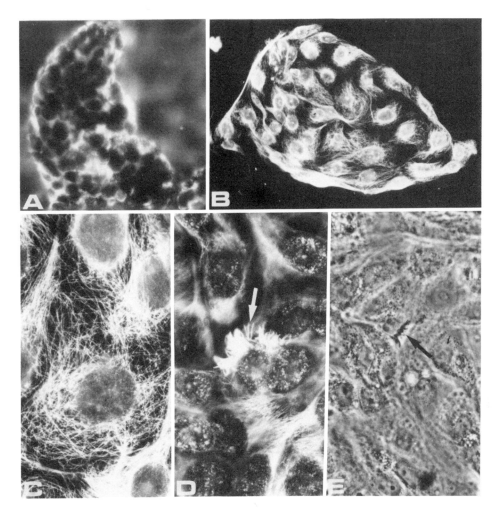

Figure 2. Cytoplasmic microtubules in human endometrial epithelial cell cultures visualized with a monoclonal antibody (New England Nuclear) after fixation and permeabilization. A: Explant (×1150) showing tubulin concentrated at the cell periphery. B: Cell island (×710). C: High magnification in the plane of the nucleus of well-flattened cells in an outgrowth (×2850). D: Near the plane of the apical cell surface, various features can be distinguished, including speckles and prominent cilia on a minority of cells (arrow) (×2850). The cilia are always confined to one restricted area of the cell and are clustered or organized in rows. Asynchronously beating cilia (arrow) can also be seen in phase contrast (E; ×1840) in cultures established from proliferative or early secretory tissue. Micrographs by S. Campbell.

phological evidence of decidualization (Glasser *et al.,* 1987). In the human, decidualized stromal cells also coexpress vimentin and desmin (Khong *et al.,* 1986). Some stromal cells contain only vimentin; these may be of lymphoid or myeloid origin. Therefore, it is important to note that the acquisition of epithelial-type characteristics by decidual cells (discussed in Sections 4 and 6) does not extend to the expression of cytoplasmic cytokeratins (Kisalus *et al.,* 1987a). Vascular endothelial cells contain largely vimentin-type subunits, whereas extra-villous cytotrophoblast contains keratin. Thus antikeratin antibodies are useful cytological tools for the identification of trophoblast in the placental bed (Bulmer and Johnson, 1985; Bulmer *et al.,* 1986; Khong *et al.,* 1986).

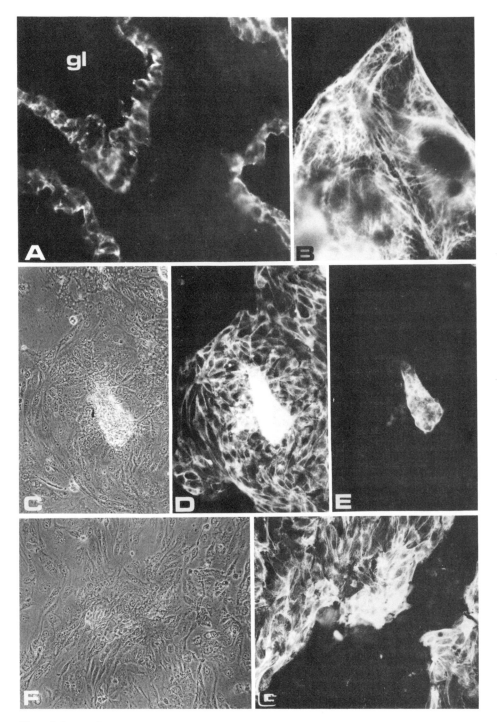

Figure 3. Immunofluorescence of keratin intermediate filaments in human endometrial tissue and cell cultures using monoclonal antibody clone 80 (Sanbio), which recognizes a broad spectrum of keratin polypeptides. A: Glandular epithelial cells in the tissue are keratin-positive; stromal cells are uniformly negative (×350) (gl, gland). B: High magnification (×1840) of epithelial cells in an outgrowth from explant culture showing the cytoplasmic distribution. Note the perinuclear basket of filaments and the concentration of keratin at adjacent cell edges where desmosomes occur. C: Phase contrast of an epithelial explant and its surrounding outgrowth.

Table 1. Intermediate Filament Polypeptides[a]

Peptide	Molecular weight	Found in
Vimentin	57,000	Mesenchyme-derived cells and many cell lines; fibroblasts, astrocytes, chondrocytes, muscle cells, endothelial cells, macrophages, lymphocytes, some epithelial cells; decidual cells
Desmin	54,000	Muscle cells, some endothelial cells, some mesenchyme-derived cell lines; decidual cells
Glial fibrillary acidic (GFA) protein	51,000	Astrocytes
Neurofilament triplet	68,000, 145,000, 200,000	Peripheral and central neurons
Keratins	40,000–68,000 (~30 different polypeptides)	Epithelial cells

[a]All intermediate filament subunit polypeptides possess structurally conserved features, the most notable of which is a central domain comprising a seven-residue "heptad" repeat (mainly hydrophobic amino acids in positions 4 and 7) that can form an α-helical coiled coil. This gives rise to morphologically indistinguishable polymers. The N- and C-terminal domains, however, are highly type-specific. The keratin family is divided into two groups: type I keratins are larger and more basic, whereas type II keratins are smaller and more acidic. At least one keratin polypeptide of each type must be expressed to allow filament formation (Moll *et al.*, 1982, 1983; Steinert *et al.*, 1985).

2.2. Oncogene Products

Evidence is accumulating that estrogen can induce expression of oncogenes in rat uterus (Murphy *et al.*, 1987; Travers and Knowler, 1987). This concept carries important implications for the control of cell proliferation in both the normal endometrium and neoplasia. Thus, administration of E_2 to prepubertal ovariectomized rats gives rise to a substantial (three- to eightfold) rise in c-*myc* mRNA (2.4 kb) after 3–4 hr. The maximal level of mRNA is three- to sixfold higher than that observed in normal adult rats in diestrus or proestrus–estrus, and during the normal cycle the level of c-*myc* mRNA is constant. Using a probe for a related protooncogene, N-*myc*, Murphy *et al.* (1987) showed a more rapid increase in the complementary mRNA of sixfold over the first 15 min of E_2 treatment to a maximum of ninefold at 30–60 min. These results were obtained under stringent hybridization conditions in Northern blotting and relate to a transcript of 3 kb. Under conditions of reduced stringency, another 2.2-kb transcript is detectable, and it too increases rapidly after stimulation with E_2. In contrast, *ras*[Ha] mRNA levels increase to a maximum at about 8 hr after hormone administration (Travers and Knowler, 1987).

Production of the chromatin-associated protein encoded by c-*myc* is associated in other systems with the diversion of cells from differentiative to proliferative phenotypes (Zimmerman *et al.*, 1986). The function of the protein encoded by *ras*[Ha] is likely to be associated with

All the cells are keratin-positive, both in the outgrowth (D; fluorescence in the plane of the substratum; note the peripheral accumulations of cytoplasmic filaments) and in the explant (E; higher plane of focus in which fluorescence from the outgrowth is lost). The substratum (C, top left) contains "matrigel," an extract of the mouse EHS tumor enriched in basal laminal macromolecules. F,G: Phase and fluorescence of a mixed culture of endometrial epithelial and stromal cells. The latter are keratin-negative. C–G: ×455. Micrographs B–G by S. Campbell.

signal transduction (Hanley and Jackson, 1987). Studies of the influence of growth factors on endometrial cell growth and proliferation are still at a formative stage; reports of the existence in endometrial cells of both growth factor receptors (Sheets *et al.*, 1985; Chegini *et al.*, 1986) and intracellular products including oncogene-encoded proteins that participate in signal transduction following receptor binding are certain to stimulate further research in this exciting area.

2.3. The 24k Protein

McGuire and co-workers have reported a series of studies of an estrogen-induced cytoplasmic protein of 24,000 daltons, which they identified initially in the human breast cancer cell line MCF-7 (Edwards *et al.*, 1980). Monoclonal antibodies to the protein (Ciocca *et al.*, 1982) bind to normal estrogen target organs as well as to some tumors but not to estrogen-receptor-negative tissues (Ciocca *et al.*, 1983a). In human uterus, the protein shows an interesting menstrual cycle dependence of expression (Ciocca *et al.*, 1983b). It appears in glandular epithelial cells in the late proliferative phase, decreasing after ovulation. In superficial epithelium it also appears in the late proliferative phase but increases to a peak of expression in the midsecretory phase before declining. Stromal cells do not show any immunoreactivity until predecidual changes are evident, and in fully differentiated decidual stromal cells staining is intense (Ciocca *et al.*, 1983a; McCrae *et al.*, 1986).

In each case, the product is located intracellularly, and in some late-secretory-phase glands it appears concentrated in apical swellings (Ciocca *et al.*, 1983b). These findings support the idea that in endometrium, progesterone as well as estrogen may play a role in regulating expression of 24k. Regional and microregional variation is also observed as with other hormonally controlled responses in the tissue. No function has yet been ascribed to the protein. However, amino acid sequence data obtained via an MCF-7 cell cDNA library suggest a homology with the low-molecular-weight heat shock proteins of *Drosophila* (Moretti-Rojas *et al.*, 1988).

3. Cell Surface

Interstitial implantation consists of a sequence of processes in which initial apposition and attachment of the embryo to uterine luminal epithelium is followed by penetration first of the cell layer and then of the basement membrane. This process involves intimate contact between embryonic and maternal cell surfaces. Molecular studies of the epithelial cell surface (as well as that of the trophoblast) are therefore important in furthering understanding of implantation. The idea of a defined, hormonally controlled period of endometrial receptivity for implantation preceded and followed by phases of refractoriness has evolved from studies of rodents and other animals (Psychoyos, 1986) and is a potentially important consideration in human embryo replacement. Indirect evidence thus suggests the probable existence of hormone-dependent changes in cell surface composition in endometrial epithelium at the time of implantation. These might involve either the removal of factors that inhibit implantation or the expression of new cell surface components the function of which is to bind trophoblast, or both (Denker, 1978, 1983). However, the molecular analysis of endometrial epithelial cell surfaces is in its infancy. Still less information is available about the surfaces of stromal cells, and these are not discussed further. The discussion of epithelial cells can be divided into considerations associated with cellular location (glands versus uterine lining and region of uterine corpus), cell polarity, and hormone-dependent compositional alterations.

All epithelial cells show compositional variations in cell surface among apical, lateral, and basal domains (Van Meer and Simons, 1986; Matlin and Simons, 1984). Variations of this sort in human endometrial epithelium are illustrated in Fig. 4. These reflect functional differences: the basal domain is responsible for anchoring the cell to the underlying matrix and for the receptivity of the cell to signals emanating from the stroma or vasculature. The lateral domain is responsible for cell–cell adhesion within the epithelium. The apical domain is involved in the control of secretory processes, the activities of cilia and microvilli, endocytosis or pinocytosis of luminal components, and interactions with the embryo. Compositional differences between apical and basolateral domains are maintained by tight junctions, which prevent the diffusion of membrane glycoproteins from apical to basolateral domains and vice versa (Wynn, 1977; Pinto da Silva and Kachar, 1982; Griepp *et al.,* 1983; Cornillie *et al.,* 1985; Tabibzadeh *et al.,* 1986). Glycolipid diffusion is also restricted (Spiegel *et al.,* 1985).

3.2. Cell Location

Various pieces of histochemical evidence support the proposition that cell surface compositional differences occur between epithelium in luminal lining and glands. In human pro-

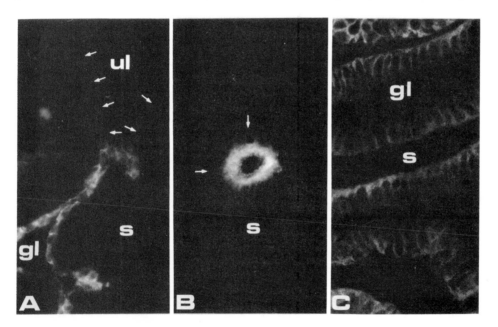

Figure 4. Immunofluorescence of human endometrium after staining with three different monoclonal antibodies recognizing cell surface-associated epitopes. A: DH71 binds to an apically distributed component in glandular epithelium throughout the menstrual cycle. The epitope is absent from luminal epithelium. The micrograph shows the abrupt termination of staining at the narrow neck of a gland. Arrows indicate the apical surface of the luminal epithelium (ul, uterine lumen). ×730. B: F51 binds to an apical epitope in glandular and luminal epithelial cells that is present in proliferative phase (shown) but disappears from most cells in secretory phase. The arrows indicate the base of the gland cells. ×360. C: CC25 binds to a basolaterally expressed epitope present on both glandular and luminal epithelial cells. This marker is absent in the proliferative phase and appears in the early secretory phase. ×730. gl, Gland lumen; s, stroma (Aplin and Seif, 1987). Taken together these observations show that endometrial epithelial cells are polarized into apical and basolateral domains, that cell surface composition differs between glandular and luminal cells, and that surface composition changes during the cycle. Micrographs by M. Seif.

liferative-phase endometrium, soy bean agglutinin, which binds to glycans containing nonreducing terminal N-acetylgalactosamine, stains cells of the lining epithelium but not those of glands (Lee and Damjanov, 1985). Twenty-one other fluorescent lectins stained luminal and glandular epithelium with equal intensity, suggesting many conserved glycoprotein and glycolipid oligosaccharides. A monoclonal antibody has also been isolated that binds to an epitope present on glandular but not luminal epithelial cells (M. W. Seif, personal communication; Fig. 4). In each case, the binding of the reporter molecule ceases abruptly at the openings of glands. An antigen specific to luminal epithelial cells of the pregnant rabbit has been identified with the aid of a monoclonal antibody by Lampelo *et al.* (1986). These data establish the principle that epithelial cells involved in embryo attachment express surface components additional to, or different from, those required in glandular sites. In addition, ciliated cells in rabbit luminal epithelium have been found to differ from nonciliated cells by virtue of the presence of binding sites for the lectin from *Dolichus biflorus* (DBA) (Anderson *et al.*, 1986), the absence of binding sites for wheat germ agglutinin (Anderson *et al.*, 1986; Thie *et al.*, 1986), and the absence of binding sites for polycationic ferritin (Anderson and Hoffman, 1984). In the mouse, a class of high-molecular-weight asparagine-linked lactosaminoglycans has been demonstrated on the surface of epithelial cells that is largely absent from stromal cells (Dutt *et al.*, 1987).

3.3. Hormone-Dependent Alterations

Alterations in endometrial cell surface composition during the reproductive cycle were first detected ultrastructurally using techniques for the visualization of anionic sites or glycocalyx on apical surfaces of epithelial cells. Alterations in glycocalyx have also been reported on the basis of light microscopy of periodic acid–Schiff-stained tissue or lectin histochemistry. The observations, discussed in the following paragraphs, are significant in relation to the concept of a period of receptivity for blastocyst attachment. However, it is noted that none of these techniques allows a definitive distinction to be made between molecules integral to the plasma membrane and those associated with it. In particular, carbohydrate-directed stains used at the light-microscopic level cannot distinguish highly glycosylated secretions from apical plasma membrane, and even at the TEM level, the distinction may not be unequivocal. Secretory components have been shown to associate with the apical surface of glandular and luminal epithelial cells (see Section 5) and are often quantitatively the dominant glycosylated species in human secretory-phase epithelium. Further biochemical characterization of the cell surface is required.

Hewitt *et al.* (1979) reported that binding sites for polycationic ferritin at physiological pH and ionic strength are associated with the apical microvilli of rat endometrial epithelial cells in estrus. Binding persists on days 2 and 3 of pregnancy but at day 4 is greatly reduced, suggesting a loss of surface anionic sites. No binding is detectable at day 6. These changes were suggested to reduce coulombic repulsion between the embryo and the endometrial surface. The microvillous glycocalyx also undergoes changes during this period, becoming globular at day 2 and then decreasing progressively, so that on day 6 little is visible. Similar changes occur in pseudopregnancy, and the alterations occur both near to and distant from the implantation site. In mice, the thickness of the glycocalyx also decreases on day 4 and especially day 5 of pregnancy. Loss of the glycocalyx appears to occur partly through endocytosis of cell surface. These changes occur both at and between implantation sites (Chávez and Anderson, 1985).

Morris and Potter (1984) studied surface charge in mouse endometrial epithelial cells by allowing cell aggregates (''vesicles'') to interact with diethylaminoethyl-Sephadex beads in the presence of increasing concentrations of a competing polyanion, dextran sulfate. Attachment of the cells to the beads could be prevented by sialidase pretreatment or by increasing the dextran sulfate concentration above a threshold level that proved to be four times greater than the threshold for inhibition of attachment of beads to blastocysts. However, the uterine epithelium showed a 50% reduction in surface negative charge at the time of implantation (day 4.5) as compared with the previous day. The results suggest that a reduction in coulombic repulsion between the blastocyst and the endometrium occurs at the receptive stage but do not obviate the requirement for more specific (and as yet unknown) adhesion mechanisms.

In the rabbit, binding of polycationic ferritin (abolished by treating the cells with sialidase) is markedly reduced by the second day of pregnancy and absent by day 6 (Anderson and Hoffman, 1984). These changes occur in ovariectomized, estradiol-treated as well as pseudopregnant animals. Fibrillar glycocalyx visualized by the periodic acid–alkaline bismuth method is abundant in estrus and up to the sixth day of pregnancy but disappears by day 7.5. In the human, surface glycocalyx increases in quantity in the early secretory phase, but with a concomitant loss of negative charge (Jansen et al., 1985).

Several groups have detected alterations in the patterns of lectin binding to endometrial epithelium at different stages of the reproductive cycle. In the human, peanut agglutinin, which binds to certain galactose-containing glycans, stains many apical epithelial cell domains in proliferative and early secretory phases, but staining disappears by late secretory phase (Bychkov and Toto, 1986). However, in glands of early pregnancy, binding increases. Similarly, soy bean agglutinin and *Vicia villosa* agglutinin, both of which recognize oligosaccharides containing N-acetylgalactosamine, bind to glands in pregnancy but not in the proliferative or secretory phase (Lee and Damjanov, 1985; Yen et al., 1986). Conversely, *Lens culinaris* lectin, for which the corresponding inhibitory monosaccharide is mannose, binds to proliferative-phase glands but not to those of early pregnancy (Lee and Damjanov, 1985). As yet, qualitative light-microscopic studies in the human have not detected changes in composition of apical epithelial cell surfaces specific to the time of implantation.

In equids, localized domains of lectin binding have been detected in the endometrial epithelium shortly before implantation (pregnancy day 33 in the mare). Thus, wheat germ agglutinin (WGA) binds to areas about ten cells in diameter while not binding to adjacent parts of the luminal epithelium or glandular epithelium (Whyte and Robson, 1984; Whyte and Allen, 1985). In early pregnancy, this binding extends across the surface epithelium and into glands. However, it is not yet clear how the localized domains of WGA-positive cells are positioned with respect to the implanting blastocyst. In the mouse, the fucose-specific lectin from *Ulex europaeus* (UEA-I) binds nonpregnant uterine epithelium, and the sites disappear in pregnancy (Lee et al., 1983). This finding contrasts with the lack of UEA-I binding in human endometrium (Lee and Damjanov, 1985). Four other lectins (*Ricinus communis* I, *Maclura pomifera*, wheat germ, and *Bauhinia purpurea*) also show pregnancy-specific alterations in binding in mouse endometrium, but 15 do not (Lee et al., 1983). Binding of *Ricinus communis* agglutinin I to the nonreducing terminal galactose of the mouse microvillous surface increases as the thickness of the glycocalyx decreases (Chávez and Anderson, 1985). Administration of a monoclonal antiprogesterone antibody at 32 hr post-coitum blocks pregnancy and leads to a detectable diminution in abundance of glycoconjugates containing galactose as monitored by binding of peanut agglutinin. No change was observed in WGA binding to endometrium, although binding sites were abolished in the ampullary region of the oviduct (Whyte et al., 1987).

In a detailed study of rabbit endometrium, Anderson et al. (1986) have combined light- and electron-microscopic localization of lectin binding sites at the microvillous membrane with SDS-PAGE and blotting analysis of luminal surface glycoproteins and their lectin-binding properties. Glycoproteins were specifically solubilized by introducing buffered 1% Triton X-100 with protease inhibitors into washed uterine lumens. This interesting procedure appears not to disrupt tight junctions, extract basolateral cell surface, or alter intracellular structure as judged by TEM but partially dissolves the apical surface. It should be stressed that the results represent an incomplete analysis of apical cell surface glycoproteins, since components tightly bound to cytoskeleton have been shown in many systems not to be solubilized under these conditions (see, for example, Prives *et al.*, 1982; Jung *et al.*, 1984), and it seems from TEM of extracted tissue that this is also the case in the present study. However, a good correlation was obtained between the biochemical and morphological observations. Thus, succinyl wheat germ agglutinin binding is absent in estrous animals but present at day 7 of pseudopregnancy on both the microvillous and intervillous glycocalyces. Little or no binding of succinyl-WGA can be observed to blots of estrus-phase detergent extracts, but several prominent glycoprotein bands appear in extracts made in pseudopregnancy, including a broadly running component of M_r 80–86,000. This glycoprotein is also present in sterile horns (pregnancy, unilateral tubal ligation) but is greatly reduced in extracts made from implantation sites.

Binding of *Ricinus communis* agglutinin (RCA I) also increases from estrus to day 7 of pseudopregnancy, and the corresponding Western blot shows a large increase in lectin-binding glycoproteins. In this case, sialidase treatment of the tissue restores much of the binding. The corresponding blot demonstrates that the increase of RCA I binding in pseudopregnancy can be explained in part by desialylation of components that are actually present in estrus; however, new glycoprotein components also appear at the apical surface. These include a component of M_r 58,000 that lacks affinity for con A, RCA I, or WGA, one of M_r 42,000 that binds WGA and RCA I, and one of M_r 24,000 that binds WGA. In each case, the results from pseudopregnancy extracts match those of the ligated horn in pregnancy, whereas implantation sites yield lower recoveries of the pregnancy-specific component.

Lampelo *et al.* (1985) isolated plasma membranes from curettings of rabbit endometrium and also demonstrated compositional differences in receptive and nonreceptive stages. Ricketts *et al.* (1984) cultured rabbit endometrial epithelial cells for 3 days *in vitro*, after which surface radioiodination was used to demonstrate differences between cells obtained at day 4 and day 6.5 of pregnancy.

3.4. Preparation for Implantation

It has been consistently demonstrated using a variety of approaches that changes in the apical surface of luminal epithelial cells in endometria of several species occurs in a manner that suggests preparation for implantation. Many of these changes occur solely in response to maternal factors and are not dependent on the presence of an embryo. However, it is likely that this preparation of the endometrium, which allows it to achieve a receptive state, takes place as a prelude to more localized surface changes that occur in response to, or are affected directly by, the apposing blastocyst. The most clear-cut demonstration of this phenomenon is the appearance of a protease (blastolemmase) at implantation sites in rabbit and other species (Denker, 1983). This enzyme, which probably originates in the embryo, may function to aid hatching of the blastocyst but may also effect local biochemical modifications of the endometrium. At any rate, implantation is prevented by protease inhibitors (Denker, 1982).

4. Extracellular Matrix

4.1. Interstitial Components

Stromal fibroblasts, which from the early proliferative phase display prominent rough endoplasmic reticulum and Golgi complexes, are probably largely responsible for the production of the collagenous extracellular matrix that accompanies tissue thickening in the human (Wienke *et al.*, 1968; Cornillie *et al.*, 1985). Similarly, mouse endometrial fibroblasts in estrus express ultrastructural features consistent with a secretory phenotype and are intimately associated with bundles of fibrils displaying the cross-banding pattern associated with collagen (64-nm periodicity) (Zorn *et al.*, 1986). However, it cannot be assumed that epithelial cells do not also contribute to the extracellular matrix of stroma as well as to the basal lamina (see, for example, Aplin *et al.*, 1985). It is likely that vascular smooth muscle and endothelial cells deposit their own characteristic matrices in endometrium as in other tissues.

Matrix production in the human stroma results in the appearance in the midproliferative phase of reticulin fibers (Dallenbach-Hellweg, 1981), which become denser and thicker towards ovulation. Fibril production continues into the early secretory phase (More *et al.*, 1974). Immunofluorescence studies (Aplin *et al.*, 1988) show the presence of stromal collagens type III, V, and VI (Figs. 5 and 6; Table 2). The stroma is also rich in collagen type I, which is extractable from the uterus in large quantities (Abedin *et al.*, 1982). Collagen type V epitopes are masked in the proliferative phase, a phenomenon also observed in other tissues (Linsenmayer *et al.*, 1983) and thought to be the result of lateral-chain associations with other major collagens, principally type I.

The ubiquitous extracellular glycoprotein fibronectin, which contains a collagen binding site capable of interacting with any of the major interstitial collagens (Owens and Baralle, 1986), is also associated with the dense proliferative-phase matrix in humans and estrus-phase stroma in rodents (Grinnell *et al.*, 1982; Glasser *et al.*, 1987; Aplin *et al.*, 1988). Fibronectin also interacts with glycosaminoglycans and may play a role in matrix organization. Fibronectin is produced by human endometrial stromal (but not epithelial) cells in culture (Siegfried *et al.*, 1984).

Beginning in the midsecretory phase, a series of processes occurring in the stromal extracellular matrix contributes significantly to predecidual changes and, in the event of pregnancy, to decidualization.

With the addition of immunocytochemical techniques for the sensitive detection of matrix molecules to previous light- and electron-microscopic data, these alterations can be seen as a logical and coherent program of tissue remodeling. Investigations into the molecular mechanisms of this transformation are, however, at an early stage. At day 21, the stroma becomes more edematous, and fibrillar components including interstitial collagens are more loosely organized (Wynn, 1977; Dallenbach-Hellweg, 1981; Aplin *et al.*, 1988) as the tissue prepares to accept the implanting blastocyst. Thus arises the important question of whether this transformation is the result of a controlled and limited dissolution of fibrillar elements, a switch in stromal cells from production of fibrillar components to more highly hydrated glycosaminoglycans (GAGs) and proteoglycans (PGs) (Scott and Haigh, 1985), or a combination of the two processes. At present, only a partial answer can be given.

Collagen breakdown occurs by limited extracellular proteolysis followed by ingestion by scavenging cells and further intracellular breakdown. Tissue collagenase activity may be regulated by the concentration of the enzyme (Hembry *et al.*, 1986) or by the occurrence of inhibitors and activators (Woessner, 1977).

The correlation between rapid matrix remodeling and the occurrence of infiltrating cells has been pointed out (Padykula, 1980) in connection with uterine involution, and macrophages have been shown to be capable of matrix degradation (Nathan, 1987). Progesterone inhibits uterine collagenase activity and can be shown to delay or prevent postpartum changes in the rat uterus (Tansey and Padykula, 1978).

Considerable morphological evidence exists to support the notion that both fibroblasts (Wienke *et al.*, 1968; Zorn *et al.*, 1986) and macrophages (Parakkal, 1969) are active in the internalization and breakdown of banded fibrillar collagens. In the human, collagen-containing lysosomes are prominent in stromal cells by day 25 of the menstrual cycle (Wienke *et al.*, 1968; Cornillie *et al.*, 1985), suggesting that some breakdown is occurring, but fibrillar collagens are still present in extracellular matrix between decidual cells at 10 weeks of gestation (Wynn, 1977). Intracellular vesicles containing collagen are visible on day 2 of

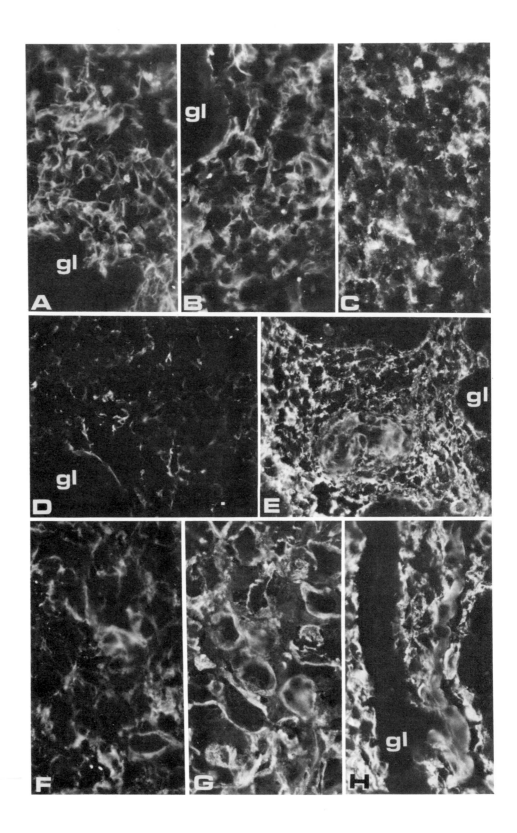

pregnancy in the mouse, and the extracellular fibril density is markedly reduced by day 4 (Zorn *et al.*, 1986), although no such reduction is evident around blood vessels or glands. By day 6 (after implantation on day 5), the fibril density is again increasing, although with a greater heterogeneity in fibril diameter, including the appearance of thick (68- to 300-nm diameter) fibrils. In the rat, stromal cells appear to be involved simultaneously in collagen production and resorption during the estrous cycle; an increased rate of breakdown in diestrus, as indicated by the presence of collagen in acid-phosphatase-containing vesicles, results in a lower fibril density in proestrus (van Veen and Peereboom-Stegeman, 1987).

Collagen self-association is suggested to begin in intracellular "filamentous bodies," which then fuse with the plasma membrane to release collagen into the extracellular space, where further polymerization occurs. Bundles of striated fibrils, sometimes sequestered in deep invaginations of the plasma membrane, persist in the rat primary decidual zone (Parr *et al.*, 1986). Consistent with these findings, collagen types I, III, and V are readily detected by immunofluorescence throughout the stroma in human secretory-phase endometrium notwith-standing a decrease in matrix density (Fig. 5). The channels and spaces between decidual cells in the first trimester also contain the major collagens and fibronectin, and the type V collagen epitopes are no longer masked, suggesting a reduction in interchain associations (Kisalus *et al.*, 1987a; Aplin *et al.*, 1988). Collagen types I, III, and V have been immunoprecipitated from the culture medium of explanted first-trimester decidua (Kisalus *et al.*, 1987a), a finding that demonstrates the continuing production of these species despite the overall reduction in fibril density.

Immunocytochemical studies of type VI collagen (Aplin *et al.*, 1988) reveal a different pattern of behavior (Fig. 6). Local diminution of staining in some areas of the stromal mesh is already noticeable in the midsecretory phase. This process continues in the late secretory phase, becoming more widespread, so that while blood vessel walls retain type VI, areas of stromal matrix away from glands become weakly stained or unstained. The marker is at this stage retained in stromal areas beneath glandular basal laminas. In fully decidualized stroma, type VI collagen is found only in vessel walls and, occasionally, as sparsely distributed large fibrils close to vessels. Menstrual-phase tissue shows a similar distribution (Fig. 6).

Qualitative studies therefore suggest that the major fibrillar collagens are reorganized with some breakdown, and quantitative estimates made during *in vitro* decidualization of rat stromal cells suggest that the rates of production of collagen type I and fibronectin are reduced (S. R. Glasser, personal communication). In contrast, extensive degradation of type VI collagen occurs until it eventually disappears from decidual stroma. Type VI collagen consists of short-triple-helical segments interrupted by nonhelical domains. The three polypeptide chains are disulfide linked (Table 2). This configuration is in contrast to the simple, uninterrupted triple-helical structure of types I, III, and V, and it confers on type VI collagen a different spectrum of sensitivity to proteases. Thus, for example, type VI is sensitive to bacterial collagenase only after reduction and alkylation, and it is insensitive to mammalian collagenase (Ayad *et al.*, 1985; Rauterberg *et al.*, 1986). Current data therefore engender the hypothesis that a type-VI-specific protease may be active in endometrial stroma beginning in the midsecretory phase.

Figure 5. Immunofluorescence of human endometrium and decidua stained with antibodies to interstitial matrix components. A: Polyclonal antibody to collagen type III, proliferative phase, showing staining in the stroma. B: Antitype III, midsecretory phase. C: Polyclonal antitype V collagen, late secretory phase tissue after treatment with acetic acid, which is required to solvate and unmask the antigen. D: Monoclonal antifibronectin, pro-liferative phase, showing a delicate network of stromal fibers. E: Polyclonal antifibronectin, late secretory phase, showing abundant staining throughout the stroma. F: Antitype III collagen, decidua, showing pericellular and intercellular staining in an area of enlarged differentiated decidual cells. G: A similar area stained with polyclonal antifibronectin. The distribution is similar to that of type III collagen. H: Antifibronectin staining in an area of stroma containing poorly differentiated cells. All ×360. Anticollagen antibodies from S. Ayad. gl, Glands.

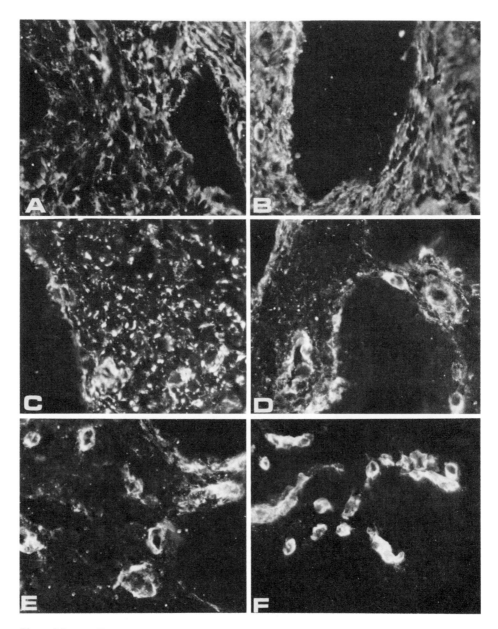

Figure 6. Immunofluorescence of type VI collagen in human endometrium and decidua using monoclonal antibody ST-1 produced by M. Seif. ST-1 binds to the 140,000-molecular-weight subunit of type VI collagen. A,B: Proliferative phase. C: Midsecretory phase. D: Late secretory phase. E: Menstrual phase. F: First-trimester decidua (all ×360). The fibrillar matrix found throughout the stroma in the proliferative phase is rich in type VI collagen. In the midsecretory phase some condensation has occurred, and by late secretory phase many deeper areas of stroma lack the marker, which is still retained beneath glandular basement membranes and in vessel walls. Menstrual-phase endometrium and decidua show similar patterns of distribution, the type VI collagen being retained for the most part only in vessel walls. The fields shown are representative; however, significant microregional variation occurs in the rate of clearance (Aplin *et al.*, 1988).

Table 2. Some Components of Extracellular Matrix with Review References

Name	Properties	Cloning/sequencing
Interstitial components		
Fibronectin	460,000 (two similar disulfide-linked subunits)	Kornblihtt *et al.* (1985)
	Carries binding sites for cells and matrix molecules (collagens, glycosaminoglycans, fibrin); also occurs in some basement membranes (Hynes and Yamada, 1982)	Skorstengaard *et al.* (1986) Differential splicing from a single gene gives rise to several closely related polypeptides
Collagen type I	$[\alpha_1(I)]_2 \alpha_2(I)$; molecular weight 300,000 Quantitatively dominant fibrillar collagen Triple-helical monomers polymerize extracellularly to banded fibrils (Hay, 1981; Marchi and LeBlond, 1983)	Ramachandran and Reddi (1976) Cheah (1985)
Collagen type II	$[\alpha_1(II)]_2$; the major cartilage collagen	Cheah (1985)
Collagen type III	$[\alpha_1(III)]_3$; disulfide-linked subunits; can form heterofibrils with type I (Henkel and Glanville, 1982)	Cheah (1985)
Collagen type V	$\alpha_1(V)\alpha_2(V)\alpha_3(V)$ or $[\alpha_1(V)]_2 \alpha_2(V)$ or $[\alpha_1(V)]_3$ (Abedin *et al.*, 1981); can form heterofibrils with type I (Linsenmeyer *et al.*, 1983)	Weil *et al.* (1987)
Collagen type VI[a]	$[\alpha_1(VI)]_2 \alpha_2(VI)$; molecular weights, $\alpha_1(VI)$ chain 140,000, $\alpha_2(V)$ chain 240,000; the trimer contains three short helical domains interrupted by nonhelical regions; more highly glycosylated than other collagens (Rauterberg *et al.*, 1986; Trüeb and Winterhalter, 1986)	
Chondroitin and dermatan sulfate proteoglycans	Structures based on large (molecular weight 200,000–300,000) core proteins (Heinegård *et al.*, 1985; Hassell *et al.*, 1986) to which are attached polysaccharides based on the repeat units $\{4glcUA\beta_1$— $3galNAc\beta_1\}$ or $\{4idUA\alpha_1$—$3galNAc\beta_1\}$ with 4- or 6-O-sulfate substituents on the amino sugars; highly hydrated; some self-aggregate; some associate with other matrix components including collagen (Scott and Haigh, 1985) and fibronectin (Schmidt *et al.*, 1987); glycoprotein-type (N- or O-linked) glycans also present	See Hassell *et al.* (1986)
Keratan sulfate	Polysaccharide of repeating $\{4glcNAc\beta_1$— $3gal\beta_1\}$ with sulfate at some C_6 positions, attached to a core protein of 40,000–55,000 molecular weight	
Hyaluronic acid	Polysaccharide of repeating $\{4glcUA\beta_1$— $3glcNAc\beta_1\}$; high molecular weight ($\sim10^6$) (Hay, 1981); binds to a class of large chondroitin sulfate proteoglycans (Heinegård *et al.*, 1985)	
Basal lamina components		
Laminin	Glycoprotein of three disulfide-linked subunits: A chain (440,000), B_1 (225,000), and B_2 (205,000); some structural features (epitopes) are tissue-specific; carries bind-	Sasaki *et al.* (1987); Barlow *et al.* (1984)

(continued)

Table 2. (*Continued*)

Name	Properties	Cloning/sequencing
	ing sites for cells, sulfated GAGs, type IV collagen (Kleinman *et al.,* 1985; Von der Mark and Kühl, 1985)	
Entactin/nidogen	Self-aggregating protein; 150,000 form may be processes to 100,000, 80,000, and 45,000 products; larger forms bind laminin, fibronectin, type IV collagen (Carlin *et al.,* 1981; Dziadek *et al.,* 1985)	
Collagen type IV	$[\alpha_1(IV)]_2 \alpha_2(IV)$; 540,000; other polypeptides may also occur; self-aggregates to form networks; binds laminin, heparan sulfate proteoglycan, fibronectin (Laurie *et al.,* 1986)	Blumberg *et al.* (1987); Sakurai *et al.* (1986)
Heparan sulfate proteoglycans	Polysaccharide $\{glcNAc\alpha_1$—$4glcUA\beta\}$, $\{glcNSO_3\alpha_1$—$4glcUA\beta\}$, $\{glcNSO_3\alpha_1$—$4idUA\alpha\}$; O-sulfates may occur at the 3 and/or 6 positions of $glcNSO_3$, the 6 positions of glcNAc, the 2 positions of the uronic acids (Gallagher *et al.,* 1986); several related core proteins have been isolated, all apparently derived from a precursor of 400,000 molecular weight; each carries three or four polysaccharide chains (Ledbetter *et al.,* 1987; Hassell *et al.,* 1986)	

[a]Collagen types VII–XIII have not been studied in the uterus.

In other tissue locations, type VI collagen has been suggested to function as a microfibrillar network connecting the large fibrils of the major collagens (Bruns *et al.,* 1986). Specific cleavage of such cross links might allow local expansion and hydration of the interstitium while retaining the support provided by collagens I, III, and V. This result could give rise to facilitated penetration of interstitially migrating trophoblast as well as maternal bone-marrow-derived cell populations. Local swelling, however, implies the existence of GAGs and PGs as hydrated, space-filling molecules (Scott and Haigh, 1985). Few data are yet available on the molecular composition of endometrial ground substance. It is therefore very interesting that in the mouse, a specific five- to sixfold increase occurs in the synthesis of hyaluronate by stromal cells on the day of implantation (Carson *et al.,* 1987).

4.2. Basal Laminal Components

In his ultrastructural studies of human decidua, Wynn (1974, 1977) noted the appearance of a pericellular matrix around stromal cells, the characteristics of which resemble those of basal lamina. This finding has been substantiated by immunocytochemical as well as biochemical studies (Wewer *et al.,* 1985; Faber *et al.,* 1986; Ksalus *et al.,* 1987a; Aplin *et al.,* 1988; Fig. 7). Similar observations have been reported in mouse (Wewer *et al.,* 1986) and rat (Parr *et al.,* 1986; Glasser *et al.,* 1987). In the proliferative phase, the basal laminal components entactin, laminin, type IV collagen, and heparan sulfate proteoglycan as well as a family of glycoproteins (major components 180,000, 165,000, and 135,000) recognized by monoclonal antibody G71 (which was raised to endometrial epithelial cells; Aplin and Seif, 1985)

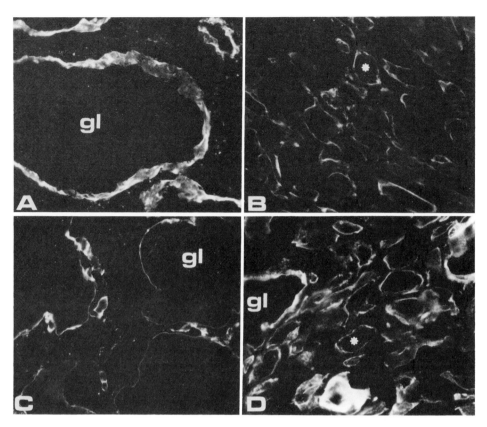

Figure 7. Immunofluorescence of basement membrane in human endometrium and decidua. A: Heparan sulfate proteoglycan (HSPG) visualized with a polyclonal antibody to the core protein in the proliferative phase. B: Monoclonal anti-HSPG, first-trimester decidua. C: Type IV collagen visualized with a monoclonal antibody in midsecretory phase. D: Type IV collagen in first-trimester decidua. In endometrium only glandular and vascular basement membranes are visible. In decidua prominent auras surround the enlarged decidual cells (e.g., asterisks) (×360). Antibodies to HSPG from P. Brenchley. Monoclonal antitype IV collagen from Sanbio. gl, Glands.

are all confined to glandular and luminal epithelial basement membranes and blood vessel walls (Fig. 7).

However, in the early secretory phase of the cycle, these components begin to appear in stromal cells. Thus, laminin is detectable in the cytoplasm of stromal cells (Faber *et al.,* 1986) and is then secreted to form small pericellular deposits. At the same time, expression of a cell surface laminin receptor (68,000 daltons) occurs for the first time in stromal cells. Heparan sulfate proteoglycan expression may be slightly retarded relative to laminin, but by the late secretory phase it and the other aforementioned components are all present in the predecidual pericellular matrix. The expression of basal laminal components by stromal cells is correlated with morphological features of decidualization. Thus, small elongated fibroblastic cells sometimes lack any trace of the markers in late-secretory-phase stroma and even in decidua of late first trimester. Enlarged polygonal decidual or predecidual cells can, in contrast, develop a full pericellular aura of basal lamina. In late secretory phase or first-trimester decidua, cells can usually be found exhibiting various stages of expression between these two extremes. Metabolic labeling of short-term organ cultures and cell cultures followed by immunoprecipitation from culture medium confirms that laminin is being produced, along with entactin, type IV collagen, heparan sulfate proteoglycan, a chondroitin sulfate proteoglycan, and fibronectin

(Wewer *et al.*, 1986; Kisalus *et al.*, 1987a). It was suggested that the relatively low yields in immunoprecipitation of the 400,000-dalton A chain of laminin result from the activity of endogenous proteases. Endometrial stromal cells from the nonpregnant mouse produce the same components in culture, suggesting that decidual differentiation can occur *in vitro* (Wewer *et al.*, 1986).

4.3. Functional Significance of Matrix Reorganization

Available evidence suggests that the process of matrix remodeling in decidualization occurs by a combination of degradation of stromal fibrillar components and production of new molecules including glycosaminoglycans and components of basal lamina. Individual decidual cells appear to be sequestered within an aura of basal lamina through which protrude cell processes containing prominent secretory bodies (Wynn, 1977; Kisalus *et al.*, 1987a,b). In the intercellular spaces and channels is a loose interstitial matrix containing fibronectin, the major fibrillar collagens, proteoglycans, and glycosaminoglycans. Some of these features are shown in Fig. 8.

Further characterization of this matrix is required, since it is the substrate through which trophoblast and cells of the immune system migrate. Indeed, these cells may themselves contribute to the matrix. Fibronectin, the various collagen types, and laminin have all been shown to promote adhesion, shape change, and migration of various cell types (Aplin and Hughes, 1982), and it is likely that interstitially migrating cytotrophoblast bears cell surface receptors for several different matrix molecules. Studies of the composition and structure of decidual extracellular matrix provide no support for the idea that, in humans, trophoblastic invasion is restricted or limited by the matrix; on the contrary, many of the features of the decidual transformation might be designed to encourage trophoblast penetration. Instead, it may be necessary to examine the matrix and humoral environment of the inner myometrium to discover limits to invasion; these may be provided by the physical barrier of a denser matrix or signals that convert migrating cytotrophoblast into stationary giant cells. Such signals could be humoral or might originate in the matrix environment itself, which has been shown to be an important factor in cellular differentiation (Bissell *et al.*, 1982).

The function of the decidual pericellular basal lamina remains a matter for speculation.

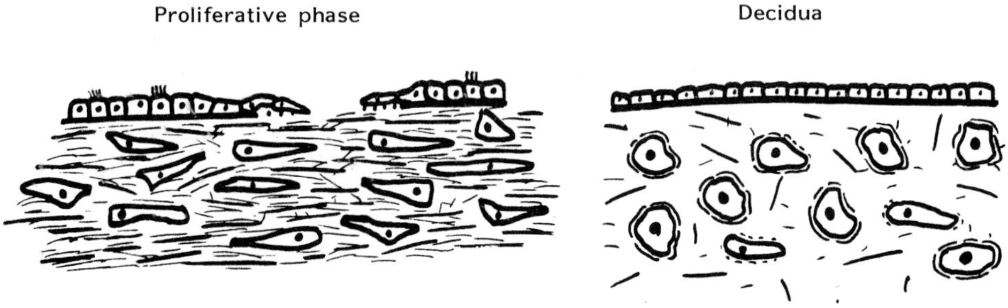

Proliferative phase   Decidua

Figure 8. A comparison of extracellular matrices in human proliferative-phase endometrium and decidua. In the proliferative phase, epithelial cells initially migrate across the denuded stroma. The basal lamina is replaced. Stromal cells produce a densely packed fibrillar extracellular matrix rich in collagens I, III, V, and VI and fibronectin. In decidua, stromal cells produce "auras" of basal lamina but also continue to manufacture interstitial components. The interfibrillar cross-linker collagen type VI is now absent, allowing the major fibrils to separate. The matrix is more hydrated. These changes might give access to migratory cell populations—bone marrow derived or trophoblast.

Given the evidence for secretion of soluble macromolecules, some of which escape from decidua into amniotic fluid (see Section 5), as well as the presence of prominent discontinuities, it is unlikely that it acts as a barrier to diffusion of solutes. It is possible that it may act to organize and tether interstitial matrix components. A specialized matrix structure may be required that is resistant to breakdown by trophoblast (Glass *et al.*, 1983). Its existence almost certainly indicates that the decidual cell population is static or nonmotile, since auras without enclosed cells are not observed. Thus, these cells may synthesize and deposit an extracellular matrix that provides a statis framework for the migratory trophoblast and bone-marrow-derived cell populations of the decidua.

5. Secretory Components

The importance of studying endometrial secretions is clear in the light of evidence that blastocyst development is influenced by the uterine milieu (Alden, 1942; Adams, 1958; Murray *et al.*, 1971; Daniel, 1972). More recent molecular studies also suggest that after implantation, the maternofetal relationship is dependent on paracrine interactions with the surrounding decidua (Bell, 1986; Bell and Smith, 1988) and that decidual products transfer into the fetal compartment.

Studies of the protein composition of uterine flushings established that changes occur during the reproductive cycle (Hirsch *et al.*, 1976; Surani, 1977; MacLaughlin *et al.*, 1986). It was pointed out, however, that the methodology in use might lead, at least in rodents, to damage of the epithelium and leaching of tissue and blood constituents (Martin, 1984). It has also been shown that, in rodents, uterine epithelial cells are active in endocytosis of macromolecules at both their apical and basal surfaces and that endocytosis is under progestational control (Parr and Parr, 1986). Evidence also exists for transcytosis from basal to apical epithelium, thus providing a mechanism whereby macromolecules from blood may gain access to the uterine lumen (Katz *et al.*, 1983; Parr and Parr, 1986). Plasma components have indeed been found in uterine flushings or luminal fluid (McLaughlin *et al.*, 1986).

With these methodological factors in mind, several groups attempted to develop experimental approaches to analyze secretory components originating in endometrium. Use of radiolabeled amino acid precursors in short-term incubations of human endometrial tissue fragments *in vitro* showed that menstrual-cycle-dependent alterations in the secretory profile occur and that changes can be induced by addition of estrogen or progesterone to the incubation medium (Strinden and Shapiro, 1983; Mulholland and Villee, 1984; Bell *et al.*, 1986a; Wheeler *et al.*, 1987; see also Maudelonde and Rochefort, 1987). On two-dimensional electrophoresis, 20–30 different proteins could be detected among the secretions in different species, including rabbit, mouse, rat, and human. Results from different laboratories cannot readily be compared if gel electrophoretic characterization is used exclusively, since different electrophoretic systems give different apparent molecular weights, so this discussion includes components of which further biochemical characterization has been attempted or for which specific antibody probes are available.

5.1. Uteroglobin

The best-characterized uterine secretory protein is uteroglobin, first identified in rabbits (Beier, 1968). The gene, of which there is one copy, has been isolated and cloned, and the amino acid sequence determined (Ponstingl *et al.*, 1978; Atger *et al.*, 1980, 1981). The protein consists of two identical subunits of 70 amino acids between which two disulfide bonds can form. The molecular weight is 15,782. Crystals have been produced of this oxidized version of uteroglobin, and the structure determined to 1.34-Å resolution (Morize *et al.*, 1987); 76% of the amino acid residues are in α helices, of which there are four per monomer. The most notable feature is the existence of a cavity (15.6 × 9 Å) between the two subunits, which probably forms the binding site for progesterone (Beato and Beier, 1978; Tancredi *et al.*, 1982). However, progesterone and its metabolites bind only to the reduced form of uteroglobin (Tancredi *et al.*, 1982), and the complexes have not yet been crystallized.

Synthesis of uteroglobin in endometrium is induced by progesterone and progestins (Beier, 1968; Bullock and Conell, 1973), which both increase the level of specific mRNA and influence posttranscriptional events so that uteroglobin production increases threefold more than the level of its mRNA (Loosfelt *et al.*, 1981; Tsai *et al.*, 1983). These effects have been reproduced in part using cultured rabbit endometrial epithelial cells (Rajkumar *et al.*, 1983a,b). The protein is detected in uterine flushings between days 3 and 8 of pregnancy (Bullock and Conell, 1973; Beier, 1976; Daniel, 1976). It is produced by nonciliated epithelial cells in which uteroglobin-containing secretory granules accumulate in apical bulges (Aumüller *et al.*, 1985). Mosaicism is evident, with some cells containing a few apical granules and others containing much greater immunoreactive deposits occupying most of the cytoplasm as visualized in the light microscope (Kirchner, 1976). Uteroglobin is also produced in other tissues including lung, prostate, and fallopian tube (Kirchner and Schroer, 1976; Muller, 1983; Aumüller *et al.*, 1985), where the hormonal dependence of expression is quite different. It has also been detected within the blastocyst (Kirchner, 1976). In addition to binding to progesterone, uteroglobin has been shown to inhibit trypsin (Beier, 1976) and to block antigenicity of blastocysts and sperm *in vitro* (Mukerjee *et al.*, 1982, 1983), but its function in the uterus is not yet clear.

5.2. *Iron-Binding Secretory Products*

Uteroferrin is a lavender-colored iron-containing basic glycoprotein secreted by pig endometrium (Chen *et al.*, 1973). Like uteroglobin, it is induced by progesterone, the rate of secretion rising to 2 g per day in midpregnancy. It accounts for 15% of the total protein secreted by the endometrium 15 days after estrus. Sodium dodecylsulfate-PAGE gives an estimated molecular weight of 35,000 with 12.5% carbohydrate by weight, including an asparagine-linked high-mannose glycan that contains the nonreducing terminal unit -man-P_i-glcNAc (Baumbach *et al.*, 1984). It has been suggested that uteroferrin may be related to the lysosomal glycoprotein enzymes that use phosphomannosyl residues as an "address" for intracellular transport from the Golgi complex (Geuze *et al.*, 1985). Uteroferrin is associated with phosphatase activity with a pH optimum of 4.9 (Schlosnagle *et al.*, 1974).

Since it is detected in allantoic fluid between days 30 and 60 of pregnancy, the function of uteroferrin may be connected with the transfer of iron across the chorioallantois. This idea is supported by experiments in which radioiodinated uteroferrin was injected into pig umbilical vein in midpregnancy. The protein is taken up rapidly by reticuloendothelial cells in the fetal liver by a mechanism that depends on binding of the uteroferrin oligosaccharide to the cell surface (Saunders *et al.*, 1985). Production of uteroferrin occurs in nonciliated cells of the glandular epithelium, where it progresses from the rough endoplasmic reticulum to the Golgi complex and then via condensing vacuoles to secretory vacuoles and into the glandular lumens. It is seen overlying placental areolae and within large absorptive chorionic epithelial cells, where it immunolocalizes to small vesicles and tubules as well as larger vacuoles (Raub *et al.*, 1985). This evidence points to a pathway of transfer of the glycoprotein from endometrial secretions to fetal blood and, presumably as a source of iron, to fetal liver.

An estrogen-stimulated secretory product of murine endometrial cells has been isolated and characterized by Teng *et al.* (1986). It is a highly basic (pI 10) glycoprotein of one polypeptide chain (70,000 molecular weight on gels) carrying asparagine-linked carbohydrate, and it is suggested that it originates in the epithelium. Antibody to the glycoprotein, which is one of the most abundant species found in uterine flushings and supernatants from labeled explant cultures, has been used to isolate cDNA from an expression library derived from uterine mRNA. The deduced amino acid sequence (with a molecular weight of 75,000 not including carbohydrate) is that of murine lactotransferrin, another member of the iron-binding family of proteins (Pentecost and Teng, 1987). Levels of the mRNA increase 300-fold after 3 days of exposure of mice to estrogen; in contrast, rat uterine tissue fails to show a response. In the human, lactotransferrin has been detected by immunohistochemical methods in secretory-phase endometrium (Tourville *et al.*, 1970). In other tissues, secretion has been reported to be under the control of hormones other than estrogen, for example, by prolactin in the mammary gland (Green and Pastewka, 1978).

5.3. Prolactin

Prolactin has been identified as a secretory product of human endometrium (Heffner *et al.*, 1986) and decidua (Riddick *et al.*, 1978) in metabolic labeling experiments using [^{35}S]methionine and [^{3}H]glucosamine with explant cultures, confirming other immunochemical and biochemical evidence for its presence in the tissue (see Healy and Hodgen, 1983; Bell, 1986). Messenger RNA and cDNA for decidual prolactin have been isolated, and the deduced amino acid sequence is identical to that of pituitary prolactin (Takahashi *et al.*, 1984). Prolactin is characteristic of late secretory endometrium, none being detectable in tissue samples obtained prior to day 22 of the normal cycle (Maslar and Riddick, 1979). Immunohistochemical studies have demonstrated prolactin in the cytoplasm of decidualized stromal cells of late-secretory-phase endometrium (Kauma and Shapiro, 1986; McRae *et al.*, 1986), although it has also been detected within glandular epithelial cells (McRae *et al.*, 1986).

The dependence of prolactin production on progesterone has been demonstrated in an endometrial organ culture system, in which prolactin secretion correlates with the onset of morphological decidualization (Daly *et al.*, 1983), and withdrawal of progesterone from late-secretory-phase cultures leads to the cessation of prolactin production (Riddick and Daly, 1982). Control of prolactin production in decidua, where cAMP inhibits synthesis and release, is clearly different from that operating in the anterior pituitary (Handwerger *et al.*, 1984, 1987). Prolactin may be produced in both a glycosylated and a nonglycosylated form, the former showing an approximate apparent molecular weight of 25,000 on SDS-PAGE (Heffner *et al.*, 1986; Lee and Markov, 1986), and a switch to lower levels of glycosylation may occur during gestation (Lee and Markov, 1986), so that quantitative measures of prolactin, including those depending on antibodies, must be evaluated in terms of the ability to detect both forms.

Prolactin is found in amniotic fluid, where its concentration is up to 100-fold greater than in maternal blood. The concentration in amniotic fluid rises to a maximum at 18 weeks of gestation, falling in later pregnancy. The detection of prolactin in fetal membranes is consistent with its originating in decidua before crossing the chorioamnion (Healy *et al.*, 1977; Frame *et al.*, 1979). Its function is presumably that of a paracrine hormone, acting either at the chorioamnion [where receptors have been found (Herington *et al.*, 1980)] or the fetus; it has been suggested that it plays a role in the control of electrolyte exchange across the amniochorion, influences synthesis of prostaglandins, and modulates surfactant production by type II pneumocytes of fetal lung (Healy and Hodgen, 1983). Evidence for the first of these functions has been obtained: patients with chronic idiopathic polyhydramnios show a reduction in binding of prolactin to the chorion laeve receptor (Healy *et al.*, 1983).

5.4. Diamine Oxidase

Diamine oxidase (DAO) has been detected in human decidua, where immunohistochemical techniques show it to be localized within the cytoplasm of stromal cells in both first-trimester and term tissue (Weisburger *et al.*, 1978; Lin *et al.*, 1978). Its status as a secretory product of decidual cells is supported by several lines of evidence, including the presence of enzyme activity in culture supernatants obtained after incubating first-trimester decidual tissue *in vitro* (Holinka and Gurpide, 1984). In pregnancy, serum levels increase progressively to a maximum at approximately 22 weeks of gestation, followed by a leveling off or slight fall in activity later in pregnancy (see Máslinski *et al.*, 1985; Bell, 1986). Diamine oxidase activity is also detectable in amniotic fluid and in chorioamnion (Southren *et al.*, 1965).

The products of deaminative oxidation of polyamines have been thought to play a role in the control of cell proliferation and immunoregulation (Máslinski *et al.*, 1985). Diamine oxidase levels are generally elevated in hypertrophic and hyperplastic tissues (Perin *et al.*, 1985). However, it is also possible that diamine oxidase functions to protect fetal tissues against endogenous histamine, putrescine, and polyamines (Máslinski *et al.*, 1985).

5.5. α_2-PEG

Several groups have independently identified a dimeric glycoprotein of subunit molecular weight 28,000 in human endometrium. It has been called α-uterine protein (AUP: Sutcliffe *et al.*, 1980a, 1982) and progestagen-associated endometrial protein (PEP: Joshi *et al.*, 1980a,b, 1981; Joshi, 1983). Recent evidence suggests similarity or identity among AUP, PEP, and the secretory endometrial glycoprotein pregnancy-associated α_2-globulin (α_2-PEG: Bell *et al.*, 1985a,b, 1986a). Both PEP and α_2-PEG are also immunologically cross-reactive with placental protein 14 (PP14: Bohn *et al.*, 1982; Bell and Bohn, 1986; Julkunen *et al.*, 1986) and chorionic α_2-microglobulin (CAG-2: Petrunin *et al.*, 1980).

The PEP was initially identified in supernatants from endometrial homogenates (Joshi *et al.*, 1980a,b) and subsequently found to rise to a concentration peak at weeks 14–15 of pregnancy (Joshi *et al.*, 1981). Immunohistochemical studies suggest that it originates in endometrial epithelial cells (Mazurkiewicz *et al.*, 1981), and both immunohistochemical and biochemical data confirm the enhanced rate of synthesis in progestin-dominated glands (Joshi *et al.*, 1980a; Mazurkiewicz *et al.*, 1981).

These results are largely consistent with the findings of Bell *et al.* (1985a,b, 1986a) on α_2-PEG, which they identified as the major labeled product secreted into culture medium by mid- and late-secretory-phase endometrial tissue in short-term (24-hr) explant culture, accounting for as much as 35% of total incorporated [^{35}S]methionine; α_2-PEG is produced in quantities two orders of magnitude greater than prolactin, which is therefore quantitatively minor (Bell *et al.*, 1987). Several isoforms of α_2-PEG are detected in isoelectric focusing with an average pI of 4.7, and some molecular weight heterogeneity is evident in SDS-PAGE (Bell *et al.*, 1985b); this may derive partly from amino acid sequence variations and partly from oligosaccharide microheterogeneity (S. C. Bell, unpublished observations). Little α_2-PEG is detected in the proliferative or early secretory phase. The main site of production has been thought (on the basis of monoclonal antibody immunohistochemistry) to be in glandular epithelial cells, which secrete α_2-PEG into luminal spaces (Bell and Smith, 1988). It is detected in uterine flushings (Bell and Doré-Green, 1987). Thus, as with prolactin, production is not simply related to progesterone concentration, and addition of progesterone to endometrial explant cultures does not affect its rate over 24 hr (Bell *et al.*, 1986a). In pregnancy, glandular epithelial cells of the decidua spongiosa continue to synthesize and secrete α_2-PEG, and during the first trimester production decreases, correlating with the morphological attenuation of the glands (Bell *et al.*, 1985b).

The related proteins α_2-PEG, PEP, AUP, and PP14 have all been detected in amniotic fluid, with maximal concentrations occurring early in the second trimester (Sutcliffe *et al.*, 1978; Joshi *et al.*, 1980c; Bohn *et al.*, 1982; Bell *et al.*, 1986b). In maternal serum, the concentration peak occurs between 5 and 10 weeks of gestation, although levels are approximately 100-fold lower than in amniotic fluid, where absolute concentrations are in the range of several tens of micrograms per milliter (Bell, 1986). No α_2-PEG is detected in fetal plasma. These temporal profiles support the notion that synthesis occurs in maternal decidual tissue, with transfer across the corioamnion required for entry into the fetal compartment. They also suggest that the function of α_2-PEG is related not to implantation but rather to placentation or embryogenesis. Any functional analysis must also take account of the presence of α_2-PEG in male seminal plasma (Bell and Patel, 1987).

N-Terminal amino acid sequences have been determined for PP14 (Huhtala *et al.*, 1987) and α_2-PEG (Bell and Smith, 1988; Bell *et al.*, 1987) and are identical in at least the first 15 positions. The sequence shows a significant similarity with horse β-lactoglobulin: 22 of the first 37 N-terminal amino acids are identical, and 14 of the remaining 15 residues result from single base-pair mutations. Lower degrees of sequence identity are found with cow, buffalo, and sheep β-lactoglobulins. β-Lactoglobulin shows significant sequence similarity with serum retinol-binding protein (Pervais and Brew, 1985) and contains a binding site for vitamin A. Structural and sequence similarities have been observed in several other proteins (Sawyer, 1987). The family probably shares a structural motif of eight strands of antiparallel β-sheet covering the binding site (Papiz *et al.*, 1986). Thus, α_2-PEG may be a human homologue of β-lactoglobulin, and the possibility exists that it may function in transporting vitamin A (or another hydrophobic effector molecule) to the fetal compartment during early gestation. The observation of abortion in maternal vitamin A deficiency (Takahashi *et al.*, 1975) is consistent with a fetal requirement for an exogenous supply of the vitamin. It has also been reported (Bolton *et al.*, 1987) that PP14 has immunosuppressive properties in the mixed lymphocyte reaction.

5.6. α_1-PEG

Bell *et al.* (1985a,b; 1986a,b) have studied a human endometrial secretory product that they have called α_1-PEG. Like α_2-PEG, it is detected in supernatants from short-term explant culture of endometrium. Its apparent approximate molecular weight is 36,000 (gel permeation) or 32,000 (SDS-PAGE), and it contains a single subunit, exhibiting more than one isoelectric point variant. The α_1-PEG production is notably elevated in late-secretory-phase supernatants, and secretion continues to increase in the first and early second trimester of pregnancy, when it appears to originate in decidualized stromal cells and represents the major secretory product.

It is immunochemically related to placental protein 12 (PP12), first described by Bohn *et al.* (Bohn and Kraus, 1980; Rosen, 1986; Bell and Bohn, 1986), and chorionic α_1-microglobulin (CAG-1) or placental-specific α_1-microglobulin (PAMG-1) (Petrunin *et al.*, 1978); thus, as expected, explants of endometrium and decidua incorporate radiolabeled precursors into secreted, immunoprecipitable PP12 (Rutanen *et al.*, 1985, 1986; Bell and Bohn, 1986). In endometrium, PP12 appears in glandular epithelium starting 4 days after ovulation (Wahlström and Seppälä, 1984) and can be induced *in vivo* and *in vitro* by progesterone. The PP12 immunostaining in midsecretory endometrium is confined to glandular epithelial cytoplasm and is not noticeable in association with the prominent secretory material appearing at this stage in gland lumens. On the basis of present information about the cellular origin of PP12/α_1-PEG, expression may switch from epithelial to stromal cells as decidual differentiation occurs. However, it is quantitatively minor in endometrium, becoming a major secretory product in the first and second trimesters of pregnancy.

The PP12/α_1-PEG is found in amniotic fluid and serum (male and both nonpregnant and pregnant female). Pregnancy serum concentrations, which reach a maximum of 120 ng/ml at 15–20 weeks of gestation, are three orders of magnitude lower than those found in amniotic fluid, where, similarly, concentrations rise to a maximum in the late second trimester and diminish slowly in the third trimester (see Bell, 1986). As with prolactin, diamine oxidase, and α_2-PEG, the data suggest transfer of α_1-PEG across the chorioamnion.

Both PP12 and α_1-PEG have been shown to bind somatomedin C, otherwise known as insulinlike growth factor 1 (IGF-1) (Koistinen et al., 1986; Bell and Smith, 1988) with high affinity (K_d 10^{-9} M). Furthermore, the N-terminal amino acid sequence of PP12 is identical with that of a somatomedin-binding protein (SmBP) isolated from amniotic fluid (Povoa et al., 1984; Koistinen et al., 1986). The SmBP and α_1-PEG also migrate similarly in SDS-PAGE (apparent approximate molecular weight 32,000). This apparent identity and the ubiquity of SmBP in body tissues (Nissley and Rechler, 1984) probably account for the detection of PP12 in other tissue locations (see Seppälä et al., 1984; Rosen, 1986; Bell and Smith, 1988). The findings also pose interesting questions regarding the function of α_1-PEG/PP12, which may be supposed to be either a carrier molecule for assisting the entry of IGF-1 into the fetal compartment or part of a system for local control of growth factor activity. It is not yet known whether decidua produces IGF-1; however, IGF-1 receptors have been detected in trophoblast (Marshall et al., 1974), an observation that raises the possibility that decidua may play a role in the paracrine control of trophoblastic proliferation by modulating the levels of free and sequestered (SmBP-bound) growth factor at the maternofetal interface.

5.7. High-Molecular-Weight Components

Many studies of uterine flushings and culture supernatants have relied on analysis by SDS-PAGE, which, especially at acrylamide concentrations in excess of 7%, is not well suited to detection of glycoprotein components with molecular weight greater than 300,000 or those showing considerable microheterogeneity of the carbohydrate prosthetic groups. (These characteristics might, by analogy with other tissues, be expected to apply to secretory mucins). However, Murray et al. (1985, 1986) noted the specific appearance of one or two high-molecular-weight protein bands in gels of uterine flushings from ovariectomized cats treated with 17β-estradiol (cat uterine protein—estrogen dependent, CUPED). They had molecular weights greater than 330,000 and disappeared in E_2-primed animals after 4 days' treatment with progesterone. The proteins could be pelleted from distilled water and then redissolved in a high-salt buffer for chromatography. They were eluted from a column of Sepharose 6B in the void volume, and this partially pure fraction was used to make an antiserum. The antiserum reacted in blots with both high-molecular-weight components. The antigens, the relationship of which is not clear, have been localized immunocytochemically to secretory granules present in endometrial epithelial cells and the uterine lumen (Murray and Verhage, 1985) and are therefore epithelial secretory products.

A menstrual-cycle-dependent sialoglycoprotein of high molecular weight has also been identified by Aplin, Seif, and co-workers (Seif et al., 1988). Mice were immunized with epithelial cell aggregates derived from endometrial glands, and a panel of monoclonal antibodies was derived and epitopes selected on the basis of variations in expression during the menstrual cycle (Aplin and Seif, 1985, 1987). One antibody, D9B1, binds to a glycoprotein that appears in endometrial epithelial cells in early secretory phase, 2 days after the LH peak (Seif et al., 1988; unpublished results). Based on immunohistochemical analysis of luminal secretions, it is largely absent in the proliferative phase, peaks after ovulation, and then declines slowly during the late secretory phase (Fig. 9). It appears to be produced in surface as well as glandular epithelial cells, including ciliated cells, which also reach a numerical maximum in the early part of the secretory phase (Masterson et al., 1975). The glycoprotein is secreted across the apical surface and into the glandular and uterine lumens, where it accumulates. It also becomes associated in many cells with the apical surface; this phenomenon has been observed in both tissue sections (Fig. 9) and cultures of endometrial epithelium (Fig. 10), where it associates with apical cilia and microvilli (Campbell et al., 1988). Production of the

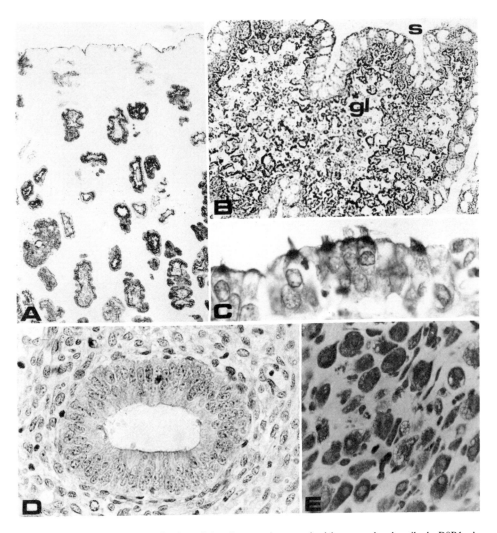

Figure 9. Immunoperoxidase localization of the glycoprotein recognized by monoclonal antibody D9B1. A: Late-secretory-phase endometrium showing antigen in gland cells and secretions and at the apical surface of luminal epithelium. Dense staining of the apical surface of glandular epithelial cells can also be discerned. The stroma is unstained. ×28. B: Detail of a gland showing cytoplasmic antigen in the epithelium and heavily stained secretions. ×350. s, Stroma; gl, gland lumen. C: Some ciliated cells carry the antigen both in association with the apical cap and in the cytoplasm. ×700. D: A typical proliferative phase gland with no staining. ×350. E: Decidual stroma of the first trimester showing antigen in cytoplasmic locations. At this stage most glands lack any cytoplasmic or luminal antigen. ×350. C, D, and E have nuclear counterstaining. Micrographs by M. Seif.

antigen by endometrial epithelial cells cultured in the absence of added hormones ceases rapidly, but some antigen persists in association with the cell surface for at least a week. Intercellular variations in expression (mosaicism) are evident in both tissue and culture (Fig. 10). In acrylamide-gradient Western blots of endometrial homogenates, D9B1 recognizes principally a high-molecular-weight component running with an apparent molecular weight in excess of 500,000, together with a minor product of approximately 400,000. Binding of the monoclonal antibody is readily abolished by treating tissue with bacterial sialidase, which suggests that sialic acid may contribute to the epitope. The subunit structure of the glycoprotein is unknown.

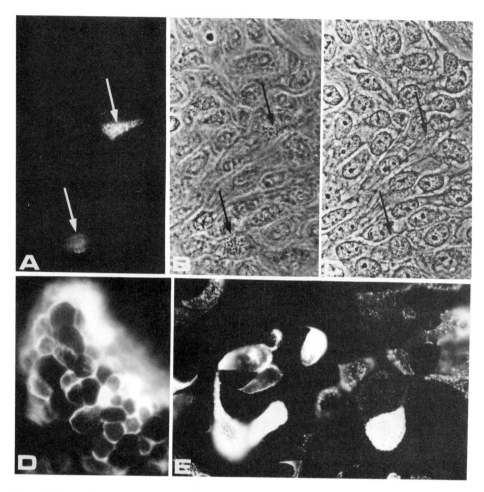

Figure 10. Immunofluorescence of the glycoprotein carrying the D9B1 epitope in proliferative- and early-secretory-phase explant cultures of endometrial epithelial cells. A: Proliferative phase. Isolated cells are positive, including ciliated cells (arrow; cf. Fig. 9C). This probably represents "carryover" from the preceding cycle. Some ciliated cells, however, are negative. B: Phase contrast in the plane of the cell apices demonstrating cilia. C: Phase contrast in the nuclear plane. D: Early-secretory-phase explant in which mosaicism is clearly demonstrated. E: Outgrowth from the same culture; mosaicism is retained (the field is confluent, and there are numerous negative cells) after 3 days in culture, but production slows in the absence of hormonal stimulation. The visible antigen is mainly cell surface associated and is retained particularly on microvilli and cilia. All ×1800. Micrographs by S. Campbell.

The antigen is also produced in decidua. By the late first trimester, it has almost disappeared from endometrial epithelium; however, production occurs in decidualizing stromal cells (Fig. 9), and it is still present at term. It can also be seen in more restricted distributions in predecidualized endometrial stroma in the late secretory phase. In Western blots, the epitope-bearing molecule appears identical to the major endometrial component. The details of hormonal control of expression remain to be elucidated, as does the function of the antigen and its role in implantation and placentation.

Another family of high-molecular-weight molecules that has been studied express the carbohydrate antigen CA125, recognized by monoclonal antibody OC125. This antigen occurs normally in certain glycoproteins of milk and amniotic fluid (Hanisch *et al.*, 1985) and is also found at the surface of various carcinoma cells (Kabawat *et al.*, 1983). Western blots of reduced amniotic fluid show two immunoreactive proteins of approximate molecular weights 240,000 and 180,000 (O'Brien *et al.*, 1986). Immunohistochemical data suggest expression of the CA125 epitope at endometrial epithelial cell surfaces at very low levels (Kabawat *et al.*, 1983); antigen can also be detected by immunoassay in endometrial and decidual cell culture supernatants (Bischof *et al.*, 1986) and in considerable amounts in decidual tissue homogenates (O'Brien *et al.*, 1986).

5.8. Other Glycoproteins

Among normal plasma proteins found in endometrium, immunoglobulin A has interesting properties. As expected, it is detected in stromal plasma cells and vascular lumens and faintly throughout the stroma. However, its expression in the endometrial epithelium as assayed by immunoperoxidase histochemistry shows a strong menstrual cycle dependency. In the proliferative and early secretory phases it is weakly detected in some gland cells and secretions, but in the midsecretory phase IgA is prominent in both glandular epithelial cells and luminal secretions. This pattern is observed in both basal and functional layers (Suzuki *et al.*, 1984).

The IgA in secretions is found in complex with a glycoprotein called secretory component, which originates in the epithelial cells and acts as a receptor for transepithelial transport. Secretory component (SC) is detectable in the glandular cells of the endometrial basalis in the proliferative and early secretory phases and more weakly in the functionalis. In the midsecretory phase intracellular staining is elevated, and SC is also found in the gland secretions, with microheterogeneity in adjacent glands (Suzuki *et al.*, 1984).

In addition to uteroglobin, two glycoprotein components of rabbit uterine flushings have been studied by Kirchner and co-workers (Thie *et al.*, 1984). Antibodies were raised to an α_2-glycoprotein and another β_2-glycoprotein, each of higher molecular weight than uteroglobin. Immunofluorescence studies demonstrate that both components are localized in the apical region of a specific ciliated epithelial cell population. The staining appears 7 days post-coitum, when the formation of syncytium is well advanced in the epithelium. This process appears specifically to exclude the positively staining ciliated cells.

Several groups have studied a family of pregnancy-related glycoproteins with structural features closely related to the protease inhibitor α_2-macroglobulin (α_2m), which is a tetramer of molecular weight about 700,000. Pregnancy zone protein (PZP; also called α_2-PAG or pregnancy-associated α_2-glycoprotein) is elevated in maternal serum. It shares extensive sequence homology with α_2-macroglobulin, and the two share common epitopes, but the native form of PZP appears to be mainly dimeric (Sottrup-Jensen *et al.*, 1984). Complexes of PZP and α_2m with proteases compete for the same fibroblast surface receptors, after which receptor-mediated endocytosis and intracellular degradation occur (Van Leuven *et al.*, 1986). Immunohistochemical studies suggest that related antigens may be produced by B lymphocytes in humans and by decidual cells in rodents, where the decidua is rich in immunoreactive products (Bell, 1979; Horne *et al.*, 1983; Panrucker *et al.*, 1983; Waites *et al.*, 1985), also known as decidualization-associated protein (DAP) or α-macrofetoprotein.

The glycoprotein pregnancy-associated plasma protein A (PAPP-A; Lin *et al.*, 1974) is also a tetramer of molecular weight $\sim$800,000, some of the structural features of which have been likened to α_2-macroglobulin (Sutcliffe *et al.*, 1980b). It has been aroused interest as a possible product of endometrium and decidua, but the most reliable data suggest production by syncytiotrophoblast (Lin and Halbert, 1976; Wahlström *et al.*, 1981; Chemnitz *et al.*, 1986). In addition to inhibiting granulocyte elastase, PAPP-A has affinity for heparin and complement component 3, suggesting that it might be a regulatory molecule involved in coagulation or complement function (Rosen, 1986).

6. Concluding Remarks

Analysis of intracellular and extracellular structural components—cytoskeleton and extracellular matrix—that are widespread in other tissues has begun to be extended to give insights into the organization of endometrium and decidua (Sections 2 and 4). The appropriate tools are also now largely available to analyze the more tissue-specific soluble secretions of endometrium (Section 5). However, the composition of the cell surface, which is so important in the process of implantation, is likely to be refractory to many current experimental approaches, since important molecules may be both tissue-specific and of low relative abundance. Thus, the further development of *in vitro* and *in vivo* models of implantation is needed so that molecular (e.g., immunochemical) probes of function may be utilized.

Table 3. Molecular Markers of Differentiative Events in Human Endometrium, Including Some Speculation Based on Observations in Other Species or Preliminary Data

	Proliferative		Mid- and mid–late secretory		First-trimester decidua	
	Epithelial	Stromal	Epithelial	Stromal	Epithelial	Stromal
Intracellular	24k heat-shock protein (gland cells)		24k heat-shock protein (luminal cells)			24k heat-shock protein
Intermediate filaments	Keratin	Vimentin	Keratin	Vimentin	Keratin	Vimentin Desmin
Extracellular matrix	Regeneration of basal lamina	Production of interstitial components (collagens I, III, V, VI, fibronectin, proteoglycans)		Reduced rate of interstitial collagen production; increased production of hyaluronic acid(?) Matrix reorganization including some breakdown (type VI collagen)		Basal lamina and interstitial matrix production and appearance of auras
Secretory products	Limited carryover of secretions from previous (nonconception) cycle		Secretory phenotype: high-molecular-weight glycoprotein, α_2-PEG, prolactin (from day 22); loss of some surface markers; appearance of new components; changes in glycosylation			Secretory phenotype: α_1-PEG, diamine oxidase, prolactin, high-molecular-weight glycoprotein
Cell surface				Further changes in glycosylation		

The phenotypic plasticity of endometrial cells is in one sense a barrier to this development, but it is also a phenomenon intimately related to tissue requirements for normal reproduction and therefore of great interest. Histologists have characterized decidualization as a process of "epithelialization" of the stroma. This term now has a partial biochemical vindication, since decidual cells have been demonstrated to produce "epithelial-type" (i.e., basement membrane) matrix macromolecules (Section 4.2). There is also limited evidence to suggest that expression of certain soluble secretory products may switch from the endometrial epithelium (and uterine lumen) in the secretory phase to the decidual stromal cell (and extracellular space) in pregnancy, thus coinciding in each case with the embryonic milieu (Table 3). Though the data re largely preliminary, these products might include prolactin (Section 5.3), α_1-PEG (Section 5.6), and the high-molecular-weight glycoprotein recognized by monoclonal antibody D9B1 (Sections 5.7; Fig. 9). There is circumstantial evidence that endometrial secretory products are important for fetal well-being; the detection of several endometrially derived components (prolactin, α_1-PEG, α_2-PEG, diamine oxidase) in amniotic fluid is consistent with the idea that human placentation has a deciduochorial as well as a hemochorial component, at least in the first trimester.

However, the phenotype of differentiated stromal cells of decidua is more correctly viewed as embodying a program of gene expression tailored for a specific set of functional requirements (Table 3). It includes production of both basement membrane and interstitial matrix macromolecules as well as the intermediate filament proteins vimentin and desmin. The latter is of particular interest since it is otherwise associated with myogenic cells. The absence from decidual cells of intermediate filament polypeptides of the keratin family, which are normally associated with epithelial cells, may be related to an absence of certain filament-associated intercellular junctional structures such as spot desmosomes and hemidesmosomes and to the absence of cell polarity.

Studies of hormone-responsive products demonstrate forcibly that similar or idential genes are controlled by quite different mechanisms in different tissue locations (for example, prolactin in pituitary and decidua; lactotransferrin in breast and endometrium; α_2-PEG in seminal plasma and endometrium; uteroglobin in lung, prostate, and endometrium). This statement also applies to different cell populations within the same tissue; for example, in early-proliferative-phase endometrium, epithelial cells engage in synthesis of basal lamina on the recently denuded stroma, whereas later in the cycle, decidualizing stromal cells produce a closely related structure. It is clear that an important task of future studies will be to unravel the molecular mechanisms responsible for the control of gene expression. However, it is the end products of the differentiative cycle that ultimately affect the process of reproduction, and the discovery of the diversity, nature, and function of products of endometrium will undoubtedly begin to influence clinical practice in forthcoming decades.

ACKNOWLEDGMENTS. I am grateful to Drs. M. W. Seif and S. Campbell for providing micrographs; to Drs. M. W. Seif, P. Brenchley, and S. Ayad for antibodies; to Dr. S. C. Bell for discussion and critical comments; and to Drs. S. R. Glasser, W. L. McGuire, and S. C. Bell for supplying data prior to publication.

7. References

Abedin, M. Z., Ayad, S., and Weiss, J. B., 1981, Type V collagen: The presence of appreciable amounts of α_3(V) chains in uterus, *Biochem. Biophys. Res. Commun.* **102**:1237–1245.

Abedin, M. Z., Ayad, S., and Weiss, J. B., 1982, Isolation and characterisation of cysteine-rich collagens from bovine placental tissues and uterus and their relationship to types IV and V collagens, *Biosci. Rep.* **2**:493–502.

Adams, C. E., 1958, Egg development in the rabbit: The influence of post-coital ligation of the uterine tube and of ovariectomy, *J. Endocrinol.* **16**:283–293.

Alden, R. H., 1942, Aspects of the egg–ovary–oviduct relationship in the albino rat. II. Egg development within the oviduct, *J. Exp. Zool.* **90**:171–175.

Anderson, T. L., and Hoffman, L. H., 1984, Alterations in epithelial glycocalyx of rabbit uteri during early pseudopregnancy and pregnancy, and following ovariectomy, *Am. J. Anat.* **171**:321–334.

Anderson, T. L., Olson, G. E., and Hoffman, L. H., 1986, Stage-specific alterations in the apical membrane glycoproteins of endometrial epithelial cells related to implantation in rabbits, *Biol. Reprod.* **34**:701–720.

Aplin, J. D., and Hughes, R. C., 1982, Complex carbohydrates of the extracellular matrix, *Biochim. Biophys. Acta* **694**:375–418.

Aplin, J. D., and Seif, M. W., 1985, Basally located epithelial cell surface component identified by a novel monoclonal antibody technique, *Exp. Cell Res.* **160**:550–555.

Aplin, J. D., and Seif, M. W., 1987, A monoclonal antibody to a cell surface determinant in human endometrial epithelium: Stage-specific expression in the menstrual cycle, *Am. J. Obstet. Gynecol.* **156**:250–255.

Aplin, J. D., Campbell, S., and Allen, T. D., 1985, The extracellular matrix of human amniotic epithelium: Ultrastructure, composition and deposition, *J. Cell Sci.* **79**:119–136.

Aplin, J. D., Charlton, A. K., and Ayad, S., 1988, An immunohistochemical study of human endometrial extracellular matrix during the menstrual cycle and first trimester of pregnancy, *Cell Tissue Res.* **253**:231–240.

Atger, M., Perricaudet, M., Toillais, P., and Milgrom, E., 1980, Bacterial cloning of the rabbit uteroglobin structural gene, *Biochem. Biophys. Res. Commun.* **93**:1082–1088.

Atger, M., Atger, P., Toillais, P., and Milgrom, E., 1981, Cloning of rabbit genomic fragments containing the uteroglobin gene, *J. Biol. Chem.* **256**:5970–5972.

Aumüller, G., Seitz, J., Heyns, W., and Kirchner, C., 1985, Ultrastructural localisation of uteroglobin immunoreactivity in rabbit lung and endometrium, and rat ventral prostate, *Histochemistry* **83**:413–417.

Ayad, S., Chambers, C. A., Shuttleworth, C. A., and Grant, M. E., 1985, Isolation from bovine elastic tissues of collagen type VI and characterisation of its form *in vivo*, *Biochem. J.* **230**:465–474.

Barlow, D. P., Green, N. M., Kurkinen, M., and Hogan, B. L. M., 1984, Sequencing of laminin B chain cDNAs reveals C-terminal regions of coiled coil alpha helix, *EMBO J.* **3**:2355–2362.

Baumbach, G. A., Saunders, P. T. K., Bazer, F. W., and Roberts, R. M., 1984, Uteroferrin has asparagine-linked high mannose-type oligosaccharides that contain mannose 6-phosphate, *Proc. Natl. Acad. Sci. U.S.A.* **81**:2985–2989.

Beato, M., and Beier, H. M., 1978, Characteristics of the purified uteroglobin-like protein from rabbit lung, *J. Reprod. Fertil.* **53**:305–314.

Beier, H. M., 1968, Uteroglobin: A hormone sensitive endometrial protein involved in blastocyst development, *Biochim. Biophys. Acta* **160**:289–291.

Beier, H. M., 1976, Uteroglobin and related biochemical changes in the reproductive tract during early pregnancy in the rabbit, *J. Reprod. Fertil. [Suppl.]* **25**:53–69.

Bell, S. C., 1979, Immunochemical identity of "decidua-associated protein" and α_2 acute phase macroglobulin in the pregnant rat, *J. Reprod. Immunol.* **1**:193–206.

Bell, S. C., 1986, Secretory endometrial and decidual proteins: Studies and clinical significance of a maternally derived group of pregnancy-associated serum proteins, *Hum. Reprod.* **1**:129–143.

Bell, S. C., and Bohn, H., 1986, Immunochemical and biochemical relationship between human pregnancy-associated secreted α_1- and α_2-globulins (α_1- and α_2-PEG) and the soluble placental proteins 12 and 14 (PP12 and PP14), *Placenta* **7**:283–294.

Bell, S. C., and Doré-Green, F., 1987, Detection and characterisation of human secretory "pregnancy-associated" endometrial α_2-globulin (α_2-PEG) in uterine luminal fluid, *J. Reprod. Immunol.* **11**:13–29.

Bell, S. C., and Patel, S. R., 1987, Immunochemical detection, physicochemical characterisation and levels of pregnancy-associated endometrial α_2-globulin (α_2-PEG) in seminal plasma of men, *J. Reprod. Fertil.* **80**:31–42.

Bell, S. C., and Smith, S., 1988, The endometrium as a paracrine organ, in: *Contemporary Obstetrics and Gynaecology*, Vol. 17, part 2 (G. V. P. Chamberlain, ed.), Butterworths, London, pp. 273–299.

Bell, S. C., Patel, S., Hales, M. W., Kirwan, P. H., and Drife, J. O., 1985a, Immunochemical detection and characterisation of pregnancy-associated endometrial α_1- and α_2-globulins secreted by human endometrium and decidua, *J. Reprod. Fertil.* **74**:261–270.

Bell, S. C., Hales, M. W., Patel, S., Kirwan, P. H., and Drife, J. O., 1985b, Protein synthesis and secretion by the human endometrium and decidua during early pregnancy, *Br. J. Obstet. Gynaecol.* **92**:793–803.

Bell, S. C., Patel, S. R., Kirwan, P. H., and Drife, J. O., 1986a, Protein synthesis and secretion by the human endometrium during the menstrual cycle and the effect of progesterone *in vitro*, *J. Reprod. Fertil.* **77**:221–231.

Bell, S. C., Hales, M. W., Patel, S. R., Kirwan, P. H., Drife, J. O., and Milford-Ward, A., 1986b, Amniotic fluid levels of secreted pregnancy-associated endometrial α_1- and α_2-globulins (α_1- and α_2-PEG), *Br. J. Obstet. Gynaecol.* **93:**909–915.

Bell, S. C., Keyte, J. W., and Waites, G. T., 1987, Pregnancy-associated endometrial α_2-globulin (α_2-PEG), the major secretory protein of the luteal phase and first trimester pregnancy endometrium, is not glycosylated prolactin but related to β-lactoglobulins, *J. Clin. Endocrinol. Metab.* **65:**1–5.

Bischof, P., Tseng, L., Brioschi, P. A., and Herrmann, W. L., 1986, Cancer antigen 125 is produced by human endometrial stromal cells, *Hum. Reprod.* **1:**423–426.

Bissell, M. J., Hall, H. G., and Parry, G., 1982, How does the extracellular matrix direct gene expression? *J. Theor. Biol.* **99:**31–68.

Blumberg, B., Mackrell, A. J., Olson, P. F., Kurkinen, M., Munson, J. M., Natzle, J. E., and Fessler, J. H., 1987, Basement membrane procollagen IV and its specialized carboxyl domain are conserved in *Drosophila,* mouse and human, *J. Biol. Chem.* **262:**5947–5950.

Bohn, H., and Kraus, W., 1980, Isolierung und Characterisierung eines neuen plazentaspezifischen Proteins (PP12), *Arch. Gynaecol.* **229:**279–291.

Bohn, H., Kraus, W., and Winckler, W., 1982, New soluble placental tissue proteins: Their isolation, characterisation, localization and quantification, *Placenta (Suppl.)* **4:**67–81.

Bolton, A. E., Pockley, A. G., Clough, K. J., Mowles, E. A., Stoker, R. J., Westwood, O. M. R., and Chapman, M. G., 1987, Identification of placental protein 14 as an immunosuppressive factor in human reproduction, *Lancet* **1:**593–595.

Bruns, R. R., Press, W., Engvall, E., Timpl, R., and Gross, J., 1986, Type VI collagen in extracellular, 100 nm periodic filaments and fibrils: Identification by immunoelectron microscopy, *J. Cell Biol.* **103:**393–404.

Bullock, D. W., and Conell, K. M., 1973, Occurrence and molecular weight of rabbit uterine "blastokinin," *Biol. Reprod.* **9:**125–132.

Bulmer, J. N., and Johnson, P. M., 1985, Antigen expression by trophoblast populations in the human placenta and their possible immunobiological relevance, *Placenta* **6:**127–140.

Bulmer, J. N., Wells, M., Bhabra, K., and Johnson, P. M., 1986, Immunohistological characterisation of endometrial gland epithelium and extravillous fetal trophoblast in third trimester human placental bed tissues, *Br. J. Obstet. Gynaecol.* **93:**823–832.

Bychkov, V., and Toto, P. D., 1986, Lectin binding to normal human endometrium, *Gynecol. Obstet. Invest.* **22:**29–33.

Campbell, S., Aplin, J. D., Seif, M. W., Richmond, S., Haynes, P., and Allen, T. D., 1988, Expression of a secretory product of microvillous and ciliated cells of the human endometrial epithelium *in vivo* and *in vitro, Hum. Reprod.* (in press).

Carlin, B., Jaffe, R., Bender, B., and Chung, A. E., 1981, Entactin, a novel basal lamina-associated sulphated glycoprotein, *J. Biol. Chem.* **256:**5209–5216.

Carson, D. D., Dutt, A., and Tang, J.-P., 1987, Glycoconjugate synthesis during early pregnancy: Hyaluronate synthesis and function, *Dev. Biol.* **120:**228–235.

Chávez, D. J., and Anderson, T. L., 1985, The glycocalyx of the mouse uterine luminal epithelium during estrus, early pregnancy and the pre-implantation period and delayed implantation. 1. Acquisition of RCA-1 binding sites during pregnancy, *Biol. Reprod.* **32:**1135–1142.

Cheah, K. S., 1985, Collagen genes and inherited connective tissue disease, *Biochem. J.* **229:**287–303.

Chegini, N., Rao, C. V., Wakim, N., and Sanfilippo, J., 1986, Binding of ^{125}I-epidermal growth factor in human uterus, *Cell Tissue Res.* **246:**543–548.

Chemnitz, J., Folkerson, J., Teisner, B., Sinosich, M. J., Tornehave, D., Westergaard, J. G., Bolton, A. E., and Grudzinskas, J. G., 1986, Comparison of different antibody preparations against PAPP-A for use in localization and immunoassay studies, *Br. J. Obstet. Bynaecol.* **93:**916–923.

Chen, T. T., Bazer, F. W., Cetorelli, J. J., Pollard, W. E., and Roberts, R. M., 1973, Purification and properties of a progesterone-induced basic glycoprotein from the uterine fluid of pigs, *J. Biol. Chem.* **248:**8560–8566.

Ciocca, D. R., Adams, D. J., Bjercke, R. J., Edwards, D. P., and McGuire, W. L., 1982, Immunohistochemical detection of an estrogen-related protein by monoclonal antibodies, *Cancer Res.* **42:**4256–4258.

Ciocca, D. R., Adams, D. J., Edwards, D. P., Bjercke, R. J., and McGuire, W. L., 1983a, Distribution of an estrogen-induced protein with a molecular weight of 24,000 in normal and malignant human tissues and cells, *Cancer Res.* **43:**1204–1210.

Ciocca, D. R., Asch, R. H., Adams, D. J., and McGuire, W. L., 1983b, Evidence for modulation of a 24k protein in human endometrium during the menstrual cycle, *J. Clin. Endocrinol. Metab.* **57:**496–499.

Cooke, P. S., Uchima, F. A., Fujii, D. K., Bern, H. A., and Cunha, G. R., 1986, Restoration of normal morphology and estrogen responsiveness in cultured vaginal and uterine epithelia transplanted with stroma, *Proc. Natl. Acad. Sci. U.S.A.* **83:**2109–2113.

Cooke, P. S., Fujii, D. K., and Cunha, G. A., 1987, Vaginal and uterine stroma maintain their inductive properties following primary culture, *In Vitro Cell Dev. Biol.* **23:**159–166.

Cornillie, F. J., Lauweryns, J. M., and Brosens, I. A., 1985, Normal human endometrium. An ultrastructural survey, *Gynecol. Obstet. Invest.* **20:**113–129.

Dallenbach-Hellweg, G., 1981, *Histopathology of the Endometrium*, 3rd ed., Springer-Verlag, Berlin.

Daly, D. C., Maslar, I. A., and Riddick, D. H., 1983, Prolactin production during *in vitro* decidualization of proliferative endometrium, *Am. J. Obstet. Gynecol.* **145:**672–678.

Daniel, J. C., 1972, Preliminary attempts to terminate pregnancy by immunological attack on uterine protein, *Experientia* **28:**700–701.

Daniel, J. C., 1976, Blastokinin and analogous proteins, *J. Reprod. Fertil. [Suppl.]* **25:**71–83.

Daya, S., Clark, D. A., Chaput, A., Devlin, C., and Jarrell, J., 1985, Suppressor cells in human decidua, *Am. J. Obstet. Gynecol.* **151:**267–270.

Denker, H.-W., 1978, The role of trophoblastic factors in implantation, in: *Novel Aspects of Reproductive Physiology* (C. H. Spilman and J. W. Wilks, eds.), Spectrum, New York, pp. 181–212.

Denker, H.-W., 1982, Proteases of the blastocyst and of the uterus, in: *Proteins and Steroids in Early Pregnancy* (H. M. Beier and P. Karlson, eds.), Springer-Verlag, Berlin, pp. 183–208.

Denker, H.-W., 1983, Basic aspects of ovoimplantation, *Obstet. Gynecol. Annu.* **12:**15–42.

DiPasquale, A., 1975, Locomotory activity of epithelial cells in culture, *Exp. Cell Res.* **94:**191–215.

Dutt, A., Tang, J.-P., and Carson, D. D., 1987, Lactosaminoglycans are involved in uterine epithelial cell adhesion *in vitro*, *Dev. Biol.* **119:**27–37.

Dziadek, M., Paulsson, M., and Timpl, R., 1985, Identification and interactive repertoire of large forms of the basement membrane protein nidogen, *EMBO J.* **4:**2513–2518.

Edwards, D. P., Adams, D. J., Savage, N., and McGuire, W. L., 1980, Estrogen induced synthesis of specific proteins in human breast cancer cells, *Biochem. Biophys. Res. Commun.* **93:**804–812.

Faber, M., Wewer, U. M., Berthelsen, J. G., Liotta, L. A., and Albrechtsen, R., 1986, Laminin production by human endometrial stromal cells relates to the cyclic and pathologic state of the endometrium, *Am. J. Pathol.* **124:**384–391.

Frame, L. T., Wiley, L., and Rogol, A. D., 1979, Indirect immunofluorescent localisation of prolactin to the cytoplasm of decidua and trophoblast cells in human placental membranes at term, *J. Clin. Endocrinol. Metab.* **49:**435–437.

Gallagher, J. T., Lyon, M., and Steward, W. P., 1986, Structure and function of heparan sulphate proteoglycans, *Biochem. J.* **236:**313–325.

Geuze, H. J., Slot, J. W., Strous, G. J. A. M., Hasilik, A., and von Figura, K., 1985, Possible pathways for lysosomal enzyme delivery, *J. Cell Biol.* **101:**2253–2262.

Glass, R. H., Aggeler, J., Spindle, A., Pedersen, R. A., and Werb, Z., 1983, Degradation of extracellular matrix by mouse trophoblast outgrowths: A model for implantation, *J. Cell Biol.* **96:**1108–1116.

Glasser, S. R., 1985, Laboratory models of implantation, in: *Reproductive Toxicology* (R. L. Dixon, ed.), Raven Press, New York, pp. 219–238.

Glasser, S. R., and Julian, J., 1986, Intermediate filament protein as a marker of uterine stromal cell decidualisation, *Biol. Reprod.* **35:**463–474.

Glasser, S. R., Lampelo, S., Munir, M. I., and Julian, J., 1987, Expression of desmin, laminin and fibronectin during *in situ* differentiation (decidualisation) of rat uterine stromal cells, *Differentiation* **35:**132–142.

Green, M. R., and Pastewka, J. V., 1978, Lactoferrin is a marker for prolactin response in mouse mammary explants, *Endocrinology* **103:**1510–1513.

Griepp, E. B., Dolan, W. J., Robbins, E. S., and Sabatini, D. D., 1983, Participation of plasma membrane proteins in formation of tight junctions by cultured epithelial cells, *J. Cell Biol.* **96:**693–702.

Grinnell, F., Head, J. R., and Hoffpanir, J., 1982, Fibronectin and cell shape *in vivo*. Studies on the endometrium during pregnancy, *J. Cell Biol.* **94:**597–606.

Guest, J. F., Elder, M. G., and White, J. O., 1986, Application of two dimensional electrophoresis to characterise hormonally sensitive proteins in the normal and abnormal uterus, *Electrophoresis* **7:**512–518.

Handwerger, S., Barry, S., and Conn, P. M., 1984, Different subcellular storage sites for decidual and pituitary-derived prolactin: Possible explanation for differences in regulation, *Mol. Cell. Endocrinol.* **37:**83–87.

Handwerger, S., Hamman, I., Costello, A., and Markoff, E., 1987, cAMP inhibits the synthesis and release of prolactin from human decidual cells, *Mol. Cell. Endocrinol.* **50:**99–106.

Hanisch, F. G., Uhlenbruck, G., Dienst, C., Stottrop, M., and Hippanf, E., 1985, Ca125 and Ca19-9: Two cancer-associated sialylsaccharide antigens on a mucus glycoprotein from human milk, *Eur. J. Biochem.* **149:**323–330.

Hanley, M. R., and Jackson, T., 1987, The *ras* gene. Transformer and transducer, *Nature* **328:**668–669.

Hassell, J. R., Kimwa, J. H., and Hascall, V. C., 1986, Proteoglycan core protein families, *Annu. Rev. Biochem.* **55:**539–567.

Hay, E. D., 1981, Extracellular matrix, *J. Cell Biol.* **91:**205s–223s.

Healy, D. L., and Hodgen, G. D., 1983, The endocrinology of human endometrium, *Obstet. Gynecol. Surv.* **38:**509–530.

Healy, D. L., Muller, H. K., and Burger, H. G., 1977, Immunofluorescence localisation of prolactin to human amnion, *Nature* **265:**642–644.

Healy, D. L., Herington, A. L., and O'Herlihy, C., 1983, Chronic polyhydramnios: Evidence for a defect in the chorion laeve receptor for lactogenic hormones, *J. Clin. Endocrinol. Metab.* **56:**520–525.

Heffner, L. J., Iddenden, D. A., and Lyttle, C. R., 1986, Electrophoretic analysis of secreted human endometrial proteins: Identification and characterisation of luteal phase products, *J. Clin. Endocrinol. Metab.* **62:**1288–1295.

Heimann, R., Rice, R. H., Gross, M. K., and Coe, E. L., 1985, Estrogen receptor expression in serially cultivated rat endometrial cells: Stimulation by forskolin and cholera toxin, *J. Cell. Physiol.* **123:**197–200.

Heinegård, D., Björne-Persson, A., Cöster, L., Franzén, A., Gardell, S., Malmström, A., Paulsson, M., Sandfalk, R., and Vogel, K., 1985, The core proteins of large and small interstitial proteoglycans from various connective tissues form distinct subgroups, *Biochem. J.* **230:**181–194.

Hembry, R. M., Murphy, G., Cawston, T. E., Dingle, J. T., and Reynolds, J. J., 1986, Characterisation of a specific antiserum for mammalian collagenase from several species: immunolocalisation of collagenase in rabbit chondrocytes and uterus, *J. Cell Sci.* **81:**105–123.

Henkel, W., and Glanville, R. W., 1982, Covalent cross-linking between molecules of collagen types I and III. The involvement of the N-terminal non-helical regions of the $\alpha 1(I)$ and $\alpha 1(III)$ chains, *Eur. J. Biochem.* **122:**205–213.

Herington, A. C., Graham, J., and Healy, D. L., 1980, The presence of lactogen receptors in human chorion laeve, *J. Clin. Endocrinol. Metab.* **51:**1466–1468.

Hewitt, K., Beer, A. E., and Grinnell, F., 1979, Disappearance of anionic sites from the surface of the rat endometrial epithelium at the time of blastocyst implantation, *Biol. Reprod.* **21:**691–707.

Hirsch, P. J., Fergusson, I. L. C., and King, R. J. B., 1976, Protein composition of human endometrium and its secretion at different stages of the menstrual cycle, *Ann. N.Y. Acad. Sci.* **286:**233–248.

Holinka, C. F., and Gurpide, E., 1984, Diamine oxidase activity in human decidua and endometrium, *Am. J. Obstet. Gynecol.* **150:**359–363.

Horne, C. H. W., Armstrong, S. S., Thomson, A. W., and Thompson, W. D., 1983, Detection of pregnancy-associated α_2-glycoprotein (α_2-PAG), an immunosuppressive agent, in IgA-producing plasma cells and in body secretions, *Clin. Exp. Immunol.* **51:**631–638.

Huhtala, M.-L., Seppälä, M., Närvänen, A., Palomäki, P., Julkunen, M., and Bohn, H., 1987, Amino acid sequence homology between human placental protein 14 and β-lactoglobulins from various species, *Endocrinology* **120:**2620–2622.

Hynes, R. O., and Yamada, K. M., 1982, Fibronectins: Multifunctional modular glycoproteins, *J. Cell Biol.* **95:**369–377.

Jansen, R. P. S., Turner, M., Johannisson, E., Landgren, B.-M., and Diczfalusy, E., 1985, Cyclic changes in human endometrial surface glycoproteins: A quantitative histochemical study, *Fertil. Steril.* **44:**85–91.

Joshi, S. G., 1983, A progestagen-associated protein of the human endometrium: Basic studies and potential clinical applications, *J. Steroid. Biochem.* **19:**751–757.

Joshi, S. G., Ebert, K. M., and Swartz, D. P., 1980a, Detection and synthesis of a progestagen-dependent protein in human endometrium, *J. Reprod. Fertil.* **59:**273–285.

Joshi, S. G., Ebert, K. M., and Smith, R. A., 1980b, Properties of the progestagen-dependent protein of the human endometrium, *J. Reprod. Fertil.* **59:**287–296.

Joshi, S. G., Smith, R. A., and Stokes, D. K., 1980c, A progestagen-dependent endometrial protein in human amniotic fluid, *J. Reprod. Fertil.* **60:**317–321.

Joshi, S. G., Bank, J. F., and Szarowski, D. H., 1981, Radioimmunoassay for a progestagen-associated protein of the human endometrium, *J. Clin. Endocrinol. Metab.* **52:**1185–1192.

Julkunen, M., Raikar, R. S., Joshi, S. G., Bohn, H., and Seppälä, M., 1986, Placental protein 14 and progestagen-dependent endometrial protein are immunologically indistinguishable, *Hum. Reprod.* **1:**7–8.

Jung, G., Helm, R. M., Carraway, C. A. C., and Carraway, K. L., 1984, Mechanism of con A-induced anchorage of the major cell surface-associated glycoproteins to the submembranous cytoskeleton in 13762 ascites mammary adenocarcinoma cells, *J. Cell Biol.* **98:**179–187.

Kabawat, W. E., Bast, R. C., Welch, W. R., Knapp, R. C., and Colvin, R. B., 1983, Immunopathologic characterization of a monoclonal antibody that recognizes common surface antigens of human ovarian tumors of serous endometrioid and clear cell types, *Am. J. Clin. Pathol.* **79**:98–104.

Katz, J., Kirsch, L., Levitz, M., Nathoo, S. A., and Seiler, S., 1983, Estrogen-stimulated uptake of plasminogen by the mouse uterus, *Endocrinology* **112**:856–861.

Kauma, S., and Shapiro, S. S., 1986, Immunoperoxidase localisation of prolactin in endometrium during normal menstrual, luteal phase defect and corrected luteal phase defect cycles, *Fertil. Steril.* **46**:37–41.

Khong, T. Y., Lane, E. B., and Robertson, W. B., 1986, An immunocytochemical study of fetal cells at the maternal–placental interface using monoclonal antibodies to keratin, vimentin and desmin, *Cell Tissue Res.* **246**:189–195.

Kirchner, C., 1976, Uteroglobin in the rabbit. I. Intracellular localisation in the oviduct, uterus and preimplantation blastocyst, *Cell Tissue Res.* **170**:415–424.

Kirchner, C., and Schroer, H. G., 1976, Uterine secretion-like proteins in the seminal plasma of the rabbit, *J. Reprod. Fertil.* **47**:325–330.

Kirk, D., and Alvarez, R. B., 1986, Morphologically stable epithelial vesicles cultured from normal human endometrium in defined media, *In Vitro Cell Dev. Biol.* **22**:604–614.

Kirk, D., and Irwin, J. C., 1980, Normal human endometrium in cell culture, *Methods Cell Biol.* **21B**:51–77.

Kirk, D., King, R. J. B., Heyes, J., Peachey, L., Hirsch, P. J., and Taylor, R. W. T., 1978, Normal human endometrium in cell culture. I. Separation and characterisation of epithelial and stromal components *in vitro*, *In Vitro* **14**:651–662.

Kisalus, L. L., Herr, J. C., and Little, C. D., 1987a, Immunolocalisation of extracellular matrix proteins and collagen synthesis in first trimester human decidua, *Anat. Rec.* **218**:402–415.

Kisalus, L. L., Nunley, W. C., and Herr, J. C., 1987b, Protein synthesis and secretion in human decidua of early pregnancy, *Biol. Reprod.* **36**:785–798.

Kleinman, D., Sharon, Y., Sarov, I., and Insler, V., 1983, Human endometrium in cell culture: A new method for culturing human endometrium as separate epithelial and stromal components, *Arch. Gynecol.* **234**:103–112.

Kleinman, H. K., Cannon, F. B., Laurie, G. W., Hassell, J. R., Aumailley, M., Terranova, V. P., Martin, G. R., and Dubois-Dalcq, M., 1985, Biological activities of laminin, *J. Cell Biochem.* **27**:317–326.

Koistinen, R., Kalkkinen, N., Huhtala, M.-L., Seppälä, M., Bohn, H., and Rutanen, E.-M., 1986, Placental protein 12 is a decidual protein that binds somatomedin and has an identical N-terminal amino acid sequence with somatomedin-binding protein from human amniotic fluid, *Endocrinology* **118**:1375–1378.

Kornblihtt, A. R., Umezawa, K., Vibe-Pedersen, K., and Baralle, F. E., 1985, Primary structure of human fibronectin: Differential splicing may generate at least 10 polypeptides from a single gene, *EMBO J.* **4**:1755–1759.

Lala, P. K., Kearns, M., Parhar, R. S., Scodrase, J., and Johnson, S., 1986, Immunological role of the cellular constituents of the decidua in the maintenance of semiallogeneic pregnancy, *Ann. N.Y. Acad. Sci.* **476**:183–205.

Lampelo, S. A., Ricketts, A. P., and Bullock, D. W., 1985, Purification of rabbit endometrial plasma membranes from receptive and non-receptive uteri, *J. Reprod. Fertil.* **75**:475–484.

Lampelo, S. A., Anderson, T. L., and Bullock, D. W., 1986, Monoclonal antibodies recognise a cell surface marker of epithelial differentiation in rabbit endometrium, *J. Reprod. Fertil.* **78**:663–672.

Laurie, G. W., Bing, J. T., Kleinman, H. K., Hassell, J. R., Aumailley, M., Martin, G. R., and Feldman, R. J., 1986, Localisation of binding sites for laminin, heparan sulphate, proteoglycans and fibronectin in basement membrane (type IV) collagen, *J. Mol. Biol.* **189**:205–216.

Ledbetter, S. R., Fisher, L. W., and Hassell, J. R., 1987, Domain structure of the basement membrane heparan sulphate proteolgycan, *Biochemistry* **26**:988–995.

Lee, D. W., and Markov, E., 1986, Synthesis and release of glycosylated prolactin by human decidua *in vitro*, *J. Clin. Endocrinol. Metab.* **62**:990–994.

Lee, M.-C., and Damjanov, I., 1985, Pregnancy-related changes in the human endometrium revealed by lectin histochemistry, *Histochemistry* **82**:275–280.

Lee, M.-C., Wu, T.-C., Wai, Y.-J., and Damjanov, I., 1983, Pregnancy-related changes in mouse oviduct and uterus revealed by differential binding of fluoresceinated lectins, *Histochemistry* **79**:365–375.

Lin, C.-W., Chapman, C. M., DeLellis, R. A., and Kirley, S., 1978, Immunofluorescent staining of histaminase (diamine oxidase) in human placenta, *J. Histochem. Cytochem.* **26**:1021–1025.

Lin, T. M., and Halbert, S. P., 1976, Placental localization of human pregnancy-associated plasma proteins, *Science* **193**:1249–1252.

Lin, T. M., Halbert, S. P., Kiefer, D., Spellacy, W. N., and Gall, S., 1974, Characterization of four human pregnancy-associated plasma proteins, *Am. J. Obstet. Gynecol.* **118**:223–236.

Lindenberg, S., Lauritsen, J. G., Nielsen, M. H., and Larsen, J. F., 1984, Isolation and culture of human endometrial cells, *Fertil. Steril.* **41:**650–652.

Linsenmayer, T. F., Fitch, J. M., Schmid, T. M., Zak, N. B., Gibney, E., Sanderson, R., and Mayne, R., 1983, Monoclonal antibodies against chicken type V collagen: Production, specificity and use for immunocytochemical localization in embryonic cornea and other organs, *J. Cell Biol.* **96:**124–132.

Loosfelt, H., Fridlansky, F., Savouret, J.-F., Atger, M., and Milgrom, E., 1981, Mechanism of action of progesterone in the rabbit endometrium. Induction of uteroglobin and its mRNA, *J. Biol. Chem.* **256:**3465–3470.

MacLaughlin, D. T., Santoro, N. F., Bauer, H. H., Lawrence, D., and Richardson, G. S., 1986, Two-dimensional gel electrophoresis of endometrial protein in human uterine fluids: Qualitative and quantitative analysis, *Biol. Reprod.* **34:**579–585.

Marchi, F., and LeBlond, C. P., 1983, Collagen biogenesis and assembly into fibrils as shown by ultrastructural and [^{3}H]proline radioautographic studies on the fibroblasts of the rat foot pad, *Am. J. Anat.* **168:**167–197.

Marshall, R. N., Underwood, L. E., Voina, S. J., Fonshee, D. B., and Van Wyke, J. J., 1974, Characterization of the insulin and somatomedin C receptors in human placental cell membranes, *J. Clin. Endocrinol. Metab.* **39:**283–289.

Martin, L., 1984, On the source of uterine "luminal fluid" proteins in the mouse, *J. Reprod. Fertil.* **71:**73–80.

Maslar, I. A., and Riddick, D. H., 1979, Prolactin production by human endometrium during the menstrual cycle, *Am. J. Obstet. Gynecol.* **135:**751–754.

Máslinski, C., Biegalski, T., Fogee, W. A., and Kitler, M. E., 1985, Diamine oxidase in developing tissues, in: *Structure and Function of Amine Oxidases* (B. Mondovi, ed.), CRC Press, Boca Raton, FL, pp. 179–186.

Masterson, R., Armstrong, E. M., and More, I. A. R., 1975, The cyclical variation in the percentage of ciliated cells in the normal human endometrium, *J. Reprod. Fertil.* **42:**537–540.

Matlin, K. S., and Simons, K., 1984, Sorting of an apical plasma membrane glycoprotein occurs before it reaches the cell surface in cultured epithelial cells, *J. Cell Sci.* **99:**2131–2139.

Maudelonde, T., and Rochefort, H., 1987, A 51k progestin-regulated protein secreted by human endometrial cells in primary culture, *J. Clin. Endocrinol. Metab.* **64:**1294–1301.

Mazurkiewicz, J. E., Bank, J. F., and Joshi, S. G., 1981, Immunocytochemical localization of a progestagen-associated endometrial protein in the human decidua, *J. Clin. Endocrinol. Metab.* **52:**1006–1008.

McRae, M. A., Newman, G. R., Walker, S. M., and Jasani, B., 1986, Immunohistochemical identification of prolactin and 24k protein in secretory phase endometrium, *Fertil. Steril.* **45:**643–648.

Misrahi, M., Atger, M., and Milgrom, E., 1987, A novel progesterone-induced messenger RNA in rabbit and human endometria. Cloning and sequence analysis of the complementary DNA, *Biochemistry* **26:**3975–3982.

Moll, R., Franke, W. W., Schiller, D. L., Geiger, B., and Krepler, R., 1982, The catalog of human cytokeratins: Patterns of expression in normal epithelia, tumors and cultured cells, *Cell* **31:**11–24.

Moll, R., Levy, R., Czernobilsky, B., Hohlweg-Majert, P., Dallenbach-Hellweg, G., and Franke, W. W., 1983, Cytokeratins of normal epithelia and some neoplasms of the female genital tract, *Lab. Invest.* **49:**599–610.

More, I. A. R., Armstrong, E. M., Larty, M., and McSeveney, D., 1974, Cyclical changes in the ultrastructure of the normal endometrial stromal cell, *Br. J. Obstet. Gynaecol.* **81:**337–347.

Moretti-Rojas, I., Fuqua, S. A. W., Montgomery, R. A., and McGuire, W. L., 1988, A cDNA for the estradiol-regulated 24k protein: Control of mRNA levels in MCF-7 cells, *Breast Cancer Res. Treat.* **11:**155–164.

Morize, I., Surcouf, E., Vaney, M. C., Epelboim, Y., Buehner, M., Fridlansky, F., Milgrom, E., and Mornon, J. P., 1987, Refinement of the L222$_1$ crystal form of oxidised uteroglobin at 1.34 Å resolution, *J. Mol. Biol.* **194:**725–741.

Morris, J. E., and Potter, S. W., 1984, A comparison of developmental changes in surface charge in mouse blastocysts and uterine epithelium using DEAE beads and dextran sulphate *in vitro*, *Dev. Biol.* **103:**190–199.

Mukherjee, A. B., Ulane, R. E., and Agrawal, A. K., 1982, Role of uteroglobin and transglutaminase in masking antigenicity of implanting rabbit embryos, *Am. J. Reprod. Immunol.* **2:**135–141.

Mukherjee, D. C., Agrawal, A. K., Marjunath, R., and Mukherjee, A. B., 1983, Suppression of epididymal sperm antigenicity in the rabbit by uteroglobin and transglutaminase *in vitro*, *Science* **219:**989–991.

Mulholland, J., and Villee, C. A., 1984, Proteins synthesized by the rat endometrium during early pregnancy, *J. Reprod. Fertil.* **72:**395–400.

Muller, B., 1983, Genital tract proteins in the male rabbit. I. Localisation of uteroglobin, *Andrologia* **15:**380–384.

Murphy, L. J., Murphy, L. C., and Friesen, H. G., 1987, Estrogen induction of N-*myc* and c-*myc* proto-oncogene expression in the rat uterus, *Endocrinology* **120:**1882–1888.

Murray, F. A., Bazer, F. W., Rundell, J. W., Vincent, C. K., Wallace, H. D., and Warnick, A. C., 1971, Developmental failure of swine embryos restricted to the oviductal environment, *J. Reprod. Fertil.* **24**:445–448.

Murray, M. K., and Verhage, H. G., 1985, The immunocytochemical localisation of a cat uterine protein that is estrogen dependent (CUPED), *Biol. Reprod.* **32**:1229–1235.

Murray, M. K., Verhage, H. G., Buhi, W. C., and Jaffe, R. C., 1985, The detection and purification of a cat uterine secretory protein that is estrogen dependent (CUPED), *Biol. Reprod.* **32**:1219–1227.

Murray, M. K., Verhage, H. G., and Jaffe, R. C., 1986, Quantification of an estrogen-dependent cat uterine protein (CUPED) in uterine flushings of estrogen- and progesterone-treated ovariectomised cats by radioimmunoassay, *Biol. Reprod.* **35**:531–536.

Nathan, C. F., 1987, Secretory products of macrophages, *J. Clin. Invest.* **79**:319–326.

Nissley, S. P., and Rechler, M. M., 1984, Insulin-like growth factors: Biosynthesis, receptors and carrier proteins, in: *Hormonal Proteins and Peptides*, Vol. XII (C. Hoa Li, ed.), Academic Press, New York, pp. 127–203.

O'Brien, T. J., Hardin, J. W., Bannon, G. A., Norris, J. S., and Quirk, J. G., 1986, CA125 antigen in human amniotic fluid and fetal membranes, *Am. J. Obstet. Gynecol.* **155**:50–55.

Oksenberg, J. R., Mor-Yosef, S., Persitz, E., Schenker, Y., Mozes, E., and Brautbar, C., 1986, Antigen-presenting cells in human decidual tissue, *Am. J. Reprod. Immunol. Microbiol.* **11**:82–88.

Owens, R. J., and Baralle, F. E., 1986, Exon structure of the collagen binding domain of human fibronectin, *FEBS Lett.* **204**:318–322.

Padykula, H., 1980, Uterine cell biology and phylogenetic considerations: An interpretation, in: *Endometrium* (F. A. Kimball, ed.), Spectrum, New York, pp. 25–42.

Panrucker, D. E., Lai, P. C. W., and Lorscheider, F. L., 1983, Distribution of acute phase α_2 macroglobulin in rat fetomaternal compartments, *Am. J. Physiol.* **245**:E138–E142.

Papiz, M. Z., Sawyer, L., Eliopoulos, E. C., North, A. C. T., Findlay, J. B. C., Sivaprasadarao, R., Jones, T. A., Newcomer, M. E., and Kraulis, P. J., 1986, The structure of β-lactoglobulin and its similarity to plasma retinol-binding proteins, *Nature* **324**:383–385.

Parakkal, P., 1969, Involvement of macrophages in collagen resorption, *J. Cell Biol.* **41**:345–354.

Parr, M. B., and Parr, E. L., 1986, Endocytosis in the rat uterine epithelium at implantation, *Ann. N.Y. Acad. Sci.* **476**:110–121.

Parr, M. B., Tung, H. N., and Parr, E. L., 1986, The ultrastructure of the rat primary decidual zone, *Am. J. Anat.* **176**:423–436.

Pentecost, B. T., and Teng, C. T., 1987, Lactotransferrin is the major estrogen inducible protein of mouse uterine secretions, *J. Biol. Chem.* **262**:10134–10139.

Perin, A., Sessa, A., and Desiderio, M. A., 1985, Diamine oxidase in regenerating and hypertrophic tissues, in: *Structure and Function of Amine Oxidases* (B. Mondovi, ed.), CRC Press, Boca Raton, FL, pp. 179–186.

Pervais, S., and Brew, K., 1985, Hology of β-lactoglobulin, serum retinol-binding protein and protein HC, *Science* **228**:335–337.

Petrunin, D. D., Gryaznova, I. M., Petrunina, Y. A., and Tatarinov, Y. S., 1978, Comparative immunochemical and physiochemical characteristics of human chorionic α_1- and α_2-microglobulins, *Bull. Exp. Biol. Med. USSR* **5**:658–661.

Petrunin, D. D., Kozljaeva, G. A., Mesrjankina, N. V., and Shevchenko, O. P., 1980, Detection of chorionic α_2-microglobulin in the endometrium in the secretory phase of the menstrual cycle and in the male sperm, *Akush. Ginekol. (Mosk.)* **3**:22–23.

Pinto da Silva, P., and Kachar, B., 1982, On tight junction structure, *Cell* **28**:441–450.

Ponstingl, H., Nieto, A., and Beato, M., 1978, Amino acid sequence of progesterone-induced rabbit uteroglobin, *Biochemistry* **17**:3908–3912.

Povoa, G., Enberg, G., Jornvall, H., and Hall, K., 1984, Isolation and characterisation of a somatomedin-binding protein from midterm human amniotic fluid, *Eur. J. Biochem.* **144**:199–204.

Prives, J., Fulton, A. B., Penman, S., Daniels, M. P., and Christian, C. N., 1982, Interaction of the cytoskeletal framework with acetylcholine receptor on the surface of embryonic muscle cells in culture, *J. Cell Biol.* **92**:231–236.

Psychoyos, A., 1986, Uterine receptivity for nidation, *Ann. N.Y. Acad. Sci.* **476**:36–42.

Rajkumar, K., Bigsby, R., Lieberman, R., and Gerschenson, L. E., 1983a, Uteroglobulin production by cultured rabbit uterine epithelial cells, *Endocrinology* **112**:1490–1498.

Rajkumar, K., Bigsby, R., Lieberman, R., and Gerschenson, L. E., 1983b, Effect of progesterone and 17β-estradiol on production of uteroglobulin by cultured rabbit uterine epithelial cells, *Endocrinology* **112**:1499–1505.

Ramachandran, G. N., and Reddi, A. H. (eds.), 1976, *Biochemistry of Collagen*, Plenum Press, New York.

Raub, T. J., Bazer, F. W., and Roberts, R. M., 1985, Localization of the iron transport glycoprotein, uteroferrin, in the porcine endometrium and placenta by using immunocolloidal gold, *Anat. Embryol.* **171:**253–258.

Rauterberg, J., Jander, R., and Troyer, D., 1986, Type VI collagen. A structural glycoprotein with a collagenous domain, in: *Frontiers of Matrix Biology,* Vol. 11 (L. Robert, ed.), S. Karger, Basel, pp. 90–109.

Ricketts, A. P., Scott, D. W., and Bullock, D. W., 1984, Radioiodinated surface proteins of separated cell types from rabbit endometrium in relation to the time of implantation, *Cell Tissue Res.* **236:**421–429.

Riddick, D. H., and Daly, D. C., 1982, Decidual prolactin production in human gestation, *Semin. Perinatol.* **6:**229–237.

Riddick, D. H., Luciano, A. A., Kusmik, W. E., and Maslar, I. P., 1978, *De novo* synthesis of prolactin by human decidua, *Life Sci.* **23:**1913–1921.

Rosen, S. W. (ed.), 1986, New placental proteins: Chemistry, physiology and clinical use, *Placenta* **7:**575–594.

Rutanen, E. M., Koistinen, R., Wahlström, T., Bohn, H., Ranta, T., and Seppälä, M., 1985, Synthesis of placental protein 12 by human decidua, *Endocrinology* **116:**1304–1309.

Rutanen, E. M., Koistinen, R., Sjoberg, J., Julkunen, M., Wahlström, T., Bohn, H., and Seppälä, M., 1986, Synthesis of placental protein 12 by human endometrium, *Endocrinology* **118:**1067–1071.

Sakurai, Y., Sullivan, M., and Yamada, Y., 1986, α_1-Type IV collagen gene evolved differently from fibrillar collagen genes, *J. Biol. Chem.* **261:**6654–6657.

Sananes, N., Weiller, S., Baulieu, E.-E., and Le Goascogne, C., 1978, *In vitro* decidualisation of rat endometrial cells, *Endocrinology* **103:**86–95.

Sasaki, M., Kato, S., Kohno, K., Martin, G. R., and Yamada, Y., 1987, Sequencing of the cDNA encoding the laminin B_1 chain reveals a multidomain protein containing cysteine-rich repeats, *Proc. Natl. Acad. Sci. U.S.A.* **84:**935–939.

Saunders, P. T. K., Renegar, R. H., Raub, T. J., Baumbach, G. A., Atkinson, P. H., Bazer, F. W., and Roberts, R. M., 1985, The carbohydrate structure of porcine uteroferrin and the role of the high mannose chains in promoting uptake by the RES cells of the fetal liver, *J. Biol. Chem.* **260:**3658–3663.

Sawyer, L., 1987, One fold among many, *Nature* **327:**659.

Schlosnagle, D. C., Bazer, F. W., Tsibris, J. C. M., and Roberts, R. M., 1974, An iron-containing phosphatase induced by progesterone in the uterine fluids, *J. Biol. Chem.* **249:**7574–7579.

Schmidt, G., Robenek, H., Harrach, B., Glössl, J., Nolte, V., Hörmann, H., Richter, H., and Kresse, H., 1987, Interaction of small dermatan sulfate proteoglycan from fibroblasts with fibronectin, *J. Cell Biol.* **104:**1683–1691.

Scott, J. E., and Haigh, M., 1985, Proteoglycan-type I collagen fibril interactions in bone and non-calcifying connective tissues, *Biosci. Rep.* **5:**71–82.

Seif, M. W., Aplin, J. D., Foden, L. J., and Tindall, V. R., 1988, A novel approach for monitoring the endometrial cycle and detecting ovulation, *Am. J. Obstet. Gynecol.* (in press).

Seppälä, M., Wahlström, T., Koskimies, A. I., Tenhunen, A., Rutanen, E. M., Koistinen, R., Huhtaniemi, I., Bohn, H., and Stenman, U.-H., 1984, Human pre-ovulatory follicular fluid, luteinized cells of hyperstimulated pre-ovulatory follicles and corpus luteum contain placental protein 12, *J. Clin. Endocrinol. Metab.* **58:**505–510.

Sheets, E. E., Tsibris, J. C. M., Cook, N. I., Virgin, S. D., DeMay, R. M., and Spellacy, W. N., 1985, *In vitro* binding of insulin and epidermal growth factor to human endometrium and endocervix, *Am. J. Obstet. Gynecol.* **133:**60–65.

Siegfried, J. M., Nelson, K. G., Martin, J. L., and Kaufman, D. G., 1984, Histochemical identification of cultured cells from human endometrium, *In Vitro* **20:**25–32.

Skorstengaard, K., Jensen, M. S., Sahl, P., Petersen, T. E., and Magnusson, S., 1986, Complete primary structure of bovine plasma fibronectin, *Eur. J. Biochem.* **161:**441–453.

Sottrup-Jensen, L., Folkerson, J., Kristensen, T., and Tack, B. F., 1984, Partial primary structure of human pregnancy zone protein: Extensive sequence homology with human α_2-macroglobulin, *Proc. Natl. Acad. Sci. U.S.A.* **81:**7353–7357.

Southren, A. L., Kobayashi, Y., Brenner, P., and Weingold, A. B., 1965, Diamine oxidase activity in human maternal and fetal plasma and tissues at parturition, *J. Appl. Physiol.* **20:**1048–1051.

Spiegel, S., Blumenthal, R., Fishman, P. H., and Handler, J. S., 1985, Gangliosides do not move from apical to basolateral plasma membrane in cultured epithelial cells, *Biochim. Biophys. Acta* **821:**310–318.

Steinert, P. M., Steven, A. C., and Roop, D. R., 1985, The molecular biology of intermediate filaments, *Cell* **42:**411–419.

Strinden, S. T., and Shapiro, S. S., 1983, Progesterone-altered secretory proteins from cultured human endometrium, *Endocrinology* **112:**862–870.

Surani, M. A. H., 1977, Qualitative and quantitative examination of the proteins of rat uterine luminal fluid during pro-oestrus and pregnancy and comparison with those of serum, *J. Reprod. Fertil.* **50**:281–287.

Sutcliffe, R. G., Brock, D. J. H., Nicholson, L. V. B., and Dunn, E., 1978, Fetal- and uterine-specific antigens in human amniotic fluid, *J. Reprod. Fertil.* **54**:86–90.

Sutcliffe, R. G., Bolton, A. E., Sharp, F., Nicholson, L. V. B., and Mackinnon, R., 1980a, Purification of human alpha uterine protein, *J. Reprod. Fertil.* **58**:435–442.

Sutcliffe, R. G., Kukulska-Langlands, B. M., Coggins, J. R., Hunter, J. B., and Gore, C. H., 1980b, Studies on human pregnancy-associated plasma protein A. Purification by affinity chromatography and structural comparison with α_2-macroglobulin, *Biochem, J.* **191**:799–809.

Sutcliffe, R. G., Joshi, S. G., Paterson, W. F., and Bank, J. F., 1982, Serological identity between human alpha uterine protein and human progestagen-dependent endometrial protein, *J. Reprod. Fertil.* **65**:207–209.

Suzuki, M., Ogawa, M., Tamada, T., Nagura, H., and Watanabe, K., 1984, Immunohistochemical localisation of secretory components and IgA in the human endometrium in relation to the menstrual cycle, *Acta Histochem. Cytochem.* **17**:223–229.

Tabibzadeh, S. S., Gerber, M. A., and Satyaswaroop, P. G., 1986, Induction of HLA-DR antigen expression in human endometrial epithelial cells *in vitro* by recombinant γ-interferon, *Am. J. Pathol.* **125**:90–96.

Takahashi, H., Nabeshima, Y., Ogata, K., and Takeuchi, S., 1984, Molecular cloning and nucleotide sequence of DNA complementary to human decidual prolactin mRNA, *J. Biochem. (Tokyo)* **95**:1491–1499.

Takahashi, Y. I., Smith, J. E., Winick, M., and Goodman, D. S., 1975, Vitamin A deficiency and fetal growth and development in the rat, *J. Nutr.* **105**:1299–1310.

Tancredi, T., Temussi, P. A., and Beato, M., 1982, Interaction of oxidised and reduced uteroglobin with progesterone, *Eur. J. Biochem.* **122**:101–104.

Tansey, T. R., and Padykula, H. A., 1978, Cellular responses to experimental inhibition of collagen degradation in the postpartum rat uterus, *Anat. Rec.* **191**:287–296.

Teng, C. T., Walker, M. P., Bhattacharyya, S. N., Klapper, D. G., DiAugustine, R. P., and McLachlan, J. A., 1986, Purification and properties of an oestrogen-stimulated mouse uterine glycoprotein, *Biochem. J.* **240**:413–422.

Thie, M., Bochskanl, R., and Kirchner, C., 1984, Purification and immunohistology of a glycoprotein secreted from the rabbit uterus before implantation, *Cell Tissue Res.* **237**:155–160.

Thie, M., Bochskanl, R., and Kirchner, C., 1986, Glycoproteins in rabbit uterus during implantation, *Histochemistry* **84**:73–79.

Tourville, D. R., Ogra, S. S., Lippes, J., and Tomasi, T. B., 1970, The human female reproductive tract: Immunohistological localization of γA, γG, γM, secretory "pieces," and lactoferrin, *Am. J. Obstet. Gynecol.* **108**:1102–1108.

Travers, M. T., and Knowler, J. T., 1987, Estrogen-induced expression of oncogenes in the immature rat uterus, *FEBS Lett.* **211**:27–30.

Trüeb, B., and Winterhalter, K., 1986, Type VI collagen is composed of a 200 kd subunit and two 140 kd subunits, *EMBO J.* **5**:2815–2819.

Tsai, M.-J., Bullock, D. W., and Woo, S. L. C., 1983, Hormonal regulation of rabbit uteroglobin gene transcription, *Endocrinology* **112**:871–876.

Van Leuven, F., Cassiman, J. J., and Van der Berghe, H., 1986, Human pregnancy zone protein and α_2-macroglobulin. High affinity binding of complexes to the same receptor on fibroblasts and characterisation by monoclonal antibodies, *J. Biol. Chem.* **261**:16622–16625.

Van Meer, G., and Simons, K., 1986, The function of tight junctions in maintaining differences in lipid composition between apical and basolateral cell surface domains of MDCK cells, *EMBO J.* **5**:1455–1464.

van Veen, H. A., and Peereboom-Stegeman, J. H. J. C., 1987, The influence of the estrous cycle on the volume density and appearance of collagen containing vacuoles in fibroblasts of the rat uterus, *Virchows Arch. [B]* **53**:23–31.

Vladimirsky, F., Chen, L., Amsterdam, A., Zur, U., and Lindner, H. R., 1977, Differentiation of decidual cells in cultures of rat endometrium, *J. Reprod. Fertil.* **49**:61–68.

Von der Mark, K., and Kühl, U., 1985, Laminin and its receptor, *Biochim. Biophys. Acta* **823**:147–181.

Wahlström, T., and Seppälä, M., 1984, PP12 is induced in the endometrium by progesterone, *Fertil. Steril.* **41**:781–784.

Wahlström, T., Teisner, B., and Folkersen, J., 1981, Tissue localisation of pregnancy-associated plasma protein A (PAPP-A) in normal placenta, *Placenta* **2**:253–258.

Waites, G. T., Udagawa, Y., Armstrong, S. S., Sewell, H. F., Bell, S. C., and Thomson, A. W., 1985, Immunohistochemical localisation of mouse α_1-pregnancy associated protein (α_1-PAP) in pregnant mice: Relationship between serum α_1-PAP levels and incidence of positive cells, *J. Reprod. Immunol.* **8**:173–185.

Weil, D., Bernard, M., Gargano, S., and Ramirez, F., 1987, The pro α_2(V) collagen gene is evolutionarily related to the major fibril-forming collagens, *Nucleic Acids Res.* **15**:181–198.

Weisburger, W. R., Mendelsohn, G., Eggleston, J. C., and Baylin, S. B., 1978, Immunohistochemical localisation of histaminase (diamine oxidase) in decidual cells of human placenta, *Lab. Invest.* **38**:703–706.

Wewer, U. M., Faber, M., Liotta, L. A., and Albrechtsen, R., 1985, Immunochemical and ultrastructural assessment of the nature of the pericellular basement membrane of human decidual cells, *Lab. Invest.* **53**:624–633.

Wewer, U. M., Damjanov, A., Weiss, J., Liotta, L. A., and Damjanov, I., 1986, Mouse endometrial stromal cells produce basement membrane components, *Differentiation* **32**:49–58.

Wheeler, C., Komm, B. S., and Lyttle, C. R., 1987, Estrogen regulation of protein synthesis in the immature rat uterus: The effects of progesterone on proteins released into the medium during *in vitro* incubations, *Endocrinology* **120**:919–923.

Whyte, A., and Allen, W. R., 1985, Equine endometrium at preimplantation stages of pregnancy has specific glycosylated regions, *Placenta* **6**:537–542.

Whyte, A., and Robson, T., 1984, Saccharides localised by fluorescent lectins on trophectoderm and endometrium prior to implantation in pigs, sheep and equids, *Placenta* **5**:533–540.

Whyte, A., Tang, C., Rutter, F., and Heap, R. B., 1987, Lectin-binding characteristics of mouse oviduct and uterus associated with pregnancy block by autologous antiprogesterone monoclonal antibody, *J. Reprod. Immunol.* **11**:209–220.

Wienke, E. C., Cavazos, F., Hall, D. G., and Lucas, F. V., 1968, Ultrastructure of the human endometrial stromal cell during the menstrual cycle, *Am. J. Obstet. Gynecol.* **102**:65–77.

Woessner, J. F., 1977, A latent form of collagenase in the involuting rat uterus and its activation by a serine proteinase, *Biochem. J.* **161**:535–543.

Wynn, R. M., 1974, Ultrastructural development of the human decidua, *Am. J. Obstet. Gynecol.* **118**:652–670.

Wynn, R. M., 1977, Histology and ultrastructure of the human endometrium, in: *Biology of the Uterus* (R. M. Wynn, ed.), Plenum Press, New York, pp. 341–376.

Yen, Y., Lee, M.-C., Salzmann, M., and Damjanov, I., 1986, Lectin binding sites on human endocervix: A comparison with secretory and proliferative endometrium, *Anat. Rec.* **215**:262–266.

Zimmerman, K. A., Yancopoulos, G. D., Collum, R. G., Smith, R. K., Kohl, N. E., Denis, K. A., Nau, M. M., Witte, O. N., Toran-Allerand, D., Gee, C. E., Minna, J. D., and Alt, F. W., 1986, Differential expression of *myc* family genes during development, *Nature* **319**:780–783.

Zorn, T. M. T., Bevilacqua, E. M. A. F., and Abrahamson, P. A., 1986, Collagen remodeling during decidualization in the mouse, *Cell Tissue Res.* **244**:443–448.

Cell Biology of the Endometrium

WENDELL W. LEAVITT

The uterus is an extremely dynamic organ the normal function of which is orchestrated by a regular procession of cellular and molecular events that occur in response to changing levels of ovarian hormones secreted during the female reproductive cycle. This is well exemplified by the human menstrual cycle as depicted in Figs. 1 and 2. The menstrual cycle is named for the one overt indication of the cyclic nature of female reproductive function, that is, the periodic discharge of blood from the vagina, which results from sloughing of the endometrium. The average menstrual cycle is 28 days in length. The first part of the cycle, the proliferative phase, is the phase when follicles grow. Ovulation occurs about midway through the cycle (day 14), and the remainder of the cycle, the secretory phase, reflects corpus luteum function.

The various events that occur during the menstrual cycle can be correlated with the pattern of ovarian and pituitary hormone secretion (Figs. 1 and 2). Ovarian function is under the control of the anterior pituitary hormones LH and FSH. The principal target of FSH in the ovary is the granulosa cell of the follicle. Early in the cycle (day 6), one follicle is selected to develop while others become atretic. This dominant follicle becomes the primary source of the rising level of estradiol during the follicular phase of the cycle. Near the middle of the cycle, an ovulatory surge of gonadotropin is triggered by the rising tide of estrogen. The LH surge causes ovulation and luteinization of follicle cells to form the corpus luteum. In a nonpregnant cycle, the corpus luteum secretes progesterone (and some estrogen) for about 2 weeks and then regresses. The regression of the corpus luteum (luteolysis) and the decline in progesterone and estrogen secretion lead to menstruation. Luteinizing hormone maintains luteal function during the menstrual cycle, but the lutein cells become refractory to LH after about 14 days (Knobil, 1980). However, if pregnancy results, human chorionic gonadotropin (hCG) is secreted and rescues the corpus luteum so that progesterone secretion is extended during early pregnancy.

Thus, cyclic mechanisms are utilized to prepare the endometrium for sperm transport as well as the nurture and implantation of the early embryo. In an infertile cycle, regressive

WENDELL W. LEAVITT ● Departments of Biochemistry and Obstetrics and Gynecology, Texas Tech University Health Sciences Center, Lubbock, Texas 79430.

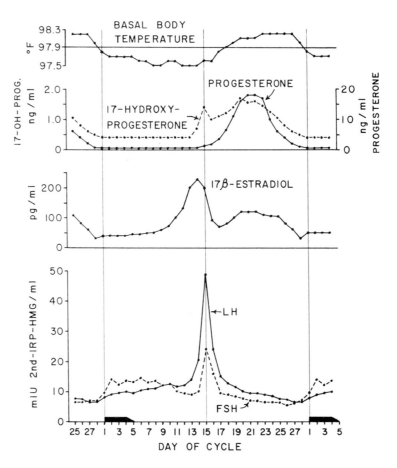

Figure 1. Representative basal body temperature and serum concentrations of gonadotropins (LH and FSH) and sex steroids (17β-estradiol, progesterone, and 17-hydroxyprogesterone) during the normal 28-day human menstrual cycle. The vertical line indicates the midcycle LH peak; shaded bars at the bottom designate the time of menses. (From Midgley *et al.*, 1973.)

changes in the uterine wall eliminate the transient endometrial tissue that was produced in preparation for a possible pregnancy. Although endometrial regression results in loss of the upper layer of tissue (functionalis), germinal cells in the basal layer are carried over into the next cycle, where they regenerate the upper layer of tissue in response to the next round of hormonal stimulation (Ferenczy, 1980; Padykula *et al.*, 1984).

The uterus is a heterogeneous organ consisting of several characteristic cell types, including luminal and glandular epithelial cells, stromal cells, fibroblasts, two or more layers of smooth muscle, and vascular elements (Bartelmez, 1957; Noyes *et al.*, 1950). The ovarian steroid hormones estrogen and progesterone cause profound changes in the growth and function of all uterine cell types, and the specific biochemical changes associated with the uterotrophic action of these hormones are of interest (Whitehead *et al.*, 1981). However, most of the studies to date have been done on the whole uterus, and the results present only a composite picture of the steroid-induced changes occurring in the different cell types. Consequently, much of the available information is of limited value because different uterine cells often respond in opposite ways to a given steroid hormone or to a combination of hormones (Finn and Martin, 1974; McCormack and Glasser, 1980; Quarmby and Korach, 1984). Thus, it is mandatory that we consider the mechanism ·of hormone action in individual cell types.

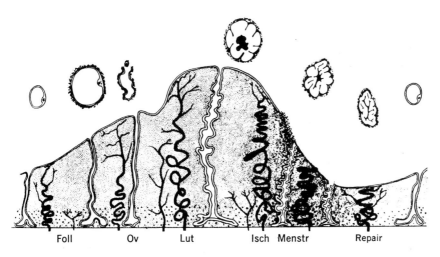

| Foll | Ov | Lut | Isch | Menstr | Repair |

Figure 2. Endometrial changes during a typical menstrual cycle with ovarian events superimposed at the top. During the follicular phase (Foll), the endometrium proliferates and thickens with elongation of uterine glands and spiral artery development. Ovulation (Ov) of the follicle shifts the steroidogenic pattern from one of estrogen domination to one of progesterone domination during the luteal phase (Lut). In the early luteal phase, there is further thickening of the endometrium, marked growth of coiled arteries, and further development of uterine glands. As luteal function diminishes at the end of the cycle, progesterone withdrawal leads to a reduction in endometrial thickness associated with loss of extracellular matrix and regressive changes in the spiral arteries, causing ischemia (Isch) and finally sloughing of the upper layer (functionalis) of the endometrium at menstruation (Menstr). (From Bartelmez, 1957.)

    The essential role of ovarian steroid hormones in the preparation of the endometrium for blastocyst implantation is well established. Estrogen and progesterone control the proliferation of luminal and glandular epithelium as well as stromal cells. The sequence and timing of steroid hormone action are important for the development of uterine sensitivity, i.e., the capacity of the endometrium to produce the implantation reaction. Uterine sensitization takes place during the first few days following ovulation, when the corpus luteum develops and secretes progesterone. During this period, the pattern of endometrial cell division is directed by hormones (Finn and Martin, 1974) and perhaps growth factors (Sirbasku and Benson, 1979), and in the mouse, for example, estrogen stimulates proliferation of luminal and glandular epithelial cells whereas progesterone controls the replication of stromal cells (Martin *et al.*, 1983). Progesterone action is essential for the development of endometrial sensitivity in all species examined, and in some species, e.g., mouse and rat, estrogen secretion is required immediately before the time of implantation in addition to progesterone. Once the rodent uterus has been programmed (sensitized) to respond, a variety of stimuli, including the blastocyst, can elicit a decidual cell reaction (DCR) when applied to the endometrium. The transformation of stromal cells into decidual cells occurs in response to either blastocyst implantation or various artificial stimuli (Shelesnyak, 1986). In contrast, the human endometrium normally shows development of decidual cells during the luteal phase of the menstrual cycle in the absence of implantation.

    The formation of new organs in the adult animal is rare. The liver is capable of new growth following partial hepatectomy, but most organs lose the ability to regenerate in the adult. The uterus of the pregnant animal presents an interesting exception to this rule in that it has the capacity to form an implantation chamber and subsequently a placenta. In this context, we are interested in learning how the ovarian steroid hormones direct the development of those uterine cells destined to form the early placenta (Kearns and Lala, 1982).

1. Mechanism of Hormone Action

1.1. General Mechanism of Hormone Action

Since hormones travel in the blood from their glands of origin to their "target" tissues, all cells are exposed to all hormones. Yet under normal circumstances, target cells respond only to their appropriate hormones. Such specificity of hormone action appears to reside in the capacity of "receptors" in the target cell to recognize the hormonal signal. We may define a hormone receptor then as a unique molecule in or on a cell that interacts with a hormone in a highly specific manner so that a characteristic response or group of responses is initiated. Receptors are now equated with sites in or on a cell that specifically bind to a hormone with a high degree of specificity and high affinity.

In producing their biological effects, hormones appear to commandeer and redirect certain of the normal regulatory processes that control cellular activities. They may do so by (1) controlling the formation or liberation of some intracellular second messenger such as cyclic adenosine monophosphate (cAMP), calcium (Ca^{2+}), or the triphosphoinositide derivatives inositol triphosphate (IP_3) and diacylglycerol (DG), (2) controlling the protein synthetic apparatus, thus causing cells to make new kinds of proteins or increased amounts of certain proteins already in production, or (3) controlling the movements of molecules across the plasma membrane, thus regulating the availability of substrates, ions, and cofactors. Clearly, these mechanisms are not mutually exclusive, and no one of them alone can account for all the actions of a given hormone (see Walker, 1983; Martin, 1987, for a detailed account of metabolic effects of hormones).

1.2. Polypeptide Hormones

Most polypeptide hormones (e.g., FSH and LH) are known to act by way of receptors located in the target cell membrane (Fig. 3). Hormone binding to the receptor activates a signal pathway that ultimately regulates a cellular process such as secretion, contraction, metabolism, or growth. This process depends on a series of proteins in the cell membrane that transduce the message to an intracellular enzyme, which forms the second messenger(s). The types of second messengers are surprisingly small, but the known messengers are capable of regulating a great variety of responses depending on the target cell involved. Two major signal pathways are now established. One employs the second messenger cAMP, and the other uses a combination of messengers including Ca^{2+} ion, IP_3, and DG. In both pathways, the receptor molecule at the cell surface communicates via a G protein (GTP-binding protein) complex with the amplifier enzyme located on the inner surface of the cell membrane. The enzyme converts highly phosphorylated precursor molecules into second messengers. For example, adenylate cyclase converts ATP to cAMP, and phospholipase C breaks down a membrane lipid phosphatidylinositol-4,5-biphosphate (PIP_2) into DG and IP_3. The liberation of the intracellular second messenger can then lead to either a direct effect of the messenger molecule or an indirect effect first triggered by activation of a specific protein kinase. The catalytic subunit of the protein kinase phosphorylates a key regulatory protein, which then mediates the response. Diacylglycerol is an activator of protein kinase C, which phosphorylates specific proteins in the cell membrane and cytoplasm, and these phosphorylated proteins may then exert specific cellular actions; IP_3 mobilizes Ca^{2+} ions from intracellular stores in the endoplasmic reticulum, and free Ca^{2+} functions as a messenger for a number of responses, such as contraction, secretion, and protein kinase activation.

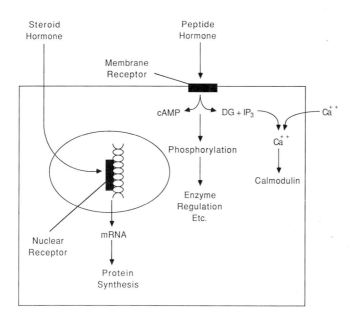

Figure 3. General mechanism of hormone action in a uterine target cell. Steroid hormones act through intra-cellular receptors located in the target cell nucleus. Polypeptide hormones act through membrane receptors on the cell surface. See text for details.

1.3. Steroid Hormones

Steroid hormones utilize a mechanism of action that is quite different from that observed with the polypeptide hormones. Steroid hormones such as estradiol and progesterone have their receptors localized to a large extent in the target cell nucleus (Fig. 3). The free steroid appears to enter the cell by diffusion, and, once it is inside the cell, steroid binding to the receptor activates the receptor protein to a form that binds tightly to DNA. Interaction of the activated hormone–receptor complex with the genome somehow stimulates gene transcription and formation of messenger RNA (mRNA) molecules, which, when translocated to the cytoplasm, are translated into proteins required for the characteristic cellular response. Thus, it appears that the steroid hormone functions to trigger the activation step that is necessary to bind the active form of the receptor protein to the responsive (acceptor) sites in the nuclear chromatin.

We shall see that it is the interaction of the activated receptor protein with nuclear acceptor sites that appears responsible for stimulating gene expression, RNA synthesis, and the formation of hormone-dependent protein species. The identity of the nuclear acceptors is not yet certain; they may be nonhistone (acid) proteins, DNA sites, or both. In addition, the details of the nuclear events regulated by the steroid–receptor complex are not yet known. Although the specific metabolic steps in the mechanism of steroid hormone action are still not clear, it is established that hormone-induced target cell responses are mediated by the stimulation of protein synthesis. Furthermore, the appearance of steroid-induced proteins is preceded by quantitative as well as qualitative changes in RNA synthesis.

Support for a primary effect of steroid hormones on nuclear gene transcription is provided by the ability of actinomycin D and other inhibitors of RNA synthesis to block hormone-induced cell responses (Segal *et al.,* 1977). Furthermore, RNA fractions obtained from the hormone-stimulated target tissue are capable of mimicking the action of the hormone when applied to hormone-deprived target tissue (Segal *et al.*, 1977). Thus, many of the cellular responses elicited by steroid hormones can be traced back to a modification of RNA metabolism. Steroid hormones are known to stimulate the formation of heterogeneous nuclear RNA, and in many cases this is followed by the increased production of ribosomal (r) RNA and often transfer (t) RNA (O'Malley and Means, 1974). The transport of these RNA species from the nucleus to the cytoplasm makes available the synthetic machinery needed for protein production. However, an increase in the amount of rRNA and tRNA does not necessarily account for the ability of steroid hormones to stimulate selectively the production of unique protein species. This aspect of steroid hormone action can be attributed to the formation of specific mRNA molecules. Recent experiments have conclusively demonstrated that the intracellular concentration of specific mRNA molecules increases coincident with or somewhat earlier than the observed fluctuations in the rate of specific protein synthesis (O'Malley *et al.*, 1979).

The avian oviduct has served as a valuable model for the elucidation of molecular events involved with ovarian steroid hormone action (Chambon *et al.*, 1984). This target organ synthesizes and secretes specific protein products in response to hormone action, and a primary effect of the hormone is to trigger transcriptional and translational processes leading to the synthesis of these secretory proteins. For example, estrogen (DES) priming of the immature chick stimulates the growth and development of the oviduct. Three oviductal cell types (ciliated, tubular gland, and goblet cells) differentiate during the first few days of estrogen exposure, and estrogen-dependent proteins, e.g., ovalbumin from tubular gland cells, appear subsequently during treatment. Protein synthesis is maintained by continued estrogen treatment and declines rapidly on estrogen withdrawal. Estrogen action is mediated by the estrogen receptor system, and the stimulation of ovalbumin synthesis appears to involve nuclear binding of receptor–hormone complex → increased number of initiation sites for RNA polymerase → enhanced RNA polymerase activity → synthesis of heterogeneous (h) RNA for ovalbumin → processing of hRNA → polysome formation → translation of mRNA → ovalbumin synthesis (O'Malley *et al.*, 1979).

Progesterone specifically induces avidin synthesis by goblet cells in the estrogen-primed chick oviduct. Biochemical studies support the concept that progesterone acts via a specific receptor system to promote selective gene action, specific mRNA production, and the *de novo* synthesis of avidin (O'Malley and Means, 1974). Schrader and O'Malley (1978) established that purified progesterone receptor preparations possess the ability to stimulate RNA initiation sites in oviduct chromatin. Oviduct progesterone receptor consists of A and B ''subunits,'' each of which binds progesterone with equal affinity and specificity. According to the Schrader and O'Malley model, the A subunit binds preferentially to DNA, whereas the B subunit has a selective affinity for nonhistone acidic proteins (AP) in the chromatin. They proposed that during hormone action the B subunit binds to AP sites, and the A subunit and its association with DNA sites may stimulate gene transcription leading to the hormonal response. According to this scheme, the B subunit acts as a ''specifier'' to direct the receptor–hormone complex to acceptor sites, which are postulated to be located proximally to the gene destined to be regulated by the A subunit (Schrader *et al.*, 1981).

The rat uterus has been used commonly for the study of molecular mechanisms attendant on estrogen action, and the concepts and views emerging from studies with this system are covered in several reviews (Segal *et al.*, 1977; Jensen, 1979; Walters, 1985). Estrogen activates a number of cellular processes leading to cell growth (RNA and protein synthesis) and cell division (DNA synthesis). There has been a tendency to emphasize one aspect (cell growth) of the uterotrophic action of estrogen at the expense of the other (cell replication). Thus, there is less known about the mitogenic effect of estrogen than about RNA and protein responses (Martin *et al.*, 1983). This can be attributed in part to the popular hypothesis that early molecular events (RNA and/or protein synthesis) were necessary for the late uterotrophic response (cell growth and hyperplasia) to estrogen action. However, evidence is lacking to support the idea that the late response is dependent on a pivotal regulatory event produced during the early response. Although a specific induced protein (IP) was identified during early stages of estrogen action, the IP turned out to be creatine kinase, and it does not appear to mediate the late response (Kaye and Reiss, 1980; Reiss and Kaye, 1981).

Much of our thinking about estrogen action in the uterus has been influenced by evidence derived from other systems. For example, the action of the steroid hormone ecdysone in insects (e.g., *Drosophila*) is known to involve an early primary response and a delayed secondary response (Alberts *et al.*, 1983). Some of the primary-response gene products (proteins) stimulate (derepress) secondary-response genes, and others shut off (repress) the primary-response genes. Temporal studies of chromosome puffing in the polytene chromosomes of *Drosophila* illustrate a characteristic pattern of puffing with time of hormone action. This has led to the concept of receptor-regulated gene networks, which mediate the primary and secondary responses that together constitute the characteristic macromolecular response of the target cell (Yamamoto, 1983).

Although early and late responses to estrogen action in the rodent uterus have been documented over the years (Segal *et al.*, 1977; Walters, 1985), they have not been reduced to the specific gene products that may be involved in regulating early and late hormone-dependent gene expression. Although we know more about estrogen action in the control of egg white protein synthesis in the chick oviduct, we know relatively little about the control of specific gene expression in the uterus. Recent studies have demonstrated that specific proteins are synthesized and secreted by the endometrium in response to steroid hormone action, and in the following sections we review the evidence for marker proteins in the uterus because these may be especially useful in unraveling the mechanism of hormone action in endometrial target cells. Evidence is accumulating that steroid hormones stimulate growth factor production (Murphy *et al.*, 1987b; Sirbasku and Benson, 1979), growth factor receptors (Mukku and Stancel, 1985), and protooncogene expression (Murphy *et al.*, 1987a) in the uterus. Further work is needed in this area to determine the role of various autocrine or paracrine growth factors and their receptors in the control of endometrial growth and development (Evans *et al.*, 1981).

1.4. Estrogen Marker Proteins

In addition to the multitude of estrogen-responsive tissue proteins including RNA polymerase, ornithine decarboxylase, induced protein (IP) (Segal *et al.*, 1977), peroxidase (Lyttle and DeSombre, 1979; Anderson *et al.*, 1984), progesterone receptor (Leavitt *et al.*, 1977), and others (Duttel *et al.*, 1986; Kneifel *et al.*, 1982; Lejeune *et al.*, 1985), specific secretory products have now been identified that may serve as markers for hormone action (DeSombre and Kuivanen, 1985). Estrogen action stimulates the synthesis and secretion of a 115,000- and a 65,000-dalton protein from the rat uterus (Komm *et al.*, 1985, 1986). Both proteins appear to be subunits of a larger protein having a molecular weight of 180,000, and this protein appears to be specific to the uterus and to be produced by epithelial cells (Lyttle *et al.*, 1987). In the rat estrous cycle, peak production occurs at estrus, and in the immature female, synthesis of the marker protein is stimulated by estrogen and inhibited by progesterone action (Lyttle *et al.*, 1987; Wheeler *et al.*, 1987). An estrogen-dependent secretory protein has been characterized for the cat (Murray *et al.*, 1985).

1.5. Progesterone Marker Proteins

1.5.1. Uteroglobin

As reviewed by Bullock *et al.* (1987), the endometrial protein uteroglobin is a major constituent of uterine fluid before implantation in the rabbit (Krishnan and Daniel, 1967;

Beier, 1968). Uteroglobin (UG) is induced by progesterone action via a selective increase in the rate of transcription of the UG gene (Muller and Beato, 1980; Shen *et al.*, 1983). Although the function of UG is not clear, it provides an excellent marker for studies of progesterone action at the molecular level (Shead *et al.*, 1981; Savouret and Milgrom, 1983; Cato and Beato, 1985). Progesterone, like other steroid hormones, is thought to act via a specific cellular receptor (Loosfelt *et al.*, 1981b, 1984, 1986). Stimulation of UG gene transcription by progesterone occurs in uterine epithelial cells (Ricketts *et al.*, 1983; Warembourg *et al.*, 1986). Uteroglobin is expressed constitutively in the lung (Savouret *et al.*, 1980), where progesterone is ineffective (Bullock, 1977) and glucocorticoids are active in this regard (Lombardero and Nieto, 1981).

The effects of estrogen on UG gene transcription need to be clarified (Suske *et. al.*, 1983). Estrogen increases the steady-state concentration of UG mRNA, as does progesterone (Loosfelt *et al.*, 1981a,b), but without a corresponding increase in UG protein. Thus, the increase in mRNA with estrogen may be a posttranscriptional phenomenon (Shen *et al.*, 1983).

Although the concentration of nuclear progesterone receptor (Rp) correlates closely with the increase in conalbumin mRNA in response to progesterone in the chick oviduct system (Mulvihill and Palmiter, 1980), such a direct relationship does not exist in the case of rabbit uteroglobin (Torkkeli, 1980). When the concentration of UG mRNA is high in early pregnancy, nuclear Rp concentration is low (Young *et al.*, 1981). The relationship between progesterone receptor and UG mRNA is reversed when estradiol exerts an antagonistic effect on UG induction by progesterone (Isomaa *et al.*, 1979; Neulen *et al.*, 1982). Continued treatment with progesterone leads to a decline in UG gene transcription (Shen *et al.*, 1983) without a loss of progesterone receptor (Rahman *et al.*, 1981; Isotalo, 1983). Thus, a cause-and-effect relationship between the progesterone receptor and the stimulation of UG gene transcription remains to be established.

A direct action of progesterone is suggested by the kinetics of induction: an increase in UG mRNA can be detected within 2 hr of progesterone treatment (Heins and Beato, 1981; Loosfelt *et al.*, 1981b). Further evidence has come from studies of the binding of progesterone receptor to defined sequences of UG DNA. Using an assay based on binding of protein–DNA complexes to nitrocellulose filters, Bailly *et al.* (1983) reported specific binding of the receptor to sequences within the promoter region (-395 to $+9$) of the UG gene. This result is similar to the finding of receptor binding in promoter regions of other steroid-regulated genes such as ovalbumin (Compton *et al.*, 1982) and chicken lysozyme (von der Ahe *et al.*, 1985). In the case of the chicken lysozyme gene, which is also stimulated by glucocorticoids, the binding site for the progesterone receptor is in the same region as that for the glucocorticoid receptor. However, these studies were done with impure receptor preparations, making it uncertain that binding to DNA in the filter assay was the result of receptor binding and not the binding of another protein. When purified progesterone receptor became available (Logeat *et al.*, 1985b), Bailly *et al.* (1986) repeated their earlier study of receptor binding to the UG promotor region and found a receptor binding site about 2.6 kb upstream from the transcription start site. This region of the UG gene had previously been reported to contain a binding site for the glucocorticoid receptor (Cato *et al.*, 1984). Overlap of binding sites for these two receptors also exists in the mouse mammary tumor virus promoter and the chicken lysozyme promoter (von der Ahe *et al.*, 1985), although the progesterone and glucocorticoid receptors have different contact points in the lysozyme promoter, only one of which is shared (von der Ahe *et al.*, 1986).

The observation that progesterone and glucocorticoid receptors both bind to regions far upstream of the UG gene is of interest. Both receptors are present in the lung and the uterus, but glucocorticoid is active in lung and progesterone in the uterus. One possible explanation for this difference in hormone sensitivity would be the existence of a regulatory factor in addition to the receptor. If this factor were tissue-specific, e.g., appearing in the uterus and not in the lung, it might account for the activity of progesterone receptor on UG expression in the uterus; the progesterone receptor would not be active in the lung where this factor was not present (Bullock *et al.,* 1987).

1.5.2. Progestin-Dependent Endometrial Protein

A hormone-dependent endometrial protein designated progesterone-dependent endometrial protein (PEP) has been isolated and characterized from human uterus (Joshi *et al.,* 1980; Joshi, 1983). The PEP is a glycoprotein (molecular weight ~47,000) that is synthesized in endometrial glands and secreted into the blood. Its synthesis increases dramatically during pregnancy as indicated by a more than 1000-fold greater PEP concentration in the decidua (Joshi, 1987). The PEP is not synthesized by the immature placenta but binds to placental cell membranes.

In normally cycling women, the serum PEP concentration increases in an exponential manner during the late luteal phase. In cycling infertile women, a direct relationship was found to exist between the serum PEP levels attained in the late luteal phase and endometrial development, the serum levels being subnormal in women with an inadequate endometrium (Joshi *et al.,* 1986).Menstrual cycles that are anovulatory or with a corpus luteum defect are associated with low luteal-phase serum PEP levels. In both pre- and postmenopausal women, serum PEP levels increase following a progestin challenge, demonstrating that PEP is indeed a progestin-dependent protein. Very low luteal-phase serum PEP levels are encountered in some women who do not conceive following *in-vitro* fertilization and embryo transfer, suggesting that endometrial inadequacy may be the cause of failure in this procedure. Serum PEP levels are markedly higher in patients who receive luteal-phase progestin support than in those with no support. In women in whom implantation occurs, serum PEP levels increase sharply within 5 days. The PEP levels peak within 4 weeks of conception. The levels remain more or less steady for 10–12 weeks post-conception and rapidly decline thereafter. The PEP has also been detected in the peritoneal fluid of women. In women with moderate to severe endometriosis, the PEP concentration in peritoneal fluid is ten-fold higher than in women with mild endometriosis or in control subjects. In some patients with primary endometrial cancer, treatment with a progestin results in a significant change in the PEP concentration in the endometrial tumor and/or the serum.

Although the role of PEP in pregnancy is not known, measurements of PEP in serum or peritoneal fluid offer a practical means to assess endometrial responses to endogenous and exogenous progesterone and progestins in infertile women, habitual aborters, patients with endometriosis, and those with endometrial hyperplasias or neoplasias (Joshi, 1987). This method is minimally invasive, quantitative, and simple enough to be used on a repetitive basis in large-scale clinical trials.

1.5.3. Other Proteins in the Human

Research on endometrial function and implantation has led to the identification of a number of proteins in the human endometrium. The names vary, depending on the investigators who conducted the research and the tissue used for the isolation of a given protein (Table 1).

Evidence for endometrial synthesis and/or secretion has been obtained for prolactin (Heffner *et al.,* 1986), diamine oxidase, alkaline phosphatase, placental protein 12 (PP12), placental protein 14 (PP14), progesterone-dependent endometrial protein (PEP), and 17 endometrial proteins designated as EP1–17. Of the latter, over 60% of radiolabeled [35S]methionine is incorporated by decidua into EP14 and EP15 or α_1-PEG and α_2-PEG *in vitro.*

In addition, many other proteins have been isolated from the endometrium. These include α-uterine protein (AUP), chorionic α_2-microglobulin (CAG-2), pregnancy-associated plasma

Table 1. Proteins Detected in the Human Endometrium

Abbreviation[a]	Full name	Reference(s)
PRL	Prolactin	Bell, 1986
DAO	Diamine oxidase	Bell, 1986
	Alkaline phosphatase	Bell, 1986
PP12*	Placental protein 12	Rutanen *et al.*, 1986
		Seppala *et al.*, 1985
		Koistinen *et al.*, 1986
EP14*	Endometrial protein 14	Bell, 1986
α_1-PEG*	α_1-Pregnancy associated endometrial protein	Bell, 1986
IGF-bp*	34K IGF-binding protein	Koistinen *et al.*, 1986
PEP**	Progestagen-dependent endometrial protein	Joshi *et al.*, 1980
PP14**	Placental protein 14	Julkunen *et al.*, 1986a,b,c
EP15**	Endometrial protein 15	Bell, 1986
AUP**	Alpha uterine protein	Bell, 1986
CAG-2**	Chrionic α_2-microglobulin	Bell, 1986
α_2-PEG**	α_2-Pregnancy-associated endometrial globulin	Bell, 1986
	β-Lactoglobulin homologue**	Huhtala *et al.*, 1986
PAPP-A	Pregnancy-associated plasma protein-A	Sjoberg *et al.*, 1984
PP5	Placental protein 5	Butzow *et al.*, 1986
EP1–17	Endometrial proteins 1–17	Bell, 1986
17-HSD	17β-Hydroxysteroid dehydrogenase	Tseng and Gurpide, 1975, 1979

[a]Asterisks indicate names likely to be synonyms.

protein-A (PAPP-A), placental protein 5 (PP5), placental protein 10 (PP10), and a number of other proteins (Strinden and Shapiro, 1983).

Comparative studies indicate that there are close similarities among some of the proteins. Thus, PP12, EP14, and α_1-PEG are closely related to one another (Bell, 1986), and so are PP14, EP15, α_2-PEG, CAG-2, PEP, and AUP (Bell, 1986; Julkunen *et al.*, 1986a). Many of the proteins appear in other tissues as well: PP12 has been found in the syncytiotrophoblast, follicular fluid, luteinized granulosa cells, fallopian tube, fetal liver, hyperplastic nodules of cirrhosis, and hepatoma cells (Rutanen *et al.*, 1986; Seppala *et al.*, 1985), and PP14 in the placenta, follicular fluid, fallopian tube, seminal plasma, and seminal vesicles (Seppala *et al.*, 1985; Julkunen *et al.*, 1986b). Those that are significantly produced and secreted by decidualized endometrium (e.g., PP12 and PP14) appear in high concentrations in amniotic fluid. However, amniotic fluid levels of PP5, PP10, and PAPP-A are low, suggesting that they are not major secretory endometrial proteins.

The N-terminal amino acid sequence of PP12 appears identical with the 34K somatomedin-binding protein of the human amniotic fluid, and PP12 binds somatomedin or insulinlike growth factor 1 (IGF-I) (Koistinen *et al.*, 1986). Thus, PP12 is the 34K IGF-binding protein (IGF-bp). The N-terminal sequence of PP14 indicates homology to β-lactoglobulin of various species (Huhtala *et al.*, 1987) but not to uteroglobin (Huhtala *et al.*, 1986). Lactoglobulins are produced by the mammary gland and are usually found in species that transfer immunoglobulins via colostrum to their young. Therefore, it is not surprising that PP14 occurs in human milk. Experiments on the incorporation of labeled [^{35}S]methionine into both IGF-bp and β-lactoglobulin substantiate the synthesis of these proteins by the endometrium *in vitro*. However, their occurrence in other tissues clearly indicates that they are not specific for the endometrium. Therefore, it would seem appropriate to name them according to biological action or function rather than after an odd physicochemical property or one of the multiple sites of synthesis. Examples of the recommended type of nomenclature are endometrial prolactin, endometrial diamine oxidase, and endometrial IGF-bp (Seppala *et al.*, 1987).

The importance of any of the endometrial proteins for implantation has not yet been clarified. The endometrial tissue concentration of IGF-bp rises sharply after ovulation, and progesterone stimulates the endometrial synthesis of IGF-bp (Rutanen *et al.*, 1986). In women participating in an *in-vitro* fertilization program whose cycles are stimulated with clomiphene and hMG, both IGF-bp and β-lactoglobulin are found in the endometrium at the time of expected embryo transfer. In a normal ovulatory cycle, the endometrial tissue concentration of β-lactoglobulin rises slowly, and so do its circulating levels, which remain high for the first days of the next cycle (Julkunen *et al.*, 1986a). Because tissue concentrations of both IGF-bp and β-lactoglobulin are related to the action of progesterone, they may serve as useful indicators of endometrial protein synthesis during normal and abnormal progesterone secretion in an aging uterus and during treatment with various progestagens.

Human uterine luminal fluid contains over two dozen proteins distinct from those of serum as detected by two-dimensional gel electrophoresis and silver staining of the proteins (MacLaughlin *et al.*, 1986). Most of these uterine fluid proteins can be detected *in vitro* by radiolabeled methionine incorporation studies, and the majority of these products are epithelial in origin (MacLaughlin *et al.*, 1986), but some are produced by decidual cells as well (Daly *et al.*, 1983). The major recognizable menstrual cycle phase-dependent change in the protein pattern in two-dimensional gels was the appearance of a protein group (number 27) of approximately 25,000 molecular weight and pI of 5.8–6.3 (MacLaughlin *et al.*, 1987). This group of proteins was found in nearly all mid- and all late-secretory-phase fluids or culture media and in none obtained earlier in the cycle. As yet, it is not known which of these proteins are induced by estrogen and which by progestin action (Bell *et al.*, 1986). However, protein group 27 appears to be different from other proteins produced by human endometrium, such as PEP (Joshi, 1987) and secretory component (Sullivan *et al.*, 1984). The human decidua is an active secretory tissue, producing prolactin (Daly *et al.*, 1983; Hoehner-Celniker *et al.*, 1984), PAPP-A, PP12 (see Table 1), and several other as yet unidentified products (Kisalus *et al.*, 1987).

1.5.4. Other Species

A progesterone-dependent secretory protein has been characterized from the cat endometrium (Boomsma and Verhage, 1987), and it has a molecular mass of 30,000 daltons and isoelectric point of 6.5–7.0 on two-dimensional gel electrophoresis.

The uterus of the pig secretes large amounts of protein in response to progesterone (Roberts *et al.*, 1986, 1987). Estrogen alone has little effect but in combination with progesterone is synergistic at low doses and inhibitory at high doses. The responses of the uterus to progesterone action are delayed and require prolonged hormone treatment. The proteins secreted by the uteri of most species are believed to play some role in the nutritional and developmental support of the conceptus, particularly during early pregnancy. Such a role is likely to be of greater importance in species such as the pig, which has noninvasive epitheliochorial placentation. Of the uterine secretions of the pig, the best-characterized is uteroferrin, a purple-colored iron-containing acid phosphatase that functions to transport iron across the placenta. Three polypeptides associated with uteroferrin are immunologically related to one another and appear to have arisen from a single precursor polypeptide. Their function is unknown. A family of plasmin/trypsin inhibitors that show sequence homology with bovine pancreatic trypsin inhibitor (aprotinin) has been characterized and appears to control intrauterine proteolytic events initiated by the conceptuses. Several other proteins are secreted in response to progesterone, but these remain to be characterized further.

Recent evidence indicates that the sheep embryo secretes a protein called ovine trophoblast protein-1 (oTP-1), which, through an antiluteolytic mechanism mediated by the uterus, allows establishment of pregnancy in the ewe (Bazer *et al.*, 1987). Of interest is the fact that oTP-1 (M_r 16,000, pI 5.5) is structurally similar to α-interferon and thus may act as a local immune modulator in pregnancy (Imakawa *et al.*, 1987).

1.5.5. Decidualization Marker Proteins

In addition to the decidual markers produced by the human, a 43,000-dalton protein appears to be produced and secreted by decidual tissue in the rat (Jacobs and Lyttle, 1987), but the role of this protein is not known at present. Also, there is evidence of embryo–uterine interaction in the proteins produced at the time of implantation in the rat (Surani, 1975, 1976, 1977) and the mouse (Nieder *et al.*, 1987). Mouse decidual cells synthesize a basement-membrane type of extracellular matrix consisting of laminin, entactin, fibronectin, type IV collagen, and heparan sulfate proteoglycan (Wewer *et al.*, 1986). In the rat, the intermediate-filament proteins vimentin and desmin are produced by decidualizing stromal cells, and desmin production may serve as a useful marker of decidualization in the rat (Glasser and Julian, 1986).

Implantation of the blastocyst in the wall of the sensitized uterus leads to proliferation of the underlying endometrial stromal cells to form the decidua (Finn and Martin, 1974). The decidual cell reaction can be induced experimentally to form ''deciduoma'' in the absence of a fertilized ovum by traumatization of the endometrium during the sensitive period (Shelesnyak, 1986). A unique feature of the deciduomal reaction in the rodent uterus is that progesterone is required for the initial stromal cell response and for the maintenance of the proliferated state of the endometrium (Astwood, 1939). Thus, the artificially decidualized hamster uterus is an ideal model system for studying the biochemical changes and alterations in specific gene expression during proliferation and differentiation of a progesterone-dominated tissue independent of estrogen action (Leavitt *et al.*, 1986).

Decidualization of the rodent uterus is a classic response to progesterone action (Astwood, 1939), and in the hamster, decidual cell growth and differentiation are absolutely dependent on progesterone (Harper, 1970; Blaha and Leavitt, 1978). Multiple progesterone-dependent changes occur in the synthesis of nuclear and cytosolic proteins in the hamster deciduoma (MacDonald *et al.*, 1983a), and there is evidence for specific alterations in endometrial protein composition during deciduomal morphogenesis (Bell, 1979; Denari *et al.*, 1976; Leavitt *et al.*, 1985a; Lejeune *et al.*, 1982; Umapathysivam and Jones, 1978). Presumably, hormone action is mediated by the progesterone receptor system present in hamster decidual tissue, and the estrogen receptor system is down-regulated during decidualization (Leavitt *et al.*, 1986). Our studies suggest that progesterone action in the decidualized uterus differs somewhat from that in the chick oviduct. In the latter model system, progesterone effects on specific gene expression are largely dependent on estrogen-induced cytodifferentiation and growth of the oviduct (O'Malley and Means, 1974). In contrast, growth and differentiation of the decidualized hamster uterus depend primarily on progesterone, which controls this process through bidirectional changes in uterine gene expression (MacDonald *et al.*, 1983a). Alterations occur in the protein composition of deciduomal tissue during differentiation, and these proteins can serve as markers of decidualization and be used to study decidual cells under conditions of cell culture. Attempts to study decidualization *in vitro* were limited to morphological and ultrastructural descriptions (Bell and Searle, 1981; Sananes *et al.*, 1978; Vladirmirsky *et al.*, 1977), but we have identified 11 nuclear and five cytosolic deciduomal proteins that can serve as specific indicators of the differentiated state of the decidual cell (Leavitt *et al.*, 1985a).

As part of our ongoing studies of decidual cell function, we became interested in the possibility that decidual cells may produce marker proteins that can be detected in the blood. Several serum proteins increase in titer during pregnancy (Hau, 1986, Seal and Doe, 1965), but the role of the decidua in the production of pregnancy proteins is not clear. Therefore, we have tested the hypothesis that decidual cells either secrete or signal the production of certain serum proteins in the hamster. Measurement of serum CBG by equilibrium binding using either [³H]progesterone or [³H]cortisol in conjunction with ion-exchange chromatography showed that decidualization increased serum CBG levels. Two-dimensional gel electrophoresis (O'Farrell, 1975) revealed that a 60,000-dalton protein increases markedly in the serum of the pseudopregnant (PSP) hamster soon after artificial induction of decidualization on PSP day 4 (Fig. 4). The 60-kilodalton (kDa) serum protein remains low in nondecidualized PSP, cyclic, or ovariectomized–estrogen/progesterone-primed animals, but it increases in the pregnant animal.

A photoaffinity labeling procedure was used to bind covalently [³H]androsta-4, 6-diene-17β-olone to CBG (Gray *et al.*, 1987). Fluorography of two-dimensional gels run under denaturing conditions established that the 60-kDa protein did not bind steroid as did CBG (69 kDa). To determine whether decidual cells could induce the 60-kDa and CBG proteins, different numbers of decidual cells were injected intraperitoneally into PSP recipients. A single injection of 50×10^6 cells induced both serum proteins within 48 hr, whereas the same number of fetal fibroblasts was ineffective (Leavitt *et al.*, 1987). Thus, these results demonstrate that hamster decidual cells induce a 60-kDa protein of unknown function and serum CBG. Since the decidual cell itself does not appear to be the source of either protein, it follows that decidual cells signal the synthesis and secretion of these proteins elsewhere in the body, most likely in the liver.

Since the liver is known to produce CBG (Weiser *et al.*, 1979; Khan *et al.*, 1984), we isolated hepatocytes from pregnant and nonpregnant hamsters and labeled liver proteins with [³⁵S]methionine in a manner similar to that used with decidual cells. Of considerable interest

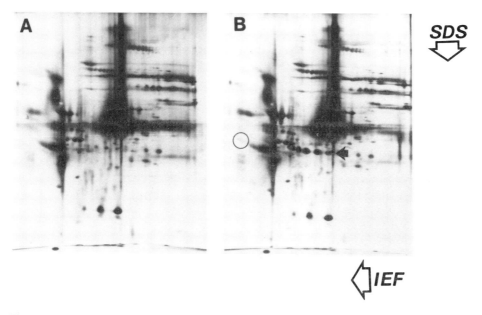

Figure 4. Two-dimensional gel analysis of serum proteins in nondecidualized (A) and decidualized (B) animals on PSP day 8. Decidualization was induced on day 4. Gels were prepared using pH 3.5–10 ampholytes in the IEF dimension and 10% polyacrylamide in the second dimension (SDS). Proteins were stained with the Gelcode system. The position of CBG (M_r 69,000, pI 4) is shown by the circle, and the 60-kDa protein (five spots with pI 5.6–6.1) is identified by the arrow in panel B.

was the finding that hepatocytes from the pregnant animal secreted significantly greater amounts of labeled CBG and the 60-kDa protein than did hepatocytes from the nonpregnant hamster (Fig. 5). Similar results were obtained in comparing hepatocytes from decidualized and nondecidualized PSP animals. These findings indicate that the liver is the principal source of the CBG and 60-kDa proteins that increase in response to decidualization of the hamster uterus. Furthermore, decidual cells appear to produce a signal that stimulates the liver to synthesize and secrete CBG and the 60-kDa protein. To our knowledge, this is the first demonstration that the decidual cell regulates serum CBG and other proteins in this manner. More importantly, these and other results suggest that an endocrine feedback relationship may exist between the decidual cell (maternal portion of the placenta) and hepatocyte (liver) in early pregnancy. Thus, the two liver proteins, CBG and 60-kDa protein, may act back at the decidual cell or elsewhere in the body during gestation in the hamster (Fig. 6).

We have begun to examine the possibility of feedback of CBG on decidual tissue. To prove a feedback role for CBG, it must first be established that CBG occurs in decidual tissue. We have studied the occurrence of CBG in the cytosol and nuclear and membrane fractions of different tissues during decidualization in the hamster (Selcer and Leavitt, 1987). In all tissues, the cytosol fraction contained considerably more CBG than did the nuclear and membrane fractions. Cytosol CBG was highest in deciduoma and myometrium, half as high in liver and kidney, and one-fifth as high in muscle and small intestine. Serum CBG increased seven-fold from day 4 to day 9 in the decidualized hamster but not in the nondecidualized, sham-operated hamster. In all tissues, serum CBG is correlated with cytosol CBG, but the high levels of CBG in uterine tissues do not appear to be explained by serum contamination because whole-body perfusion with buffered saline fails to remove the majority of cytosol CBG. The CBG content of deciduoma and myometrium exceeds that of the other tissues examined, and all three

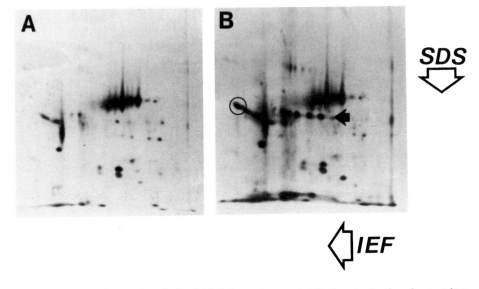

Figure 5. Two-dimensional gel analysis of labeled proteins secreted by hepatocytes in primary culture. Hepatocytes were isolated from nonpregnant (proestrus) and pregnant (day 14) hamsters, plated in 60-mm culture dishes coated with Cell-Tak, and grown in defined medium for 24 hr. Labeling was with [^{35}S]methionine. Equal volumes of medium (100 μl) were loaded on each gel. However, incorporation of labeled methionine into TCA-precipitable protein was greater in panel B (pregnant) than in panel A (nonpregnant). The positions of CBG (circle) and 60-kDa protein (arrow) are shown in panel B.

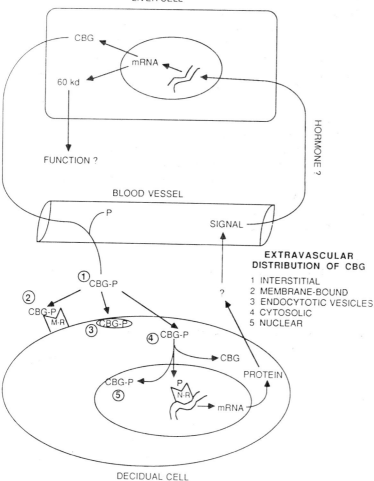

Figure 6. Proposed decidua–hepatic endocrine axis. In this model, the decidual cell produces a signal (hormone) that stimulates the hepatocyte to synthesize and secrete CBG and 60-kDa protein. The CBG has a potential feedback action at the level of the decidual cell either at membrane sites or within the cell, perhaps to deliver steroid (P) to intracellular receptors. A function for the 60-kDa protein is not yet established.

subcellular fractions of these uterine tissues contain CBG. However, the cytosol fraction accounts for over 99% of the CBG detected in the uterus.

These results confirm and extend our earlier study of progesterone-binding components in decidualized hamster uterus (Do and Leavitt, 1978). Two distinct progesterone-binding proteins are present in uterine cytosol. Component 1 has the properties expected of a progesterone receptor (hormonal binding specificity, low capacity, and heat lability), whereas component 2 is a CBG-like binder (binding affinity for cortisol and progesterone, high capacity, and heat stability). On the basis of this evidence, a model of progesterone action was proposed (Leavitt *et al.*, 1978) in which progesterone leaves the vascular space bound to component 2 (CBG). Thus, the extravascular distribution of CBG has been confirmed, and our recent results show that CBG is bound to the cell membrane and nuclear fractions of uterine tissue, albeit in smaller quantities than are found in the cytosol fraction (Selcer and Leavitt, 1987). This finding suggests that CBG distribution may extend beyond the interstitial space and into the decidual cell.

Recent studies using immunocytochemical techniques have demonstrated an intracellular localization of CBG in several rat tissues, including liver, kidney, uterus, thyroid, and pituitary (Kuhn *et al.*, 1986). Intracellular CBG could arise from *de novo* synthesis or sequestration from the circulation. That the CBG in deciduomal cytosol is derived from the blood is supported by the strong correlation that exists between tissue CBG and serum CBG levels (Selcer and Leavitt, 1987). Furthermore, decidual cells in culture do not synthesize and secrete labeled CBG during incubation with [^{35}S]methionine under conditions in which hepatocytes do produce labeled CBG (Fig. 5). The CBG found in cytosol does not represent contamination from blood during tissue fractionation, because *in situ* vascular perfusion prior to tissue removal had no significant effect on cytosol CBG titers in either deciduoma or myometrium (Do and Leavitt, 1978). Thus, the bulk of cytosol CBG in deciduoma is derived from blood and localized in the extravascular space. Since the extravascular space is composed of interstitial and cellular compartments, our results suggest that either or both of these compartments may concentrate CBG during the decidualization process, as depicted in Fig. 6.

Recent evidence suggests that CBG may function to transport steroid hormones from the serum to the target cell (Siiteri *et al.*, 1982). Our findings lend additional support for a cellular transport function of CBG, especially in the uterus, where a preferential uptake of CBG seems to occur in decidual and myometrial tissues. At the level of the target cell, CBG may function to maintain a high local concentration of progesterone for subsequent binding to intracellular progesterone receptors (Fig. 6), and in the case of decidual cells, such a finding may be very important because hamster decidual tissue is dependent on this hormone for its growth and maintenance. Exactly how CBG may deliver steroid hormones to the target cells is not known. However, our results suggest that membrane and nuclear binding of CBG may occur, and it remains to be determined whether specific binding sites for CBG exist in decidual cells, as appears to be the case in prostate and pituitary cells (Perrot-Applanat *et al.*, 1984; Hryb *et al.*, 1986).

The 60-kDa protein has not yet been identified, but its level in serum rises markedly during pregnancy. Although the function of the 60-kDa protein is not known, it certainly appears to be a marker for decidualization and early pregnancy in the hamster. The pregnancy marker proteins described for other species (Hau, 1986) are thought to be produced by either uterine or placental tissues. To our knowledge, this is the first example of a pregnancy protein derived from liver. Even more interesting is the possibility that the production of 60-kDa protein is controlled by an endocrine mechanism that becomes operative during the development of decidual cells in the early implantation site. Additional work is necessary to determine the nature of the endocrine signal produced by the decidual cell and the possible feedback effects of the 60-kDa protein on the decidua (Fig. 6) and other sites in the maternal and fetal compartments.

2. Steroid Receptors

2.1. Receptor Distribution

Early models of estrogen action suggested that unoccupied estrogen receptors are located in the cytoplasm of the target cell (Gorski *et al.*, 1968; Jensen *et al.*, 1968). Binding of estradiol was thought to stimulate a temperature-dependent translocation of the hormone–receptor complex into the nucleus, where transformation (activation) of the receptor into a conformation that binds tightly to DNA occurs (Yamamoto and Alberts, 1972; Grody *et al.*,

1982). The translocation or two-step model was generally accepted until 1984, when two new approaches revealed that estrogen receptors were predominantly nuclear proteins. The development of specific receptor antibodies (Greene and Jensen, 1982) permitted the immunocytochemical localization of receptor in intact tissue (King and Greene, 1984; McClellan *et al.*, 1984), and centrifugal enucleation of target cells following pretreatment with cytochalasin allowed the separation of cellular cytoplasm (cytoplasts) from nuclei (Welshons *et al.*, 1984; Gravanis and Gurpide, 1986). Both techniques showed that most receptor, including the unoccupied form, was distributed primarily in the target cell nucleus (Welshons *et al.*, 1985). Thus, the estrogen receptor appears to reside in the target cell nucleus, and the unoccupied (unactivated) receptor is now thought to be bound with low affinity to some nuclear component (Hansen and Gorski, 1985, 1986; Gorski *et al.*, 1986). The unoccupied receptor is readily extracted during tissue homogenization in dilute aqueous buffers, whereas the occupied receptor is not. The estrogen–receptor complex can be extracted in buffers containing high salt concentration (0.4 M KCl) or other reagents (Thomas and Leung, 1984; Geier *et al.*, 1985).

2.2. Receptor Assays

Although several methods have been used for the study of uterine steroid receptors (Sherman and Stevens, 1984), few of these procedures permit the simultaneous analysis of estrogen and progesterone receptors in cell nuclei and cytosol (Chamness *et al.*, 1975). The original assay developed for estrogen receptor utilized a Tris-EDTA (TE) buffer, which does not permit adequate progesterone receptor recovery. Receptor stability is improved by addition of glycerol and monothioglycerol to the TE buffer system (Leavitt *et al.*, 1974). In addition, the nuclear exchange procedure developed for the assay of total estrogen receptor is performed with nuclear suspensions (Anderson *et al.*, 1972), and this approach is not suitable for the assay of nuclear progesterone receptor because hormone–receptor complex is rapidly lost from nuclei even at low temperature (Walters and Clark, 1978). Nuclear estrogen receptor can be measured after KCl extraction from the nuclear fraction (Zava *et al.*, 1976), and this procedure gives good receptor recovery and assay precision. Furthermore, good recovery of nuclear progesterone receptor can be achieved by extraction of nuclei with Tris buffer containing glycerol and 0.5 M KCl (Chen and Leavitt, 1979).

On the basis of these considerations, an assay was developed appropriate for studying the subcellular distribution of estrogen and progesterone receptors in uterine tissues during the estrous cycle and pregnancy (Evans *et al.*, 1980). Cytosol and nuclear KCl extracts are prepared from fresh tissue. Cytosol receptors are assayed at 0°C for 16–18 hr, which provides the total progesterone receptor (Leavitt *et al.*, 1974) and the unoccupied estrogen receptor (Okulicz *et al.*, 1981a). Total estrogen receptor can be determined by exchange assay at 30°C for 1 hr, and occupied estrogen receptor is estimated from the difference between total and unoccupied receptor (Okulicz *et al.*, 1981a). The solubilized nuclear receptors are measured by exchange assay performed at 30°C for 1 hr in the case of estrogen receptor (Evans *et al.*, 1980) and at 0°C for 16–18 hr for progesterone receptor (Chen and Leavitt, 1979). The nuclear exchange assays measure total receptor and also permit estimation of unlabeled steroid in the nuclear KCl extract (Chen and Leavitt, 1979).

New assay methods were needed for the study of occupied and unoccupied forms of nuclear estrogen receptor. A significant problem with the KCl procedure was that it underestimated occupied estrogen receptor. Recently, we succeeded in developing conditions for the low-temperature exchange assay of nuclear estrogen receptor using 10 mM pyridoxal phosphate (PLP) (Okulicz *et al.*, 1983). Greater recovery of occupied receptor can be achieved with the PLP assay done at low temperature than with the KCl procedure. Total estrogen receptor is measured by [^{3}H]estradiol exchange in 10 mM PLP at 0°C at 0°C for 18 hr (Okulicz *et al.*, 1983). Unoccupied estrogen receptor is determined at 0°C for 2 hr in the presence of

Table 2. Conditions for the Assay of Estrogen (Re) and Progesterone (Rp) Receptors

	KCl (0.5 M)[a]	NaSCN (0.5 M)[b]	PLP (10 mM)[c]
Total Re	30°C, 1 hr	0°C, 24 hr	0°C, 24 hr
Unoccupied Re	0°C, 24 hr	No	0°C, 2 hr[d] (+ glycerol)
Occupied Re	Yes	No	Yes
Total Rp	0°C, 24 hr	No	0°C, 24 hr[e]

[a]Evans *et al.*, 1980.　　　　　　　[d]Leavitt and Okulicz, 1985a.
[b]Sica *et al.*, 1981.　　　　　　　　[e]Chen *et al.*, 1981.
[c]Okulicz *et al.*, 1983.

glycerol, which blocks dissociation of occupied receptor (Leavitt and Okulicz, 1985a). Occupied receptor equals total estrogen receptor minus the unoccupied sites. We had previously shown that PLP could be used to extract and measure nuclear progesterone receptor (Chen *et al.*, 1981). Thus, the PLP assay permits the simultaneous measurement of total progesterone receptor as well as occupied and unoccupied forms of estrogen receptor (Table 2).

Routinely, receptor assays are conducted using fresh tissue or cells, which are homogenized in the appropriate buffer with a Polytron Pt-10 (Brinkman Instruments, Westbury, NY). Care is taken to maintain the samples at 0–4°C at all times. Cytoplasmic and nuclear fractions are separated by centrifugation of the homogenate at 800 x *g* for 10 min. The low-speed cytoplasmic fraction is centrifuged at high speed (170,000 x *g*) for 30 min to prepare cytosol and a high-speed pellet. The high-speed pellet containing the membrane fraction is homogenized in TMG (50 mM Tris-maleate, 5 mM $MnCl_2$, 1% gelatin, pH 7.6) buffer for assay of membrane receptors such as the oxytocin receptor (Leavitt, 1985b). Cytosol and nuclear extract are used for steroid receptor assay using conventional saturation and Scatchard plot analysis (Scatchard, 1949) of binding data (Fig. 7).

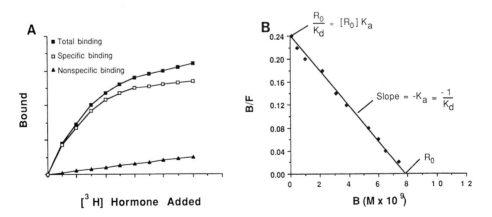

Figure 7. Saturation analysis of steroid receptors using [³H]ligand. Specific binding is the difference between total and nonspecific binding (A), and specific binding results are subjected to Scatchard plot analysis (B). The receptor concentration (Ro) is obtained from the intercept on the *x*-axis, and the slope (-K_a) is a measure of receptor affinity.

Much has been learned about the macromolecular events regulated by steroid hormones in target cells that synthesize and secrete hormone-specific protein products, and we understand some of the details about the hormonal regulation of egg white proteins in the avian oviduct and uteroglobin in the mammalian uterus. Progesterone action can be attributed to the regulation of gene expression and the formation of specific messenger RNA molecules for these export proteins. However, the nature of the interaction between the receptor–hormone complex and the acceptor (effector) sites in the target cell nucleus that control gene expression remains largely unknown (Fig. 3).

For our purposes, the acceptor site is defined as a low-capacity, high-affinity, target-tissue-specific domain that preferentially binds a single class of steroid hormone receptors. Spelsberg and colleagues have shown that avian oviduct acceptor sites exhibit these properties (Spelsberg *et al.*, 1983). Therefore, we have applied methods developed by this group to investigate uterine acceptor sites for the progesterone receptor (Rp). To validate the acceptor site assay, we prepared chick oviduct Rp and chromatin in the manner described by Spelsberg *et al.* (1983) and used the avian system as a reference standard for our characterization of hamster uterine Rp acceptor sites.

Hamster Rp binding to hamster crude chromatin or DNA resulted in a binding capacity and affinity similar to that observed with the avian system (Cobb and Leavitt, 1987a). Like chick Rp, hamster Rp binds to acceptor sites in crude chromatin in a saturable and high-affinity manner. Figure 8 shows that hamster uterine Rp binds to target tissue (deciduoma or uterus) chromatin at a 50% higher level than it binds to nontarget tissue (small intestine) chromatin, suggesting that Rp acceptor sites are tissue specific. Evidence for species specificity is provided in Fig. 8, which shows that the level of hamster Rp binding to hamster nontarget tissue acceptor sites occurs at the same low level as hamster Rp binding to avian target tissue (chick oviduct) acceptor sites. On the basis of these studies, it appears that hamster Rp acceptor sites, like avian acceptor sites, are saturable, high affinity, tissue specific, and species specific.

Having examined the binding properties of Rp acceptor sites in crude chromatin, we asked what nuclear components made up the acceptor site. Were the sites discrete, extractable proteins, were they specific DNA sequences, or were they a complex assembly of protein and DNA? To address these questions, we extracted chromatin with 0–6 M guanidine hydrochloride (GuHCl), a reagent that extracts histones and neutral chromatin protein at [GuHCl] < 1 M and extracts increasing amounts of acidic nonhistone protein at increasingly higher concentrations (Fig. 9). The matrix remaining after GuHCl extraction is referred to as nucleoacidic protein (NAP) chromatin. Binding of Rp to chromatin increased as increasing concentrations of GuHCl were used for extraction. However, if GuHCl concentrations >4 M were used, Rp binding to the extracted chromatin decreased (Cobb and Leavitt, 1987a).

These results are consistent with earlier studies of the chick oviduct, which have been used to construct a model for Rp–chromatin interactions. In that model, low concentrations of GuHCl strip inhibitory "masking proteins" from acceptor sites, allowing association of increasing amounts of Rp with acceptor sites. High (>4 M) GuHCl concentrations extract the acceptor sites themselves, thus reducing Rp binding to chromatin (Fig. 9). A large portion of Rp binding to NAP may represent nonspecific binding rather than binding to a finite number of Rp acceptor sites (Cobb and Leavitt, 1987b). Thus, the binding of activated Rp to crude chromatin may represent the actual acceptor sites in target cell nuclei. Since the high level of Rp binding sites in NAP chromatin may be an extraction artifact, the proposed involvement of masking proteins in regulating the availability of acceptor sites should be viewed with caution.

As an alternative to acceptor site regulation, changes in the Rp molecule itself may be important (Cobb and Leavitt, 1987b). The Rp isolated from hamster uteri on days 1–4 of the estrous cycle was incubated with crude chromatin, NAP chromatin, and DNA. The apparent

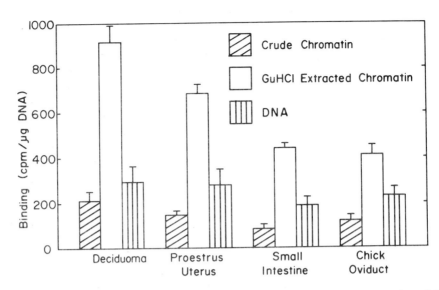

Figure 8. Hamster progesterone receptor binding to chromatin, 4 M GuHCl-extracted chromatin, and DNA prepared from hamster deciduoma, proestrus uterus, small intestine, and chick oviduct. From Cobb and Leavitt (1987a).

level of Rp binding to crude chromatin and NAP chromatin increased 2.5-fold from day 1 to day 4, but Rp binding to DNA remained constant. This observation suggests that ovarian-cycle-dependent changes occur in the unactivated Rp that affect its interactions with chromatin, and these changes disappear when receptor is activated. The three matrices, crude chromatin-cellulose, NAP chromatin-cellulose, and DNA-cellulose, bind activated Rp in a KC1-extractable manner (Cobb and Leavitt, 1987b). Although NAP chromatin displayed increased salt-resistant Rp binding, such binding was not sensitive to competition with various forms of hormone–Rp complex, and it was unaffected by Rp activation state. These findings indicate that the previous concept of Rp acceptor sites in chromatin should be expanded to include another level of control that appears to involve the receptor protein itself (Dougherty *et al.*, 1982; Logeat *et al.*, 1985a).

2.4. Estrogen–Progestin Interactions

One hormone may act to alter the expression of a second hormone, and the modulation of estrogen action by progesterone in female target organs is a classic example of this phenomenon. Progesterone and estrogen exert opposing effects on the estrogen receptor (Re) and progesterone receptor (Rp) systems. Estrogen up-regulates the Re and Rp systems by stimulation of macromolecular synthesis, leading to accumulation of available receptor sites in the target cell (Leavitt *et al.*, 1977, 1979, 1983). In contrast, progesterone down-regulates both the Re and Rp systems by processes that are not fully understood (Katzenellenbogen, 1980). Interaction of progesterone with its receptor causes loss of Rp sites by an unknown mechanism in conjunction with receptor activation and binding in the target cell nucleus (Milgrom *et al.*, 1973; Leavitt *et al.*, 1974). Furthermore, it is well established that progesterone modifies estrogen-stimulated responses in the uterus.

In recent years, attempts have been made to elucidate the molecular basis for the interaction between progesterone and estrogen. Progesterone antagonism of cytoplasmic Re replenishment was described in studies with the rat uterus (Hseuh *et al.*, 1976; Clark *et al.*, 1977; Bhakoo and Katzenellenbogen, 1977). When estradiol and progesterone were administered simultaneously to estrogen-primed rats, the cytosol Re replenishment response that is normally observed 12–24 hr after estradiol treatment was reduced (Bhakoo and Katzenellenbogen, 1977). The progesterone-induced decline of cytosol Re was correlated with reduced nuclear Re retention and diminished uterotrophic response to secondary estradiol stimulation (Clark *et al.*, 1977). A mechanism was proposed for progesterone antagonism of estrogen action based on the premise that inhibition of cytosol Re replenishment would limit the quantity of Re available for binding with hormone and thus blunt the uterine response to estrogen stimulation (Clark *et al.*, 1977). We now know that this is not the case (Leavitt *et al.*, 1983), and recent studies done with the hamster and rat have provided further insight into the mechanism of progesterone regulation of the Re system.

In order to understand how progesterone (P) action is mediated, we must first review Re dynamics (Fig. 10). Estrogen (E) action in target tissues occurs when E enters the cell, binds to its high-affinity, ligand-specific, low-capacity receptor protein (Re), which is loosely associated with various nuclear components (Gorski *et al.*, 1984, 1986). After E binds to Re, the ReE complex is rapidly modified or "activated" (Grody *et al.*, 1982; Skafar and Notides,

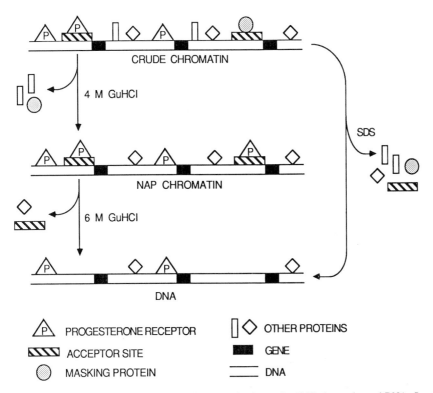

Figure 9. A model for progesterone receptor binding to crude chromatin, NAP chromatin, and DNA. See text for details.

1985), changing its physicochemical properties with an increase in affinity for nuclear binding sites, called acceptor sites, which are believed to be composed of DNA and chromatin proteins (Spelsberg *et al.*, 1983). By convention, the loosely bound ReE complex is referred to as cytosolic ReE, since it is found in the cytosolic fraction after tissue homogenization (Grody *et al.*, 1982). The tightly bound ReE complex is referred to as nuclear ReE, since its removal from the nuclear fraction requires extraction with high salt concentration, pyridoxal 5'-phosphate, or thiocyanate (Walters, 1985). A similar scheme is believed to apply to P and its receptor, Rp (Grody *et al.*, 1982). Retention of ReE by nuclear binding sites has been correlated with an increase in the transcription (Taylor and Smith, 1981) and translation of Rp, Re, oxytocin receptor proteins in the uterus (Leavitt *et al.*, 1983), egg white proteins in the chick oviduct (Mulvihill and Palmiter, 1977), and a host of other E-induced proteins. Decrease in ReE retention is similarly correlated with decreased levels of these proteins (Anderson *et al.*, 1975; O'Malley *et al.*, 1979; Chuknyiska and Roth, 1985).

In order to address the question of how P controls the Re system, we first review pertinent physiological studies that suggested ways to design experiments to address this question. The first line of evidence comes from the estrogen-dominated uterus that one finds during the hamster estrous cycle, and we review the acute effects of P on Re in the proestrus hamster uterus. The second line of evidence comes from the P-dominated myometrium and relates to pregnancy maintenance and to the mechanism of parturition at the end of pregnancy. The third line of evidence has to do with recent studies that we have done on Re synthesis and degradation in uterine decidual cells, as measured by the density-shift method. Finally, acceptor site studies, using methods adapted from Spelsberg *et al.* (1983), have permitted us to identify a binding site in uterine chromatin that seems to qualify as an Re acceptor site. We discovered a very rapid effect of P on the regulation of these acceptor sites in the proestrus hamster uterus (Cobb and Leavitt, 1985).

2.5. Hamster Estrous Cycle

In the 4-day estrous cycle of the hamster (Fig. 11), there is a preovulatory surge of P secretion on the day of proestrus (day 4), as occurs in other rodent species such as the rat and

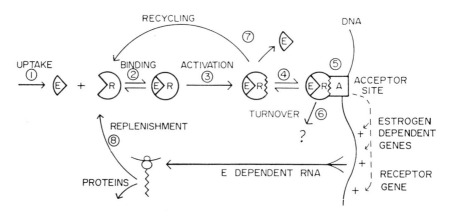

Figure 10. Estrogen receptor dynamics in a uterine target cell. Steps are (1) hormone uptake by the cell, (2) binding to unoccupied receptor, (3) receptor activation, (4) binding to acceptor sites, (5) receptor retention, (6) receptor processing, (7) receptor recycling, and (8) receptor replenishment. Abbreviations: E, estradiol-17β; R, estrogen receptor; A, nuclear acceptor site. Adapted from Leavitt (1985a).

mouse. As estrogen secretion increases during follicular development on days 2–4 of the cycle, there is an increase in uterine nuclear Re levels and also an induction of Rp, reflecting the up-regulation of receptors that one sees with E action in the uterus. Down-regulation begins with preovulatory P secretion at midcycle. One sees a very rapid effect of P on the Rp system, and the net result in terms of Rp levels is the down-regulation of Rp. There is also a loss of nuclear Re at midcycle, and we became interested in the cause of this down-regulation. The possibilities were that this was a result of (1) estrogen withdrawal, (2) P action, or (3) a combination of both. As reviewed elsewhere (Leavitt *et al.*, 1983), we found that the rapid decrease in the nuclear Re was really the result of P action and not estrogen withdrawal. This observation prompted our interest in what P was doing at the level of the target cell nucleus. Thus, we designed experiments to determine which form of Re might be regulated, and, using conventional receptor assays as well as new assays developed to optimize the recovery of occupied Re (Okulicz *et al.*, 1983), we found, using the E-dominated uterus, that there was a very rapid and selective effect of P treatment on the occupied form of nuclear Re (Okulicz *et al.*, 1981a,c; Leavitt and Okulicz, 1985). This was of considerable interest because it suggested that P controlled the biologically important form of the receptor, i.e., nuclear occupied Re. Furthermore, in temporal studies, P had a very rapid effect on the occupied form of nuclear Re occurring within 2 to 4 hr (Okulicz *et al.*, 1981a,b).

These and other studies (Evans and Leavitt, 1980) suggest that P acts by way of its receptor system, perhaps to induce some RNA or protein, which then either produces a new

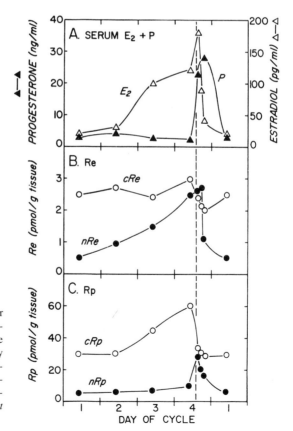

Figure 11. Serum steroid–uterine receptor relationships during the hamster estrous cycle. The dashed vertical line indicates the time of the critical period for the ovulatory surge of gonadotropin. Abbreviations: c, cytosol; E_2, estradiol-17β; n, nuclear; P, progesterone; Re, estrogen receptor; Rp, progesterone receptor. Adapted from Leavitt *et al.* (1983).

factor or activates a preexisting factor, which we call the estrogen receptor regulatory factor (ReRF) (Okulicz *et al.*, 1981c; MacDonald *et al.*, 1982, 1983b). We first proposed that this factor might act to stimulate degradation of the occupied form of the nuclear Re (Leavitt *et al.*, 1983). Since we have not been able to prove that this factor acts directly on the receptor (Leavitt, 1985a,c), an alternative hypothesis is that the factor may act on what the hormone–receptor complex is associated with in the chromatin, i.e., the nuclear acceptor site.

It is hoped that information derived from studies of the rodent uterus will shed light on the mechanisms controlling receptor site availability in the human uterus, where fluctuations in Re and Rp levels occur during the menstrual cycle (Flickinger *et al.*, 1977; Robel *et al.*, 1981). However, it should be emphasized that experimental evidence is needed from other species in order to demonstrate the generality of the down-regulation phenomenon. This is especially true in species of lower vertebrates that do not utilize embryo or egg retention in the reproductive process.

2.6. Pregnancy

We were also interested in receptor regulation during pregnancy, when Re and Rp are chronically down-regulated (Leavitt, 1985a,b), and in particular, what happens when P is withdrawn, in terms of the recovery of the Re system and estrogen-dependent proteins. In this situation, ovariectomized animals were given Silastic pellets containing E and P, which maintain blood levels of E and P equivalent to those present during normal pregnancy. The plan was to maintain E levels at a steady state, so that the only hormone that changes at time zero, on removal of the P pellet, is the fall in serum P. Within 4 to 8 hr of P withdrawal, there is a significant recovery of nuclear Re and cytosol Re (Leavitt, 1985a,b; Leavitt *et al.*, 1985b). Thus, under steady-state E exposure, the recovery of Re is accompanied by an increase in estrogen-dependent proteins such as Rp in the cytosol fraction and the oxytocin receptor in the membrane fraction. These observations are consistent with the idea that P down-regulates the nuclear Re chronically, and in the withdrawal paradigm, we see a recovery not only of the occupied nuclear Re from extremely low levels within 4 hr but also a significant recovery of occupied cytosol Re (Leavitt, 1985a,b). Thus, the situation here may not be exactly equivalent to a reversal of the acute down-regulation that we see in response to P action in the estrogen-primed uterus, but a similar phenomenon seems to be operative. This provides further support for the ReRF hypothesis that P induces something that controls the occupied form of Re, perhaps by regulation of Re retention on the nuclear acceptor sites. Clearly, the hormone withdrawal studies show that this effect is reversed rapidly when P is removed from the target cell.

2.7. Density-Shift Studies

In primary cultures of hamster decidual cells (Leavitt *et al.*, 1985a), the up- and down-regulation of receptors can be studied easily because the cells will grow in either the presence or absence of P under the culture conditions (Leavitt and Takeda, 1986). If cells are grown in the presence of P, and then P is withdrawn at time zero, both Rp and Re recover within 8 to 16 hr (Leavitt and Takeda, 1986). Next, these cells were used to study the effect of P on Re dynamics, and this was accomplished using the density-shift method to measure Re synthesis and degradation.

Figure 12 outlines how this experiment is conducted. First, the cells are grown in the absence of hormones. Then Re is charged with unlabeled E, and at time zero the cells are exposed to dense amino acids (containing ^2H, ^{13}C, ^{15}N). The dense amino acids are incorporated into the proteins being synthesized under these conditions. Since the Re is one of the

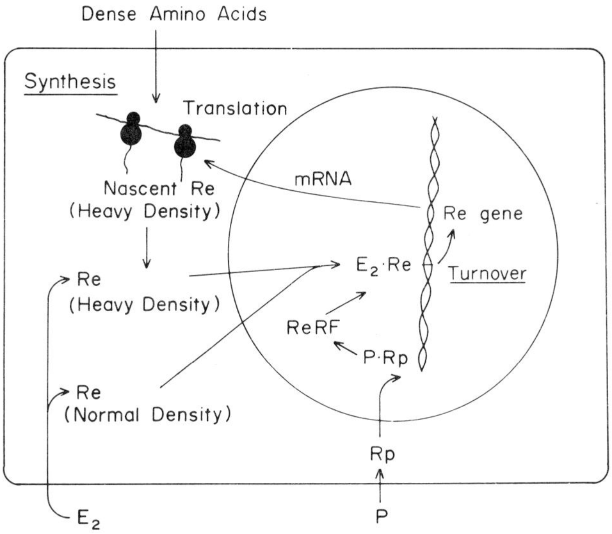

Figure 12. Outline of density-shift experiment using decidual cell cultures. Decidual cells are first grown in the absence of hormone, and then the cells are incubated with unlabeled estradiol (E_2) to charge Re. At time zero, the cells are incubated in medium enriched with dense amino acids that contain the heavy isotopes ^2H, ^{13}C, and ^{15}N. Two hormonal regimens were compared: E_2 alone versus E_2 plus P. At various times of incubation, the nuclear Re was extracted and labeled by exchange with [^{125}I]estradiol, and the Re of normal density (4 S) and heavy density (6 S) were determined by density-gradient centrifugation. The rate of disappearance of normal-density Re provides the measure of Re degradation, and the rate of appearance of heavy-density Re represents Re synthesis.

proteins that is synthesized, it incorporates the heavy amino acids, producing the so-called "heavy" form of Re that is identified by sucrose gradient centrifugation (Eckert *et al.*, 1984). The Re of normal density is the receptor that was present at the start of the experiment, and the decay of the normal-density form of the Re determines how fast the receptor protein is being degraded. The rate of appearance of the heavy-density form of Re is a measure of how fast the receptor is being synthesized. Experiments were done in which the cells were exposed to E or E plus progestin (either P or the synthetic progestin R5020) during incubation with dense amino acids. Figure 13 depicts the gradient results. The Re of normal density is labeled with [^{125}I]estradiol, and it sediments at 4 S under these conditions. Within 3 hr, the heavy-density form of Re is seen at 6 S, and with time, the 6 S peak increases as the heavy amino acids are incorporated into the newly synthesized receptor. The 4 S peak decreases with time of incubation, and this decline represents the preexisting receptor being degraded under these experimental conditions.

When cells exposed to E alone and to E plus progestin are compared, at 1 hr there is no difference in the Re profile, but by 3 hr both Re peaks are substantially reduced with E plus progestin. By 9 hr the progestin effect is clear. From the loss of the 4 S normal-density peak, we can calculate Re turnover, and within 3 hr, P causes a significant enhancement of the Re turnover (Fig. 14). The data from the second peak, when corrected for the difference in receptor turnover, provide a measure of Re synthesis (Schimke, 1975). With E alone, the rate of Re synthesis increases by 9 hr, when there is a significant difference in Re synthesis between E alone and E plus progestin (Fig. 14). What is the interpretation of these results? First, there is a rapid effect of P on Re turnover, within 3 hr, and this effect is maintained through the period studied. Under these culture conditions, progestin does not change Re

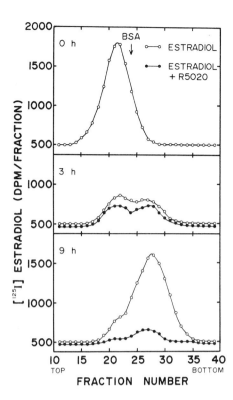

Figure 13. Sedimentation profiles of nuclear Re as determined by the density-shift technique. Decidual cell cultures were incubated with either 1 nM estradiol (open circles) or 1 nM estradiol plus 10 nM R5020 (closed circles) in the presence of heavy amino acids, as depicted in Fig. 12. After 3, 6, and 9 hr of incubation, nuclear Re was extracted and labeled with [^{125}I]estradiol, and the heavy- and normal-density forms of Re were separated by density-gradient centrifugation. Bovine serum albumin (BSA) was used as a sedimentation marker (4.6 S). From Takeda and Leavitt (1986).

synthesis. What progestin appears to do is block E-induced Re synthesis, which is the so-called replenishment response that one sees with E action (Fig. 10). However, this happens subsequent to the P-induced change in Re turnover. Thus, this experiment demonstrates that the first effect of P is on receptor degradation, and there is a secondary, later response on Re synthesis that may be a consequence of the earlier effect on Re turnover (Takeda and Leavitt, 1986).

How can we explain P-induced Re degradation? Since we have not been able to show that P induces a factor that directly acts on the receptor, there must be something else involved. The missing link appears to be the nuclear acceptor sites for Re. Figure 15 shows acceptor site binding curves as determined with techniques that we have developed, using uterine chromatin derived from the proestrus hamster uterus. The proestrus uterus is an estrogen-dominated tissue, and the chromatin is prepared and coupled to cellulose for binding to labeled ReE complex that is also derived from the proestrus uterus. If we treat the proestrus animal for 2 hr with P *in vivo* and then harvest the chromatin in the same way and perform a binding assay with the same labeled ReE preparation, we find a substantial decrease in the binding of hormone–receptor complex to chromatin (Fig. 15). This difference in the binding capacity of control and P-treated chromatin can be accounted for by specific saturable binding sites, since the binding can be inhibited competitively by unlabeled ReE complex (Fig. 15). A similar loss of Re acceptor sites is observed on the day of proestrus, before and after the endogenous preovulatory P surge, as compared with 2 hr and 4 hr of P treatment before the time of the P surge. The Re–acceptor binding results suggest that P acts either at the level of the ReE complex as it exists on acceptor sites or on the acceptor site itself (Fig. 10).

We have attempted to determine whether P-dependent modification of the receptor protein could account for decreased nuclear retention. Ovariectomized hamsters were treated with E and P implants for 15 days. This hormonal regimen is similar to that which occurs during the 16-day gestation period of the hamster. On day 15, P implants were removed from one group and left in the other group, and the E implants remained in both groups. Activated cytosolic

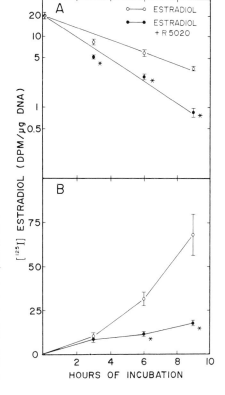

Figure 14. Estrogen receptor (Re) degradation (A) and synthesis (B) as influenced by progesterone action in decidual cells. The half-life ($t_{1/2}$) of nuclear Re was determined from the regression lines calculated from the normal-density (4 S) Re peak (see Fig. 13). The $t_{1/2}$ of nuclear Re was 3.9 hr for cells incubated with E_2 (open circles), and progestin treatment (closed circles) shortened the $t_{1/2}$ of Re to 1.9 hr. Synthesis of Re was calculated from the size of the heavy-density (6 S) peak using the formula: $K_s = K_d \cdot R_t/(1 - e^{-kdt})$, where K_s is the synthesis rate, $K_d = 0.693/t_{1/2}$, and R_t is the Re value (DPM/μg DNA) at time t. With this approach, the corrected synthesis ($K_s \cdot t$) of nuclear Re was calculated and plotted in panel B. From Takeda and Leavitt (1986).

ReE was prepared from both groups and then incubated with proestrus uterine chromatin to ascertain whether differences existed in the ability of these receptor preparations to bind to Re acceptor sites. The saturation profile of P-withdrawn ReE was identical to that of P-treated ReE, indicating no effect on the receptor protein. In contrast, P action *in vivo* significantly decreases nuclear retention of ReE. These studies suggest that the receptor itself is not the

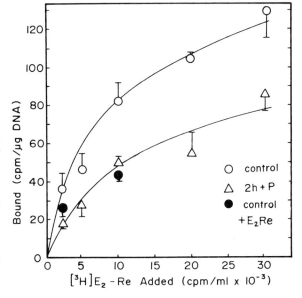

Figure 15. Progesterone (P)-induced depletion of nuclear Re acceptor sites from uterine chromatin. Proestrus hamsters were treated for 2 hr with 5 mg P (triangles) or oil vehicle (control, open circles). Chromatin was isolated and linked to cellulose as described by Spelsberg *et al.* (1983). Then, binding assays were performed at 0°C using different concentrations of [³H]-E_2-Re complex prepared from uterine cytosol (obtained from control animals) and concentrated by ammonium sulfate (45%) precipitation prior to assay. A competition experiment was done using a fivefold excess of radioinert E_2-Re complex (closed circles).

substrate for the P-induced activity (factor) and that nuclear receptor loss occurs by an alternative mechanism at the level of the chromatin acceptor sites (Fig. 10).

In summary, P selectively down-regulates the occupied form of nuclear Re, and there is a rapid depletion of nuclear acceptor sites within 2 hr. Progesterone stimulates Re turnover within 3 hr, and subsequently P inhibits E-induced Re synthesis at 9 hr. Thus, we propose that it is the P-induced depletion of nuclear acceptor sites that appears to enhance nuclear Re turnover (Fig. 10) and thus interrupt at least some aspects of E-dependent gene transcription. Our working hypothesis is that P somehow blocks or alters the high-affinity acceptor sites for Re, and this, then, leads to an enhancement of Re turnover. This model requires a rather rapid mechanism for degrading receptor, at least as we recognize it from steroid binding studies, and P appears to increase the half-time of Re turnover from 4 hr to 2 hr. Thus, our studies show that P doubles the Re degradation rate by some mechanism that stimulates the already rapid turnover ($t_{1/2} = 4$ hr) of the Re protein in the target cell nucleus. The amino-terminal amino acid composition of a protein appears to determine the protein's half-life (Bachmoir *et al.*, 1986; Dice, 1987), and proteins with PEST regions rich in proline (P), glutamic acid (E), serine (S), and threonine (T) are rapidly degraded in eukaryotic cells (Rogers *et al.*, 1986). Recent information on the amino acid sequence of the human Re (S. Greene *et al.*, 1986; G. L. Green *et al.*, 1986) supports the idea that the rapid turnover of nuclear Re could be related to the amino acid composition of one or more regions of the receptor protein. Exactly how the P-induced loss of nuclear acceptor sites relates to Re degradation remains to be determined.

It is important to emphasize that in all studies to date, nuclear ReE levels were measured using labeled-steroid binding assays. These assays are designed to detect only those receptor forms capable of binding ligand. With this in mind, the possibility had to be considered that the apparent loss of nuclear Re by P action may affect only ligand–Re binding while leaving the remainder of the receptor intact. Decreased ligand binding could be caused either by interaction of another protein with the receptor, by changes in the conformation of the receptor, or by covalent modification of the receptor protein (Milgrom, 1981; Dickerman and Kumar, 1982). Since nuclear ReE complexes from P-treated cells have no detectable physicochemical differences from those from control cells (Leavitt, 1985a), such modification of Re would have to be subtle, perhaps involving phosphorylation of a single key amino acid residue.

Work of Auricchio and colleagues (Migliaccio *et al.*, 1982, 1984; Auricchio *et al.*, 1981a,b) demonstrated that an Re tyrosine residue is a substrate for endogenous nuclear phosphatase and cytosolic kinase action. Tyrosine phosphorylation has been implicated as a key regulatory event in cellular differentiation and growth. Phosphorylation of Re tyrosine residues enhances Re estrogen-binding capacity without altering Re affinity for ligand. These investigators observed an apparent "inactivation" or loss of E-binding capacity that was attributable to dephosphorylation of a receptor tyrosine residue(s). They proposed that, *in vivo,* a nuclear phosphatase causes an apparent loss of Re by inhibiting ligand–receptor interaction. A potential involvement of phosphorylation in Re regulation was also demonstrated by Moudgil and Eessalu (1980). In their studies, incubation of cytosol ReE with ATP at 0–4°C for 1 hr enhanced ReE binding to nuclei and DNA-cellulose. When a nonhydrolyzable ATP analogue was substituted for ATP in the incubation, no enhanced activation was observed. Similarly, Fleming *et al.* (1982) showed that cGMP, ATP, and GTP, but not cAMP, increased the apparent recovery of ReE from nuclei. They proposed that a cGMP-dependent protein kinase was involved in Re activation. Unfortunately, no effect of receptor dephosphorylation on DNA–Re interactions has yet been demonstrated.

Although binding assays are a useful approach to the study of ReE turnover, they provide little information about putative non-ligand-binding forms of Re. Monsma *et al.* (1984) used tamoxifen aziridine to label covalently the receptor and follow its degradation. The loss of covalently bound ligand was assumed to parallel loss of Re. Surprisingly, the loss of the ligand binding site and the loss of immunoreactive Re protein occurred simultaneously (Monsma *et al.,* 1984). This suggests that significant changes in the tertiary structure of the receptor accompany degradation or inactivation of the functional ligand binding site (Sherman and Stevens, 1984). On this basis, antibodies to receptor may prove very useful in the detection of receptor products formed during Re processing in the nucleus. Certainly, monoclonal antibodies to conformation-dependent epitopes will provide information about how receptor structure changes under various experimental conditions (Greene, 1984).

Recent studies indicate that quaternary changes in receptor structure may be even more significant than tertiary changes in regulating Re function. Immunocytochemical analyses of receptor forms occurring during short-term (30-min) or longer-term (6-hr) E exposure revealed only one form of nuclear receptor in short-term E-treated cells (Kasid *et al.,* 1984; Jakesz *et al.,* 1983). This Re form was an activated monomer (4 S) showing rapid ligand dissociation (half-time 8.5 min). After longer exposure to E, nuclei contained both the monomeric form and an activated 8.8 S dimer. The dimer elutes differently from hydroxylapatite and has a slower dissociation rate (216 min) than the monomeric form. There does not appear to be a differential turnover of different Re forms in MCF-7 cells. Monsma *et al.* (1984) allowed cells to incorporate heavy amino acids (^{13}C, ^{15}N, ^{2}H) into Re, which was first charged with ligand and then covalently cross-linked to adjacent macromolecules. Only one major receptor form, a 130,000-Da homodimer, was evident, and the subunits of the homodimer were degraded simultaneously. Gorski's (Sakai and Gorski, 1984) and Notides' (Notides *et al.,* 1981, 1985) laboratories have provided additional information regarding monomer–dimer interactions, and both groups present evidence for dimer interactions with DNA, although they disagree on the sequence of events involved and the significance of receptor dimerization to hormone action.

2.8. A Unifying Concept

It is generally believed that a relationship must exist between the number of nuclear receptor sites and hormone-dependent gene transcription (Anderson *et al.,* 1974; Mulvihill and Palmiter, 1977; Chambon *et al.,* 1984). However, evidence is needed to verify that such a relationship actually exists (Yamamoto and Alberts, 1976), and in the case of estrogen, it is not certain whether hormone action is the result of receptor binding and retention by nuclear acceptor sites (Kon and Spelsberg, 1982; Ruh and Spelsberg, 1983; Spelsberg *et al.,* 1983), receptor "processing" in the nucleus (Horwitz and McGuire, 1978,b, 1980), or other events (Skafar and Seaver; 1985, Gorski *et al.,* 1986). Thus, we need to learn more about nuclear receptor retention and processing in order to learn how hormone action is mediated at the level of gene expression.

We have been unable to detect physicochemical modifications in the nuclear Re that would inhibit its retention and accelerate its turnover rate (Leavitt, 1985a,c). Therefore, it is likely that the P-induced decrease in nuclear ReE retention results from a change in the nuclear acceptor site for receptor rather than a change in the receptor itself. If the nuclear Re acceptor site were lost, receptor might be more susceptible to proteolysis. The idea that P modulates nuclear ReE–chromatin interactions is consistent with previous reports that steroid hormones cause numerous changes in various chromatin proteins (Horton and Szego, 1984), including histone acetylation (Libby, 1972; Pasqualini *et al.,* 1981), induction and synthesis of nonhistone acidic chhromosomal proteins (Cohen and Hamilton, 1975; Gilmour, 1981), increased DNAse I sensitivity (Keller *et al.,* 1975; Cushing *et al.,* 1985), and other changes in chromatin conformation (Bloom and Anderson, 1979; Chambon *et al.,* 1984).

In order to consider how P action might alter the nuclear Re binding site, it is first necessary to understand the characteristics of that site. Proposed nuclear ReE binding sites include the nuclear matrix (Alexander *et al.,* 1987; Barrack and Coffey, 1980, 1983), DNA (Burch and Weintraub, 1983; Renkawitz *et al.,* 1984; von der Ahe *et al.,* 1986; Mulvihill *et al.,* 1982; Lai *et al.,* 1983), basic nonhistone chromatin proteins (Puca *et al.,* 1975), and acidic nonhistone chromatin proteins (Kon and Spelsberg, 1982; Ross and Ruh, 1984; Toyoda *et al.*, 1985; Singh *et al.*, 1986).

Because ReE possesses the ability to activate and develop an increased affinity for DNA, earlier investigators proposed that the nuclear binding site for the receptor was DNA. This hypothesis has been tested by several investigators who used recombinant DNA technology to clone E-dependent genes (Jost *et al.*, 1984, 1985; Zwelling *et al.*, 1983). Although a detailed account of this gene regulatory structure is beyond the scope of this discussion, we can consider the enhancer and promoter regions and their putative role in ReE binding (Chambon *et al.*, 1984). An illustration of their spatial relationship is provided in Fig. 16. From 3' (right) to 5' (left), the entire gene and its regulatory elements consist of a 3' flanking region, the transcript and its intervening sequences, a cap site or "start" site proximal to the transcript, a 30-base-pair "spacer," the TATA box, a 70- to 90-base-pair "spacer," a polymorphic GC-rich sequence, another "spacer" region of greatly varying length, an "enhancer" sequence, and finally, the remainder of the 5' flanking region. The enhancer sequences are 76-base-pair repeats and are located not only in the 5' flanking region but also within the 3' flanking region, in the intervening sequences, and proximal (110 bp from the cap site) and distal (several hundred to several thousand bp from the cap site) to the regulated gene. Each of these regions may contain specific sequences to which regulatory components of the transcriptional machinery bind (Chandler *et al.*, 1983; Emerson *et al.*, 1985). The ReE may be a part of that machinery, and several of these sequences have been implicated as the receptor binding site. Estrogen receptors bind to regulatory sequences in the vitellogenin gene (Jost *et al.*, 1984) and the prolactin gene (Maurer, 1985). Other steroid receptors have been shown to bind primarily but not exclusively to the 5' flanking regions of the hormone-responsive gene (Karin *et al.*, 1984a,b; Payvar *et al.*, 1983; Mulvihill *et al.*, 1982). The receptor appears to interact with enhancer sequences that may be located at varying distances from the transcription initiation site (Fig. 16).

Recent studies (Green and Chambon, 1986) indicate that steroid hormone receptors belong to a family or regulatory proteins whose ability to control gene expression is activated by the binding of hormone (Fig. 17). The control of gene expression by these receptor proteins may be achieved by the interaction of *trans*-acting proteins with the *cis*-acting DNA-promoter elements including the steroid receptor. Sequence homology is apparent among selected regions of several steroid receptors (Conneely *et al.*, 1986; Greene *et al.*, 1986) and the thyroid hormone receptor with the v-*erb*-A oncogene (Fig. 17). Thus, these receptor proteins may have evolved from a common ancestral receptor gene, and the DNA binding domain appears to be conserved in all of them. The hormone-binding region is located near the carboxy terminus, and the amino terminus appears to vary considerably in the different receptors.

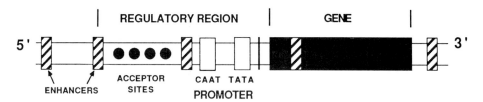

Figure 16. Structural organization of hormone-regulated gene. The 5' flanking region contains regulatory elements such as promoter sequences (CAAT, TATA, CAP) and other sequences that recognize receptor and acceptor site proteins. Enhancer sequences appear to occur at various locations in the 5' flanking region, in the 3' flanking region, and internally in the structural gene. Acceptor proteins are thought to bind to specific sequences in the regulatory region (adjacent to enhancers?), and receptor binding to the acceptor sites is believed to cause looping of the DNA, which appears to be necessary for active gene transcription.

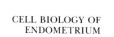

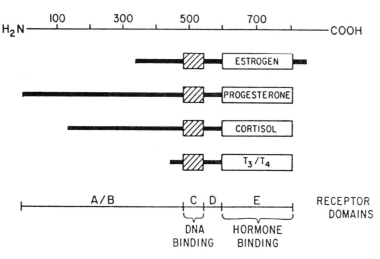

Figure 17. Schematic comparison of steroid and thyroid (T_3/T_4) hormone receptors' predicted amino acid sequences as deduced from cloning and sequence analysis of appropriate complementary DNA. The steroid receptor can be divided into six regions. Region E, the hormone-binding domain (which lies in the carboxyl portion of the receptor), and particularly region C, the DNA-binding domain (approximately 66 amino acid residues with two pairs of cysteines), have a significant (17% and 45–55%, respectively) structural homology, and regions A/B (the immunogenic domain) and the hydrophilic region D have little or no significant homology. Sequence comparisons have revealed similarities between the protein product of the v-*erb*-A oncogenes and all of these receptors. Thus, the steroid receptors, probably also including the 1,25-dihydroxyvitamin D_3 receptor, and the thyroid receptor all may have evolved from a common ancestral gene. From Norman and Litwack (1987).

Although these speculations are intriguing, it is unlikely that the complex actions of steroid hormones can be completely explained by receptor binding to specific DNA sequences. As Lin and Riggs (1975) and von Hippel *et al.* (1984) have pointed out, the specific binding of a protein with DNA requires a very high affinity for the specific sequence in order to overcome the large amount of nonspecific binding to DNA. In the case of steroid receptors, it is not certain that the binding affinity for DNA sequences is high enough to account for gene regulatory responses. Thus, a more complex interaction of receptor with acceptor proteins and DNA seems more likely.

How could receptor–acceptor site interaction stimulate gene transcription, and how could its absence diminish transcription rates? Electron micrographs of estrogen-stimulated chick oviduct chromatin show that the chromatin is arranged in multiple "loops" with attachment points near the chromosomal matrix. These loops are DNAse I hypersensitive, contain nascent RNA transcripts, and do not appear in the E-withdrawn state. The attachment sites of these loops to the nuclear matrix contain a number of transcriptionally related proteins such as topoisomerases (Cockerill and Garrard, 1986), and these also may contain steroid hormone receptor binding sites. A functional model for loop formation has been proposed by O'Malley *et al.* (1983). The basis of their model was the finding that actively transcribed genes existed as "loops" and that the loops were intimately associated with the nuclear matrix. They proposed that within the loops, each E-dependent gene contained a consensus sequence that, when associated with ReE, stimulates transcription. The loop was then specifically attached to proteins of the nuclear matrix for continued stimulation of gene transcription.

A simple P-dependent event such as dephosphorylation of an acceptor protein could trigger a cascade that would produce significant changes in overall chromatin conformation and gene transcription. It may be pertinent that Rp is associated with a 90-kDa protein that may contain protein kinase activity (Garcia *et al.*, 1983), although it is equally likely that Rp may activate or modulate another factor(s) responsible for acceptor protein modification (Sullivan *et al.*, 1986). As the Rp rapidly turns over (Horwitz *et al.*, 1985), modification of acceptor proteins ceases, and the original conformation of the nuclear ReE binding site is restored by synthesis of new acceptor proteins or perhaps by some reverse reaction (phosphorylation?). Thus, the model allows for reversibility and recovery of P-dependent down-regulation of nuclear ReE. Of course, one should keep in mind that the down-regulated condition may be the normal or resting state and not an inhibited state.

In summary, we have observed that progesterone acts, via its nuclear receptor, to decrease rapidly the level of occupied nuclear Re, to increase the rate of nuclear receptor turnover, and to reduce rapidly the number of nuclear acceptor sites for Re. We propose that progesterone activates a factor (ReRF) that, in turn, modifies the acceptor site for Re. Such modification is thought to impede receptor association and to prevent conformational changes in chromatin required to form transcriptionally active chromatin loops. Because non-chromatin-bound nuclear estrogen receptor is not afforded protection by its association with other chromatin components, it is more susceptible to either general or specific proteolysis, and its turnover rate increases greatly. Although we have advanced this hypothesis from the available evidence, it remains to be tested experimentally and will likely be modified as new information is generated from future experiments in this exciting field of research. New approaches using new probes for the receptor protein (Greene, 1984; Logent *et al.*, 1981, 1983) and the receptor genes (Maxwell *et al.*, 1987; White *et al.*, 1987) will undoubtedly provide new knowledge about the mechanisms controlling receptor site availability. Although we have begun to understand how hormones turn genes on, we do not understand how hormone-dependent gene expression is turned off. We hope that the material presented in this chapter will direct attention to new studies of this important question.

ACKNOWLEDGMENTS. The author is grateful to Dr. Kyle W. Selcer and Dr. Andrea D. Cobb for helpful discussions and assistance with the figures, and he is eternally indebted to Mrs. Constance Leavitt for the skillful preparation of the manuscript. Studies from the author's laboratory were supported by NIH grant HD18712 and NSF grant DCB8502702.

3. References

Alberts, B., Bray, D., Lewis J., Raff, M., Roberts K., and Watson, J. D., 1983, *Molecular Biology of the Cell,* Garland Publishing, New York, London.

Alexander, R. B., Greene, G. L., and Barrack, E. R., 1987, Estrogen receptors in the nuclear matrix: Direct demonstration using monoclonal antireceptor antibody, *Endocrinology* **120**:1851–1857.

Anderson, J. N., Clark, J. H., and Peck, E. J., Jr., 1972, Oestrogen and nuclear binding sites: Determination of specific sites by [³H]-oestradiol exchange, *Biochem. J.* **126**:561–567.

Anderson, J. N., Peck, E. J., Jr., and Clark, J. H., 1974, Nuclear receptor–estradiol complex: A requirement for uterotrophic responses, *Endocrinology* **95**:174–178.

Anderson, J. N., Peck, E. J., Jr., and Clark, J. H., 1975, Estrogen-induced uterine responses and growth: Relationship to receptor estrogen binding by uterine nuclei, *Endocrinology* **96**:160–167.

Anderson, W. A., Ahluwalia, B. S., Westney, L. S., Burnett, C. C., and Ruchel, R., 1984, Cervical mucus peroxidase is a reliable indicator for ovulation in humans, *Fertil. Steril.* **41**:697–702.

Astwood, E. B., 1939, An assay method for progesterone based upon the decidual cell reaction in the rat, *J. Endocrinol.* **1**:49–55.

Auricchio, F., Migliaccio, A., and Rotondi, A., 1981a, Inactivation of oestrogen receptor *in vitro* by nuclear dephosphorylation, *Biochem. J.* **194**:569–574.

Auricchio, F., Migliaccio, A., Castoria, G., Lastoria, S., and Schiavone, E., 1981b, ATP-dependent enzyme activating hormone binding of estradiol receptor, *Biochem. Biophys. Res. Commun.* **101**:1171–1178.

Bachmoir, A., Finley, D., and Varshovksy, A., 1986, *In vivo* half life of a protein is a function of its amino-terminal residue, *Science* **234**:179–186.

Bailly, A., Atger, M., Atger, P., Carbon, M.-A., Alizon, M., VuHai, M. T., Logeat, F., and Milgrom, E., 1983, The rabbit uteroglobin gene: Structure and interaction with the progesterone receptor. *J. Biol. Chem.* **258**:10384–10390.

Bailly, A., LePage, C., Rauch, M., and Milgrom, E., 1986, Sequence-specific DNA binding of the progesterone receptor to the uteroglobin gene: Effects of hormone, antihormone and receptor phosphorylation, *EMBO J.* **5**:3235–3242.

Barrack, E. R., and Coffey, D. S., 1980, The specific binding of estrogens and androgens to the nuclear matrix of sex hormone responsive tissues, *J. Biol. Chem.* **255**:7265–7275.

Barrack, E. R., and Coffey, D. S., 1983, The role of the nuclear matrix in steroid hormone action, in: *Biochemical Actions of Hormones,* Volume 10 (G. Litwack, ed.), Academic Press, New York, pp. 23–90.

Bartelmez, G. W., 1957, The phases of the menstrual cycle and their interpretation in terms of the pregnancy cycle, *Am. J. Obstet. Gynecol.* **74**:931–955.

Bazer, F. W., Vallet, J. L., Ashworth, C. J., Anthony, R. V., and Roberts, R. M., 1987, The role of ovine conceptus secretory proteins in the establishment of pregnancy, in: *Cell and Molecular Biology of the Uterus* (W. W. Leavitt, ed.), Plenum Press, New York, pp. 221–235.

Beier, H. M., 1968, Uteroglobin: A hormone-sensitive endometrial protein involved in blastocyst development, *Biochim. Biophys. Acta* **160**:289–298.

Bell, S. C., 1979, Synthesis of decidualization-associated protein in tissues of the rat uterus and placenta during pregnancy, *J. Reprod. Fertil.* **56**:255–262.

Bell, S. C., 1986, Purification of human secretory pregnancy-associated endometrial α_2-globulin (α_2-PEG) from cytosol of first trimester pregnancy endometrium, *Hum. Reprod.* **1**:313–318.

Bell, S. C., and Searle, R. F., 1981, Differentiation of decidual cells in mouse endometrial cell cultures, *J. Reprod. Fertil.* **61**:425–433.

Bell, S. C., Patel, S. R., Kirwan, P. U., and Drife, J. O., 1986, Protein synthesis and secretion by the human endometrium during the menstrual cycle and the effect of progesterone *in vitro, J. Reprod. Fertil.* **77**:221–231.

Bhakoo, H., and Katzenellenbogen, B. S., 1977, Progesterone modulation of estrogen-stimulated uterine biosynthetic events and estrogen receptor levels, *Mol. Cell. Endocrinol.* **8**:121–134.

Blaha, G. C., and Leavitt, W. W., 1978, Deciduomal responses in the uteri of ovariectomized golden hamster, comparing progesterone and three closely related steroids applied *in utero, Biol. Reprod.* **18**:441–447.

Bloom, K. S., and Anderson, J. N., 1979, Conformation of ovalbumin and globin genes in chromatin during differential gene expression, *J. Biol. Chem.* **254**:10532–10539.

Boomsma, R. A., and Verhage, H. G., 1987, Detection of a progesterone-dependent secretory protein synthesized by cat endometrium, *Biol. Reprod.* **37**:117–126.

Bullock, D. W., 1977, *In vitro* translation of messenger RNA for a uteroglobin-like protein from rabbit lung, *Biol. Reprod.* **17**:104–110.

Bullock, D. W., Lamb, D. J., Rider, V. C., and Kima, P. E., 1987, The rabbit progesterone receptor and uteroglobin gene expression, in: *Cell and Molecular Biology of the Uterus* (W. W. Leavitt, ed.), Plenum Press, New York, pp. 79–97.

Burch, J. B. E., and Weintraub, H., 1983, Temporal order of chromatin structural changes associated with activation of the major chicken vitellogenin gene, *Cell* **33**:65–76.

Butzow, R., Alfthan, H., Julkunen, M., Rutanen, E. M., Bohn, H., and Seppala, M., 1986, Human endometrium and menstrual fluid contain placental protein 5 (PP5), *Hum. Reprod.* **1**:287–289.

Cato, A. C. B., and Beato, M., 1985, The hormonal regulation of uteroglobin gene expression, *Anticancer Res.* **5**:65–82.

Cato, A. C. B., Geisse, S., Wentz, M., Westphal, H. M., and Beato, M., 1984, The nucleotide sequences recognized by the glucocorticoid receptor in the rabbit uteroglobin gene region are located far upstream from the initiation of transcription, *EMBO J.* **3**:2771–2782.

Chambon, P., Dierich, A., Gaub, M., Jokowler, S., Jongstra, J., Krust, A., LePennec, J., Oudet, P., and Reudelhuber, T., 1984, Promoter elements of genes coding for proteins and modulation of transcription by estrogen and progesterone, *Recent Prog. Horm. Res.* **40**:1–42.

Chamness, G. C., Hutt, K., and McGuire, W. L., 1975, Protamine-precipitated estrogen receptor: A solid-phase ligand exchange assay, *Steroids* **25**:627–635.

Chandler, V. L., Maler, B. A., and Yamamoto, K. R., 1983, DNA sequences bound specifically by glucocorticoid receptor *in vitro* render a heterologous promoter hormone responsive *in vivo, Cell* **33**:489–499.

Chen, T. J., and Leavitt, W. W., 1979, Nuclear progesterone receptor in the hamster uterus: Measurement by [^{3}H]progesterone exchange during the estrous cycle, *Endocrinology* **104**:1588–1597.

Chen, T. J., MacDonald, R. G., Robidoux, W. F., Jr., and Leavitt, W. W., 1981, Characterization and quantification of pyridoxal 5'-phosphate-extracted nuclear progesterone receptor, *J. Steroid Biochem.* **14**:1023–1028.

Chuknyiska, R. S., and Roth, G. S., 1985, Decreased estrogenic stimulation of RNA polymerase II in aged rat uteri is apparently due to reduced nuclear binding of receptor–estradiol complexes, *J. Biol. Chem.* **260:**8661–8663.

Clark, J. H., Hseuh, A. J. W., and Peck, E. J., Jr., 1977, Regulation of estrogen receptor replenishment by progesterone, *Ann. N.Y. Acad. Sci.* **286:**161–178.

Cobb, A., and Leavitt, W. W., 1985, Progesterone rapidly decreases the number of chromatin binding sites for nuclear estrogen receptor in the mammalian uterus, *J. Cell. Biol.* **101:**202a.

Cobb, A. D., and Leavitt, W. W., 1987a, Characterization of nuclear acceptor sites for mammalian progesterone receptor: Comparison with the chick oviduct system, *Gen. Comp. Endocrinol.* **67:**214–220.

Cobb, A. D., and Leavitt, W. W., 1987b, Characterization of nuclear binding sites for different forms of uterine progesterone receptor, *Mol. Cell. Endocrinol.* **52:**51–61.

Cockerill, P. N., and Garrard, W. T., 1986, Chromosomal loop anchorage of the kappa immunoglobulin gene occurs next to the enhancer in a region containing topoisomerase II sites, *Cell* **44:**273–282.

Cohen, M. E., and Hamilton, T. H., 1975, Effect of estradiol-17β on the synthesis of specific uterine nonhistone chromosomal proteins, *Proc. Natl. Acad. Sci. U.S.A.* **72:**4346–4350.

Compton, J. G., Schrader, W. T., and O'Malley, B. W., 1982, Selective binding of chicken progesterone receptor A subunit to a DNA fragment containing ovalbumin gene sequences, *Biochem. Biophys. Res. Commun.* **105:**96–103.

Conneely, O. M., Sullivan, W. P., Toft, D. O., Birnbaumer, M., Cook, R. G., Maxwell, B. L., Zarucki-Schulz, T., Greene, G. L., Schrader, W. T., and O'Malley, B. W., 1986, Molecular cloning of the chicken progesterone receptor, *Science* **233:**767–770.

Cushing, C. L., Bambara, R. A., and Hilf, R., 1985, Interactions of estrogen–receptor and antiestrogen–receptor complexes with nuclei *in vitro*, *Endocrinology* **116:**2419–2430.

Daly, D. C., Maslar, I. A., and Riddick, D. H., 1983, Prolactin production during *in vitro* decidualization of proliferative endometrium, *Am. J. Obstet. Gynecol.* **145:**672–678.

Denari, J. H., Germino, N. I., and Romer, J. M., 1976, Early synthesis of uterine proteins after decidual stimulus in the pseudo-pregnant rat, *Biol. Reprod.* **15:**1–8.

DeSombre, E. R., and Kuivanen, P. C., 1985, Progestin modulation of estrogen-dependent marker protein synthesis in the endometrium, *Sem. Oncol.* **12:**6–11.

Dice, J. F., 1987, Molecular determinants of protein half-lives in eukaryotic cells, *FASEB J.* **1:**349–357.

Dickerman, H. W., and Kumar, S., 1982, The polynucleotide binding sites of estradiol receptor complexes, in: *Hormones and Cancer* (W. W. Leavitt, ed.), Plenum Press, New York, pp. 1–18.

Do, Y. S., and Leavitt, W. W., 1978, Characterization of a specific progesterone receptor in decidualized hamster uterus, *Endocrinology* **102:**443–451.

Dougherty, J. J., Puri, R. K., and Toft, D. O., 1982, Phosphorylation *in vivo* of chicken oviduct progesterone receptor, *J. Biol. Chem.* **257:**14226–14230.

Dutt, A., Tang, J., Welply, J. K., and Carson, D. D., 1986, Regulation of N-linked glycoprotein assembly in uteri by steroid hormones, *Endocrinology* **118:**661–668.

Eckert, R. L., Mullick, A., Rorke, E. A., and Katzenellenbogen, B. S., 1984, Estrogen receptor synthesis and turnover in MCF-7 breast cancer cells measured by a density shift technique, *Endocrinology* **114:**629–637.

Emerson, B. M., Lewis, C. D., and Felsenfeld, G., 1985, Interaction of specific nuclear factors with the nuclease-sensitive region of the chicken adult β-globin gene: Nature of the binding domain, *Cell* **41:**21–30.

Evans, M. I., Hager, L. J., and McKnight, G. S., 1981, A somatomedin-like peptide hormone is required during the estrogen-mediated induction of ovalbumin gene transcription, *Cell* **25:**187–193.

Evans, R. W., and Leavitt, W. W., 1980, Progesterone inhibition of uterine nuclear estrogen receptor: Dependence on RNA and protein synthesis, *Proc. Natl. Acad. Sci. U.S.A.* **77:**5856–5860.

Evans, R. W., Chen, T. J., Hendry, W. J. III, and Leavitt, W. W., 1980, Progesterone regulation of estrogen receptor in the hamster uterus during the estrous cycle, *Endocrinology* **107:**383–390.

Ferenczy, A., 1980, Regeneration of the human endometrium, in: *Progress in Surgical Pathology*, Volume 1 (C. M. Genoglio and L. M. Wolff, eds.), Masson, New York, pp. 157–177.

Finn, C. A., and Martin, L., 1974, The control of implantation, *J. Reprod. Fertil.* **39:**195–206.

Fleming, H., Blumenthal, R., and Gurpide, E., 1982, Effects of cyclic nucleotides on estradiol binding in human endometrium, *Endocrinology* **111:**1671–1677.

Flickinger, G. L., Elsner, C., Illingworth, D. V., Muerhler, E. K., and Mikhail, G., 1977, Estrogen and progesterone receptors in female genital tract of humans and monkeys, *Ann. N.Y. Acad. Sci.* **286:**180–189.

Garcia, T., Tuohima, P., Mester, J., Buchon, T., Renoir, J., and Baulieu, E., 1983, Protein kinase activity of purified components of the chicken oviduct progesterone receptor, *Biochem. Biophys. Res. Commun.* **113:**960–966.

Geier, A., Haimsohn, M., Beeny, R., and Lunenfeld, B., 1985, Physical–chemical properties of the estrogen receptor solubilized by micrococcal nuclease, *J. Steroid Biochem.* **23:**137–143.

Gilmour, S., 1981, The role of acidic proteins in gene regulation, in: *Acidic Proteins of the Nucleus* (I. L. Cameron and J. R. Jeter, Jr., eds.), Academic Press, New York, pp. 297–316.

Glasser, S. R., and Julian, J., 1986, Intermediate filament protein as a marker of uterine stromal cell decidualization, *Biol. Reprod.* **35:**463–474.

Gorski, J., Toft, D., Shyamala, G., Smith, D., and Notides, A., 1968, Hormone receptors: Studies on the interaction of estrogen with the uterus, *Recent Prog. Horm. Res.* **24:**45–80.

Gorski, J., Welshons, W., and Sakai, D., 1984, Remodeling the estrogen receptor model, *Mol. Cell. Endocrinol.* **36:**11–15.

Gorski, J., Welshons, W., Sakai, D., Hansen, J., Walent, J., Kassis, J., Shull, J., Stack, G., and Campen, C., 1986, Evolution of a model of estrogen action, *Recent Prog. Horm. Res.* **42:**297–329.

Gravanis, A., and Gurpide, E., 1986, Enucleation of human endometrial cells: Nucleo-cytoplasmic distribution of DNA polymerase α and estrogen receptor, *J. Steroid Biochem.* **24:**469–474.

Gray, G. O., Rundle, S., and Leavitt, W. W., 1987, Purification and partial characterization of a corticosteroid-binding globulin from hamster serum, *Biochim. Biophys. Acta* **926:**40–53.

Green, S., and Chambon, P., 1986, A superfamily of potentially oncogenic hormone receptors, *Nature* **324:**615–617.

Green, S., Walter, P., Kumar, V., Krust, A., Bornert, J. M., Argos, P., and Chambon, P., 1986, Human oestrogen receptor cDNA: Sequence, expression and homology of v-*erb*-A, *Nature* **320:**134–139.

Greene, G. L., 1984, Application of immunochemical techniques to the analysis of estrogen receptor structure and function, in: *Biochemical Actions of Hormones,* Volume 11 (G. Litwack, ed.), Academic Press, New York, pp. 207–239.

Greene, G. L., and Jensen, E. V., 1982, Monoclonal antibodies as probes for estrogen receptor detection and characterization, *J. Steroid Biochem.* **16:**353–359.

Greene, G. L., Gilna, P., Waterfield, M., Baker, A., Hort, Y., and Shine, J., 1986, Sequence and expression of human estrogen receptor complementary DNA, *Science* **231:**1150–1154.

Grody, W. W., Schrader, W. T., and O'Malley, B. W., 1982, Activation, transformation, and subunit structure of steroid hormone receptors, *Endocrine Rev.* **3:**141–163.

Hansen, J. C., and Gorski, J., 1985, Conformational and electrostatic properties of unoccupied and liganded estrogen receptors determined by aqueous two-phase partitioning, *Biochemistry* **24:** 6078–6085.

Hansen, J. C., and Gorski, J., 1986, Conformational transitions of the estrogen receptor monomer, *J. Biol. Chem.* **261:**13990–13996.

Harper, M. J. K., 1970, Hormonal control of the deciduomal response of the golden hamster uterus, *Anat. Rec.* **167:**225–230.

Hau, J. (ed.), 1986, *Pregnancy Proteins in Animals,* Walter de Gruyter, Berlin.

Heffner, L. J., Iddenden, D. A., and Lyttle, C. R., 1986, Electrophoretic analyses of secreted human endometrial proteins: Identification and characterization of luteal phase prolactin, *J. Clin. Endocrinol. Metab.* **62:**1288–1295.

Heins, B., and Beato, M., 1981, Hormonal control of uteroglobin secretion and preuteroglobin mRNA content in rabbit endometrium, *Mol. Cell. Endocrinol.* **21:**139–148.

Hochner-Celniker, R. D., Rop, M., Eldor, A., Segal, S., Polti, Z., Fuks, Z., and Vodlavsky, I., 1984, Growth characteristics of human first trimester decidual cells cultured in serum-free medium: Production of prolactin, prostaglandins and fibronectin, *Biol. Reprod.* **31:**827–836.

Horton, M. J., and Szego, C. M., 1984, Chromatin proteins of rat preputial-gland: Acute changes in response to estrogen, *Int. J. Biochem.* **16:**447–460.

Horwitz, K. B., and McGuire, W. L., 1978a, Actinomyocin D prevents nuclear processing of estrogen receptor, *J. Biol. Chem.* **253:**6319–6322.

Horwitz, K. B., and McGuire, W. L., 1978b, Nuclear mechanisms of estrogen action: Effects of estradiol and anti-estrogens on estrogen receptors in nuclear processing, *J. Biol. Chem.* **253:**8185–8191.

Horwitz, K. B., and McGuire, W. L., 1980, Nuclear estrogen receptors. Effects of inhibitors on processing and steady state levels, *J. Biol. Chem.* **255:**9699–9705.

Horwitz, K. B., Wei, L., Selacek, S. M., and D'Arville, C. N., 1985, Progestin action and progesterone receptor structure in human breast cancer: A review, *Recent Prog. Horm. Res.* **41:**249–316.

Hryb, D. J., Khan, M. S., Romas, N. A., and Rosner, W., 1986, Specific binding of human corticosteroid-binding globulin to cell membranes, *Proc. Natl. Acad. Sci. U.S.A.* **83:**3253–56.

Hseuh, A. J. W., Peck, E. J., Jr., and Clark, J. H., 1976, Control of uterine estrogen receptor levels by progesterone, *Endocrinology* **98:**438–444.

Huhtala, M. L., Kalkkinen, N., Palomaki, P., Julkunen, M., Bohn, H., and Seppala, M., 1986, XIV Annual Meeting of International Society for Oncodevelopment, *Biol. Med. Abstr.* 96.

Huhtala, M. L., Seppala, M., Narvanen, A., Palomaki, P., Julkunen, M., and Bohn, H., 1987, Amino acid sequence homology between human placental protein 14 and β-lactoglobulins from various species, *Endocrinology* **120:**2620–2622.

Imakawa, K., Anthony, R. V., Niwano, Y., Hansen, T., Kazemi, M., Polites, H. G., Marotti, K. R., and Roberts, R. M., 1987, Ovine trophoblast protein-1 (oTP-1), a polypeptide implicated in mediating maternal recognition of pregnancy in sheep, is an interferon of the alpha class, *J. Cell Biol.* **105:**11a.

Isomaa, V., Isotalo, H., Orava, M., Torkkeli, T., and Janne, O., 1979, Changes in cytosol and nuclear progesterone receptor concentrations in the rabbit uterus and their relation to induction of progesterone-related uteroglobin, *Biochem. Biophys. Res. Commun.* **88:**1237–1304.

Isotalo, H., 1983, Regulation of uteroglobin synthesis and conservation of progesterone and estrogen receptors in immature rabbit uterus during prolonged progesterone treatment, *Biochem. Biophys. Res. Commun.* **115:**1015–1022.

Jacobs, M. H., and Lyttle, C. R., 1987, Uterine media proteins in the rat during gestation, *Biol. Reprod.* **36:**157–165.

Jakesz, R., Kasid, A., Greene, G., and Lippman, M. E., 1983, Characteristics of different cytoplasmic and nuclear estrogen receptors appearing with continuous hormonal exposure, *J. Biol. Chem.* **258:**11807–11813.

Jensen, E. V., 1979, Interaction of steroid hormones with the nucleus, *Pharmacol. Rev.* **30:**477–491.

Jensen, E. V., Suzuki, T., Kawashima, T., Stumpf, W. E., Jungblut, P. W., and DeSombre, E., 1968, A two-step mechanism for the interaction of estradiol with rat uterus, *Proc. Natl. Acad. Sci. U.S.A.* **59:**632–638.

Joshi, S. G., 1983, A progestagen-associated protein of the human endometrium: Basic studies and potential clinical applications, *J. Steroid Biochem.* **19:**751–757.

Joshi, S. G., 1987, Progestin-dependent human endometrial protein: A marker for monitoring human endometrial function, in: *Cell and Molecular Biology of the Uterus* (W. W. Leavitt, ed.), Plenum Press, New York, pp. 167–186.

Joshi, S. G., Ebert, K. M., and Smith, R. A., 1980, Properties of the progestagen-dependent protein of the human endometrium, *J. Reprod. Fertil.* **59:**287–296.

Joshi, S. G., Rao, R., Henriques, E. E., Raiker, R. S., and Gordon, M., 1986, Luteal phase concentrations of a progestagen-associated endometrial protein (PEP) in the serum of cycling women with adequate or inadequate endometrium, *J. Clin. Endocrinol. Metab.* **65:**1247–1249.

Jost, J., Seldran, M., and Geiser, M., 1984, Preferential binding of the estrogen–receptor complex to a region containing the estrogen-dependent hypomethylation site preceding the chicken vitellogenin II gene, *Proc. Natl. Acad. Sci. U.S.A.* **81:**429–433.

Jost, J., Geiser, M., and Seldran, M., 1985, Specific modulation of the transcription of cloned avian vitellogenin II gene by estradiol–receptor complex *in vitro*, *Proc. Natl. Acad. Sci. U.S.A.* **82:**988–991.

Julkunen, M., Apter, D., Seppala, M., Stenman, U. H., and Bohn, H., 1986a, Serum levels of placental protein 14 reflect ovulation in nonconceptional menstrual cycles, *Fertil. Steril.* **45:**47–50.

Julkunen, M., Raikar, R. S., Joshi, S. G., Bohn, H., and Seppala, M., 1986b, Placental protein 14 and progestagen-dependent endometrial protein are immunologically indistinguishable, *Hum. Reprod.* **1:**7–8.

Julkunen, M., Wahlstrom, T., and Seppala, M., 1986c, Human fallopian tube contains placental protein 14, *Am. J. Obstet. Gynecol.* **154:**1076–1079.

Karin, M., Eberhardt, N. L., Mellon, S. H., Malich, N., Richards, R. I., Slater, E. P., Barta, A., Martial, J. A., Baxter, J. D., and Cathala, G., 1984a, Expression and hormonal regulation of the rat growth hormone gene in transfected mouse L cells, *DNA* **3:**147–155.

Karin, M., Haslinger, A., Holtgreve, H., Richards, R. I., Krauter, P., Westphal, H. M., and Beato, M., 1984b, Characterization of DNA sequences through which cadmium and glucocorticoid hormones induce human metallothionein-II$_A$ gene, *Nature* **308:**513–519.

Kasid, A., Huff, K., Greene, G. L., and Lippman, M. E., 1984, A novel nuclear form of estradiol receptor in MCF-7 human breast cancer cells, *Science* **225:**1162–1165.

Katzenellenbogen, B. S., 1980, Dynamics of steroid hormone receptor action, *Annu. Rev. Physiol.* **42:**17–35.

Kaye, A. M., and Reiss, N., 1980, The uterine estrogen induced protein (IP): Purification, distribution and possible function, in: *Steroid Induced Uterine Proteins* (M. Beato, ed.), Elsevier, New York, pp. 3–19.

Kearns, M., and Lala, P. K., 1982, Bone marrow origin of decidual cell precursors in the pseudopregnant mouse uterus, *J. Exp. Med.* **155:**1537–1554.

Keller, R. K., Socher, S. H., Krall, J. F., Chandra, T., and O'Malley, B. W., 1975, Fractionation of chick oviduct chromatin: IV. Association of protein kinase with transcriptionally active chromatin, *Biochem. Biophys. Res. Commun.* **66:**453–459.

Khan, M. S., Aden, D., and Rosner, W., 1984, Human corticosteroid binding globulin is secreted by a hepatoma-derived cell line, *J. Steroid Biochem.* **20**:677–78.

King, W. J., and Greene, G. L., 1984, Monoclonal antibodies localize oestrogen receptor in the nuclei of target cells, *Nature* **307**:745–747.

Kisalus, L. L., Nunley, W. C., and Herr, J. C., 1987, Protein synthesis and secretion in human decidua of early pregnancy, *Biol. Reprod.* **36**:785–789.

Kneifel, M. A., Leytus, S. P., Fletcher, E., Weber, T., Mangel, W. F., and Katzenellenbogen, B. S., 1982, Uterine plasminogen activator activity: Modulation by steroid hormones, *Endocrinology* **111**:493–501.

Knobil, E., 1980, The neuroendocrine control of the menstrual cycle, *Recent Prog. Horm. Res.* **36**:53–88.

Koistinen, R., Kalkkinen, N., Huhtala, M. L., Seppala, M., Bohn, H., and Rutanen, E. M., 1986, Placental protein 12 is a decidual protein that binds somatomedin and has identical N-terminal amino acid sequence with somatomedin-binding protein from human amniotic fluid, *Endocrinology* **118**:1375–1378.

Komm, B. S., Keeping, H. S., Sabogal, G., and Lyttle, C. R., 1985, Comparison of media proteins from ovariectomized rat uteri following estrogen treatment, *Biol. Reprod.* **32**:443–450.

Komm, B. S., Rusling, D. J., and Lyttle, C. R., 1986, Estrogen regulation of protein synthesis in the immature rat uterus: The analysis of proteins released into the medium during *in vitro* incubation, *Endocrinology* **118**:2411–2416.

Kon, O. L., and Spelsberg, T. C., 1982, Nuclear binding of estrogen receptor complex: Receptor specific nuclear acceptor sites, *Endocrinology* **111**:1925–1934.

Krishnan, R. S., and Daniel, J. C., Jr., 1967, "Blastokinin": Inducer and regulator of blastocyst development in the rabbit uterus, *Science* **158**:490–492.

Kuhn, R. W., Green, A. L., Raymoure, W. J., and Siiteri, P. K., 1986, Immunocytochemical localization of corticosteroid-binding globulin in rat tissues, *J. Endocrinol.* **108**:31–36.

Lai, E. C., Riser, M. E., and O'Malley, B. W., 1983, Regulated expression of the chicken ovalbumin gene in a human estrogen-responsive cell line, *J. Biol. Chem.* **258**:12693–12701.

Leavitt, W. W., 1985a, Progesterone regulation of nuclear estrogen receptors: Evidence for a receptor regulatory factor, in: *Molecular Mechanism of Steroid Hormone Action* (V. K. Moudgil, ed.), Walter de Gruyter, Berlin, pp. 437–470.

Leavitt, W. W., 1985b, Hormonal regulation of myometrial estrogen, progesterone and oxytocin receptors in the pregnant and pseudopregnant hamster, *Endocrinology* **116**:1079–1084.

Leavitt, W. W., 1985c, Gene regulation by progesterone, in: *Handbook on Receptor Research* (F. Auricchio, ed.), Field Educational Italia Acta Medica, Rome, pp. 179–209.

Leavitt, W. W., and Okulicz, W. C., 1985a, Occupied and unoccupied estrogen receptor during the estrous cycle and pregnancy, *Am. J. Physiol.* **249**:E589–E594.

Leavitt, W. W., and Okulicz, W. C., 1985b, Progesterone control of nuclear estrogen receptor: Demonstration in hamster uterus during the estrous cycle and pseudopregnancy using a new exchange assay, *J. Steroid Biochem.* **22**:583–588.

Leavitt, W. W., and Takeda, A., 1986, Hormonal regulation of estrogen and progesterone receptors in hamster decidual cells, *Biol. Reprod.* **35**:475–484.

Leavitt, W. W., Toft, D. O., Strott, C. A., and O'Malley, B. W., 1974, A specific progesterone receptor in the hamster uterus: Physiologic properties and regulation during the estrous cycle, *Endocrinology* **94**:1041–1053.

Leavitt, W. W., Chen, T. J., Allen, T. C., and Johnston, J. O., 1977, Regulation of progesterone receptor formation by estrogen action, *Ann. N.Y. Acad. Sci.* **286**:210–225.

Leavitt, W. W., Chen, T. J., Do, Y. S., Carlton, B. D., and Allen, T. C., 1978, Biology of progesterone receptors, in: *Receptors and Hormone Action,* Volume 2, (B. W. O'Malley and L. Birnbaumer, eds.), Academic Press, New York, pp. 157–188.

Leavitt, W. W., Chen, T. J., and Evans, R. W., 1979, Regulation and function of estrogen and progesterone receptor systems, in: *Steroid Hormone Receptor Systems* (W. W. Leavitt and J. H. Clark, eds.), Plenum Press, New York, pp. 197–222.

Leavitt, W. W., MacDonald, R. G., and Okulicz, W. C., 1983, Hormonal regulation of estrogen and progesterone receptor systems, in: *Biochemical actions of Hormones,* Volume 10 (G. Litwack, ed.), Academic Press, New York, pp. 323–356.

Leavitt, W. W., MacDonald, R. C., and Shwaery, G. T., 1985a, Characterization of deciduoma marker proteins in hamster uterus: Detection in decidual cell cultures, *Biol. Reprod.* **32**:631–643.

Leavitt, W. W., Okulicz, W. C., McCracken, J. A., Schramm, W., and Robidoux, W. F., 1985b, Rapid recovery of nuclear estrogen receptor and oxytocin receptor in the ovine uterus following progesterone withdrawal, *J. Steroid Biochem.* **22**:687–691.

Leavitt, W. W., Takeda, A., and MacDonald, R. G., 1986, Progesterone regulation of protein synthesis and steroid receptor levels in decidual cells, *Ann. N.Y. Acad. Sci.* **476**:136–157.

Leavitt, W. W., Rundle, S., Thompson, K., Selcer, K. W., and Gray, G. O., 1987, Decidual cell function: Evidence for a role in the regulation of serum CBG and a 60Kda protein during early pregnancy in the hamster, in: *Cell and Molecular Biology of the Uterus* (W. W. Leavitt, ed.), Plenum Press, New York, pp. 187–205.

Lejeune, B., Lecocq, R., Lamy, F., and Leroy, F., 1982, Changes in the pattern of endometrial protein synthesis during decidualization in the rat, *J. Reprod. Fertil.* **66**:519–523.

Lejeune, B., Lamy, F., Lecocq, R., Deschacht, J., and Leroy, F., 1985, Patterns of protein synthesis in endometrial tissues from ovariectomized rats treated with oestradiol and progesterone, *J. Reprod. Fertil.* **73**:223–228.

Libby, P. R., 1972, Histone acetylation and hormone action: Early effects of oestradiol-17β on histone acetylation in rat uterus, *Biochem. J.* **130**:663–669.

Lin, S.-Y., and Riggs, A. D., 1975, The general affinity of *lac* repressor for *E. coli* DNA: Implications for gene regulation in procaryotes and eucaryotes, *Cell* **4**:107–111.

Logeat, F., VuHai, M. T., and Milgrom, E., 1981, Antibodies to rabbit progesterone receptor: Crossreaction with human receptor, *Proc. Natl. Acad. Sci. U.S.A.* **78**:1426–1430.

Logeat, F., VuHai, M. T., Fournier, A., Legrain, P., Buttin, C., and Milgrom, E., 1983, Monoclonal antibodies to rabbit progesterone receptor: Crossreaction with other mammalian progesterone receptors, *Proc. Natl. Acad. Sci. U.S.A.* **80**:6456–6460.

Logeat, F., LeCunff, M., Pamphile, P., and Milgrom, E., 1985a, The nuclear-bound form of the progesterone receptor is generated through a hormone-dependent phosphorylation, *Biochem. Biophys. Res. Commun.* **131**:421–428.

Logeat, F., Pamphile, R., Loosfelt, H., Jolivet, A., Fournier, A., and Milgrom, E., 1985b, One-step immunoaffinity purification of active progesterone receptor. Further evidence in favor of the existence of a single steroid-binding subunit, *Biochemistry* **24**:1029–1037.

Lombardero, M., and Nieto, A., 1981, Glucocorticoid and developmental regulation of uteroglobin synthesis in rabbit lung, *Biochem. J.* **200**:487–498.

Loosfelt, H., Fridlansky, F., Atger, M., and Milgrom, E., 1981a, A possible non-transcriptional effect of progesterone, *J. Steroid Biochem.* **15**:107–113.

Loosfelt, H., Fridlansky, F., Savouret, J.-F., Atger, M., and Milgrom, E., 1981b, Mechanism of action of progesterone in the rabbit endometrium: Induction of uteroglobin and its messenger RNA, *J. Biol. Chem.* **256**:3465–3471.

Loosfelt, H., Logeat, F., VuHai, M. T., and Milgrom, E., 1984, The rabbit progesterone receptor. Evidence for a single steroid-binding subunit and characterization of receptor mRNA, *J. Biol. Chem.* **259**:14196–14201.

Loosfelt, H., Atger, M., Misrahi, M., Guischon-Mantel, A., Meriel, C., Logeat, F., Benarous, R., and Milgrom, E., 1986, Cloning and sequence analysis of rabbit progesterone-receptor complementary DNA, *Proc. Natl. Acad. Sci. U.S.A.* **83**:9045–9049.

Lyttle, C. R., and DeSombre, E. R., 1979, Uterine peroxidase as a marker for estrogen action, *Proc. Natl. Acad. Sci. U.S.A.* **74**:3162–3166.

Lyttle, C. R., Wheeler, C., and Komm, B. S., 1987, Hormonal regulation of rat uterine secretory protein synthesis, in: *Cell and Molecular Biology of the Uterus* (W. W. Leavitt, ed.), Plenum Press, New York, pp. 119–136.

MacDonald, R. G., Okulicz, W. C., and Leavitt, W. W., 1982, Progesterone-induced inactivation of nuclear estrogen receptor in hamster uterus is mediated by acid phosphatase, *Biochem. Biophys. Res. Commun.* **104**:570–576.

MacDonald, R. G., Morency, K. O., and Leavitt, W. W., 1983a, Progesterone modulation of specific protein synthesis in the decidualized hamster uterus, *Biol. Reprod.* **28**:753–766.

MacDonald, R. G., Rosenberg, S. P., and Leavitt, W. W., 1983b, Localization of estrogen receptor-regulatory factor in the uterine nucleus, *Mol. Cell. Endocrinol.* **32**:301–313.

MacLaughlin, D. T., Santoro, N. F., Bauer, H. H., Lawrence, D., and Richardson, G. S., 1986, Two-dimensional gel electrophoresis of endometrial protein in human uterine fluids: Qualitative and quantitative analysis, *Biol. Reprod.* **34**:579–585.

MacLaughlin, D. T., Richardson, G. S., Santoro, N. F., Hargraves, A. A., and Bauer, H. H., 1987, Analysis of proteins secreted by the human endometrium *in vivo* and *in vitro*, in: *Cell and Molecular Biology of the Uterus* (W. W. Leavitt, ed.), Plenum Press, New York, pp. 151–165.

Martin, B. R., 1987, *Metabolic Regulation: A Molecular Approach*, Blackwell Scientific, Palo Alto, CA.

Martin, L., Finn, C. A., and Trinder, G., 1983, Hypertrophy and hyperplasia in the mouse uterus after oestrogen treatment. An autoradiographic study, *J. Endocrinol.* **56**:133–144.

Maurer, R. A., 1985, Selective binding of the estradiol receptor to a region at least one kilobase upstream from the rat prolactin gene, *DNA* **4:**1–9.

Maxwell, B. L., McDonnell, D. P., Conneely, O. M., Schulz, T. Z., Greene, G. L., and O'Malley, B. W., 1987, Structural organization and regulation of the chicken estrogen receptor, *Mol. Endocrinol.* **1:**25–35.

McClellan, M. C., West, N. B., Tacha, D. E., Greene, G. L., and Brenner, R. M., 1984, Immunocytochemical localization of estrogen receptors in the macaque reproductive tract with monoclonal antiestrophilins, *Endocrinology* **114:**2002–2014.

McCormack, S. A., and Glasser, S. R., 1980, Differential response of individual uterine cell types from immature rats treated with estradiol, *Endocrinology* **106:**1634–1649.

Midgley, A. R., Jr., Gay, V. L., Keyes, P. L., and Hunter, J. S., 1973, Human reproductive endocrinology, in: *Human Reproduction* (E. S. E. Hafez and T. N. Evans, eds.), Harper & Row, New York, pp. 201–236.

Migliaccio, A., Lastoria, S., Moncharmont, B., Rotondi, A., and Auricchio, F., 1982, Phosphorylation of calf uterus, estradiol receptor by endogenous Ca^{++}-stimulated kinase activating the hormone binding of the receptor, *Biochem. Biophys. Res. Commun.* **109:**1002–1010.

Migliaccio, A., Rotondi, A., and Auricchio, F., 1984, Calmodulin-stimulated phosphorylation of 17β-estradiol receptor on tyrosine, *Proc. Natl. Acad. Sci. U.S.A.* **81:**5921–5925.

Milgrom, E., LuuThi, M. T., Atger, M., and Baulieu, E. E., 1973, Mechanisms regulating the concentration and the conformation of progesterone receptor(s) in the uterus, *J. Biol. Chem.* **248:**6366–6374.

Milgrom, E., 1981, Activation of steroid receptor complexes, in: *Biochemical Actions of Hormones,* Volume 8 (G. Litwack, ed.), Academic Press, New York, pp. 465–492.

Monsma, F. J., Jr., Katzenellenbogen, B. S., Miller, M. A., Ziegler, Y. S., and Katzenellenbogen, J. A., 1984, Characterization of the estrogen receptor and its dynamics in MCF-7 human breast cancer cells using a covalently attaching antiestrogen, *Endocrinology* **115:**143–153.

Moudgil, V. K., and Eessalu, T. E., 1980, Activation of estradiol–receptor complex by ATP *in vitro,* FEBS Lett. **122:**189–192.

Mukku, V. R., and Stancel, G. M., 1985, Regulation of epidermal growth factor receptor by estrogen, *J. Biol. Chem.* **260:**9820–9824.

Muller, H., and Beato, M., 1980, RNA synthesis in rabbit endometrial nuclei. Hormonal regulation of transcription of the uteroglobin gene, *Eur. J. Biochem.* **112:**235–245.

Mulvihill, E. R., and Palmiter, R. D., 1977, Relationship of nuclear estrogen receptor levels to induction of ovalbumin and conalbumin mRNA in chick oviduct, *J. Biol. Chem.* **252:**2060–2068.

Mulvihill, E. R., and Palmiter, R. D., 1980, Relationship of nuclear progesterone receptors to induction of ovalbumin and conalbumin mRNA in chick oviduct, *J. Biol. Chem.* **255:**2085–2092.

Mulvihill, E. R., LePennec, J. P., and Chambon, P., 1982, Chicken oviduct progesterone receptor: Location of specific regions of high-affinity binding in cloned DNA fragments of hormone-responsive genes, *Cell* **28:**621–632.

Murphy, L. J., Murphy, L. C., and Friesen, H. G., 1987a, Estrogen induction of N-*myc* and c-*myc* proto-oncogene expression in the rat uterus, *Endocrinology* **120:**1882–1888.

Murphy, L. J., Murphy, L. C., and Friesen, H. C., 1987b, Estrogen induces insulin-like growth factor-1 expression in the rat uterus, *Mol. Endocrinol.* **1:**445–450.

Murray, M. K., Verhage, H. G., Buhi, W. C., and Jaffe, R. C., 1985, The detection and purification of a cat uterine secretory protein that is estrogen dependent (CUPED), *Biol. Reprod.* **32:**1219–1225.

Neulen, J., Beato, M., and Beier, H. M., 1982, Cytosol and nuclear progesterone-receptor concentrations in the rabbit endometrium during early pseudopregnancy under different treatments with estradiol and progesterone, *Mol. Cell. Endocrinol.* **25:**183–193.

Nieder, G. L., Weitlauf, H. M., and Suda-Hartman, M., 1987, Synthesis and secretion of stage-specific proteins by peri-implantation mouse embryos, *Biol. Reprod.* **36:**687–699.

Norman, A. W., and Litwack, G., 1987, *Hormones,* Academic Press, Orlando, FL.

Notides, A. C., Lerner, N., and Hamilton, D. E., 1981, Positive cooperativity of the estrogen receptor, *Proc. Natl. Acad. Sci. U.S.A.* **78:**4926–4930.

Notides, A. C., Susson, S., and Callison, S., 1985, An allosteric regulatory mechanism for estrogen receptor activation, in: *Molecular Mechanisms of Steroid Hormone Action* (V. K. Moudgil, ed.), Walter de Gruyter, New York, pp. 173–197.

Noyes, R. W., Hertig, A. T., and Rock, J., 1950, Dating the endometrial biopsy, *Fertil. Steril.* **1:**3–25.

O'Farrell, P. H., 1975, High resolution two-dimensional electrophoresis of proteins, *J. Biol. Chem.* **250:**4007–4021.

Okulicz, W. C., Evans, R. W., and Leavitt, W. W., 1981a, Progesterone regulation of the occupied form of nuclear estrogen receptor, *Science* **213:**1503–1505.

Okulicz, W. C., Evans, R. W., and Leavitt, W. W., 1981b, Progesterone regulation of estrogen receptor in the rat uterus. A primary inhibitory influence on the nuclear fraction, *Steroids* **37**:463–470.

Okulicz, W. C., MacDonald, R. G., and Leavitt, W. W., 1981c, Progesterone-induced estrogen receptor-regulatory factor in hamster uterine nuclei: Preliminary characterization in a cell-free system, *Endocrinology* **109**:2273–2275.

Okulicz, W. C., Boomsma, R. A., MacDonald, R. G., and Leavitt, W. W., 1983, Conditions for the measurement of nuclear estrogen receptor at low temperature, *Biochim. Biophys. Acta* **757**:128–136.

O'Malley, B. W., and Means, A. R., 1974, Female steroid hormones and target cell nuclei, *Science* **183**:610–620.

O'Malley, B. W., Roop, D. R., Lai, E. D., Nordstrom, J. L., Catterall, J. F., Swaneck, G. E., Colbert, D. A., Tsai, M. J., Dugaiczyk, A., and Woo, S. L. C., 1979, The ovalbumin gene: Organization, structure, transcription and regulation, *Recent Prog. Horm. Res.* **35**:1–146.

O'Malley, B. W., Tsai, M. J., and Schrader, W. T., 1983, Structural considerations for the action of steroid hormones in eucaryotic cells, in: *Steroid Hormone Receptors* (H. Ericksson and J. Gustafsson, eds.), Elsevier, New York, pp. 307–328.

Padykula, H. A., Coles, L. G., McCracken, J. A., King, N. W., Jr., Longcope, C., and Kaiserman-Abramof, I. R., 1984, A zonal pattern of cell proliferation and differentiation in the rhesus endometrium during the estrogen surge, *Biol. Reprod.* **32**:1103–1118.

Pasqualini, J. R., Cosquer-Clavreul, C., Vidali, G., and Allfrey, V. G., 1981, Effects of estradiol on the acetylation of histones in the fetal uterus of the guinea pig, *Biol. Reprod.* **25**:1035–1039.

Payvar, F., DeFranco, D. G., Firestone, L., Edgar, B., Wrange, D., Okret, S., Gustafsson, J.-A., and Yamamoto, K. R., 1983, Sequence-specific binding of glucocorticoid receptor to MMTV DNA at sites within and upstream of the transcribed region, *Cell* **35**:381–392.

Perrot-Applanat, M., Racadot, O., and Milgrom, E., 1984, Specific localization of plasma corticosteroid-binding globulin immunoreactivity in pituitary corticotrophs, *Endocrinology* **115**:559–569.

Puca, G. A., Nola, E., Hibner, V., Cicala, G., and Sica, V., 1975, Interaction of the estradiol receptor from calf uterus with its nuclear acceptor sites, *J. Biol. Chem.* **250**:6452–6459.

Quarmby, V. E., and Korach, K. S., 1984, Differential regulation of protein synthesis by estradiol in uterine component tissues, *Endocrinology* **115**:687–697.

Rahman, S. S., Billiar, R. B., and Little, B., 1981, Studies on the decline of uteroglobin synthesis and secretion in the rabbit uterus during the continued presence of circulating progesterone, *Endocrinology* **108**:2222–2230.

Reiss, N. A., and Kaye, A. M., 1981, Identification of the major component of the oestrogen-induced protein of the rat uterus as the BB isozyme of creatine kinase, *J. Biol. Chem.* **256**:5741–5747.

Renkawitz, R., Schutz, G., von der Ahe, D., and Beato, M., 1984, Sequences in the promoter region of the chicken lysozyme gene required for steroid regulation and receptor binding, *Cell* **37**:503–510.

Ricketts, A. P., Hagensee, M., and Bullock, D. W., 1983, Characterization in primary monolayer culture of separated cell types from rabbit endometrium, *J. Reprod. Fertil.* **67**:151–162.

Robel, P., Martel, R., and Baulieu, E. E., 1981, Estradiol and progesterone receptors in human endometrium, in: *Biochemical Actions of Hormones,* Volume 8 (G. Litwack, ed.), Academic Press, New York, pp. 493–514.

Roberts, R. M., Raub, T. J., and Bazer, F. W., 1986, Role of uteroferrin in transplacental iron transport in the pig, *Fed. Proc.* **45**:2513–2518.

Roberts, R. M., Murray, M. K., Burke, M. G., Ketcham, C. M., and Bazer, F. W., 1987, Hormonal control and function of secretory proteins, in: *Cell and Molecular Biology of the Uterus* (W. W. Leavitt, ed.), Plenum Press, New York, pp. 137–150.

Rogers, S., Wells, R., and Rechsteiner, M., 1986, Amino acid sequences common to rapidly degraded proteins: The PEST hypothesis, *Science* **234**:364–368.

Ross, P., Jr., and Ruh, T. S., 1984, Binding of the estradiol–receptor complex to reconstituted nucleoacidic protein from calf uterus, *Biochim. Biophys. Acta* **782**:18–25.

Ruh, T. S., and Spelsberg, T. C., 1983, Acceptor sites for the oestrogen receptor in hen oviduct chromatin, *Biochem. J.* **210**:905–912.

Rutanen, E. M., Koistinen, R., Sjoberg, J., Julkunen, M., Wahlstrom, T., Bohn, H., and Seppala, M., 1986, Synthesis of placental protein 12 by human endometrium, *Endocrinology* **118**:1067–1071.

Sakai, D., and Gorski, J., 1984, Estrogen receptor transformation to a high-affinity state without subunit–subunit interactions, *J. Biochem.* **23**:3541–3547.

Sananes, N., Weiller, S., Baulieu, E. E., and Le Goascogne, C., 1978, *In vitro* decidualization of rat endometrial cells, *Endocrinology* **103**:86–95.

Savouret, J.-F., and Milgrom, E., 1983, Uteroglobin: A model for the study of progesterone action in mammals, *DNA* **2**:99–107.

Savouret, J.-F., Loosfelt, H., Atger, M., and Milgrom, E., 1980, Differential hormonal control of a messenger RNA in two tissues: Uteroglobin mRNA in the lung and the endometrium, *J. Biol. Chem.* **255:** 4131–4136.

Scatchard, G., 1949, The attractions of proteins for small molecules and ions, *Ann. N.Y. Acad. Sci.* **51:**660–672.

Schimke, R. T., 1975, Methods for analysis of enzyme synthesis and degradation in animal tissues, in: *Methods in Enzymology,* Volume XL (B. W. O'Malley and J. G. Hardman, eds.), Academic Press, New York, pp. 241–266.

Schrader, W. T., and O'Malley, B. W., 1978, Molecular structure and analysis of progesterone receptors, in: *Receptors and Hormone Action,* Volume 2 (B. W. O'Malley and L. Birnbaumer, eds.), Academic Press, New York, pp. 189–224.

Schrader, W. T., Birnbaumer, M. E., Hughes, M. R., Weigel, N. L., Grody, W. W., and O'Malley, B. W., 1981, Studies on the structure and function of the chicken progesterone receptor, *Recent Prog. Horm. Res.* **37:**583–633.

Seal, U.S., and Doe, R. P., 1965, Vertebrate distribution of corticosteroid binding globulin and some endocrine effects on concentration, *Steroids* **5:**827–841.

Segal, S. J., Scher, W., and Koide, S. S., 1977, Estrogens, nucleic acids, and protein synthesis in uterine metabolism, in: *Biology of the Uterus* (R. Wynn, ed.), Plenum Press, New York, pp. 139–201.

Selcer, K. W., and Leavitt, W. W., 1987, Hamster uterine tissue concentrates CBG during decidualization, in: *Program of Annual Meeting of Endocrine Society,* The Endocrine Society, Indianapolis, p. 105.

Seppala, M., Koskimies, A. I., Tenhunen, A., Rutanen, E. M., Sjoberg, J., Koistinen, R., Julkunen, M., and Wahlstrom, T., 1985, Pregnancy proteins in seminal plasma, seminal vesicles, preovulatory follicular fluid and ovary, *Ann. N.Y. Acad. Sci.* **442:**212–226.

Seppala, M., Huhtala, M. L., Julkunen, M., Koistinen, R., and Rutanen, E. M., 1987, Uterine proteins, nomenclature determined by biological action, *Res. Reprod.* **19:**2.

Shelesnyak, M. C., 1986, A history of research on nidation, *Ann. N.Y. Acad. Sci.* **476:**5–24.

Shen, X.-Z., Tsai, M.-J., Bullock, D. W., and Woo, S. L. C., 1983, Hormonal regulation of rabbit uteroglobin gene transcription, *Endocrinology* **112:**871–876.

Sherman, M. R., and Stevens, J., 1984, Structure of mammalian steroid receptors: Evolving concepts and methodological developments, *Physiol. Rev.* **46:**83–105.

Sica, V., Weisz, A., Petrillo, A., Armetta, I., and Puca, G. A., 1981, Assay of total estradiol receptor in tissue homogenate and tissue fractions by exchange with sodium thiocyanate at low-temperature, *Biochemistry* **20:**686–693.

Siiteri, P. K., Murai, J. T., Hammond, G. L., Nisker, J. A., Raymoure, W. J., and Kuhn, R. W., 1982, The serum transport of steroid hormones, *Recent Prog. Horm. Res.* **38:** 457–510.

Singh, R. K., Ruh, M. F., Butler, W. B., and Ruh, T. S., 1986, Acceptor sites on chromatin for receptor-bound by estrogen versus antiestrogen in antiestrogen-sensitive and -resistant MCF-7 cells, *Endocrinology* **118:**1087–1095.

Sirbasku, D. L. A., and Benson, R. H., 1979, Estrogen-inducible growth factors that may act as mediators (estromedins) of estrogen promoted tumor cell growth, in: *Hormones and Cell Culture,* Volume 6, *Cold Spring Harbor Conferences on Cell Proliferation,* Cold Spring Harbor Laboratory, New York, pp. 477–497.

Sjoberg, J., Wahlstrom, T., and Seppala, M., 1984, Pregnancy-associated plasma protein-A in the human endometrium is dependent on the effect of progesterone, *J. Clin. Endocrinol. Metab.* **58:**359–362.

Skafar, D. E., and Notides, A. C., 1985, Modulation of the estrogen receptor's affinity for DNA by estradiol, *J. Biol. Chem.* **260:**12208–12215.

Skafar, D. F., and Seaver, S. S., 1985, Desensitization of the chick oviduct to estrogen: Mediation at different levels of gene expression, *Endocrinology* **116:**1755–1762.

Snead, R., Day, L., Chandra, T., Mace, M., Jr., Bullock, D. W., and Woo, S. L. C., 1981, Mosaic structure and mRNA precursors of uteroglobin, a hormone-regulated mammalian gene, *J. Biol. Chem.* **256:**11911–11918.

Spelsberg, T. C., Littlefield, B. A., Seelke, R., Martin-Dani, G., Toyoda, H., Boyd-Leinen, P., Thrall, C., and Kon, O. L., 1983, Role of specific chromosomal proteins and DNA sequences in the nuclear binding sites for steroid receptors, *Recent Prog. Horm. Res.* **39:**463–517.

Strinden, S. T., and Shapiro, S. S., 1983, Progesterone-altered secretory proteins from cultured human endometrium, *Endocrinology* **112:**862–870.

Sullivan, D. A., Richardson, G. S., MacLaughlin, D. T., and Wira, C. R., 1984, Variations in the levels of secretory component in human uterine fluid during the menstrual cycle, *J. Steroid Biochem.* **20:**509–514.

Sullivan, W. P., Beito, T. G., Proper, J., Krco, C. J., and Toft, D. O., 1986, Preparation of monoclonal antibodies to the avian progesterone receptor, *Endocrinology* **119:**1549–1557.

Surani, M. A. H., 1975, Hormonal regulation of proteins in the uterine secretion of ovariectomized rats and the implications for implantation and embryonic diapause, *J. Reprod. Fertil.* **43**:411–417.

Surani, M. A. H., 1976, Uterine luminal proteins at the time of implantation in rats, *J. Reprod. Fertil.* **48**:141–145.

Surani, M. A. H., 1977, Radiolabeled rat uterine luminal proteins and their regulation by oestradiol and progesterone, *J. Reprod. Fertil.* **50**:289–296.

Suske, G., Wenz, M., Cato, A. C. B., and Beato, M., 1983, The uteroglobin gene region: Hormonal regulation, repetitive elements and complete nucleotide sequence, *Nucleic Acids Res.* **11**:2257–2264.

Takeda, A., and Leavitt, W. W., 1986, Progestin-induced down regulation of nuclear estrogen receptor in uterine decidual cells: Analysis of receptor synthesis and turnover by the density-shift method, *Biochem. Biophys. Res. Commun.* **135**:95–104.

Taylor, R. N., and Smith, R. G., 1981, Effects of highly purified estrogen receptors on gene transcription in isolated nuclei, *Biochemistry* **21**:1781–1787.

Thomas, T., and Leung, B. S., 1984, Characterization of nuclear estradiol receptors released by micrococcal nuclease and deoxyribonuclease I, *J. Steroid Biochem.* **21**:35–42.

Torkkeli, T., 1980, Early changes in rabbit uterine progesterone receptor concentrations and uteroglobin synthesis after progesterone administration, *Biochem. Biophys. Res. Commun.* **97**:5598–5605.

Toyoda, H., Seelke, R. W., Littlefield, B. A., and Spelsberg, T. C., 1985, Evidence for specific DNA sequences in the nuclear acceptor sites of the avian oviduct progesterone receptor, *Proc. Natl. Acad. Sci. U.S.A.* **82**:4722–4726.

Tseng, L., and Gurpide, E., 1975, Induction of human endometrial estradiol dehydrogenase by progestins, *Endocrinology* **97**:825–833.

Tseng, L., and Gurpide, E., 1979, Stimulation of various 17β- and 20α-hydroxysteroid dehydrogenase activities by progestins in human endometrium, *Endocrinology* **104**:1745–1748.

Umapathysivam, K., and Jones, W. R., 1978, An investigation of decidual specific proteins in the rat, *Int. J. Fertil.* **23**:138–142.

Vladirmirsky, F., Chen, L., Amsterdam, A., Zor, U., and Lindner, H. R., 1977, Differentiation of decidual cells in cultures of rat endometrium, *J. Reprod. Fertil.* **49**:61–68.

von der Ahe, D., Janich, S., Scheidereit, C., Renkawitz, R., Schutz, G., and Beato, M., 1985, Glucocorticoid and progesterone receptors bind to the same sites in two hormonally regulated promoters, *Nature* **313**:706–708.

von der Ahe, D., Renoir, J. M., Buchou, T., Baulieu, E. E., and Beato, M., 1986, Receptors for glucocorticoid and progesterone recognize distinct features of a DNA regulatory element, *Proc. Natl. Acad. Sci. U.S.A.* **83**:2817–2821.

Von Hippel, P. H., Bear, D. G., Morgan, W. D., and McSwiggen, J. A., 1984, Protein–nucleic acid interactions in transcriptions: A molecular analysis, *Annu. Rev. Biochem.* **53**:389–446.

Walker, R., 1983, *The Molecular Biology of Enzyme Synthesis,* John Wiley & Sons, New York.

Walters, M. R., 1985, Steroid hormone receptors in the nucleus, *Endocrine Rev.* **6**:512–543.

Walters, M. R., and Clark, J. H., 1978, Stoichiometric translocation of the rat uterine progesterone receptor, *Endocrinology* **103**:1952–1955.

Warembourg, M., Tranchant, O., Atger, M., and Milgrom, E., 1986, Uteroglobin messenger ribonucleic acid: Localization in rabbit uterus and lung by *in situ* hybridization, *Endocrinology* **119**:1632.

Weiser, J. W., Do, Y. S., and Feldman, D., 1979, Synthesis and secretion of corticosteroid-binding globulin by rat liver. A source of heterogeneity of hepatic corticosteroid-binders, *J. Clin. Invest.* **63**:461–467.

Welshons, W. V., Lieberman, M. E., and Gorski, J., 1984, Nuclear localization of unoccupied oestrogen receptors, *Nature* **307**:747–749.

Welshons, W. V., Krummel, B. M., and Gorski, J., 1985, Nuclear localization of unoccupied receptors for glucocorticoids, estrogens, and progesterone in GH$_3$ cells, *Endocrinology* **117**:2140–2147.

Wewer, U. M., Damjanov, A., Weiss, J., Liotta, L. A., and Damjanov, I., 1986, Mouse endometrial stromal cells produce basement-membrane components, *Differentiation* **32**:49–58.

Wheeler, C., Komm, B. S., and Lyttle, C. R., 1987, Estrogen regulation of protein synthesis in the immature rat uterus: The effects of progesterone on proteins released into the medium during *in vitro* incubations, *Endocrinology* **120**:919–923.

White, R., Lees, J. A., Needham, M., Ham, J., and Parker, M., 1987, Structural organization and expression of the mouse estrogen receptor, *Mol. Endocrinol.* **1**:736–744.

Whitehead, M. I., Townsend, P. T., Pryse-Davies, J., Ryder, T. A., and King, R. J. B., 1981, Effects of estrogens and progestins on the biochemistry and morphology of the postmenopausal endometrium, *N. Engl. J. Med.* **305**:1599–1605.

Yamamoto, K. R., 1983, On steroid receptor regulation of gene expression and the evolution of hormone-controlled gene networks, in: *Steroid Hormone Receptors: Structure and Function* (H. Eriksson and J. A. Gustafsson, eds.), Elsevier, New York, pp. 285–306.

Yamamoto, K. R., and Alberts, B. M., 1972, *In vitro* conversion of estradiol-receptor protein to its nuclear form: Dependence on hormone and DNA, *Proc. Natl. Acad. Sci. U.S.A.* **69:**2105–2109.

Yamamoto, K., and Alberts, B. M., 1976, Steroid receptors: Elements for modulation of eukaryotic transcription, *Annu. Rev. Biochem.* **43:**721–746.

Young, C. E., Smith, R. G., and Bullock, D. W., 1981, Uteroglobin mRNA and levels of nuclear progesterone receptor in endometrium, *Mol. Cell. Endocrinol.* **22:**105–113.

Zava, D. T., Harrington, N. Y., and McGuire, W. L., 1976, Nuclear estradiol receptor in the adult rat uterus: A new exchange assay, *Biochemistry* **15:**4292–4297.

Zwelling, L. A., Kerrigan, D., and Lippman, M. E., 1983, Protein-associated intercalator-induced DNA scission is enhanced by estrogen stimulation in human breast cancer cells, *Proc. Natl. Acad. Sci. U.S.A.* **80:**6182–6186.

8

The Endometrium of Delayed and Early Implantation

RANDALL L. GIVEN and ALLEN C. ENDERS

A delay of implantation is a prominent feature in the reproductive pattern of many animals (Renfree and Calaby, 1981). It is responsible for extending the length of gestation beyond that expected, considering the size of the young at birth and the relative maturity of the neonates. It is particularly interesting since it appears to be a condition in which the development of the blastocyst is controlled by the uterus. Although the term delay of implantation suggests that the attachment of the embryo to the uterus is prevented, the prolongation can occur at any time during the preimplantation period from entry into the uterus until adhesion of the blastocyst to uterine luminal epithelium.

In carnivores, marsupials, and the roe deer the delay occurs early in the preimplantation period, for there is an extended period of quiescence in blastocyst growth followed by a period of appreciable increase in size (activation) before implantation is initiated. In the mink, repeated matings can occur during the delay period, resulting in blastocysts of different ages but in a similar developmental stage (R. Enders, 1952). In the roe deer there may be a period of slow growth during the quiescent portion followed by rapid elongation of the embryo before implantation (Short and Hay, 1966). The lactational delay is relatively short in the rat and mouse, the loss of the zona pellucida is retarded, and after an initial increase in size there is no further growth until after implantation (Surani, 1975b; Weitlauf *et al.*, 1979). Delayed implantation also can be induced experimentally in the rat and mouse by ovariectomy of the female by day 4 of pregnancy. Ordinarily delayed implantation cannot be induced experimentally in other rodents lacking a normal delay (e.g., hamster: Orsini and Meyer, 1962). The zona pellucida may be present during the entire delay period (carnivores: Wright, 1963) or may be absent for all of the delay (armadillo: A. Enders, 1966).

RANDALL L. GIVEN ● Department of Anatomy and Neurosciences, University of Texas Medical Branch, Galveston, Texas 77550. ALLEN C. ENDERS ● Department of Human Anatomy, University of California School of Medicine, Davis, California 95616.

Delayed implantation has proved to be a useful phenomenon in studies of reproduction because it permits separation of a variety of endometrial and embryonic changes preceding implantation from those of implantation. It also has a unique advantage in rats and mice in that it can be manipulated by the investigator to control more precisely developmental events in the embryo and uterus. Delayed implantation is a period in which the blastocyst is dependent on the intrauterine environment and consequently on the condition of the endometrium. Therefore, changes in the endometrium play a critical role in the survival of the embryo. The purpose of this chapter is to survey the endometrium of delayed and early implantation in several species and relate these observations to the development of the preimplantation embryo.

1. Marsupials

In the relatively short time since Sharman (1955a,b) documented the presence of delayed implantation in marsupials, a great deal has been learned concerning reproduction in this intriguing group (Tyndale-Biscoe and Renfree, 1987). Delay of implantation is confined to the macropodid marsupials (the kangaroos and wallabies) with the exception of one species, the noolbenger (honey possum, *Tarsipes spencerae:* Renfree, 1980). The patterns of reproduction within this group are extremely diverse, not only because of species variation but because of the responsiveness of the animals to local seasonal conditions (Tyndale-Biscoe *et al.*, 1974; Renfree, 1981; Tyndale-Biscoe and Renfree, 1987).

When a delay of implantation is interposed in the reproductive cycle, it is lactation-induced and apparently is produced by an interference with full luteal development. The basic pattern of delay of implantation in macropod marsupials is as follows. An ovulation occurs around the time of parturition. Following fertilization of this ovum, the cleaving zygote receives an albumin coat and egg shell membrane in the oviduct as it moves down to enter the ipsilateral uterus. It reaches the stage of a small unilaminar blastocyst and subsequently undergoes a period of quiescence. At the termination of the period of quiescence, there is a period of several days during which the activated blastocyst increases in size and number of cells prior to loss of the shell membrane and attachment to the endometrium. Because of the period of blastocyst enlargement prior to implantation, the Australian workers refer to the interposed period as "embryonic diapause" or blastocyst quiescence. It should be noted, however, that a similar period of blastocyst enlargement at the end of a period of delayed implantation is found in many carnivores and in the roe deer and is missing only in those species that do not show a marked increase in blastocyst size prior to "normal" implantation. However, in macropods conditions for activation of the blastocyst are not the same as those for subsequent maintenance of the embryo (the latter requires a fully luteal endometrium: Tyndale-Biscoe, 1970), and the postimplantation period is shorter than the "activation" period.

The two uteri of the marsupial reproductive tract are short, saccular, and fusiform in both monotocous and polytocous species. They are surprisingly similar in widely diverse marsupials, including the New World forms such as the philander opossum and the Virginia opossum, as well as in macropod and nonmacropod Australian species. However, they do not show the diversity of gross or histological structure found in Eutheria (for review, see Tyndale-Biscoe and Renfree, 1987). In nondelaying species such as the ringtail opossum (Hughes *et al.*, 1965) or in philander opossum (personal observation), the endometrium is richly glandular, composed in early pregnancy of a luminal epithelium of columnar epithelial cells that cover a series of folds into which the simple tubular and branched tubular glands enter (Fig. 1). The glands have tall columnar epithelial cells with nuclei in a distinctly basal position. Both glandular and luminal epithelia have some ciliated cells, especially in the neck region of the glands. A particularly prominent feature of pregnancy is the pronounced edema of the lamina propria of the endometrium (Padykula and Taylor, 1976). In most species the tendency toward pseudostratification of the luminal epithelium decreases as pregnancy progresses, whereas stromal edema increases.

During delayed implantation in marsupials, the endometrium is more highly developed than during anestrus but less developed than after the initiation of blastocyst activation and subsequent gestation. Tyndale-Biscoe (1963) listed the range of diameters of the anestrous uterus of the Rottnest Island wallaby, *Setonix,* as 3–5 mm and that during delay as 5–7 mm. He also reported that the endometrial glands were longer and more coiled in delay than in anestrus. The lumina of the glands were large and patent, and the epithelium was columnar with basally situated nuclei. There was apparently no structural difference in the uterus between lactating animals in delay and nonpregnant lactating animals. In early pregnancy in species with and without a quiescence, the glandular epithelium is composed of slender elongated epithelial cells, whereas the luminal epithelial cells are broader with a more centrally placed nucleus and less extensive apical cytoplasm (Figs. 1 and 2).

During delayed implantation in the tammar wallaby, *Macropus eugenii,* the uterus is smaller than after the activation of the blastocyst, and the amount and concentration of protein in the uterine secretion are less during the quiescent period (Tyndale-Biscoe *et al.,* 1974). When uterine fluids were collected from the tammar wallaby and the proteins analyzed by electrophoretic mobility, it was found that the quantities of these proteins differed from those in other body fluids and that there were uterine-specific prealbumins present (Renfree, 1973). Analysis of endometrial explants incubated in medium containing [^{3}H]leucine has shown an increase in both tissue and secreted proteins by 4 days after activation, which is 1 day before metabolic activation of the embryo begins (Shaw and Renfree, 1986). Thus, the endometrium may play an important role in altering the luminal contents and activating the quiescent embryo. Increased endometrial protein secretion also occurs following administration of progesterone and estradiol to the delayed implanting animal (Shaw and Renfree, 1986), an observation that suggests that these hormones are necessary for induction of endometrial protein secretion and proper development of the embryo.

In nondelaying marsupials such as the Virginia opossum and the phalangerid *Trichosurus,* the increase in uterine weight and secretions following ovulation is similar in pregnant and nonpregnant females (Tyndale-Biscoe *et al.,* 1974; Renfree, 1975). Although this relationship apparently holds true in the tammar wallaby during the activation phase, the further increase in uterine weight and secretions seen after attachment of the blastocyst does not occur in the contralateral uterus (Shaw and Renfree, 1986) or in nonpregnant animals under similar conditions. Consequently, this increase in weight is considered to be a response to the conceptus. An additional difference between the delaying and nondelaying species of marsupials is the greater similarity of the uterine fluids in the latter to the composition of maternal blood serum.

Glutaraldehyde-fixed portions of uteri from six red kangaroos (*Macropus rufus*) killed during the delayed implantation period were available for this study. One of the kangaroos was in the "activation" stage of blastocyst enlargement. In general, the development of the uterine glands of the red kangaroo during the delay period is greater than that of rodents during the delay period. The endometrium is moderately vascular and mildly edematous, and macrophages are common in the connective tissue (Fig. 2).

A comparison of the glandular epithelium of four animals with quiescent blastocysts with one containing an activated blastocyst showed that although both were composed of tall columnar cells, glandular cells in the latter were approximately twice as tall as those of the quiescent stage (Fig. 3). They were considerably larger than the gland cells of late pregnancy in a nondelaying species (Fig. 5). Lipid droplets are more abundant in gland cells during the quiescent period, and vacuoles are present in these cells in quiescent and activated stages. However, large granules are prominent in the cells of glandular epithelium from the activation period. With electron microscopy, both types of gland cells have appreciable granular endoplasmic reticulum, but extensive dilation of the cisternae is seen during the activation period

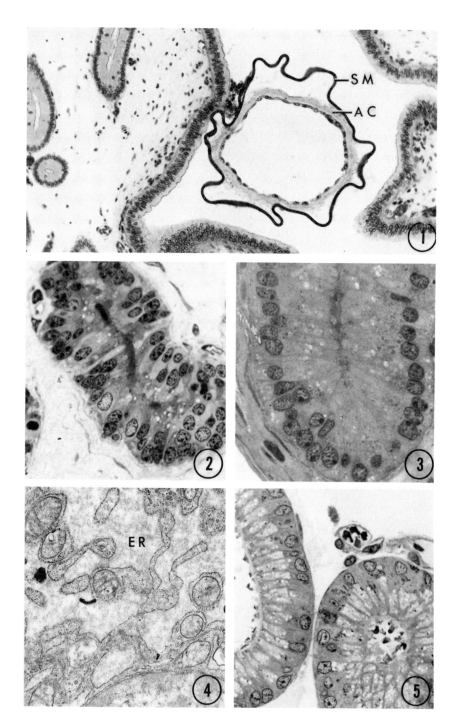

Figure 1. Micrograph of a section through a uterus from a philander opossum in early pregnancy. The blastocyst is separated from the uterine luminal epithelium by the shell membrane (SM). The zona pellucida is the thin light band between the protoderm and the albuminous coat (AC). Note the well-developed glands surrounded by edematous stroma. ×150.

Figure 2. Micrograph of a uterine gland from the red kangaroo during delayed implantation. There is a mixed population of tall columnar cells surrounding a lumen containing dense-staining extracellular material. ×630

(Fig. 4). Glandular epithelial cells at this stage also have well-developed Golgi complexes and numerous large granules containing a flocculent material of varying density. Similar changes have been noted in the uterine glands of the red-necked wallaby, *Macropus rufogriseus* (Walker and Hughes, 1981).

From the evidence concerning both uterine fluid and uterine histology, it appears that the kangaroo uterus is neither atrophic nor devoid of secretory activity during the quiescent period; instead, the gland cells have appreciably more secretory capacity during the activation stage. It is interesting that a dilated granular endoplasmic reticulum has been reported during the blastocyst-swelling stages not only in the red kangaroo but also in the roe deer, mink, and spotted skunk.

2. Roe Deer

The roe deer (*Capreolus capreolus*) is the only artiodactyl in which the existence of a delayed implantation period has been established. Short and Hay (1965, 1966) reviewed the early literature on delayed implantation in the European roe deer (Ziegler, 1843; Bischoff, 1854) and have added their own observations on this species. Aitken *et al.* (1973) and Aitken (1974a,b, 1975, 1981) confirmed the earlier findings that fertilization occurs in late July or early August, and that soon afterward the zona pellucida is lost and the blastocyst begins a period of delayed implantation lasting until late December or early January. During the delay period, the blastocyst grows slowly and shows evidence of change in the trophoblast and differentiation of the endoderm. After the period of relative quiescence, but prior to implantation, rapid elongation of the blastocyst takes place. Actual attachment of the trophoblast to the caruncles does not occur until after this increase in length. Contrary to the observations of Prell (1938) and of Stieve (1950), Short and Hay (1966) did not find any evidence of ovulation during a second rut in the fall. Some preliminary evidence reported by Lincoln and Guinness (1972) suggests that the time of implantation is not under photoperiod control, although the annual molt was advanced with altered photoperiod in the two animals observed.

The uterus of the roe deer, like that of other artiodactyls, is bicornuate. There is a relatively large region of communication between the two horns, from which the cornua pass cranially and then laterally in two broadly curved arcs. The endometrium surrounding the large lumina of the cornua is composed of irregular folds that are interrupted mesometrially by a variable number of aglandular caruncles (Fig. 6). (See Harrison and Hyett, 1954, and Harrison and Hamilton, 1952, for a structural description of the uterus in several deer species and the distribution of caruncles.)

The histological description of the roe deer uterus that follows is based on three blocks of endometrium. Two of these are from roe deer in the delay period, and one is from a roe deer with a 22-mm (early postimplantation) embryo (kindly sent to us by Dr. Roger Short); the description is also based on the findings of Aitken and Short. In delay uteri, the surface

---

Figure 3. Micrograph of a uterine gland from the red kangaroo during the stage in which the blastocyst is enlarged and activated. Note the extreme hypertrophy of the gland cells and the numerous small granules and vacuoles situated between the nuclei and the lumen. ×630

Figure 4. Electron micrograph of a gland cell from the red kangaroo during the activation stage of delayed implantation. The cisternae of endoplasmic reticulum (ER) are highly dilated and contain flocculent material. ×16,800.

Figure 5. Uterine glands from a philander opossum in late pregnancy. The stroma is highly edematous, and the apical ends of the gland cells are filled with small vacuoles. ×485.

epithelium covering the protruding caruncles is tall columnar, the basal regions of the cells are vacuolated, and the nuclei are occasionally flattened on their basal ends. The cells are not ciliated. A central vascular stalk is present in the pedicel forming the base of the caruncle. The vessels spread fanlike into the richly cellular connective tissue that underlies the surface epithelium. Neither glands nor crypts were present in caruncles of the two delay specimens, although the latter are well developed in the endometrium of the postimplantation animal (Figs. 6 and 8).

The surface epithelium of the intercaruncular endometrium is similar to that covering the caruncles, except that the columnar cells are somewhat shorter and interrupted periodically by the openings of the numerous glands. Aitken (1974a) reports that at the onset of embryonic elongation the number and diameter of the gland openings increase. The glands are simple branched-tubular structures. The necks of the individual glands are broadly dilated and contain scattered ciliated cells. The neck region is slightly coiled. It branches shortly to give rise to the fundic portions of the glands, which in turn rebranch before extending down to the myometrial surface. The fundic portions of the glands are slightly coiled and are smaller in diameter than the neck segments. The cells are low columnar with basally situated nuclei, and few cilia are present (Fig. 7). Aitken et al. (1973) noted a sharp decrease in cell height in glandular fundi at the time of embryonic elongation. Although most of the fundic glands are only slightly dilated, some individual glands are more broadly dilated. Small amounts of periodic acid–Schiff-positive material can be found throughout the glands and overlying the surface epithelium. Apical granules are also seen in many of the cells of the neck segment.

The endometrial stroma in the intercaruncular area is more edematous and less cellular than that in the caruncular pedicel (Fig. 6). Aitken et al. (1973) further noted that the endometrium is most edematous in early August, subsides gradually, and then increases again at the time of placental attachment. The endometrium is quite vascular, and the vessels in the subsurface region are moderately dilated. The connective tissue in this region is slightly more cellular.

The postimplantation endometrium is not only hypervascular and edematous but also contains glands that are highly dilated and have areas in which colloidal contents distend the lumen. The caruncles also become more vascular and develop distinctive surface crypts (Fig. 8).

Aitken et al. (1973) and Aitken (1974a, 1975, 1981) described the endometrium of the roe deer at the ultrastructural level from the time of fertilization until after implantation. They found that the most dramatic changes in the endometrium occurred at the onset of embryonic elongation, when the fundic cells of the glands are suddenly divested of the apical vesicles that accumulated during the delay period. These clear vesicles are apparently derived from the Golgi apparatus, and their release results in a marked decline in the height of these cells. The Golgi apparatus, which proliferates during the delay period, shows a marked decline by the end of the period of embryonic elongation. The endoplasmic reticulum is never well developed in this cell type and remains poorly developed during the implantation period. The fundic cells remain free of apical vesicles throughout the implantation period.

Aitken (1975) also reported that the nonciliated cells of the necks of the endometrial glands also contain clear supranuclear vesicles and more basal lipid than is seen in the cells of the gland fundi. The apical vesicles are also lost in these cells at the beginning of embryonic elongation. However, these cells do not appear as inactive as the glandular cells. The lipid material is retained, and electron-dense lyosomelike granules appear in the cells. During the early stages of implantation, the granular endoplasmic reticulum and the nuclear membrane contain moderately electron-dense material in their cisternae that could possibly be secreted. At this time granular inclusions near the apical cell membrane also appear to release material into the lumen. Lipid deposits disappear from the cells, but lysosomelike granules are still seen.

Aitken (1975) reported that at the time of release of the clear vesicles from the glandular

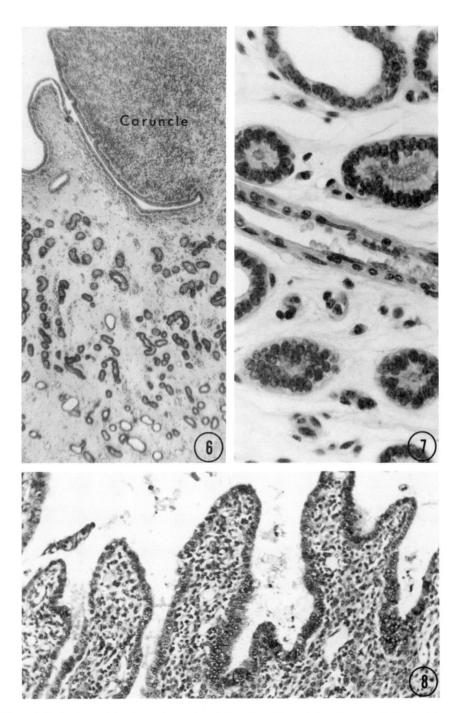

Figure 6. Section through the uterus of a roe deer during delayed implantation. The caruncle is aglandular and has relatively dense stroma. The rest of the endometrium contains numerous branched tubular glands. ×60.
Figure 7. Roe deer uterus during delayed implantation. At this magnification, the differential dilation of some of the basal endometrial glands is seen. Note the arteriole in the center of the micrograph and the edematous connective tissue. ×540.
Figure 8. Crypt formation on the caruncular surface is seen in this section of a roe deer uterus at the stage of embryonic elongation. ×160.

epithelium and during the beginning of embryonic elongation, the lumina of the necks and fundic portions of the glands are filled with clear vesicles, abundant cellular debris, and electron-dense cellular material. At implantation large amounts of this material are still present. Another phenomenon that was noted by Aitken (1974a, 1975) was the presence of large apical protrusions from the surface of the luminal and ductal epithelium at the time of embryonic elongation and implantation. These protrusions are seen in the caruncular and intercaruncular luminal epithelium and were suspected of being an apocrine-type secretion. The number of these protrusions seems to decrease later in the implantation period.

The sudden decrease in clear apical vesicles in the glandular fundi and ductal epithelia at about the time of rapid embryonic elongation led Aitken *et al.* (1973) and Aitken (1974a,b, 1981) to suggest that the material released may stimulate embryonic elongation and subsequent development. Aitken (1975) also suggested that the secretion of material from the granular endoplasmic reticulum in the neck region of the glands may not affect embryonic elongation but could possibly be a result of embryonic growth. Analysis of the uterine flushings revealed that there was a significant rise in calcium, protein, carbohydrate, and α-amino nitrogen content during embryonic elongation (Aitken, 1974a,b). Studies also indicated that there were elevated estrogen and progesterone levels during embryonic attachment (Aitken, 1974a, 1981; Hoffman *et al.*, 1978; Sempere, 1977), which may act to stimulate the secretory activity in the endometrium. However, since no change was noted in the ovaries of the roe deer during the delay period (they appear to remain active), this estrogen and progesterone rise may be a result rather than a cause of increased embryonic growth (Aitken, 1974a, 1981; Hoffman *et al.*, 1978).

3. Armadillos

Delayed implantation was first reported in the nine-banded armadillo (*Dasypus novemcinctus*) by Patterson (1913) and confirmed by Hamlett (1932a), who also pointed out that the mulita armadillo, *Dasypus hybridis,* probably has a delay of implantation (Hamlett, 1935). A series of studies established that in Texas the delay of implantation in the nine-banded armadillo lasts from the time of ovulation and mating in midsummer until implantation in November and December (A. C. Enders, 1966; Peppler and Canale, 1980) but not 22 months as stated by Michener (1986). During the delay period, the corpus luteum is somewhat active (Talmage *et al.,* 1954; Labhsetwar and Enders, 1968) and is well developed (A. C. Enders, 1966), although plasma progesterone levels remain low compared to postimplantation values (Peppler and Stone, 1976, 1980). The blastocyst remains in the fundic portion of the uterus simplex (Patterson, 1913) in a chamber bordered laterally by the openings of the oviducts and ventrally and dorsally by endometrial folds formed where the thicker endometrium of the body of the uterus overlaps the thinner endometrium of the fundus (A. C. Enders and Buchanan, 1959a).

Implantation and resumption of development are accompanied by a significant rise in plasma progesterone (Peppler and Stone, 1976, 1980). Curiously, the length of the delay period can be shortened experimentally by bilateral ovariectomy (Buchanan *et al.,* 1956; A. C. Enders and Buchanan, 1959b). Implantation occurs approximately 18 days following bilateral ovariectomy in the absence of exogenous hormones (A. C. Enders, 1966).

The endometrium of the armadillo during the delay period is richly glandular (A. C. Enders *et al.,* 1958; A. C. Enders, 1961). The luminal epithelium is pseudostratified columnar and is interrupted periodically by straight, simple tubular glands, which pass with little branching directly toward the myometrium (Fig. 9). In the body of the uterus, the glands are slightly dilated and consist of a straight neck region of columnar epithelial cells with basal nuclei, a

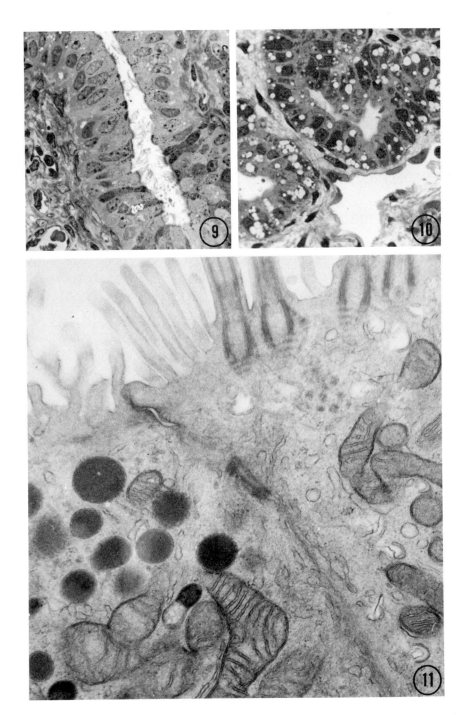

Figure 9. Glandular epithelium of an armadillo during delayed implantation. The epithelium is composed of light ciliated cells and interposed darker secretory cells. Note the dense stroma. ×485.

Figure 10. Glandular epithelium of an armadillo just after implantation. The light areas in the cells are lipid droplets, and the darker patches are glycogen. ×485.

Figure 11. Electron micrograph of two gland cells from an armadillo uterus during delayed implantation. The ciliated cell (right) has significantly smaller mitochondria than the secretory cell (left). The secretory cell contains numerous dense apical granules. ×40,500.

more tortuous suprasinusoidal portion, and a short coiled basal portion lying beneath the venous sinusoids.

During delay, lipid droplets are numerous in glandular and luminal epithelial cells but are most conspicuous in the deeper portions of the glands. Glycogen can be seen in scattered cells. Alkaline phosphatase activity is limited largely to the stroma, but acid phosphatase and esterase activity can be detected in the epithelial cells. Succinic dehydrogenase activity is readily demonstrable throughout the epithelium.

The stroma consists of loose connective tissue containing blood vessels with an unusual pattern. Coiled arterioles penetrate the basal stroma from the myometrium, with relatively straight capillaries extending toward the luminal epithelium. These capillaries ramify throughout the endometrium and pass back toward the myometrium. The capillaries enter large venous sinuses that form an anastomotic network within the body and fundus of the uterus. In turn, the sinuses are drained by numerous channels passing through the basal endometrium into the myometrium. The stroma is richly cellular rather than edematous.

In the fundic portion of the uterus, the sinuses are well developed, but the endometrium is thinner. The glands are more highly coiled and lack a distinctive neck portion. Ciliated cells are found scattered in the epithelium throughout the uterus and are common in both the glands and luminal epithelium of the fundic region (Fig. 9).

The ciliated cells are large and pale and have numerous rod-shaped mitochondria and abundant uniform long microvilli in addition to cilia (Fig. 11). Although they contain some lysosomes and a well-developed Golgi complex, there are relatively few granules in this cell type. The nonciliated "secretory" cells have numerous apical granules and larger mitochondria than those in the ciliated cells (Figs. 11 and 12). Some of the mitochondria are unusually large, having diameters several times those of mitochondria of the ciliated cells. More polyribosomes are found in the secretory cells than in the ciliated cells, and granular endoplasmic reticulum is neither dilated nor abundant. Both ciliated and secretory cells have some lipid droplets, especially basally. The surface of the secretory cells is irregular, with caveolae between microvilli and occasional larger cavities with flocculent material suggesting the release of granules.

The impression given by the cytology of the epithelial cells is that they are secretory cells producing a granular material at a relatively low rate. They do not appear inactive.

Appreciable changes in the endometrium occur at implantation. The epithelial cells store glycogen and lipid and become broader, and the sinuses enlarge (Fig. 10). Ciliated cells diminish in number. Microvilli on the glandular cells are longer, and although there is appreciable agranular endoplasmic reticulum and some strands of granular endoplasmic reticulum, there is no dilation of the latter, and the apical secretion granules disappear (Fig. 13). It should be noted that the armadillo blastocyst loses its abembryonic trophoblast shortly after attaching to the endometrium, thus inverting the yolk sac at a stage when the endoderm extends only slightly beyond the inner cell mass. Subsequent growth of the conceptus pushes the endoderm out of the fundic recess into the body of the uterus, where it is directly exposed to the patent uterine glands. There is some evidence that the fundic area and the body of the armadillo uterus are physiologically different (Buchanan, 1967).

The accumulation of glycogen and lipid in gland cells after implantation, coupled with their short stature and lack of granular endoplasmic reticulum, indicates a reduced secretory activity, although it is difficult to correlate these findings with the concurrent events of implantation. Weaker *et al.* (1981) also reported lower uptake of [^{3}H]estradiol in the endometrium of pregnant animals than in nonpregnant animals, especially in the glands and stromal tissue.

In the absence of biochemical or autoradiographic data on endometrial secretion, it is difficult to ascertain from cytological evidence alone the relative activity of the cells. In comparison with other delaying species, it can be seen that armadillo gland cells also appear to release granules that were present during delay, but unlike the mink, spotted skunk, roe deer,

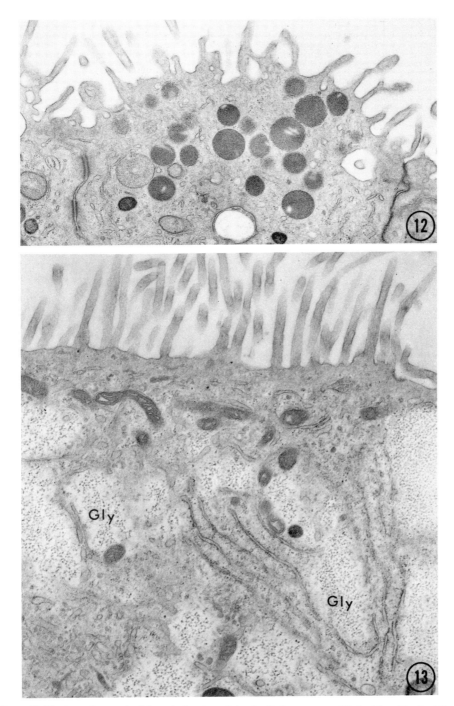

Figure 12. Electron micrograph of the apical region of gland cells from an armadillo in delayed implantation. Note irregular microvilli and numerous large secretory granules. ×24,000.

Figure 13. Electron micrograph of the apical region of a gland cell from an armadillo just after implantation. The extensive areas of glycogen granules (Gly) are partially extracted, and the microvilli are longer and more regular than before implantation. ×23,000.

or kangaroo, there is no extensive dilated endoplasmic reticulum after implantation, and the gland cells are not hypertrophied. Consequently, the ways in which the endometrium nurtures the postimplantation conceptus in the armadillo remain enigmatic despite the fact that there is extremely early yolk sac inversion in this species.

4. Insectivores and Chiroptera

Knowledge of the reproductive biology of the insectivores is limited. Vogel (1981) reviewed reproduction in these primitive mammals in which delayed implantation had been described in only two species, the Siberian mole (*Talpa altica*) and the European shrew (*Sorex araneus*). The Siberian mole has a gestation period of 9 to 10 months. A summer mating is followed by an extended delay of implantation until the next spring (Borodulina, 1951; Baevski, 1967; Judin, 1974). Brambell (1935) and Tarkowski (1957) described the presence of a delay period in the European common shrew, *Sorex araneus,* which was later confirmed by Vogel (1972). In this species a postpartum mating occurs, and the resulting pregnancy is thought to be prolonged by a delay in implantation. Although Brambell does not describe the histology of the endometrium of delay of implantation *per se,* he does describe the endometrium of the second pregnancy. As in the initial pregnancy, the endometrium undergoes a number of changes prior to the swelling of the blastocyst that occurs during implantation. Changes occurring before implantation include displacement of the nucleus of the luminal epithelial cells from a single row to multiple levels and an enhanced development of the uterine glands, which are confined to the antimesometrial portion of the endometrium. From this evidence it seems that the delay in the common shrew occurs while the endometrium is in a preimplantation condition. Brambell has also suggested that a delay may exist in the lesser shrew (Brambell, 1937; Brambell and Hall, 1936).

Early embryonic development and implantation have been reviewed in several species of Chiroptera (Rasweiler, 1979; Burns, 1981), but delayed implantation has not been studied extensively. Delayed implantation has been reported in the fruit bat, *Eidolon* (Mutere, 1967; Fayenuwo and Halstead, 1974), the Indian bat, *Rhinolophus rouxi* (Ramakrishna and Rao, 1977), and *Miniopterus* (Peyre and Herlant, 1967). In *Miniopterus* the histology and ultrastructure of delayed and implanting embryos have been described (Wallace, 1978; van der Merwe, 1982; Kimura and Uchida, 1983), but the condition of the endometrium in relation to delay and implantation has yet to be studied. The interesting climatic factors associated with the delay in these species have also been considered by Wimsatt (1975).

5. Carnivores

Delayed implantation occurs in both pinniped and fissiped carnivores. Among pinniped carnivores, it is a common feature in seals (Renfree and Calaby, 1981; Boshier, 1981; Daniel, 1981), having been reported in the common seal, *Phoca vitulina* (Fisher, 1954; Harrison, 1960, 1969), gray seal, *Halichoerus grypus* (Backhouse and Hewer, 1964; Hewer and Backhouse, 1968), cape fur seal, *Arctocephalus pusillus* (Rand, 1954), northern fur seal, *Callorhinus ursinus* (Pearson and Enders, 1951; Daniel, 1970), and elephant seal, *Mirounga leonina* (Laws, 1956). Among fissiped carnivores, a period of delayed implantation is probably the general rule in bears (Hamlett, 1935; Wright, 1981) and has been confirmed in the black bear (Wimsatt, 1963), grizzly bear (Craighead *et al.,* 1969), and polar bear (Hamlett,

1935). It is also extremely common in the mustelids (Mead, 1981) but has not been reported in any of the other fissiped families.

The uterus in carnivores is bicornuate, with the lumina of the two horns becoming confluent at the cervical region. The endometrium is generally richly glandular in adult animals and is composed of a series of longitudinal folds, usually five or more in number, that give the lumen a pentaradiate form when seen in cross section.

The glands of young animals are simple, straight, tubular sacculations arising periodically from the surface of the folds and passing parallel to one another towards the myometrium. Because of this arrangement, glands arising near the apices of the folds are longer than those at the margins and have a somewhat straighter course.

Generally, there is a short communicating portion of the gland, which is the isthmic portion; a relatively straight portion, which may be dilated during the breeding season; and an extensive body, which is often convoluted and frequently terminates in a basal coiled portion. Luminal epithelial cells are tall columnar, and the epithelium of the glands is lower. Cilia are not present in carnivore uteri.

5.1. Seals

In seals, mating may occur within a week after parturition. Each uterine horn bears a pup alternately. Thus, while one horn is in the state of postpartum reorganization, a blastocyst may well be present in the contralateral horn. The duration of lactation does not appear to affect the time of implantation; rather, current evidence suggests that the photoperiod may control the length of gestation (Temte, 1985).

Despite the widespread interest in reproduction in seals, there are relatively few observations on the endometrium. In a study of the embryology and fetal growth of the gray seal, Hewer and Backhouse (1968) observed an increasing hypertrophy of uterine glands during the period of embryonic enlargement prior to implantation. More recently, Boshier (1979, 1981) described the ultrastructure of the endometrium in two gray seals thought to be from the preimplantation period. The luminal epithelium was columnar, with prominent junctional complexes, apical Golgi complexes, and some granular endoplasmic reticulum. Mitochondria were ovoid with a dense matrix. These cells also contained some lipid and occasional clear apical vesicles. Prior to implantation, there was an increase in cell height and intracellular lipid. The glands were also more open, and they accumulated secretory material. The epithelium in glands that appeared more active also contained clear vesicles and some basal lipid. Ouellette and Ronald (1985) have described uteri of gray and harp seals during the delayed implantation period, at 2 to 2.5 months after implantation, and during postpartum reorganization. The epithelium of the delay period was similar to that previously described. The glands were surrounded by highly vascular stroma, whereas the luminal epithelium was columnar with prominent nuclei and irregular folds. The endometrium of the placental region was altered extensively by the invading trophoblast; however, the basal regions of the glands still appeared active.

Pearson and Enders (1951) reported that uterine glands of fur seals in which unattached blastocysts were found were well developed and "secreting actively." They found that both luminal and glandular epithelium was tall columnar and that the lumen usually contained both secretory material and cellular debris. In a study of the histology of the reproductive tract of the fur seal, Craig (1964) further noted that the glandular lumina contained acidophilic secretory material. With the onset of implantation, the glandular cells became more active in appearance, with coiling of the glands and dilation of the lumina with an acidophilic secretion. The necks of the gland also became more open in the uterine lumen, and the stroma more edematous. Although the pinniped endometrium appears active during the delay and implantation periods, more information is needed to characterize fully its changes.

5.2. Bears

In bears, evidence of a delay of implantation is available for most species (Wright, 1981). In addition, the giant panda (*Ailuropoda melanoleuca*), which is now regarded as an ursid, is also thought to have a delay of implantation. However, the American black bear is the only bear species in which delayed implantation has been studied extensively. Wimsatt (1963) has made detailed histological observations of endometria from the preovulatory to the postimplantation period from bears in the upper New York State area. In this species, breeding takes place in the beginning of the summer, probably by mid-June. Implantation of the blastocysts occurs in the fall; specimens from animals killed early in December are implanted. The luminal epithelium of the endometrium is composed of columnar cells with round bulging apices. Lipid droplets are present in both basal and supranuclear regions. The glands take origin from the entire endometrial surface. They have a short constricted isthmus leading into a relatively narrow straight neck segment, which joins the wider convoluted tubular secretory crypts. The secretory crypts of the glands occupy the greater width of the endometrium, extending down to the deep layers, where relatively coarse bundles of collagen and the intervascular plexus separate the stroma of the endometrium from the circular muscle layer.

Epithelial cells of the secretory crypts are tall columnar, with a rounded nucleus close to the base of the cell. Lipid droplets are present beneath and above the nucleus, but there is a clear apical region devoid of lipid droplets. Some diastase-resistant periodic acid–Schiff-positive material is sometimes present within the crypts and in the neck segments. Neck cells histologically resemble crypt cells without the apical end.

Wimsatt (1974), in a further study of the morphogenesis of fetal membranes and placenta of the black bear, states that implantation is central and superficial. Wimsatt (1963) also noted that in the uterus of a recently implanted specimen, lipid was still plentiful in the epithelium of the neck and upper crypt cells of the glands but that it had completely disappeared from the lower two-thirds of the crypts and the surface epithelium. During the implantation period, endometrial glands show further growth and hypertrophy.

5.3. Mustelids

The mustelids exhibit a wide variety of gestation periods (Mead, 1981; Renfree and Calaby, 1981). The ferret (*Mustela furo*), for example, does not delay at all. The mink (*Mustela vison*) has a short delay period of variable length, depending on how early in the breeding season the individual animal mates. The longest delay periods are exhibited by the fisher, *Martes pennanti* (Wright, 1963; Wright and Coulter, 1967), river otter, *Lutra canadensis* (Hamilton and Eadie, 1964), and individual European badgers, *Meles meles* (Canivenc and Laffargue, 1963), in which breeding occurs in the postpartum estrus with the result that animals are pregnant most of the year. In some species, such as the short-tailed weasel or stoat, *Mustela erminea,* breeding does not ordinarily occur until some time after parturition but takes place while the animal is still lactating. In the western spotted skunk, *Spilogale putorius latifrons* (Mead, 1968b), marten, *Martes americana,* American badger, *Taxidea taxus,* long-tailed weasel, *Mustela frenata,* and wolverine, *Gulo gulo* (Wright, 1963), breeding occurs at the end of the summer after the termination of lactation, and the delay period lasts until the next spring. Consequently, most of these mustelids have a relatively long delay period.

The sea otter (*Enhydra lutris*) has no distinct breeding season but breeds throughout the year (Sinha *et al.,* 1966) and has an estimated gestation period of 8 to 9 months (Barabash-Nikiforov, 1935). In a brief histological description of the sea otter uterus, Sinha *et al.* (1966) noted that the endometrium is filled with coiled glands that show secretory activity during the delay period. The endometrium of implanted animals is edematous and congested with coiled glands. In the area of the placental attachment the glands become progressively dilated and hypertrophied and appear secretory as development proceeds.

5.3.1. Badger

In the European badger bilateral ovariectomy does not result in death of the blastocysts, although histological evidence of regression of the endometrium has been reported (Harrison and Neal, 1959). Harrison (1963) has stated that the endometrium of delayed implantation in the badger does not vary throughout the delay period, although the vaginal epithelium shows structural modifications during delay. He described the mucosa as having a luminal epithelium of tall columnar cells with palely staining cytoplasm. The glands are relatively straight and exhibit little secretory activity. More recent studies by Bonnin and Canivenc (1980) demonstrate dramatic changes in the glandular epithelium at the time of implantation. During the delay period the glandular cells are pyramidal with abundant clear apical vesicles. Before implantation, the uterine glands become dilated with abundant secretory material in the lumina. The glandular cells lack the clear vesicles found previously and are now filled with glycogen granules. These changes parallel a short increase in the concentration of amino acids in uterine flushings prior to implantation.

Although Hamlett (1932b) and Wright (1966) thoroughly discussed the reproductive cycle of the American badger, there is still little information concerning the endometrium during the delay period, although it appears to be similar to the European species. We have had an opportunity to study the uteri from two animals killed during the delay period. The endometrium is glandular and highly vascular (Fig. 14). The luminal epithelial cells have extensive deposits of glycogen. The luminal epithelium extends into the neck of the gland, where a sharp transition to the neck epithelial cell type occurs (Figs. 14 and 19). The neck cells have abundant glycogen but far less than that seen in the luminal epithelium. A few sparsely filled granules are seen, and some dilated granular endoplasmic reticulum is present. The straight neck portion ends as the gland becomes more coiled, and there is a gradual transition to glandular epithelial cells, which are large with spherical nuclei situated in the lower third of the columnar cells. The apices of these gland cells are filled with a sparse flocculent material and dilated rough endoplasmic reticulum (Fig. 20). The glandular lumen contains PAS-positive material and debris. The endometrium is among the more active seen in delayed implantation.

5.3.2. Skunk

The spotted skunk (*Spilogale putorius*) is the only mustelid species that shows both obligate delay and no delay of implantation. Eastern forms (*S. putorius interrupta, S. p. ambarvalis,* and probably *S. p. putorius*) breed in April and have a gestation period of 50–65 days (Mead, 1968a), whereas the western forms (*S. p. gracilis, S. p. leucoparia, S. p. latifrons,* and *S. p. phenax*) breed in September, with parturition occurring in May (Mead, 1968b). The gestation period has been further delineated in *S. p. latifrons* into a total period of 230 to 250 days in which the delay period lasted from 200 to 220 days (Foresman and Mead, 1973). Mead (1968b) suggested that the eastern and western forms are actually distinct species.

The histological description provided here is based on delayed-implanting and implanting animals described by Sinha and Mead (1976) and tissue blocks kindly provided by Dr. Rodney

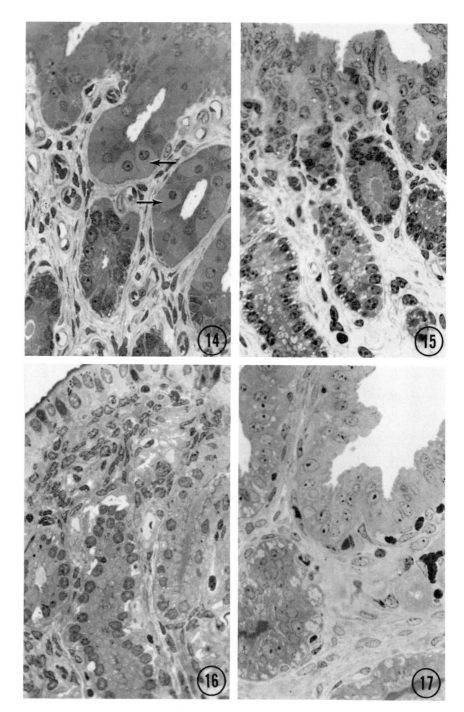

Figure 14. Uterus from a badger (*Taxidea taxus*) during delayed implantation. The large cells with the centrally situated nuclei extend from the luminal surface into the necks of the glands (arrows). It is these cells that contain masses of glycogen. ×485.

Figure 15. Uterus from a short-tailed weasel (*Mustela erminea*) during delayed implantation. As in the badger, the luminal epithelial cells are large and contain abundant glycogen. ×485.

Figure 16. Uterus of a mink (*Mustela vison*) during delayed implantation. The luminal epithelium is tall columnar, and glands are abundant. However, there is no accumulation of glycogen in the luminal cells, and the amount of glycogen in the gland cells varies during this stage. ×485.

Figure 17. Uterus of a mink at an early postimplantation stage. Note the general hypertrophy of both luminal and glandular epithelia and the subepithelial capillary plexus. ×485.

Mead. The uteri have prominent longitudinal folds covered by columnar epithelium with uterine glands that radiate from the lumen toward the myometrium for a short distance. The subepithelial region is well vascularized with numerous capillaries surrounding the glands (Fig. 18). A distinct basal zone separates the glands from the myometrium and contains connective tissue elements and blood vessels. During delayed implantation the glands contain a homogeneous electron-dense material. Although the luminal epithelium is taller than the epithelium in the necks of the glands, both epithelia have a similar ultrastructural appearance (Figs. 21 and 22). Both cell types have a round basal nucleus and a distinct supranuclear Golgi complex. Numerous mitochondria and short cisternae of granular endoplasmic reticulum are found throughout the cytoplasm. The apical border has prominent microvilli, which extend into the lumen. A layer of electron-lucent apical vesicles is located beneath the microvilli. Some lipid and glycogen accumulations are found beneath the nucleus. During delay these cells not only compose the luminal and neck epithelium of the glands but extend well into the base of the glands (Fig. 18).

The cells at the base of the glands have an active secretory appearance during delay of implantation. The entire apical region of the cells is filled with vesicles containing a flocculent electron-dense material (Fig. 23). The Golgi complex has large dilated cisternae, which occupy the supranuclear region with many large and small vesicular profiles surrounding them. Numerous dilated cisternae of granular endoplasmic reticulum are found throughout the juxtanuclear and basal regions. These cisternae are filled with a homogeneous electron-dense material. Similar profiles of granular endoplasmic reticulum are also seen in the mink, roe deer, and kangaroo.

Prior to implantation, the uterine cornua begin to enlarge, preimplantation blastocyst

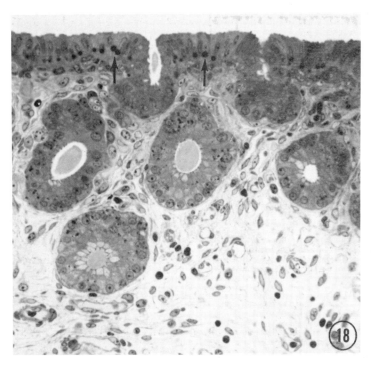

Figure 18. Uterus of a spotted skunk (*Spilogale putorius latifrons*) during delayed implantation. The luminal epithelium is tall columnar with prominent lipid droplets (arrows). The cells at the base of the glands contain numerous apical granules (compare with Fig. 23). Note that the neck epithelial cells occupy most of the gland, whereas the secretory cells are confined to the base. ×310.

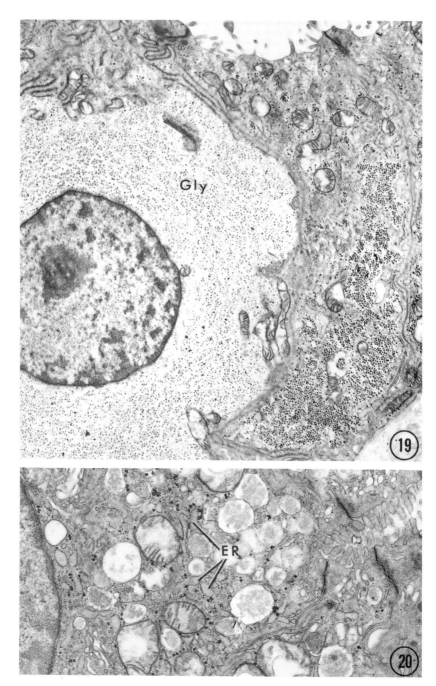

Figure 19. Electron micrograph of a badger uterus during delayed implantation. Note transition between large luminal-epithelial-type cells filled with glycogen (Gly) and the smaller more typical glandular epithelial cells at the right. ×11,700.

Figure 20. Electron micrograph of a badger uterine gland during delayed implantation. The presence of short segments of dilated endoplasmic reticulum (ER) and especially the numerous vacuoles with flocculent content suggest some secretory activity. ×16,200.

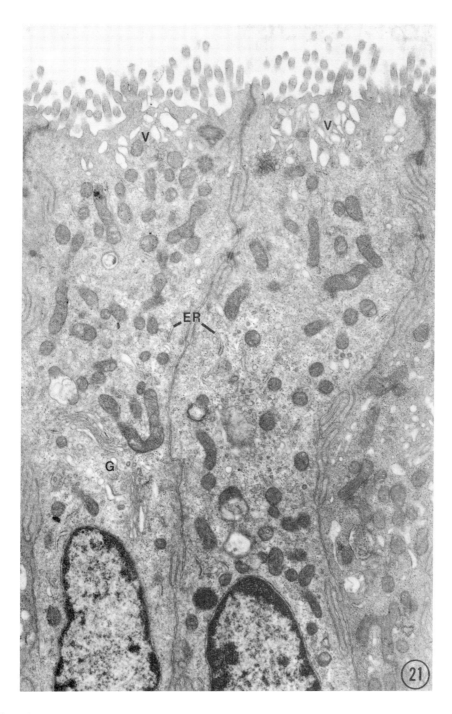

Figure 21. The apical portion of the luminal epithelium of the spotted skunk during delayed implantation is shown in this electron micrograph. Numerous apical vesicles (V) are present beneath the luminal surface. A compact Golgi complex (G) occupies the supranuclear region, and short undilated cisternae of endoplasmic reticulum (ER) are found throughout the cytoplasm. The extensive folding of lateral cell borders is characteristic. ×20,000.

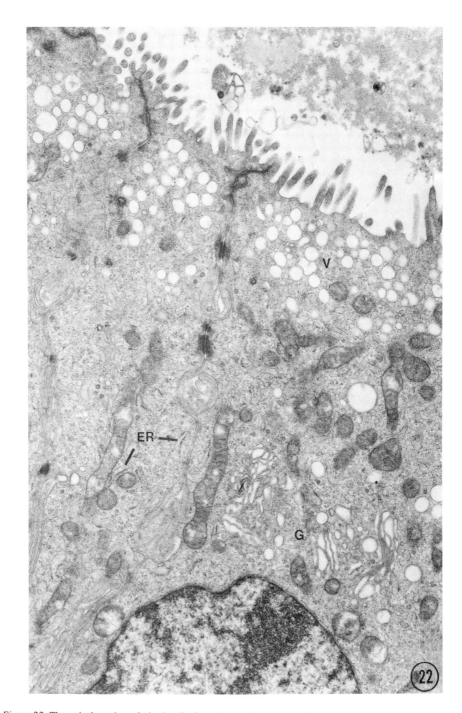

Figure 22. The apical portion of gland cells from the spotted skunk during delayed implantation. The gland lumen contains flocculent material, and a thick layer apical vesicles (V) is present beneath the microvilli. A prominent Golgi complex (G) is above the nucleus, and undilated cisternae of endoplasmic reticulum (ER) are dispersed among numerous mitochondria. ×19,000.

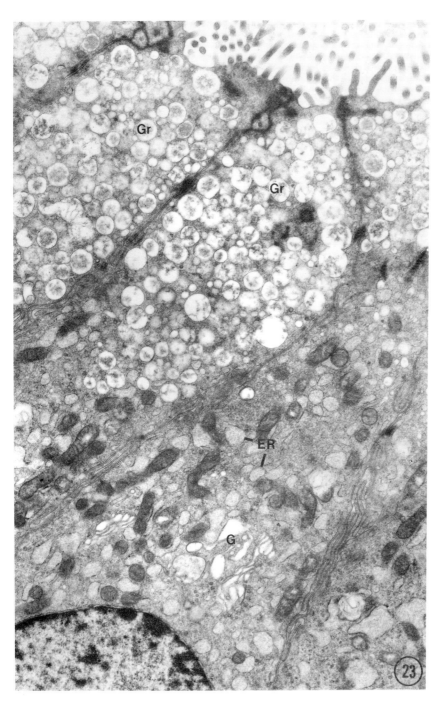

Figure 23. Cells from the base of glands in the spotted skunk during the activation period are shown. Numerous granules (Gr) filled with flocculent material occupy the apical portion of the cells. Dilated cisternae of granular endoplasmic reticulum (ER) and a compact Golgi complex (G) are above the nucleus. ×14,900.

swelling occurs, the luminal epithelial cells increase in height, and the glands deepen and contain dense secretory material. The basic ultrastructure of the luminal epithelial cells, cells in the neck region of the glands, and the basal "secretory" cells does not change during the activation period. However, the proportion of active secretory-type cells in the glandular epithelium appears to increase prior to implantation, thus giving the glands a more active appearance. After implantation, the endometrium is thick and well vascularized and continues to contain active-appearing glands (Mead, 1968a). The luminal epithelium maintains a similar ultrastructural appearance during the postimplantation period. The secretory-type glandular cells continue to appear active, with extensive areas of granular endoplasmic reticulum and extensive Golgi complexes. Thus, the endometrium maintains its active appearance into the early postimplantation period.

5.3.3. Weasel

Wright (1963) has made some preliminary observations on the histochemistry of the endometrium of the long-tailed weasel. He noted that the endometrium has glycogen in the luminal epithelium in the typical delay state. He also reported that when weasels were ovariectomized during the delay period, the endometrium underwent regression. In this sense, he believes that the uterus is not in an anestrus condition but is being maintained (possibly by the interstitial cells of the ovary). Wright (1963) also reports that, in one instance, ovariectomy resulted in death of the blastocysts.

It is interesting that Deanesly (1935), in describing the uterus of the pseudopregnant short-tailed weasel (before she ascertained that these animals had a delay period; Deanesly, 1943), described the endometrium as being in a luteal phase, exhibiting the same features as did the uteri in early implantation.

Portions of the uteri were obtained by unilateral hysterectomy from two short-tailed weasels at four times during the delay period. This endometrium showed a remarkable concentration of glycogen in the tall columnar luminal epithelial cells. The nuclei are displaced to the apical ends of the luminal epithelial cells, with the cells becoming virtual sacs of glycogen. The glands have relatively low columnar epithelial cells with little glycogen except in the neck regions, where a transition to the surface epithelium occurs. Some secretory material is present within the lumina of the glands, and supranuclear granules are present in some of the cells of the basal portions of the glands (Fig. 15).

In electron micrographs, the luminal epithelial cells are truly remarkable and appear very similar to the luminal cells of the American badger. Glycogen fills the cytoplasm except at the very apex and a thin zone at the margin of the cells (Fig. 24) (see also Schlafke et al., 1981). The microvilli are well developed and have a glycocalyx similar to that seen in the intestine. There are numerous agranular tubules in the cytoplasm adjacent to the microvilli. Mitochondria lie just below this cytoplasm and interdigitate with the glycogen-rich lower portions of the cell. A small Golgi zone is located between the apical tips and the nuclei. The few strands of granular endoplasmic reticulum present are situated largely along the margins of the cells. Ribosomes are associated with the peripheral and perinuclear regions of the cytoplasm.

In contrast to the luminal epithelial cells, the glandular epithelial cells are largely devoid of glycogen during the delay period (Fig. 25) (see also Schlafke et al., 1981). The microvilli of the cells are shorter than those of the luminal epithelial cells. Caveolae can frequently be found at the bases of these microvilli as well as at the lateral margins of the cells. A small subapical vacuolated region is apparent in many of the gland cells. The Golgi zone is more highly developed, and some of the cisternae are dilated and often show fusion with associated Golgi vesicles. The endoplasmic reticulum shows numerous small slightly dilated cisternae. Ribosomes are numerous, not only in association with the endoplasmic reticulum but also free within the cytoplasm. Mitochondria are large, but no extraordinarily large mitochondria are seen. A basolateral intercellular space is a common feature of the glandular epithelium. Some

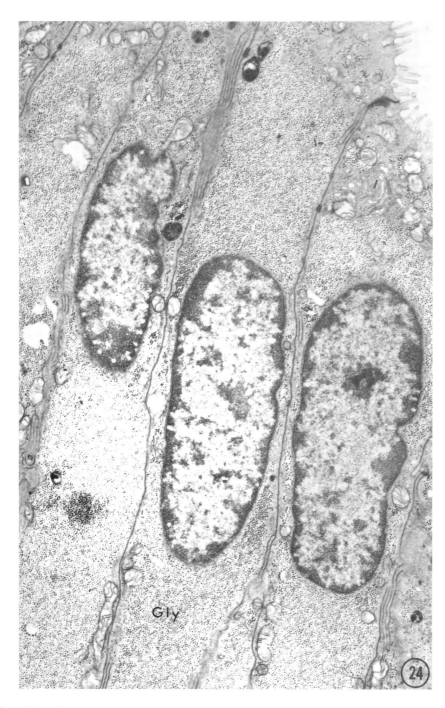

Figure 24. In this section through the uterine luminal epithelium of a weasel during delayed implantation, the cells are seen to be largely filled with fine granules of glycogen (Gly). The rest of the cytoplasmic components are largely confined to the apical, peripheral, and perinuclear regions. ×8000.

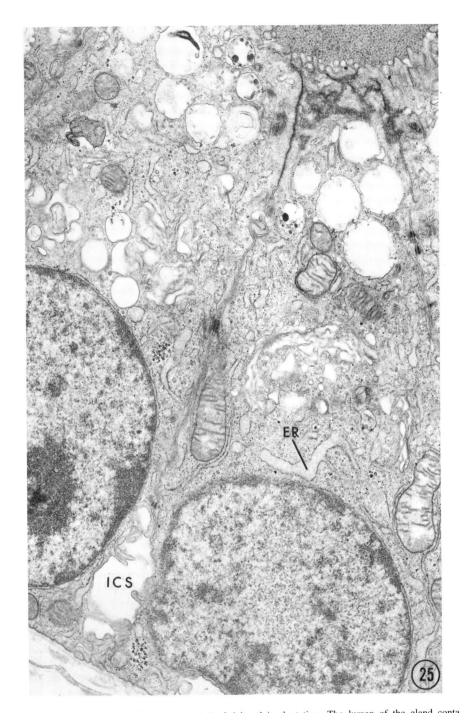

Figure 25. Weasel gland cells from the period of delayed implantation. The lumen of the gland contains granular material. A number of large vesicles are seen above the Golgi complex at the apex of the glandular cells. More basally, there is granular endoplasmic reticulum (ER) with a flocculent content. The dilated intercellular space (ICS) is characteristic. ×22,700.

glandular epithelial cells have a few lipid droplets, and most of the epithelial cells of the basal glands have large supranuclear granules that appear to be lipid pigment.

Sheldon (1972) reported that after ovariectomy during the delay period, the luminal epithelium declined sharply in height, apparently because of a loss of stored material. The glandular epithelium, however, was not so sensitive. Unlike those of the European badger, the blastocysts in this group of weasels largely deteriorated within 3 weeks, and all were fragmented by 9 weeks after ovariectomy, even though the immediate reaction was a proliferation of embryonic cell mass elements. Sheldon concluded that mitotic activity in the blastocyst was stimulated even though the uterine environment could not support further embryonic differentiation.

5.3.4. Mink

More information is available concerning the uterus of the mink than that of any of the other mustelids. The mink delay period is dependent on the time of breeding, since implantation occurs at approximately the same time in all individuals (R. K. Enders, 1952). In standard breeding practice, a single female will be bred more than once. Both superfetation and superfecundation result from multiple breeding and ovulation during the delay period (Hansson, 1947; R. K. Enders, 1956). Thus, the mink exhibits an unusual type of delay in that it occurs during the breeding season, the length of which depends on how early in the season the individual female is bred.

Histological descriptions of the mink endometrium have been given by Hansson (1947) and R. K. Enders (1952). Histochemical studies were reported by A. C. Enders (1961), R. K. Enders and A. C. Enders (1963), and Murphy and James (1974). In general, the endometrium during delay in the mink exhibits appreciable variation, especially as viewed histochemically. The luminal epithelium is columnar (Fig. 16). The surface of the luminal and glandular epithelium is covered by a periodic acid–Schiff-positive coat, and alkaline phosphatase activity is exhibited in the apices of these cells. However, the thickness of the PAS-positive coat, the extent of the alkaline phosphatase activity, and the amount of glycogen in the cells all vary during the delay period. It has been suggested (R. K. Enders and A. C. Enders, 1963) that this variation arises from the fluctuations in follicular development superimposed on the partial luteinization of the corpora lutea of delay and that the fluctuations consequently represent relative follicular or luteal ascendancy. Murphy and James (1974) agreed with R. K. Enders and A. C. Enders (1963) in regard to the variability in the presence of glycogen. However, they reported no variability in the PAS-positive material but instead saw a uniform distribution of mucosubstances.

The mink endometrium exhibits relatively little lipid or phospholipid during the delay period (A. C. Enders, 1961). Murphy and James (1974) reported hyaluronidase- and sialidase-susceptable material in cells of luminal epithelium and particularly in gland necks and gland bases during the delay period. During the delay period sulfated mucopolysaccharides were also found in luminal epithelial cells and gland necks.

The onset of implantation is reflected in the uterus by a hypertrophy of the luminal epithelial cells (Fig. 17), an increase in the alkaline phosphatase activity, a decrease in acid phosphatase activity, and a broadening of the opening of the isthmus of the glands onto the luminal epithelium. This results in a dentate appearance similar to that described in the cat in early implantation (Dawson and Kosters, 1944). Murphy and James (1974) also noted a general increase in PAS-positive diastase-resistant material but a depletion of glycogen in the uterine epithelium during the postimplantation period. Also, sulfated mucopolysaccharides appear in the glands during this period, while acidic mucopolysaccharides show no change from the delay appearance.

Electron microscopy of the mink endometrium during the delay period reveals a number of significant features. The glandular epithelial cells from the body of the glands have moderate amounts of dilated granular endoplasmic reticulum. In the apical ends of these cells are numerous membrane-bound granules that exhibit a localized region of increased density (Fig. 27). The Golgi complex is extensive. Although mitochondria are not especially abundant within the glandular cells, many of the mitochondria are unusually large and spherical, with peculiar spiral cristae. Numerous capillaries indent the glands during this period.

The luminal epithelial cells of the delay period are taller than those of the glands and have longer microvilli projecting from their conical apical borders (Fig. 26) (see also Schlafke *et al.*, 1981). The mitochondria are more normal in appearance, being rod-shaped with lamelliform cristae. There is a concentration of mitochondria in the apical region of the cell. No membrane-bound granules of the type described in gland cells are present, but a few dense pigment granules are present in the supranuclear cytoplasm. Occasionally lipid droplets are present basally. The granular endoplasmic reticulum is composed of a few undilated cisternae. Scattered membranes of agranular endoplasmic reticulum are common along the margins of the cell, both laterally and basally. A few subapical vacuoles are usually seen in these cells. The nuclei of the luminal epithelial cells are farther from the base than in glandular cells, and the Golgi zone is more compact. The cytology of the glands suggests that these cells are secreting small amounts of protein. The luminal epithelial cells, although taller, show no evidence of secretory activity but have features that are compatible with the function of absorption of luminal fluid.

The glandular epithelia during the late delay and postimplantation periods show notable changes from their earlier appearance (A. Enders *et al.*, 1963). The endoplasmic reticulum is extensively dilated, leaving only thin strands of cytoplasm between the cisternae (Figs. 28 and 29). The giant mitochondria, as well as the secretion granules, disappear. Golgi cisternae are more dilated than seen previously. During this period the luminal epithelium shows little change from its appearance in delay.

In the mustelids, the endometrium contains two to three distinct cell types during the delay period. The appearance of these cells varies somewhat among species, but all appear active during, in some cases, a long delay period. Marked changes occur at the onset of blastocyst expansion and implantation, including loss and apparent release of materials found within the cells and appearance of the characteristics of more highly secretory cells (Schlafke *et al.*, 1981). The general appearance of the endometrium also changes with increasing dilation of glands and general hypertrophy of the epithelium. In several species undergoing obligate delay, the concentration of uterine fluid protein has been shown to be low during the delay period, but it increases dramatically in the mink, northern fur seal, and western spotted skunk at about the time of implantation (Daniel and Krishman, 1969; Daniel, 1971; Mead *et al.*, 1979).

The changes in uterine histology and composition of uterine fluid are coincidental with the sharp rise in plasma progesterone levels noted at about the time of implantation in several delay species (European badger: Bonnin *et al.*, 1978; Canivenc and Bonnin, 1981; mink: Møller, 1973; northern fur seal: Daniel, 1975; spotted skunk: Mead and Eik-Nes, 1969; Mead, 1981; stoat: Gulamhusein and Thawley, 1974). However, studies of these species have shown that administration of exogenous progesterone is not sufficient to stimulate implantation (for review, see Mead, 1981; Mead *et al.*, 1981; Murphy *et al.*, 1983). Other undetermined factors produced by the corpus luteum, in addition to progesterone or estrogen, appear to be necessary for implantation to occur (Foresman and Mead, 1978; Murphy *et al.*, 1983; Mead *et al.*, 1981; Ravindra and Mead, 1984). Evidence in the mink and ferret also suggests that prolactin supports the corpus luteum and may control implantation in mustelids (Murphy, 1979; Murphy *et al.*, 1981; Martinet *et al.*, 1981). However, more information is necessary before our understanding of the interrelationship of the corpus luteum, embryo, and endometrium during the delay period and implantation is complete.

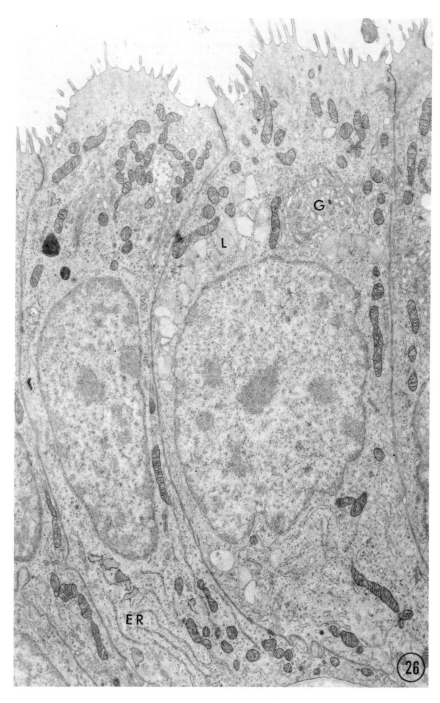

Figure 26. The tall columnar luminal epithelial cells of the endometrium of a mink in delayed implantation are shown in this micrograph. Note the rounded apical surfaces with protruding microvilli. The Golgi zones (G) are compact, and the endoplasmic reticulum (ER) is in the form of elongated undilated cisternae. A few lipid granules (L) are found in some of these cells, but no secretion granules are present. ×11,000.

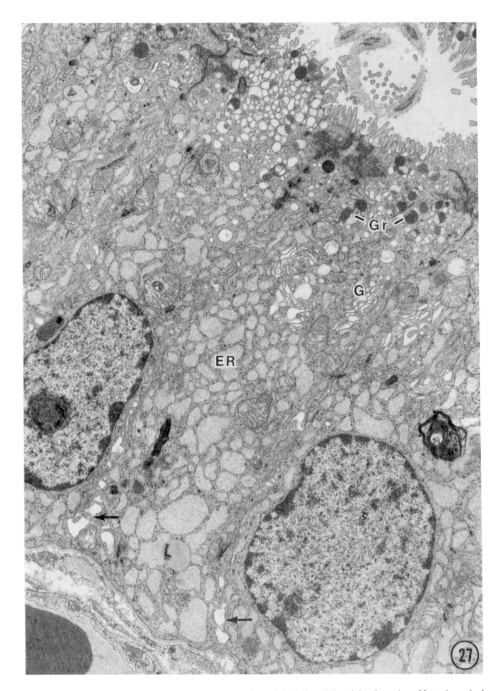

Figure 27. Glandular epithelial cells from a uterus of a mink during delayed implantation. Note the apical granules (Gr) and the extensive apical Golgi complexes (G). Dilated cisternae of endoplasmic reticulum (ER) fill much of the cell. The basolateral intercellular spaces are dilated (arrows). ×9000.

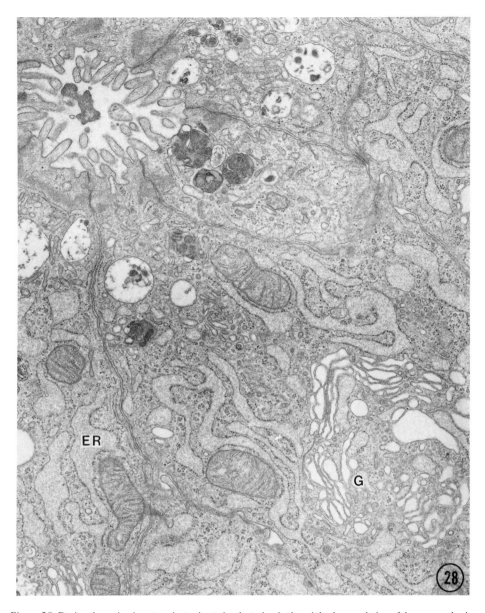

Figure 28. During the activation stage just prior to implantation in the mink, the population of dense granules in gland cells is depleted. Golgi zones (G) and cisternae of endoplasmic reticulum (ER) remain prominent. ×19,600.

6. Rodents

The subject of delayed implantation in rodents was first investigated by Lataste (1891), who noticed that when female rats were allowed to breed at the postpartum estrus, those suckling young had a longer gestation period than did mated but nonlactating females. He correctly attributed this prolongation of pregnancy to a delay in the time of implantation. Lataste also must be considered the first to study delayed implantation experimentally. He

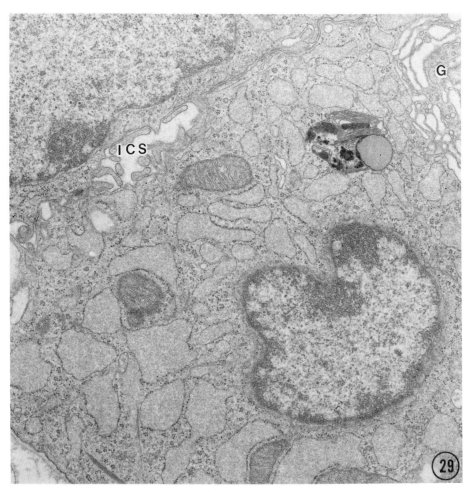

Figure 29. Basal region of an endometrial gland cell of a mink just prior to implantation. Dilated cisternae of rough endoplasmic reticulum largely fill this region of the cells. Golgi complex (G); intercellular space (ICS). ×19,600.

altered the implantation time, as judged by gestation length, both by removal of young from lactating females and by cauterization of nonlactating females. Since Lataste's time, extensive studies have been made of delayed implantation in the rat and the laboratory mouse. The gerbil has also been added to the group of laboratory animals known to have a lactational delay (Marston and Chang, 1965; Norris and Adams, 1971). Whereas limited work has been done concerning the distribution of delayed implantation in wild rodents (exceptions, in addition to Lataste's work, are reports of the vole, *Clethrionomys glareolus,* by Brambell and Rowlands, 1936; Andersson and Gustafsson, 1979; the deer mouse, *Peromyscus sp.,* by Svihla, 1932; Layne, 1968; and the northern grasshopper mouse, Egoscue, 1960), a great deal of information has been added to our understanding of the endocrine control of delay in the laboratory rat and mouse and of the blastocyst under these conditions.

Although it is clearly inaccurate to summarize all data accumulated concerning the various ways delayed implantation may be experimentally induced in the rat and mouse in one sentence, the overwhelming mass of the data suggests that delay of implantation in these species is a matter of progesterone dominance of the uterus in the absence of a sufficiency of estrogen. The delay period ends and implantation is initiated when an estrogen stimulus is given to the animal (for review, see Gidley-Baird, 1981). During the early delay period, rat and mouse blastocysts continue to grow and attain a size as great as or greater than those flushed from normal pregnant uteri at implantation (Schlafke and Enders, 1963; A. C. Enders and Schlafke, 1965; Surani, 1975a; Weitlauf *et al.*, 1979). Thus, the blastocysts can be considered "postdeveloped," as opposed to the "preswelling" condition of blastocysts in animals exhibiting central implantation.

The uterus of the myomorph rodents is relatively rich in stroma and poor in glandular epithelium compared with that of other groups exhibiting delay. The lumen is a nearly closed trench bordered by columnar epithelial cells with sparsely distributed simple coiled glands entering it. During delay there is some interdigitation of the adjacent microvilli of luminal epithelial cells of the two sides of the uterus (Hedlund and Nilsson, 1971; Martin *et al.*, 1970; Parr, 1983). A number of low longitudinal folds of endometrium are present, lending a serpentine appearance to a cross section of the lumen. An additional fold is often found in a mesometrial position, resulting in a T or inverted-L shape to the luminal cross section. When implantation follows delay, the lumen withdraws from the antimesometrial portion of the endometrium, and the "trench" becomes shorter. The epithelial "attachment reaction" becomes more pronounced, possibly after an intermediate period of transient fluid accumulation (Nilsson, 1974, 1980).

In both rat and mouse, the luminal epithelium is clearly the most abundant epithelial constituent of the endometrium. The tall columnar cells of this epithelium have abundant basal lipid droplets (Fig. 30). Glands tend to have fewer lipid droplets, although some may be present in the neck regions; in the mouse, a few droplets extend into the basal coils of the glands. The glandular epithelium is composed of more cuboidal cells than the luminal epithelium, and the nuclei are more basally situated. The lamina propria is highly vascular, with subluminal and periglandular plexuses as well as radially situated vessels throughout the highly cellular stroma (Fig. 30).

A number of studies have been concerned with the histochemistry of mouse (Hall, 1973, 1975) and rat (A. C. Enders, 1961) uteri in delay and preimplantation. Lipid, which is pronounced in luminal epithelial cells, appears to be restudied every few years (Alden, 1947; Elftman, 1958; A. Enders, 1961; Christie, 1967; Boshier and Holloway, 1973; Hall, 1975; Boshier, 1976; Boshier *et al.*, 1981). Although there is some variation in results concerning the amount of free fatty acids and lipid, most authors agree that lipid is abundant when progesterone predominates and that estrogen can produce a mobilization of the lipid (Elftman, 1963). Little or no glycogen is present in epithelial cells during delay, and alkaline phosphatase activity is very low in the epithelium, although the vascular bed is well demonstrated by this enzyme. Following an estrogen stimulus to the delay uterus, alkaline phosphatase activity appears at the luminal cell surface (Nilsson and Lundkvist, 1979). On the other hand, acid phosphatase and β-glucuronidase can be demonstrated in the apical ends of both luminal and glandular epithelial cells, especially in the area where the Golgi complex and most of the lysosomes are situated (A. C. Enders, 1961). At implantation there is a marked decrease in the β-glucuronidase activity in the luminal epithelium adjacent to the blastocyst (Roy *et al.*, 1983).

The general cytology of the epithelium of the rat uterus during delay has previously been described (Warren and Enders, 1964; A. C. Enders, 1967). Recent studies of the functional activity of the luminal epithelium have shown that it is involved in both endocytosis and exocytosis during delayed implantation. Exogenous tracers introduced into the uterine lumen are rapidly incorporated into large apical vacuoles (3 μm in diameter) (Fig. 31) formed by large ectoplasmic pinopods (Fig. 32) and into small vesicles (0.1 μm in diameter; A. C. Enders and Nelson, 1973; Parr and Parr, 1974, 1978). These vacuoles are then channeled into multivesicular bodies and lysosomes (Parr and Parr, 1978), which utilize microtubule-dependent mechanisms to move through the cells (Parr *et al.*, 1978; Parr, 1979) and may release some material along lateral intercellular borders (Enders and Nelson, 1973). Endocytosis

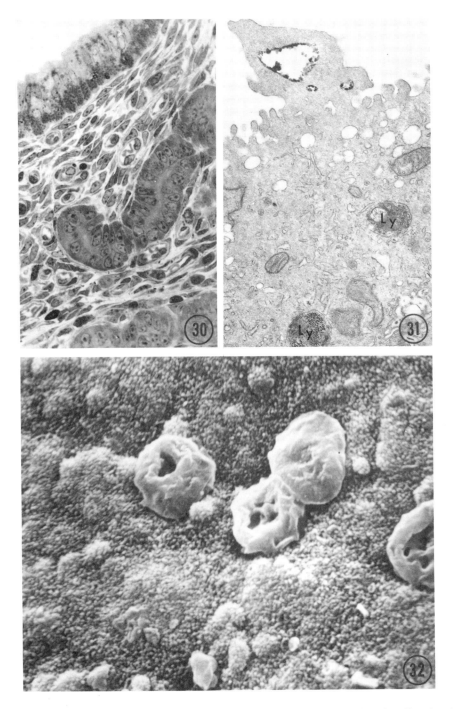

Figure 30. Light micrograph of the endometrium of a mouse on day 8 of delayed implantation. Note the tall columnar luminal epithelium containing supranuclear and subnuclear lipid. Lipid is also seen in the glandular epithelium. Note numerous capillaries closely apposed to the glandular coils. ×520.

Figure 31. Transmission electron micrograph of the uterine luminal epithelium of a rat on day 11 of delayed implantation. The edge of a large pinopod is seen on the apical surface of the cell. Peroxidase is present within vesicles in the pinopod. A few irregular strands of granular endoplasmic reticulum are present, as well as large secondary lysosomes (Ly). ×20,300.

Figure 32. Scanning electron micrograph of the luminal surface of a rat on day 11 of delay. Several pinopods are seen projecting from the microvillous surface. ×5900.

occurs under the influence of progesterone during delay and the days before normal implantation (A. C. Enders and Nelson, 1973; Parr and Parr, 1974, 1978). The administration of estrogen to the animal causes a decline in this apical endocytotic activity (Parr and Parr, 1977). Beyond the obvious function of removing uterine luminal contents prior to implantation, endocytosis may move "messengers" into the stroma or alter the composition of the epithelial cell apical membrane (Parr and Parr, 1986).

The luminal epithelium of the rat also exhibits secretory activity during the delay period. Apical vesicles, derived from the Golgi complex, are found at the apical borders of the cells (Parr, 1980, 1982a). They have membrane-staining properties similar to those of the apical cell membrane and are not involved in pinocytotic activity. Similar vesicles are also present in the luminal epithelium on day 5 of pregnancy prior to normal implantation. The number of vesicles appears to correlate with peak endocytotic activity. These vesicles may replace the apical cell membrane taken into the cells during endocytosis. Release of the vesicles could also provide a mechanism for changes in apical cell membrane prior to implantation (Parr, 1982a). Estrogen administration during the delay period causes a decline in the number of apical vesicles (Parr, 1982a). Recent studies using intraveneous administration of horseradish peroxidase have also shown uptake of tracer at the basolateral cell membrane of the luminal epithelium. Reaction product moves through the cell in tubules and small vesicles and finally accumulates at the cell apex for release by exocytosis (Parr, 1980, 1982b). This movement increases at implantation and may be one pathway for transport of plasma components into the uterine and glandular lumina. Fluorescence labeling has shown immunoglobulin within small granules in both luminal and glandular epithelium, which suggests a transport pathway through the epithelium similar to that seen using horseradish peroxidase (Parr and Parr, 1986).

The luminal epithelium of the mouse uterus during experimentally delayed implantation has also been described as having funguslike apical protrusions similar to pinopods observed in the rat by Psychoyos and Mandon (1971) and A. Enders and Nelson (1973). The protrusions make craterlike imprints in the blastocysts of delay when viewed by scanning electron microscopy (Bergstrom, 1972; Bergstrom and Nilsson, 1972). These protrusions are present throughout the experimental delay period and are active in the uptake of uterine luminal material (Parr and Parr, 1977). Both microvilli and pinopods of the luminal epithelium have a negatively charged glycoprotein cell surface coat (A. Enders and Schlafke, 1974). This cell coat appears to have a similar thickness on day 4 of pregnancy and during delay of implantation but is reduced in thickness on the day of implantation (Chavez and Anderson, 1985); however, lectin binding indicates that no change occurs in D-galactose residues during these time periods. This cell surface coat is of uniform thickness on all luminal epithelial cells including the site of blastocyst contact. In the rat, the surface coat also shows a uniform thickness on all areas, and no reduction in thickness was observed on the day of implantation. However, different techniques were used to demonstrate its presence (A. Enders et al., 1980).

The glandular epithelium of the mouse has been described at the light and ultrastructural levels during delay of implantation (Given and Enders, 1978). Simple tubular glands extend from the lumen and have a straight neck and a coiled basal region (Fig. 30). The glandular epithelium is composed of low columnar cells, which surround a narrow lumen that contains electron-dense material (Fig. 33). The cells have prominent apical microvilli, a well-developed Golgi complex lateral to the nucleus, and short cisternae of endoplasmic reticulum. Numerous electron-lucent vesicles are found along the apical borders of the cells. Multivesicular bodies are also characteristic of the apical regions of the cells. The basal regions of the cells contain lipid droplets and irregular cisternae of granular endoplasmic reticulum. The appearance of the glandular epithelium of the delayed-implanting uterus is similar to that observed in the endometrium of normally implanting animals on day 4 of pregnancy (Given and Enders, 1980).

Although many studies have been concerned with changes in the mouse uterus and blastocyst during normal implantation (Finn and Hinchliffe, 1965; Potts, 1966; Finn and McLaren, 1967; Potts and Wilson, 1967; Reinius, 1967; Potts, 1968; Wong and Dickson,

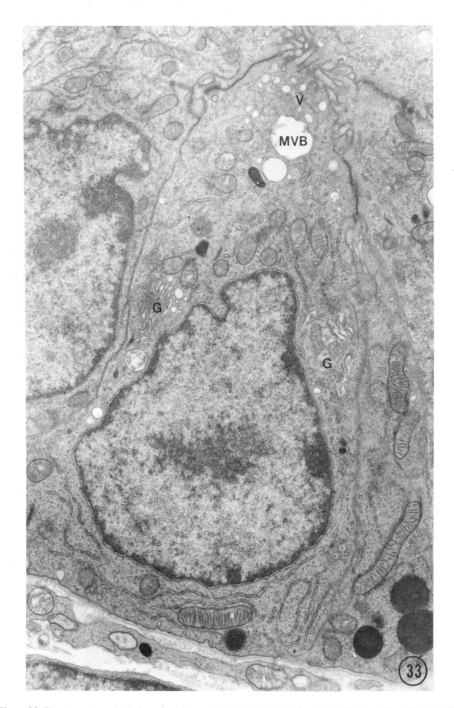

Figure 33. Electron micrograph of mouse uterine gland cell on day 8 during delayed implantation. Vesicles (V) and multivesicular bodies (MVB) occupy the apices of the cells. Prominent Golgi complexes (G) are located lateral to the nucleus. Irregular cisternae of granular endoplasmic reticulum are found throughout the cytoplasm. ×12,400.

1969; Smith and Wilson, 1971, 1974; Calarco and Epstein, 1973; Sherman and Wudl, 1976; Tachi and Tachi, 1986), the appearance of the endometrium during the implantation that follows the delay period has not been documented extensively. McLaren (1968) stated that after estrogen administration or removal of the litter during lactational delay, several changes could be seen in the mouse endometrium. These changes included the disappearance of shed zonas, the appearance of pontamine blue reactivity, stromal edema, and primary decidual formation. The same sequence of changes was seen by Finn and McLaren (1967) during normal implantation.

Nilsson (1974) has also noted some of the progressive changes seen after estrogen induction of implantation during experimental delay. The luminal epithelium lacks the large apical protrusions seen during delay, and the blastocysts are separated from the luminal epithelium by material that he considered a uterine secretion (Nilsson, 1974; Nilsson and Lundkvist, 1979) and is similar to a material seen by Potts (1968). Nilsson (1974, 1980) also noted a movement of apical vesicles toward the uterine lumen, followed by their depletion, which was interpreted as a discharge into the lumen. Subsequently, the luminal cell surface becomes progressively less microvillous and eventually closely apposed to trophoblast surface.

The glandular epithelium of the mouse undergoes several changes during implantation following the delay period (Given and Enders, 1978; Schlafke et al., 1981). Twenty-four hours following the 17β-estradiol stimulation of implantation, the glandular lumen is dilated with flocculent material. By 48 hr after 17β-estradiol administration, the glandular lumen is filled with a homogeneous electron-dense material (Fig. 34). The electron-lucent apical vesicles are no longer observed, and a new population of granules appears that contain electron-dense material similar to that seen in the lumen. The Golgi complex assumes a more apical position while the basal granular endoplasmic reticulum enlarges and has a more orderly arrangement of cisternae. These changes in the glandular epithelium are indicative of increased secretory activity. Similar changes in the glandular epithelium are also found during normal implantation on days 5 and 6 of pregnancy (Given and Enders, 1980).

Jenkinson (1913) described the uterine glands of the mouse during the implantation period as ''open glands with long necks. These secrete a coagulable, presumably proteoid material. These secretions are absorbed by the free blastocyst.'' More recent studies confirm these early impressions. The aforementioned cytological changes in the uterine glands as well as those observed during normal implantation are indicative of increased secretory activity at the time of implantation (Given and Enders, 1980). Secretory activity in the glands during the normal implantation period has been analyzed using light- and electron-microscopic autoradiography. Sites of protein and glycoprotein synthesis, intracellular transport, and release were followed using the tritiated tracers leucine, proline, and galactose (Given and Enders, 1981a,b). The amino acids were incorporated into the glandular epithelium by 20 min after intravenous administration, and labeled products were found in the glandular lumen by 45 min and at an even higher density by 90 min after administration (Given and Enders, 1981a). In vitro administration of tritiated galactose demonstrated similar rates of synthesis and secretion of glycoproteins (Given and Enders, 1981b). The rate of movement of labeled product into the glandular lumen was the same on days 4, 5, and 6 of pregnancy. Intracellular localization of labeled amino acids was initially highest over the granular endoplasmic reticulum and Golgi complex and then declined at 45 and 90 min. Localization of label over small cytoplasmic vesicles was highest at the later time intervals; thus, they appeared to be involved in intracellular transport of material to the lumen. In addition, larger apical vesicles appeared to be a transport pathway on day 5, and apical granules on day 6 of pregnancy. These pathways are similar to those seen in the luminal epithelium of the rat (Parr, 1980, 1982a,b). These observations provide the first direct evidence of the secretory capability of the uterine glands of the mouse during the periimplantation period. However, they do not provide quantitative values for production of the glands or the amount released into the uterine lumen (Given and Enders, 1981a; Schlafke et al., 1981).

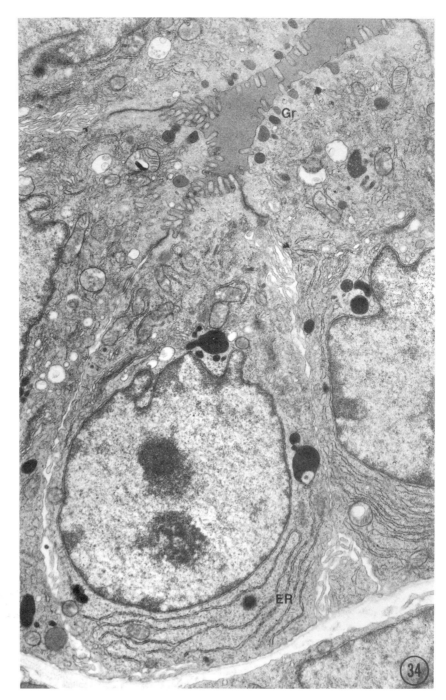

Figure 34. Uterine gland cells of mouse 48 hr after stimulation of implantation following a delay period. The gland lumen is filled with homogeneous electron-dense material. Note the absence of vesicles and presence of granules (Gr) along the apical cell border. A prominent Golgi complex and multivesicular bodies are above the nucleus. The cisternae of granular endoplasmic reticulum (ER) have an orderly arrangement at the base of the cells. ×11,900.

Changes in the composition of uterine fluid parallel the cytological changes observed in the luminal and glandular epithelium during implantation in the rat and mouse. Early studies in mice by Gwatkin (1969) reported a rise in amino acid and protein concentrations from day 3 of pregnancy until day 6. Amino acid concentration during the delay period was only slightly higher than that found on the day of implantation (day 5), and the species of amino acids present were similar at all time periods. Subsequent studies of uterine luminal proteins in both rats and mice have found that uterine protein concentration was consistently low during the delay period (Pratt, 1977; Aitken, 1977a; Surani, 1975b, 1976). Serum proteins comprise many of the proteins found during delay (Aitken, 1977a; Surani, 1975b). There is an increase in uterine protein concentration at the time of implantation both after the delay period and on day 5 or 6 (Gore-Langton and Surani, 1976; Pratt, 1977; Aitken, 1977a; Surani, 1975b, 1976, 1977a,b). Many of the proteins found at implantation appear to be of high molecular weight, uterine specific, and present only at the time of implantation (Fishel, 1979; Aitken, 1977a; Surani, 1976, 1977a,b). The appearance of these proteins is controlled by estrogen stimulation of the progesterone-dominated uterus (Fishel, 1979; Pratt, 1977; Aitken, 1977a; Surani, 1975b, 1977b). Some immunoglobulin accumulations have also been observed in the uterine lumen surrounding the blastocyst and in the uterine glands at the time of implantation (Bernard et al., 1977). Martin (1984) and Milligan and Martin (1984) have pointed out that many of the proteins reported to be present in uterine fluid may actually be from interstitial fluids that are released following damage to the luminal epithelium when collection fluid is forced through the uterine horn. The increase in serum protein at implantation reported in some studies may be the result of extensive damage to the closely apposed luminal epithelial sheets during flushing. However, other approaches that analyze protein synthesis in small pieces of endometrium (Mulholland and Villee, 1984) or isolated luminal epithelium or stroma (Lejeune et al., 1985) suggest a shift in specific uterine proteins produced at implantation compared with those of the preimplantation or delayed-implantation periods. Some proteins disappear while other proteins appear following the stimulus for implantation. Although it has been suggested that some of the proteins may be responsible for inhibition of embryonic development during delay or the metabolic stimulus at implantation (Lejeune et al., 1985), these proteins do not yet have specific known functions in the implantation process. Rather, their association with implantation is only a close temporal one.

Other studies have attempted to ascertain the specific function of some uterine fluid components. Mintz (1970) reported the presence of a factor with *in vivo* zonalytic activity in the uterine fluid of mice just before implantation. Proteinase activity in the uterine fluid during this period also was reported (Pinsker et al., 1974). Because of its temporal association with implantation, this agent was termed "implantation-inducing factor." The agent was absent during the delay period but appeared to be present after estrogen administration. Sacco and Mintz (1975) found immunologic evidence of two antigens in uterine fluid at the time of implantation, which could be these proteinases, and hypothesized that they might alter the blastocyst surface as well as help lyse the zona pellucida. An endopeptidase in rat uterine fluid that was linked to lysis of the zona pellucida has also been described (Joshi and Murray, 1974; Rosenfield and Joshi, 1977). Immunofluorescent methods have localized this factor in the glandular epithelium on days 5 and 6 of pregnancy in the rat. Hoversland and Weitlauf (1978, 1981, 1982) also described a hormone-dependent factor from the uterine fluid of mice with *in vitro* zonalytic activity that was present in ovariectomized animals given progesterone and estrogen. This factor corresponded to similar *in utero* zonalytic activity that was present when a maximum concentration of chymotrypsinlike activity was found in the uterine fluid.

Other factors in mouse uterine fluid appear to inhibit hatching of the blastocyst from the zona pellucida during delayed implantation (Aitken, 1977b). Still other components appear to be present in the uterine fluid of mice that help maintain the delayed implanting embryo in a state of metabolic quiescence. Weitlauf (1976, 1978) has reported factors in the uterine fluid of delayed-implanting animals that inhibited the RNA synthesis in blastocysts. However, these factors also were present in animals under simulated implanting conditions. More recently, O'Neill and Quinn (1983) have found that this inhibitory activity is dependent on the presence of delayed-implanting embryos in the uterine fluid. The inhibitory activity is reduced by 6 hr after estrogen administration only in the presence of blastocysts.

As can be seen, analysis of the intraluminal contents of the uterus has shown the presence of several factors that may be important in the development of the embryo and implantation. However, the precise role of these constituents and the cellular basis of their appearance remain to be determined.

7. Nonhuman Primates

Although there is no delay of implantation in primates, the time of implantation in most nonhuman primates is relatively late; that is, it varies from about 9 days after ovulation (rhesus monkey, baboon: A. Enders and Schlafke, 1986; A. Enders et al., 1983; Hendrickx, 1971) to as much as 12 days after ovulation (marmoset: Moore et al., 1985; Hearn, 1986). Since the function of the endometrium that sets it off from other mucous membranes is to receive and nurture the blastocyst, it seems particularly appropriate to describe its structure at the time of implantation and note the particular changes that occur either specifically or in response to the attaching blastocyst.

Bartelmez et al. (1951) and Bartelmez (1957), in careful studies of serially sectioned endometrium of the rhesus monkey throughout the cycle, chose to describe four separate zones. These zones are not as useful as they might be for describing the endometrium and its response to implantation, since the zones tend to blend into one another, and variation in structure, gland length, and coiling is considerable. Bartelmez refers to zone III as an intermediate zone at the time of implantation. It seems simpler to describe three zones (Fig. 35).

The *superficial zone* at the time of implantation consists of luminal epithelium and associated stroma, as in zone I of Bartelmez. In addition, this zone should include the epithelium in the surface grooves and the necks of the glands. It should be noted that most glands arise not directly from the luminal surface but from a series of grooves or crevices in the surface (Fig. 36), from each of which one or two glands arise. The epithelium of the grooves and the necks of the glands (regions with short epithelium and a more nearly closed lumen than other portions of the gland) are included in the superficial zone because this is the epithelium that responds to the blastocyst by becoming hypertrophic and polyploid, thus forming the epithelial plaque reaction (A. C. Enders et al., 1985). The stroma of this region responds to implantation by forming a ring of extreme subepithelial edema surrounding the implantation site (Figs. 37 and 38). The vessels within the superficial zone include fine juxtaluminal capillaries and the beginnings of the venular system that dilates and undergoes endothelial hypertrophy and hyperplasia during implantation.

The *principal zone* of the endometrium lies between the superficial zone and the basal convoluted zone. In this region, glands are relatively straight (Fig. 35), radiating from the lumen towards the myometrium as a series of variably wavy tubes that increase in diameter as they become deeper in the endometrium. At the time of implantation this is the thickest of the three zones. The branching of the glands that occurs in this zone is dichotomous. Most of the coiled arteries in this zone are relatively small. However, major coiled arteries may extend a short distance into the zone before giving rise to multiple branches.

The lumina of the glands are slightly open and are ovoid in cross section. Venules of this region undergo remarkable dilation during implantation and within 2 days after the initiation of implantation form a pronounced red spot within the endometrium.

The most basal zone of the endometrium is the *convoluted zone* (Fig. 35). In this region glands are irregularly coiled. In addition to some branching, the deeper portions of the glands

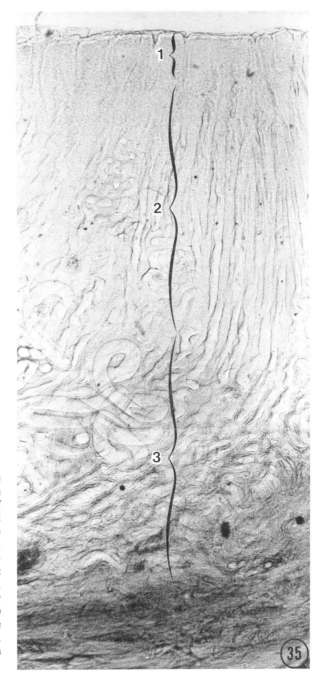

Figure 35. Thick slice through the entire thickness of the endometrium of a rhesus monkey at the time of implantation. There is a superficial portion (1) constituting the surface epithelium and subepithelial stroma. A region where the glands are relatively straight constitutes the greatest thickness of the endometrium (2), and a variable region of relatively convoluted portions of the glands (3) is adjacent to the myometrium. The coiled profiles of a large artery and, superficial to it, a smaller artery can be seen at the left. ×30.

often show a number of small short outpocketings. The ratio of area occupied by epithelial cells to that of stroma increases in the gland-rich regions of this zone. However, major coiled arteries are present, interrupting the area of glands. The venules become confluent with veins in this zone, and many lymphatic vessels are found (Fig. 39).

Bensley (1951) described mitosis during the cycle in the rhesus monkey, and more recently Padykula *et al.* (1984) have made a detailed study of the zonal pattern of [3H]thymidine incorporation around the time of ovulation. They showed that all zones at that

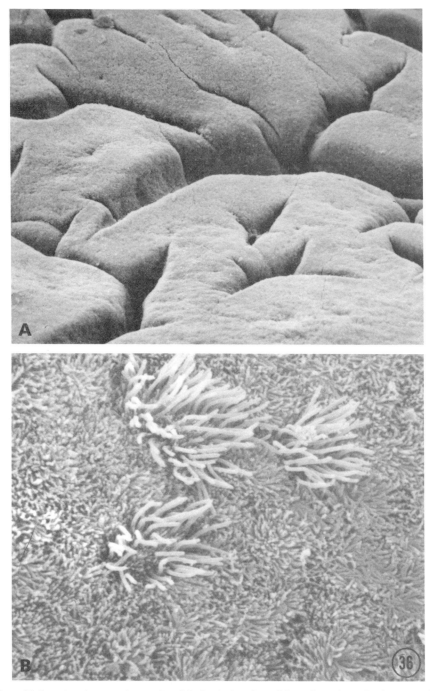

Figure 36. Scanning electron micrographs of the luminal surface of the endometrium of a rhesus monkey at implantation (day 10). A: Note that the smooth luminal surface is interrupted by grooves or crevices. One or several glands may open into a crevice. B: Most of the luminal epithelial cells have a microvillous border, but scattered cells are ciliated. A, ×190; B, ×5200.

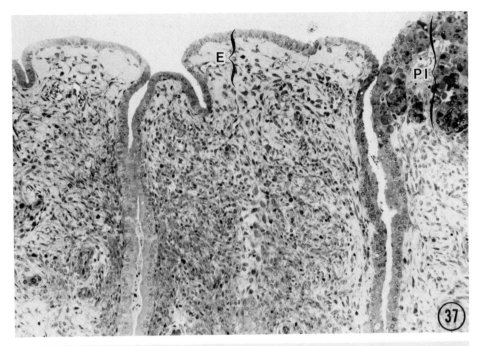

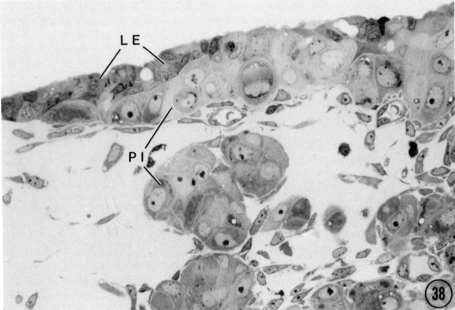

Figure 37. Endometrium adjacent to an area of implantation on day 13 of pregnancy in a rhesus monkey. At the extreme right is a region of epithelial cell hypertrophy forming a part of the epithelial plaque (P1). Peripheral to the plaque, the superficial stroma is edematous (E). Note that at the left, two glands enter a single crevice. ×115.

Figure 38. At higher magnification, it can be seen that it is the basal plaque cells (P1) that hypertrophy under the luminal epithelium (LE), whereas all of the cells hypertrophy in the necks of the glands. The stroma is edematous. ×500.

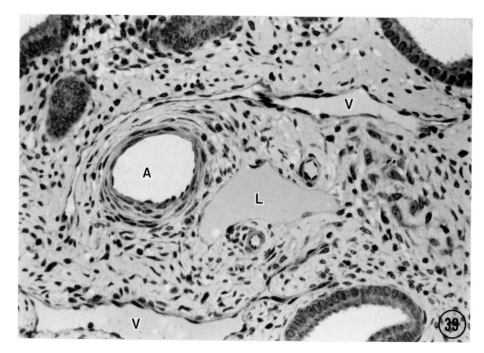

Figure 39. An artery (A), veins (V), and lymphatic vessel (L) in the basal part of the principal zone of the endometrium of a rhesus monkey. ×300.

stage had some DNA replication but suggested that, since Hartmann (1944) had shown that the entire endometrium could be reconstituted from small portions of the most basal region, most of the mitotic activity constituted transit-amplifying cells. Brenner *et al.* (1983) briefly compared the endometrium of the cynomolgus monkey with that of the rhesus and noted that they were essentially similar, showing postovulatory "stromal mitosis and enlargement, gland cell enlargement, increased glandular sacculation, spiral artery development, increased glandular secretory activity, and increased stromal edema in Zone I."

A few observations on the fine structure of some gland cells have been published (Padykula *et al.*, 1984; A. C. Enders *et al.*, 1985; Nelson, 1986), but no systematic study of the fine structure of the entire endometrium at the time of implantation has appeared.

In general the glandular epithelium of the principal zone consists primarily of secretory cells with only an occasional ciliated cell (Figs. 36 and 40). During implantation, many secretory cells contain an apical accumulation of vesicles with flocculent content (Fig. 41). In addition, there are often regions of glycogen accumulation within the cells, which may be more extensive in the cynomolgus monkey (Brenner *et al.*, 1983). The luminal epithelium consists of taller columnar cells and more numerous ciliated cells. Numerous short uniform microvilli are present on the secretory cells, although regions of microvilli are occasionally interrupted when secretory vesicles are most numerous.

Except for the stage of first adhesion of blastocyst to endometrium, which has not been described in primates, there is considerable information concerning the endometrium of the rhesus monkey during the first week of implantation. Wislocki and Streeter (1938) and Heuser and Streeter (1941) originally described the material in the Carnegie collection from this time period, and others, notably Luckett (1974), have also made use of this material. More recently A. C. Enders *et al.* (1985) have described the cytology of a series of implantation sites from the first week of postimplantation development.

In the earliest implantation stage, 9.5 days after ovulation, trophoblast had penetrated the

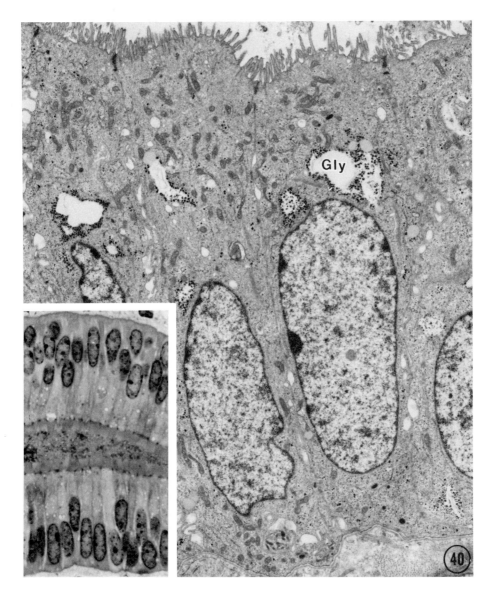

Figure 40. Glandular epithelium in the principal zone of the endometrium. The tall columnar cells contain patches of glycogen granules (Gly). Rhesus monkey, day 10 of pregnancy. ×7000; inset ×760.

luminal epithelium but not its basal lamina; the only local modification in the endometrium was an increase in the number of eosinophil leukocytes within the stroma (A. C. Enders *et al.*, 1983, 1985). However, implantation sites just ½–1 day later show a number of modifications. The most obvious is the beginning of an epithelial plaque response (Fig. 42). The first cells to show this modification are the basal cells within the uterine luminal epithelium. In addition to hyperplasia and hypertrophy, the large size of the nucleolus suggests that the cells become polyploid. During the next few days of gestation the epithelial plaque response extends into the crevices and necks of the glands, where all of the cells are involved (Fig. 38). The cells enlarge and begin to show glycogen storage.

Epithelial plaque cells also form at the secondary implantation site, where abembryonic

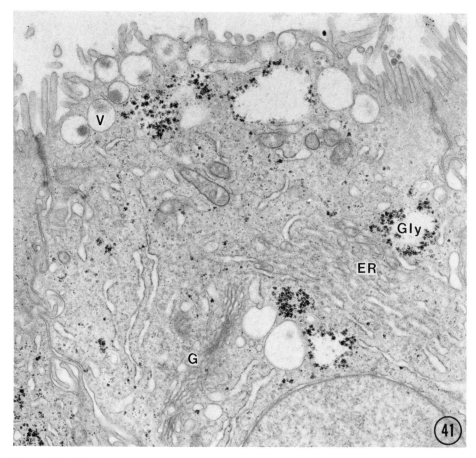

Figure 41. Apical region of an endometrial gland cell, showing vesicles (V) containing flocculent material typical of many of these cells. Note also the extensive areas of endoplasmic reticulum (ER), Golgi zones (G), and glycogen (Gly). Rhesus monkey, day 13 of pregnancy. ×15,300.

trophoblast contacts the uterus. The primary and secondary plaque regions may not center precisely on the blastocyst, and both regions usually show areas where trophoblast invasion is proceeding in the absence of plaque. Wislocki and Streeter (1938) reported that an occasional plaque area could be found removed from the implantation site, and Rossman (1940) demonstrated that a plaque reaction could be induced by trauma. Surprisingly, plaque areas persist for a relatively short time, and the degeneration of this area may begin by day 16. Epithelial plaque cells are also seen during early implantation in the baboon (Tarara *et al.*, 1987).

Another early and temporary endometrial response to implantation is extreme subepithelial edema, which results in a pad of gelatinous-looking stroma surrounding the implantation site (Fig. 37). The edematous area contains only a few scattered cells, largely fibroblasts and macrophages. During the late previllous period, the edematous region is pronounced in both rhesus monkey and baboon (Tarara *et al.*, 1987), and its reduction occurs slowly.

In the rhesus monkey, decidual transformation of endometrial stromal fibroblasts is slow, incomplete, and never produces cells quite as large as those in the human. However, by days 13 and 14, an increase in the amount of granular endoplasmic reticulum and in the number of intermediate filaments is seen within some of the fibroblast cells. Later the cells become modestly rounded, the endoplasmic reticulum becomes dilated, and some glycogen accumulates. The baboon and green monkey endometrium also shows decidualization of stromal cells;

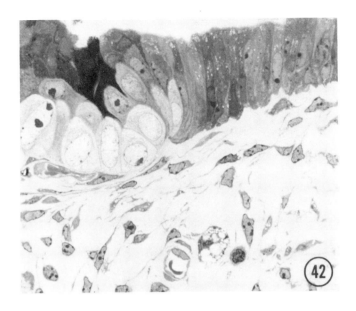

Figure 42. Margin of a region of epithelial plaque (left) adjacent to normal luminal epithelial cells (right) from an implantation site on day 10 of pregnancy in a rhesus monkey. ×760.

although the epithelioid transformation takes place in these species, the endometrium does not form a solid mass of decidual cells.

Endometrial granular cells increase in number during the first 2 weeks after implantation. These round cells, with striking accumulation of granules in the Golgi region (Cardell *et al.*, 1969), become more obvious during the second week after implantation, when they begin to accumulate glycogen. Morphologically, the cells resemble NK cells (natural killer lymphocytes), but their origin is not yet known.

Endothelial proliferation and hypertrophy are striking features of the venules of the principal zone of the endometrium (A. C. Enders *et al.*, 1985; Denker *et al.*, 1985). Numerous mitoses occur in the endothelial cells within 1 or 2 days of implantation. Subsequently, the endothelial cells of the venules hypertrophy impressively, and nuclei tend to assume a superficial position. The columnar nature of the endothelial cells gives the venules a glandular appearance. However, the polarity of the cells is reversed in that the Golgi zones are usually basal. The function of these high endothelial cells is unknown; they have also been identified in the green monkey (Owiti *et al.*, 1986) and in the baboon (Tarara *et al.*, 1987). Two or 3 days after the beginning of hypertrophy in the venules, large rounded intravascular cells appear in the coiled arteries. Many investigators believe that these cells are trophoblast cells (Ramsey *et al.*, 1976). However, they appear in patches in the slightly deeper coiled arteries instead of forming a continuous front that invades from the trophoblastic plate. Consequently, their origin remains problematic.

8. Discussion

Delayed implantation is a reproductive phenomenon found in a wide variety of mammalian species. Therefore, it is not surprising that there is variety in the endometrial structure of animals that exhibit delayed implantation. In some species the endometrium appears relatively quiescent during the portion of delayed implantation that precedes embryonic activation.

In the mouse, for example, gland lumina do not become dilated until implantation occurs. The endometria of the delay period can have a more active appearance in others. In the tammar wallaby, in which the delay period is in the anestrous season, glandular development of the uteri is greater than in nonmated animals. The weasel and badger are extraordinary in appearing to have a tremendous energy reserve in the form of glycogen in the superficial epithelium during delayed implantation. Several other species, such as the armadillo, have a highly vascular endometrium that has typical secretory glandular cells reminiscent of a preimplantation condition in nondelaying species.

It is not possible to generalize about classes of compounds found in endometrial cells during delay. Lipid is abundant in the rat and mouse in delay but is seen in abundance in the armadillo and mink only after implantation. Glycogen, which is prominent in the weasel and badger, is almost absent in several other species and appears only after implantation in the armadillo. In many species, cytological differences between luminal epithelial cells and glandular epithelial cells are rather remarkable during the delay period. In others, such as the spotted skunk, a large proportion of the glandular cells resemble luminal epithelium, while only the very basal cells appear secretory. Autoradiographic studies of mouse endometrium suggest that even though the glandular epithelia appear quiescent, they may actively secrete proteins and glycoproteins. However, information is needed in more species about the time sequence of formation, storage, and release of cellular products by both the luminal and glandular epithelium during delay and at implantation. This will provide a better understanding of the functional role of these epithelia in sustaining a diapausing blastocyst and supplying the periimplantation embryo.

Although it is obvious that the uterus controls blastocyst development during delay, it is good to see more evidence from other species, such as the roe deer and carnivores, that changes in endometrial structure coincide with blastocyst elongation (Aitken, 1974a) or activation prior to implantation. In carnivores, the presence of apical granules or vesicles, increase or dilation of the granular endoplasmic reticulum, and prominence of the Golgi complex at activation are indicative of increased secretory activity in the glands. The endometrial appearance during activation resembles that seen just before implantation in the ferret (*Mustela putorius*), which does not delay (Schlafke *et al.*, 1981). The glandular epithelium of the mouse also shows marked changes in secretory activity at implantation. In the pig, which has no delay, the glandular epithelium also shows changes similar to those in the roe deer at the time of embryonic elongation (Geisert *et al.*, 1982). The rhesus monkey, which does not delay but has a relatively late implantation, also maintains an active-appearing endometrium during the preimplantation period. However, it must be remembered that some or most of this secretory activity may not be related to implantation but to the support of the postimplantation embryo and fetal membranes.

Another encouraging trend has been the analysis of uterine fluid during delay of implantation and at implantation. Changes in the composition of uterine fluid at these times often coincide with the observed changes in the endometrium. Although some aspects of the nature of these fluids and the quantitative data can be influenced by the method of collection, data of this type and data on oxygen tension and ionic fluxes will help us understand the environment of the delayed blastocyst and changes at implantation.

The constituents of the uterine lumen in delay and nondelay species are the net result of influx and efflux (Fig. 43). Potentially, materials can enter the uterus from the oviduct (peritoneal fluid, oviductal secretions, transudates) and the endometrium (secretions by glandular and luminal epithelium, transudation from the vessels and stroma, direct diffusion of small molecules, dehiscence of luminal cells, and leukocyte migration). The blastocyst may also contribute substances acting locally (prostaglandins, proteases) and those having a more widespread effect (hormones).

On the efflux side, there is not only the possibility of direct loss from the cervix but, in

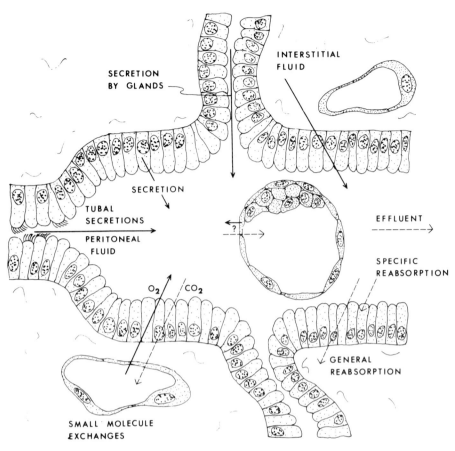

Figure 43. A diagrammatic representation of some of the possible factors responsible for maintaining the intrauterine environment during delayed implantation. The size of the uterine lumen is exaggerated in this figure so that the movement of luminal constituents can be represented.

addition, there is transudation from the lumen into stroma, pinocytosis such as that reported in the rat and mouse, and micropinocytosis, which would include specific reabsorption of selected components of uterine fluid. It is at least theoretically possible that the removal of a specific component by the blastocyst also could be significant. These constituents may be present only briefly or for more extended periods, but they all contribute to the environment of the blastocyst.

Although there are almost always alternative explantations, there seems to be increasing evidence of blastocyst-related effects during delayed implantation and implantation. The size of the corpora lutea increases in progesterone-delayed implantation when blastocysts are permitted to enter the uterus rather than prevented by ligature to the oviducts (Chatterton *et al.*, 1975). During activation, the delayed-implanting mouse blastocyst also appears to enhance the loss of inhibitory factors from uterine fluid (O'Neill and Quinn, 1983). In addition, there is evidence that the implanting blastocyst interacts with the endometrium, possibly through secreted prostaglandins or estrogen, to help initiate implantation (Dey and Johnson, 1986; Kennedy, 1983). Similarly, production of substances, possibly estrogen, by the blastocyst may be responsible for the increase in estrogen and progesterone receptors found in the implantation site of rats (Ward *et al.*, 1978; De Hertogh *et al.*, 1986).

Different aspects of intrauterine exchange have been emphasized by individual studies in particular species. Vascular exchanges are important for both oxygen and pH changes and are potentially quite variable, as seen in the rat (Yochim, 1975). The finding by several investigators that uterine specific proteins increase after the initiation of implantation following delay in rats and mice implicates endometrial secretion as an important part in the changing periimplantation environment. In a nondelay carnivore, the cat, it has been suggested that a uterine specific protein found in uterine glands and isolated from uterine fluid may be involved in implantation (Murray and Verhage, 1985). In the mink, in which the blastocyst survives in a highly variable climate during delay, including occasional augmentation by seminal fluid, specific secretion either to inhibit or to stimulate blastocyst development seems probable.

There has been a difference of opinion whether blastocysts are inhibited from further development during delay of implantation or are simply in a deficient, especially protein-deficient, environment (McLaren, 1973; Surani, 1977c). On the other hand, the increase in secretory activity in the roe deer, which undergoes a preimplantation swelling, has been interpreted as a release of accumulated secretion rather than a sudden change in nature of material synthesized (Aitken, 1974b).

Recently the role of absorption by the uterus has received considerable attention. In particular, the role that pinocytosis may play both in limiting the uterine environment and in permitting close apposition of uterus to the blastocyst has been demonstrated using tracers in the rat and mouse. These studies also indicate that the apical junctional complexes of the luminal epithelial cells are an effective barrier to larger molecules. The importance of absorption along the basal–lateral border for transport of materials to the uterine lumen has also been demonstrated. Such studies reveal the importance of the epithelium in the regulation of the uterine environment and the need for further research to understand better its function during the periimplantation period.

Evidence points to the presence of an active inhibitor in uterine fluid, at least in the rodent, that suppresses blastocyst metabolism (Weitlauf, 1976, 1978). During the quiescent period, RNA, DNA, and protein synthesis and glycolysis are all suppressed in the embryo (Sherman and Barlow, 1972; Weitlauf, 1974, 1982; Given and Weitlauf, 1981; Weitlauf *et al.*, 1979; Nieder and Weitlauf, 1984). This inhibition is lost with the stimulation of implantation in the presence of the embryo (O'Neill and Quinn, 1983). At implantation, endometrial protein secretion is altered, and it has been suggested that inhibitory proteins may be lost and stimulatory proteins appear at this time (Lejeune *et al.*, 1985).

Delay of implantation continues to be an important tool in the study of early embryonic development and implantation. In this chapter we have reviewed the endometrium of delay and the changes that occur at implantation in several species. However, this is only one facet of the research that utilizes this phenomenon. The delayed implantation model also has been used to investigate the endocrine control of implantation, blastocyst metabolism, and blastocyst–endometrial interrelationships. Although we do not know the exact nature of the control the uterus exerts on embryonic development, these areas of research will continue to expand our understanding of that control.

ACKNOWLEDGMENTS. We are happy to acknowledge the aid of the following investigators: Dr. R. K. Enders, who provided seal, mink, and marten material; Dr. P. L. Wright, who not only provided badger material but also made several live weasels available; Dr. R. A. Mead, who provided blocks of western spotted skunk material; Dr. R. V. Short, who kindly provided paraffin blocks of roe deer uterus; Dr. Hugh Tyndale-Biscoe, who provided glutaraldehyde-fixed red kangaroo material; and Dr. John Biggers, who provided some of the philander opossum material. Thanks are also extended to Thomas Blankenship for excellent technical assistance and Emily Preslar for preparation of the manuscript. Part of this work was supported by grant HD10342 from the National Institute of Child Health and Human Development.

Aitken, R. J., 1974a, Delayed implantation in roe deer (*Capreolus capreolus*), *J. Reprod. Fertil.* **39**:225–233.

Aitken, R. J., 1974b, Calcium and zinc in the endometrium and uterine flushing of the roe deer (*Capreolus capreolus*) during delayed implantation, *J. Reprod. Fertil.* **40**:333–340.

Aitken, R. J., 1975, Ultrastructure of the blastocyst and endometrium of the roe deer (*Capreolus capreolus*) during delayed implantation, *J. Anat.* **119**:369–384.

Aitken, R. J., 1977a, Changes in the protein content of mouse uterine flushings during normal pregnancy and delayed implantation, and after ovariectomy and oestradiol administration, *J. Reprod. Fertil.* **50**:29–36.

Aitken, R. J., 1977b, The culture of mouse blastocysts in the presence of uterine flushings collected during normal pregnancy, delayed implantation and pro-oestrus, *J. Embryol. Exp. Morphol.* **41**:295–300.

Aitken, R. J., 1981, Aspects of delayed implantation in the roe deer (*Capreolus capreolus*), *J. Reprod. Fertil. [Suppl.]* **29**:83–95.

Aitken, R. J., Burton, J., Hawkins, J., Kerr-Wilson, R., Short, R. V., and Stevens, D. H., 1973, Histological and ultrastructural changes in the blastocyst and reproductive tract of the roe deer (*Capreolus capreolus*), during delayed implantation, *J. Reprod. Fertil.* **34**:481–493.

Alden, R. H., 1947, Implantation of the rat egg. II. Alterations in epithelial lipids of the rat uterus under normal and experimental conditions, *Anat. Rec.* **97**:1–19.

Andersson, C. B., and Gustafsson, T. O., 1979, Delayed implantation in lactating bank voles, *Clethrionomys glareolus*, *J. Reprod. Fertil.* **57**:349–352.

Backhouse, K. M., and Hewer, H. E., 1964, Features of reproduction in the grey seal, *Med. Biol. Illus.* **14**:144–150.

Baevski, Y. B., 1967, Cytocaryometric researches on blastocyst in the mole, *Talpa altaica*, during the diapause period, *Dokl. Akad. Nauk SSSR* **176**:1198–2000.

Barabash-Nikiforov, I. I., 1935, The sea otter of the Commander Islands, *J. Mammal.* **16**:225–261.

Bartelmez, G. S., 1957, The form and the functions of the uterine blood vessels in the rhesus monkey, *Contrib. Embryol. Carnegie Inst.* **36**:153–182.

Bartelmez, G. W., Corner, G. W., and Hartman, C. G., 1951, Cyclic changes in the endometrium of the rhesus monkey (*Macaca mulatta*), *Contrib. Embryol. Carnegie Inst.* **34**:99–146.

Bensley, C. M., 1951, Cyclic fluctuations in the rate of epithelial mitosis in the endometrium of the rhesus monkey, *Contrib. Embryol. Carnegie Inst.* **34**:89–98.

Bergstrom, S., 1972, Delay of blastocyst implantation in the mouse by ovariectomy or lactation. A scanning electron microscope study, *Fertil. Steril.* **23**:548–561.

Bergstrom, S., and Nilsson, O., 1972, Ultrastructural response of blastocysts and uterine epithelium to progesterone deprivation during delayed implantation in mice, *J. Endocrinol.* **55**:217–218.

Bernard, O., Ripoche, M.-A., and Bennett, D., 1977, Distribution of maternal immunoglobulins in the mouse uterus and embryo in the days after implantation, *J. Exp. Med.* **145**:58–75.

Bischoff, T. L. W., 1854, *Entwicklingsgeschichte des Rehes*, J. Ricker'sche Buchhandlung, Giessen.

Bonnin, M., and Canivenc, R., 1980, Environmental factors involved in delayed implantation, *Prog. Reprod. Biol.* **7**:173–188.

Bonnin, M., Canivenc, R., and Ribes, C., 1978, Plasma progesterone levels during delayed implantation in the European badger (*Meles meles*), *J. Reprod. Fertil.* **52**:55–58.

Borodulina, T. L., 1951, Latent period of embryonic development in the Siberian mole, *Dokl. Akad. Nauk SSSR* **80**:689–692.

Boshier, D. P., 1976, Effects of the rat blastocyst on neutral lipids and non-specific esterases in the uterine luminal epithelium at the implantation area, *J. Reprod. Fertil.* **46**:245–247.

Boshier, D. P., 1979, Electron microscopic studies on the endometrium of the grey seal (*Halichoerus grypus*) during its preparation for nidation, *J. Anat.* **128**:721–735.

Boshier, D. P., 1981, Structural changes in the corpus luteum and endometrium of seals before implantation, *J. Reprod. Fertil. [Suppl.]* **29**:143–149.

Boshier, D. P., and Holloway, H., 1973, Effects of ovarian steroid hormones on histochemically demonstrable lipids in the rat uterine epithelium, *J. Endocrinol.* **56**:59–67.

Boshier, D. P., Holloway, H., and Millener, N. M., 1981, Triacylglycerols in the rat uterine epithelium during the oestrous cycle and early pregnancy, *J. Reprod. Fertil.* **62**:441–446.

Brambell, F. W. R., 1935, Reproduction in the common shrew (*Sorex araneus* L.). I. The oestrous cycle of the female, *Phil. Trans. R. Soc. Lond. [B]* **225**:1–50.

Brambell, F. W. R., 1937, The influence of lactation of the mammalian embryo, *Am. J. Obstet. Gynecol.* **33**:942–954.

Brambell, F. W. R., and Hall, K., 1936, Reproduction in the lesser shrew (*Sorex minutus Linnaeus*), *Proc. Zool. Soc. Lond.* 957.

Brambell, F. W. R., and Rowlands, I. W., 1936, Reproduction of the bank vole (*Evotomys glareolus*, Schreber). I. The oestrous cycle of the female, *Phil. Trans. R. Soc. Lond. [B]* **226**:71–97.

Brenner, R. M., Carlisle, K. S., Hess, D. L., Sandow, B. A., and West, B. A., 1983, Morphology of the oviducts and endometria of cynomolgus macaques during the menstrual cycle, *Biol. Reprod.* **29**:1289–1302.

Buchanan, G. D., 1967, The presence of two conceptuses in the uterus of a nine-banded armadillo, *J. Reprod. Fertil.* **13**:329–331.

Buchanan, G. D., Enders, A. C., and Talmage, R. V., 1956, Implantation in armadillos ovariectomized during the period of delayed implantation, *J. Endocrinol.* **14**:121–129.

Burns, J. M., 1981, Aspects of endocrine control of delay phenomena in bats with special emphasis on delayed development, *J. Reprod. Fertil. [Suppl.]* **29**:61–66.

Calarco, P. G., and Epstein, C. J., 1973, Cell surface changes during preimplantation development in the mouse, *Dev. Biol.* **332**:208–213.

Canivenc, R., and Bonnin, M., 1981, Environmental control of delayed implantation in the European badger (*Meles meles*), *J. Reprod. Fertil. [Suppl.]* **29**:25–33.

Canivenc, R., and Laffargue, M., 1963, Inventory of problems raised by the delayed ova implantation in the European badger (*Meles meles* L.), in: *Delayed Implantation* (A. C. Enders, ed.), University of Chicago Press, Chicago, pp. 115–125.

Cardell, R. R., Jr., Hisaw, F. L., and Dawson, A. B., 1969, The fine structure of granular cells in the uterine endometrium of the rhesus monkey (*Macaca mulatta*) with a discussion of the possible function of these cells in relaxin secretion, *Am. J. Anat.* **124**:307–340.

Chatterton, R. T., Jr., Macdonald, G. J., and Ward, D. A., 1975, Effect of blastocysts on rat ovarian steroidogenesis in early pregnancy, *Biol. Reprod.* **13**:77–82.

Chavez, D. J., and Anderson, T. L., 1985, The glycocalyx of the mouse uterine luminal epithelium during estrus, early pregnancy, the peri-implantation period, and delayed implantation. I. Acquisition of *Ricinus communis* I binding sites during pregnancy, *Biol. Reprod.* **32**:1135–1142.

Christie, G. A., 1967, Implantation of the rat embryo: Further histochemical observations on carbohydrate, RNA and lipid metabolic pathways, *J. Reprod. Fertil.* **13**:281–296.

Craig, A. M., 1964, Histology of reproduction and the estrus cycle in the female fur seal, *Callorhinus ursinus*, *J. Fish. Board. Can.* **21**:773–811.

Craighead, J. J., Hornocker, M. G., and Craighead, F. C., 1969, Reproductive biology of young female grizzly bears, *J. Reprod. Fertil. [Suppl.]* **6**:447–475.

Daniel, J. C., Jr., 1970, Dormant embryos of mammals, *Bioscience* **20**:411–415.

Daniel, J. C., Jr., 1971, Growth of the preimplantation embryo of the northern fur seal and its correlation with changes in uterine protein, *Dev. Biol.* **26**:316–322.

Daniel, J. C., Jr., 1975, Concentrations of circulating progesterone during early pregnancy in the northern fur seal, *Callorhinus ursinus*, *J. Fish. Res. Board Can.* **32**:65–66.

Daniel, J. C., Jr., 1981, Delayed implantation in the northern fur seal (*Callorhinus ursinus*) and other pinnipeds, *J. Reprod. Fertil. [Suppl.]* **29**:35–50.

Daniel, J. C., Jr., and Krishman, R. S., 1969, Studies on the relationship between uterine fluid components and the diapausing state of blastocysts from mammals having delayed implantation, *J. Exp. Zool.* **172**:267–282.

Dawson, A. B., and Kosters, B. A., 1944, Preimplantation changes in the uterine mucosa of the cat, *Am. J. Anat.* **74**:1–35.

Deanesly, R., 1935, The reproductive processes of certain mammals. IX. Growth and reproduction in the stoat (*Mustela erminea*), *Phil. Trans. R. Soc. Lond. [B]* **225**:459–492.

Deanesly, R., 1943, Delayed implantation in the stoat (*Mustela mustela*), *Nature* **151**:365–366.

De Hertogh, R., Ekka, E., Vanderheyden, I., and Glorieux, B., 1986, Estrogen and progesterone receptors in the implantation sites and interembryonic segments of rat uterus endometrium and myometrium, *Endocrinology* **119**:680–684.

Denker, H.-W., Enders, A. C., and Schlafke, S., 1985, Bizarre hypertrophy of vascular endothelial cells in rhesus monkey endometrium: Experimental induction and electron microscopical characteristics, *Verh. Anat. Ges.* **79**:545–548.

Dey, S. K., and Johnson, D. C., 1986, Embryonic signals in pregnancy, *Ann. N.Y. Acad. Sci.* **476**:49–62.

Egoscue, H. J., 1960, Laboratory and field studies of the northern grasshopper mouse, *J. Mammal.* **41**:99–110.

Elftman, H., 1958, Estrogen control of the phospholipids of the uterus, *Endocrinology* **62**:410–415.

Elftman, H., 1963, Estrogen induced changes in the Golgi apparatus and lipid of the uterine epithelium of the rat in the normal cycle, *Anat. Rec.* **146:**139–143.

Enders, A. C., 1961, Comparative studies on the endometrium of delayed implantation, *Anat. Rec.* **139:**483–497.

Enders, A. C., 1966, The reproductive cycle of the nine-banded armadillo (*Dasypus novemcinctus*), in: *Comparative Biology of Reproduction in Mammals* (I. W. Rolands, ed.), Academic Press, New York, pp. 295–310.

Enders, A. C., 1967, The uterus in delayed implantation, in: *Cellular Biology of the Uterus* (R. M. Wynn, ed.), Appleton-Century-Crofts, New York, pp. 151–186.

Enders, A. C., and Buchanan, G. D., 1959a, The reproductive tract of the female nine-banded armadillo, *Tex. Rep. Biol. Med.* **17:**323–340.

Enders, A. C., and Buchanan, G. D., 1959b, Some effects of ovariectomy and injection of ovarian hormones in the armadillo, *J. Endocrinol.* **19:**251–258.

Enders, A. C., and Nelson, D. M., 1973, Pinocytotic activity of the uterus of the rat, *Am. J. Anat.* **138:**277–300.

Enders, A. C., and Schlafke, S., 1965, The fine structure of the blastocyst: Some comparative studies, *Ciba Found. Symp.* **12:**29–59.

Enders, A. C., and Schlafke, S., 1974, Surface coats of the mouse blastocyst and uterus during the preimplantation period, *Anat. Rec.* **180:**31–46.

Enders, A. C., and Schlafke, S., 1986, Implantation in nonhuman primates and in the human, in: *Comparative Primate Biology*, Volume 3: *Reproduction and Development* (W. R. Dukelow and J. Erwin, eds.), Alan R. Liss, New York, pp. 291–210.

Enders, A. C., Buchanan, G. D., and Talmage, R. V., 1958, Histological and histochemical observations on the armadillo uterus during the delayed and post-implantation periods, *Anat. Rec.* **130:**639–657.

Enders, A. C., Enders, R. K., and Schlafke, S., 1963, An electron microscopic study of the gland cells of the mink endometrium, *J. Cell Biol.* **18:**405–418.

Enders, A. C., Schlafke, S., and Welsh, A. O., 1980, Trophoblastic and uterine luminal epithelial surfaces at the time of blastocyst adhesion in the rat. *Am. J. Anat.* **159:**59–72.

Enders, A. C., Hendrickx, A. G., and Schlafke, S., 1983, Implantation in the rhesus monkey: Initial penetration of the endometrium, *Am. J. Anat.* **167:**275–298.

Enders, A. C., Welsh, A. O., and Schlafke, S., 1985, Implantation in the rhesus monkey: Endometrial responses, *Am. J. Anat.* **173:**147–169.

Enders, R. K., 1952, Reproduction in the mink (*Mustela vison*), *Proc. Am. Phil. Soc.* **96:**691–755.

Enders, R. K., 1956, Delayed implantation in mammals, in: *Transactions of the Second Conference on Gestation* (Josiah Macy, Jr. Foundation), (C. A. Villee, ed.), Madison Publishing Co., Madison, NJ, pp. 113–130.

Enders, R. K., and Enders, A. C., 1963, Morphology of the female reproductive tract during delayed implantation in the mink, in: *Delayed Implantation* (A. C. Enders, ed.), University of Chicago Press, Chicago, pp. 129–140.

Fayenuwo, J. O., and Halstead, L. B., 1974, Breeding cycle of straw-colored fruit bat, *Eidolon helvum,* at Ile-Ife, Nigeria, *J. Mammal.* **55:**453–454.

Finn, C. A., and Hinchliffe, J. R., 1965, Histological and histochemical analysis of the formation of implantation chambers in the mouse uterus, *J. Reprod. Fertil.* **9:**301–309.

Finn, C. A., and McLaren, A., 1967, A study of the early stages of implantation in mice, *J. Reprod. Fertil.* **13:**259–267.

Fishel, S. B., 1979, Analysis of mouse uterine proteins at pro-oestrus, during early pregnancy and after administration of exogenous steroids, *J. Reprod. Fertil.* **55:**91–100.

Fisher, H. D., 1954, Delayed implantation in the harbour seal, *Phoca vitulina* L., *Nature* **173:**879–880.

Foresman, K. R., and Mead, R. A., 1973, Duration of postimplantation in a western subspecies of the spotted skunk (*Spilogale putorius*), *J. Mammal.* **54:**521–523.

Foresman, K. R., and Mead, R. A., 1978, Luteal control of nidation in the ferret (*Mustela putorius*), *Biol. Reprod.* **18:**490–496.

Geisert, R. D., Renegar, R. H., Thatcher, W. W., Roberts, R. M., and Bazer, F. W., 1982, Establishment of pregnancy in the pig. I. Interrelationships between preimplantation development of the pig blastocyst and uterine endometrial secretions, *Biol. Reprod.* **27:**925–939.

Gidley-Baird, A. A., 1981, Endocrine control of implantation and delayed implantation in rats and mice, *J. Reprod. Fertil. [Suppl.]* **29:**97–109.

Given, R. L., and Enders, A. C., 1978, Mouse uterine glands during the delayed and induced implantation periods, *Anat. Rec.* **190:**271–284.

Given, R. L., and Enders, A. C., 1980, Mouse uterine glands during the peri-implantation period. I. Fine structure, *Am. J. Anat.* **157:**169–179.

Given, R. L., and Enders, A. C., 1981a, Mouse uterine glands during the peri-implantation period. II. Autoradiographic studies, *Anàt. Rec.* **199:**109–127.

Given, R. L., and Enders, A. C., 1981b, Autoradiographic studies of mouse uterine glands during the peri-implantation period, in: *Cellular and Molecular Aspects of Implantation* (D. Bullock and S. Glasser, eds.), Plenum Press, New York, pp. 454–456.

Given, R. L., and Weitlauf, H. M., 1981, Resumption of DNA synthesis during activation of delayed implanting mouse blastocysts, *J. Exp. Zool.* **218:**253–259.

Gore-Langton, R. E., and Surani, M. A. H., 1976, Uterine luminal proteins of mice, *J. Reprod. Fertil.* **46:**271–274.

Gulamhusein, A. P., and Thawley, A. R., 1974, Plasma progesterone levels in the stoat, *J. Reprod. Fertil.* **36:**405–408.

Gwatkin, R. B. L., 1969, Nutritional requirements for post-blastocyst development in the mouse, *Int. J. Fertil.* **14:**101–105.

Hall, K., 1973, Lactic dehydrogenase and other enzymes in the mouse uterus during the peri-implantation period of pregnancy, *J. Reprod. Fertil.* **34:**79–91.

Hall, K., 1975, Lipids in the mouse uterus during early pregnancy, *J. Endocrinol.* **65:**233–243.

Hamilton, W. J., Jr., and Eadie, W. R., 1964, Reproduction in the otter, *J. Mammal.* **45:**242–251.

Hamlett, G. W. D., 1932a, The reproductive cycle in the armadillo, *Wiss. Zool.* **141:**143–157.

Hamlett, G. W. D., 1932b, Observations on the embryology of the badger, *Anat. Rec.* **53:**283–303.

Hamlett, G. W. D., 1935, Delayed implantation and discontinuous development in the mammals, *Rev. Biol.* **10:**432–447.

Hansson, A., 1947, The physiology of reproduction in mink (*Mustela vison* Schreb) with special reference to delayed implantation, *Acta Zool. Stockh.)* **28:**1–136.

Harrison, R. J., 1960, Reproduction and reproductive organs in common seals (*Phoca vitulina*), *Mammalia* **24:**372–385.

Harrison, R. J., 1963, A comparison of factors involved in delayed implantation in badgers and seals in Great Britain, in: *Delayed implantation* (A. C. Enders, ed.), University of Chicago Press, Chicago, pp. 99–114.

Harrison, R. J., 1969, Reproduction and reproductive organs, in: *The Biology of Marine Mammals* (H. T. Anderson, ed.), Academic Press, New York, pp. 253–348.

Harrison, R. J., and Hamilton, W. J., 1952, The reproductive tract and placenta and membranes of Père David's deer (*Elaphurus davidianus* Milne Edwards), *J. Anat.* **86:**203–255.

Harrison, R. J., and Hyett, A. R., 1954, The development and growth of the placentomes in the fallow deer (*Dama dama* L.), *J. Anat.* **88:**338–355.

Harrison, R. J., and Neal, E. G., 1959, Delayed implantation in the badger (*Meles meles*), *Mem. Soc. Endocrinol.* **6:** 23–25.

Hartmann, C. G., 1944, Regeneration of the monkey uterus after surgical removal of the endometrium and accidental endometriosis, *West. J. Surg. Obstet. Gynecol.* **52:**87–102.

Hearn, J. P., 1986, The embryo–maternal dialogue during early pregnancy in primates, *J. Reprod. Fertil.* **76:**809–819.

Hedlund, K., and Nilsson, O., 1971, Hormonal requirements for the uterine attachment reaction and blastocyst implantation in the mouse, hamster and guinea-pig, *J. Reprod. Fertil.* **26:**267–269.

Hendrickx, A. G., 1971, *Embryology of the Baboon,* University of Chicago Press, Chicago.

Heuser, C. H., and Streeter, G. L., 1941, Development of the macaque embryo, *Contrib. Embryol. Carnegie Inst.* **29:**15–55.

Hewer, H. R., and Backhouse, K. M., 1968, Embryology and foetal growth of the grey seal, *Halichoerus grypus, J. Zool. (Lond.)* **155:**507–533.

Hoffman, B., Barth, D., and Karg, H., 1978, Progesterone and estrogen levels in peripheral plasma of the pregnant and nonpregnant roe deer (*Capreolus capreolus*), *Biol. Reprod.* **19:**931–935.

Hoversland, R. C., and Weitlauf, H. M., 1978, The effect of estrogen and progesterone on the level of amidase activity in fluid flushed from the uteri of ovariectomized mice, *Biol. Reprod.* **19:**908–912.

Hoversland, R. C., and Weitlauf, H. M., 1981, Lysis of the zona pellucida and attachment of embryos to the uterine epithelium in ovariectomized mice treated with oestradiol-17β and progesterone, *J. Reprod. Fertil.* **62:**111–116.

Hoversland, R. C., and Weitlauf, H. M., 1982, *In vitro* zona-lytic activity in uterine fluid from ovariectomized mice treated with oestradiol-17β and progesterone, *J. Reprod. Fertil.* **64:**223–226.

Hughes, R. L., Thomson, J. A., and Owen, W. H., 1965, Reproduction in natural populations of the Australian ringtail possum, *Pseudochirus pergrinus* (Marsupialia: Phalangeridae), in Victoria, *Aust. J. Zool.* **13:**383–406.

Jenkinson, J. W., 1931, *Vertebrate Embryology*, Clarendon Press, Oxford.

Joshi, M. S., and Murray, I. M., 1974, Immunological studies of the rat uterine fluid peptidase, *J. Reprod. Fertil.* **37**:361–365.

Judin, B. S., 1974, Characteristics of the reproduction of the Siberian mole *Asioscalops altaica, Acta Theriol.* **19**:355–366.

Kennedy, T. G., 1983, Embryonic signals and the initiation of blastocyst implantation, *Aust. J. Biol. Sci.* **36**:531–543.

Kimura, K., and Uchida, T. A., 1983, Ultrastructural observations of delayed implantation in the Japanese long-fingered bat, *Miniopterus schreibersii fuliginosus, J. Reprod. Fertil.* **69**:187–193.

Labhsetwar, A. P., and Enders, A. C., 1968, Progesterone in the corpus luteum and placenta of the armadillo, *Dasypus novemcinctus, J. Reprod. Fertil.* **16**:381–387.

Lataste, F., 1891, De la variation de durée la gestation chez les mammifères et des circonstances qui déterminent ces variations, *Mem. Soc. Biol.* **43**:21–31.

Laws, R. M., 1956, The elephant seal, *Mirounga leonina,* III. Physiology of reproduction, *Falkland Isl. Depend. Surv. Sci. Rep.* **15**:1–66.

Layne, J. N., 1968, Ontogeny, in: *Biology of Peromyscus (Rodentia)* (J. A. King, ed.), American Society of Mammalogists Lawrence, KS, pp. 148–253.

Lejeune, B., Lamy, F., Lecocq, R., Deschacht, J., and Leroy, F., 1985, Patterns of protein synthesis in endometrial tissues from ovariectomized rats treated with oestradiol and progesterone, *J. Reprod. Fertil.* **73**:223–228.

Lincoln, G. A., and Guinness, F. E., 1972, Effect of altered photoperiod on delayed implantation and moulting in roe deer, *J. Reprod. Fertil.* **31**:455–457.

Luckett, W. P., 1974, Comparative development and evolution of the placenta in primates, *Contrib. Primatol.* **3**:142–234.

Marston, J. H., and Chang, M. C., 1965, The breeding, management and reproductive physiology of the Mongolian gerbil *(Meriones unguiculatus)*, *Lab. Anim. Care* **15**:34–48.

Martin, L., 1984, On the source of uterine ''luminal fluid'' proteins in the mouse, *J. Reprod. Fertil.* **71**:73–80.

Martin, L., Finn, C. A., and Carter, J., 1970, Effects of progesterone and oestradiol-17β on the luminal epithelium of the mouse uterus, *J. Reprod. Fertil.* **21**:461–469.

Martinet, L., Allais, C., and Allain, D., 1981, The role of prolactin and LH in luteal function and blastocyst growth in mink *(Mustela vison)*, *J. Reprod. Fertil. [Suppl.]* **29**:119–130.

McLaren, A., 1968, A study of blastocysts during delay and subsequent implantation in lactating mice, *J. Endocrinol.* **42**:453–463.

McLaren, A., 1973, Blastocyst activation, in: *The Regulation of Mammalian Reproduction* (S. J. Segal, R. Crozier, P. A. Corfman, and P. G. Concliffe, eds.), Charles C. Thomas, Springfield, IL, pp. 321–334.

Mead, R. A., 1968a, Reproduction in eastern forms of the spotted skunk (genus *Spilogale*), *J. Zool. (Lond.)* **156**:119–136.

Mead, R. A., 1968b, Reproduction in western forms of the spotted skunk (genus *Spilogale*), *J. Mammal.* **49**:373–390.

Mead, R. A., 1981, Delayed implantation in mustelids, with special emphasis on the spotted skunk, *J. Reprod. Fertil. [Suppl.]* **29**:11–24.

Mead, R. A., and Eik-Nes, K. B., 1969, Seasonal variation in plasma levels of progesterone in western forms of the spotted skunk, *J. Reprod. Fertil. [Suppl.]* **6**:397–403.

Mead, R. A., Rourke, A. W., and Swannack, A., 1979, Changes in uterine protein synthesis during delayed implantation in the Western spotted skunk and its regulation by hormones, *Biol. Reprod.* **21**:39–46.

Mead, R. A., Concannon, P. W., and McRae, M., 1981, Effect of progestins on implantation in the Western spotted skunk, *Biol. Reprod.* **25**:128–133.

Michener, J. A., 1986, *Texas,* Random House, New York.

Milligan, S. R., and Martin, L., 1984, The resistance of the mouse uterine lumen to flushing and possible contamination of samples by plasma and interstitial fluid, *J. Reprod. Fertil.* **71**:81–87.

Mintz, B., 1970, Control of embryo implantation and survival, in: *Advances in the Biosciences 6* (G. Raspe, ed.), Pergamon Press–Vieweg, Oxford, pp. 317–341.

Møller, O. M., 1973, The progesterone concentrations in the peripheral plasma of the mink *(Mustela vison)* during pregnancy, *J. Endocrinol.* **56**:121–132.

Moore, H. D. M., Gens, S., and Hearn, J. P., 1985, Early implantation stages in the marmoset monkey *(Callithrix jacchus)*, *Am. J. Anat.* **172**:2665–278.

Mulholland, J., and Villee, C. A., Jr., 1984, Proteins synthesized by the rat endometrium during early pregnancy, *J. Reprod. Fertil.* **72**:395–400.

Murphy, B. D., 1979, The role of prolactin in implantation and luteal maintenance in the ferret, *Biol. Reprod.* **21**:517–521.

Murphy, B. D., and James, D. A., 1974, Mucopolysaccharide histochemistry of the mink uterus during gestation, *Can. J. Zool.* **52**:687–693.

Murphy, B. D., Concannon, P. W., Travis, H. F., and Hansel, W., 1981, Prolactin: The hypohyseal factor that terminates embryonic diapause in mink, *Biol. Reprod.* **25**:487–491.

Murphy, B. D., Mead, R. A., and McKibbin, P. E., 1983, Luteal contribution to the termination of preimplantation delay in mink, *Biol. Reprod.* **28**:497–503.

Murray, M. K., and Verhage, H. G., 1985, The immunocytochemical localization of a cat uterine protein that is estrogen-dependent (CUPED), *Biol. Reprod.* **32**:1229–1231.

Mutere, F. A., 1967, The breeding biology of equatorial vertebrates: Reproduction in the fruit bat, *Eiodolon helvum,* at latitude 0°20′N, *Zoology (Lond.)* **153**:153–161.

Nelson, D. M., 1986, Morphology and glycoprotein synthesis of uterine glandular epithelium in human basal plate, *Anat. Rec.* **216**:146–153.

Nieder, G. L., and Weitlauf, H. M., 1984, Regulation of glycolysis in the mouse blastocyst during delayed implantation, *J. Exp. Zool.* **231**:121–129.

Nilsson, B. O., 1974, The morphology of blastocyst implantation, *J. Reprod. Fertil.* **39**:187–194.

Nilsson, B. O., 1980, Electron microscopic aspects of epithelial changes related to implantation, *Prog. Reprod. Biol.* **7**:70–80.

Nilsson, B. O., and Lundkvist, O., 1979, Ultrastructural and histochemical changes of the mouse uterine epithelium on blastocyst activation for implantation, *Anat. Embryol.* **155**:311–321.

Norris, M. L., and Adams, C. E., 1971, Delayed implantation in the Monogolian gerbil, *Meriones unguiculatus, J. Reprod. Fertil.* **27**:487.

O'Neill, C., and Quinn, P., 1983, Inhibitory influences of uterine secretions on mouse blastocysts decreases at the time of blastocyst activation, *J. Reprod. Fertil.* **29**:123–126.

Orsini, M. W., and Meyer, R. K., 1962, Effect of varying doses of progesterone on implantation in the ovariectomized hamster, *Proc. Soc. Exp. Biol. Med.* **110**:713–715.

Ouellette, J., and Ronald, K., 1985, Histology of reproduction in harp and grey seals during pregnancy, postparturition, and estrus, *Can. J. Zool.* **63**:1778–1796.

Owiti, G., Cukierski, M., Tarara, R. P., Enders, A. C., and Hendrickx, A. G., 1986, Early placentation in the African green monkey (*Cercopithecus aethiops*), *Acta Anat.* **127**:184–194.

Padykula, H. A., and Taylor, J. M., 1976, Cellular mechanisms involved in cyclic stromal renewal of the uterus. I. The opossum, *Didelphis virginians, Anat. Rec.* **184**:5–26.

Padykula, H. A., Coles, L. G., McCracken, J. A., King, N. W., Jr., Longcope, C., and Kaiserman-Abramof, I. R., 1984, A zonal pattern of cell proliferation and differentiation in the rhesus endometrium during the estrogen surge, *Biol. Reprod.* **31**:1103–1118.

Parr, M. B., 1979, A morphometric analysis of microtubules in relation to the inhibition of lysosome movement in the rat uterine epithelium, *Eur. J. Cell Biol.* **20**:189–194.

Parr, M. B., 1980, Endocytosis at the basal and lateral membranes of rat uterine epithelium during early pregnancy, *J. Reprod. Fertil.* **60**:95–99.

Parr, M. B., 1982a, Apical vesicles in the rat uterine epithelium during early pregnancy: A morphometric study, *Biol. Reprod.* **26**:915–924.

Parr, M. B., 1982b, Effects of ovarian hormones on endocytosis at the basal membranes of rat uterine epithelial cells, *Biol. Reprod.* **26**:909–913.

Parr, M. B., 1983, Relationship of uterine closure to ovarian hormones and endocytosis in the rat, *J. Reprod. Fertil.* **68**:185–188.

Parr, E., and Parr, M., 1974, Uterine luminal epithelium: Protrusions mediate endocytosis, not apocrine secretion, in the rat, *Biol. Reprod.* **11**:220–223.

Parr, M. B., and Parr, E. L., 1977, Endocytosis in the uterine epithelium in the mouse, *J. Reprod. Fertil.* **50**:151–153.

Parr, M. B., and Parr, E. L., 1978, Uptake and fate of ferritin in the uterine epithelium of the rat during early pregnancy, *J. Reprod. Fertil.* **52**:183–188.

Parr, M. B., and Parr, E. L., 1986, Endocytosis in the rat uterine epithelium at implantation, *Ann. N.Y. Acad. Sci.* **476**:110–121.

Parr, M. B., Kay, M. G., and Parr, E. L., 1978, Colchicine inhibition of lysosome movement in the rat uterine epithelium, *Cytobiologie* **18**:374–378.

Patterson, J. T., 1913, Polyembryonic development in *Tatusia novemcincta, J. Morphol.* **24**:559–684.

Pearson, A. K., and Enders, R. K., 1951, Further observations on the reproduction of the Alaskan fur seal, *Anat. Rec.* **111**:695–712.

Peppler, R. D., and Canale, J., 1980, Quantitative investigation of the annual pattern of follicular development in the nine-banded armadillo (*Dasypus novemcinctus*), *J. Reprod. Fertil.* **59**:193–197.

Peppler, R. D., and Stone, S. C., 1976, Plasma progesterone level in the female armadillo during delayed implantation and gestation: Preliminary report, *Lab. Anim. Sci.* **26:**501–504.

Peppler, R. D., and Stone, S. C., 1980, Plasma progesterone level during delayed implantation, gestation, and postpartum period in the armadillo, *Lab. Anim. Sci.* **30:**188–191.

Peyre, A., and Herlant, M., 1967, Ova-implantation différée et déterminisme hormonal chez le Minioptère, *Miniopterus schreibersi* K. (Chiroptère), *C.R. Sèance Soc. Biol.* **161:**1779–1782.

Pinsker, M. C., Sacco, A. G., and Mintz, B., 1974, Implantation-associated proteinase in mouse uterine fluid, *Dev. Biol.* **38:**285–290.

Potts, D. M., 1966, The attachment phase of ovoimplantation, *Am. J. Obstet. Gynecol.* **96:**1122–1128.

Potts, D. M., 1968, The ultrastructure of implantation in the mouse, *J. Anat.* **103:**77–90.

Potts, D. M., and Wilson, I. B., 1967, The preimplantation conceptus of the mouse at 90 hours post coitum, *J. Anat.* **102:**1–11.

Pratt, H. P. M., 1977, Uterine proteins and the activation of embryos from mice during delayed implantation, *J. Reprod. Fertil.* **50:**1–8.

Prell, H., 1938, Die Tragzeit des Rehes, *Zuchtungskunde* **13:**325–345.

Psychoyos, A., and Mandon, P., 1971, Scanning electron microscopy of the surface of the rat uterine epithelium during delayed implantation, *J. Reprod. Fertil.* **26:**137–138.

Ramakrishna, P. A., and Rao, K. V. B., 1977, Reproductive adaptations in the Indian rhinolphid bat, *Rhinolophus rouxi (Temminck)*, *Curr. Sci.* **42:**270–271.

Ramsey, E. M., Houston, M. L., and Harris, J. W. S., 1976, Interactions of the trophoblast and maternal tissues in three closely related primate species, *Am. J. Obstet. Gynecol.* **124:**647–652.

Rand, R. W., 1954, Reproduction in the female cape fur seal *Arctocephalus pusillus, Proc. Zool. Soc. (Lond.)* **124:**717–740.

Rasweiler, J. J. IV, 1979, Early embryonic development and implantation in bats, *J. Reprod. Fertil.* **56:**403–416.

Ravindra, R., and Mead, R. A., 1984, Plasma estrogen levels during pregnancy in the Western spotted skunk, *Biol. Reprod.* **30:**1153–1159.

Reinius, S., 1967, Ultrastructure of blastocyst attachment in the mouse, *Z. Zellforsch.* **77:**257–266.

Renfree, M. B., 1973, Proteins in the uterine secretions of the marsupial *Macropus eugenii, Dev. Biol.* **32:**41–49.

Renfree, M. B., 1975, Uterine proteins in the marsupial, *Didelphis marsupialis virginia,* during gestation, *J. Reprod. Fertil.* **42:**163–166.

Renfree, M. B., 1980, Embryonic diapause in the honey possum *Tarsipes spencerae, Search* **11:**81.

Renfree, M. B., 1981, Embryonic diapause in marsupials, *J. Reprod. Fertil. [Suppl.]* **29:**67–78.

Renfree, M. B., and Calaby, J. H., 1981, Background to delayed implantation and embryonic diapause, *J. Reprod. Fertil. [Suppl.]* **29:**1–9.

Rosenfeld, M. G., and Joshi, M. S., 1977, A possible role of a specific uterine fluid peptidase in implantation in the rat, *J. Reprod. Fertil.* **51:**137–139.

Rossman, I., 1940, The deciduomal reaction in the rhesus monkey (*Macaca mulatta*), *Am. J. Anat.* **66:**277–365.

Roy, S. K., Sengupta, J., and Manchanda, S. K., 1983, Histochemical study of β-glucuronidase in the rat uterus during implantation and pseudopregnancy, *J. Reprod. Fertil.* **68:**161–164.

Sacco, A. G., and Mintz, B., 1975, Mouse uterine antigens in the implantation period of pregnancy, *Biol. Reprod.* **12:**498–503.

Schlafke, S. J., and Enders, A. C., 1963, Observations on the fine structure of the rat blastocyst, *J. Anat.* **97:**353–361.

Schlafke, S. J., Enders, A. C., and Given, R. L., 1981, Cytology of the endometrium of delayed and early implantation with special reference to mice and mustelids, *J. Reprod. Fertil. [Suppl.]* **29:**135–141.

Sempere, A., 1977, Plasma progesterone levels in the roe deer, *Capreolus capreolus, J. Reprod. Fertil.* **5:**365–366.

Sharman, G. B., 1955a, Studies on marsupial reproduction. II. The oestrous cycle of *Setonix brachyurus, Aust. J. Zool.* **3:**44–55.

Sharman, G. B., 1955b, Studies on marsupial reproduction. III. Normal and delayed pregnancy in *Setonix brachyurus, Aust. J. Zool.* **3:**56–70.

Shaw, G., and Renfree, M. B., 1986, Uterine and embryonic metabolism after diapause in the tammar wallaby, *Macropus eugenii, J. Reprod. Fertil.* **76:**339–347.

Shelden, R. M., 1972, The fate of short-tailed weasel, *Mustela erminea,* blastocysts following ovariectomy during diapause, *J. Reprod. Fertil.* **31:**347–352.

Sherman, M. I., and Barlow, P. W., 1972, Deoxyribonucleic acid content in delayed mouse blastocysts, *J. Reprod. Fertil.* **29:**123–126.

Sherman, M. I., and Wudl, L. R., 1976, The implanting mouse blastocyst, in: *The Cell Surface in Animal Development* (G. Poste and G. R. Nicolson, eds.), North Holland, Amsterdam, pp. 81–125.

Short, R. V., and Hay, M. F., 1965, Delayed implantation in the roe deer, *Capreolus capreolus, J. Reprod. Fertil.* **9:**372–373.

Short, R. V., and Hay, M. F., 1966, Delayed implantation in the roe deer *Capreolus capreolus,* in: *Comparative Biology of Reproduction in Mammals* (I. W. Rolands, ed.), Academic Press, London, pp. 173–194.

Sinha, A. A., and Mead, R. A., 1976, Morphological changes in the trophoblast, uterus and corpus luteum during delayed implantation in the Western spotted skunk, *Am. J. Anat.* **145:**331–356.

Sinha, A. A., Conaway, C. H., and Kenyon, K. W., 1966, Reproduction in the female sea otter, *J. Wildl. Man.* **30:**121–130.

Smith, M. S. R., and Wilson, I. B., 1971, Histochemical observations on early implantation in the mouse, *J. Embryol. Exp. Morphol.* **25:**165–174.

Smith, A. F., and Wilson, I. B., 1974, Cell interaction at the maternal–embryonic interface during implantation in the mouse, *Cell Tissue Res.* **152:**525–542.

Stieve, H., 1950, Anatomische-biologische Untersuchungen über die Fortpflanzungstätigkeit des europäischen Rehes (*Capreolus capreolus capreolus* L.), *Z. Mikrosk. Anat. Forsch.* **55:**427–530.

Surani, M., 1975a, Zona pellucida denudation, blastocyst proliferation and attachment in the rat, *J. Embryol. Exp. Morphol.* **33:**343–353.

Surani, M., 1975b, Hormonal regulation of proteins on the uterine secretion of ovariectomized rats and the implications for implantation and embryonic diapause, *J. Reprod. Fertil.* **43:**411–417.

Surani, M. A. H., 1976, Uterine luminal proteins at the time of implantation in rats, *J. Reprod. Fertil.* **48:**141–145.

Surani, M. A. H., 1977a, Qualitative and quantitative examination of the proteins of rat uterine luminal fluid during pro-oestrus and pregnancy and comparison with those of serum, *J. Reprod. Fertil.* **50:**281–287.

Surani, M. A. H., 1977b, Radiolabelled rat uterine luminal proteins and their regulation by oestradiol and progesterone, *J. Reprod. Fertil.* **50:**289–296.

Surani, M. A. H., 1977c, Cellular and molecular approaches to blastocyst uterine interactions at implantation, in: *Development in Mammals,* Volume 1 (M. H. Johnson, ed.), Elsevier/North Holland, Amsterdam.

Svihla, A., 1932, *A Comparative Life History Study of the Mice of the Genus Peromyscus,* University of Michigan Museum of Zoology, Ann Arbor.

Tachi, C., and Tachi, S., 1986, Macrophages and implantation, *Ann. N.Y. Acad. Sci.* **476:**158–182.

Talmage, R. V., Buchanan, G. D., Kraintz, F. W., Lazo-Wasem, E. A., and Zarrow, M. X., 1954, The presence of a functional corpus luteum during delay implantation in the armadillo, *J. Endocrinol.* **11:**44–49.

Tarara, R. P., Enders, A. C., Hendrickx, A. G., Gulamhusein, N., Hodges, J. K., Hearn, J. P., Eley, R. B., and Else, J. G., 1987, Early implantation and embryonic development of the baboon: Stages 5, 6 and 7, *Anat. Embryol.* **176:**267–275.

Tarkowski, A. K., 1957, Studies on reproduction and prenatal morality of the common shrew (*Sorex araneus* L.). Part II. Reproduction under natural conditions, *Ann. Univ. Mariae Curie-Sklodowska* **10:**177–244.

Temte, J. L., 1985, Photoperiod and delayed implantation in the northern fur seal (*Callorhinus ursinus*), *J. Reprod. Fertil.* **73:**127–131.

Tyndale-Biscoe, C. H., 1963, The role of the corpus luteum in the delayed implantation of marsupials, in: *Delayed Implantation* (A. C. Enders, ed.), University of Chicago Press, Chicago, pp. 15–32.

Tyndale-Biscoe, C. H., 1970, Resumption of development by quiescent blastocysts transferred to primed, ovariectomized recipients in the marsupial, *Macropus eugenii, J. Reprod. Fertil.* **23:**25–32.

Tyndale-Biscoe, H., and Renfree, M., 1987, *Reproductive Physiology of Marsupials,* Cambridge University Press, New York.

Tyndale-Biscoe, C. H., Hearn, J. P., and Renfree, M. B., 1974, Control of reproduction in macropodid marsupials, *J. Endocrinol.* **63:**589–614.

van der Merwe, M., 1982, Histological study of implantation in the Natal clinging bat (*Miniopterus schreibersii natalensis*), *J. Reprod. Fertil.* **65:**319–323.

Vogel, P., 1972, Beitrag zur Fortpflanzungsbiologie der Gattungen *Sorex, Neomys, und Crodidura* (*Soricidae*), *Verh. Naturf. Ges. (Basel)* **82:**165–192.

Vogel, P., 1981, Occurrence and interpretation of delayed implantation in insectivores, *J. Reprod. Fertil. [Suppl.]* **29:**51–60.

Walker, M. T., and Hughes, R. L., 1981, Ultrastructural changes after diapause in the uterine glands, corpus luteum and blastocyst of the red-necked wallaby, *Macropus rufogriseus banksianus, J. Reprod. Fertil.* *[Suppl.]* **29:**151–158.

Wallace, G. I., 1978, A histological study of the early stages of pregnancy in the bent-winged bat (*Miniopterus schreibersii*) in northeastern New South Wales, Australia (30°27′S), *J. Zool.* **185:**519–537.

Ward, W. F., Frost, A. G., and Ward-Orsini, M., 1978, Estrogen binding by embryonic and interembryonic segments of the rat uterus prior to implantation, *Biol. Reprod.* **18:**598–601.

Warren, R. H., and Enders, A. C., 1964, An electron microscope study of the rat endometrium during delayed implantation, *Anat. Rec.* **148:**177–195.

Weaker, F. J., Villareal, C., and Sheridan, P. J., 1981, Localization of ^{3}H-estradiol in the uterus of pregnant and non-pregnant armadillos, *Cell Tissue Res.* **220:**773–780.

Weitlauf, H. M., 1974, Metabolic changes in the blastocysts of mice and rats during delayed implantation, *J. Reprod. Fertil.* **39:**213–224.

Weitlauf, H. M., 1976, Effect of uterine flushings on RNA synthesis by ''implanting'' and ''delayed implanting'' mouse blastocysts *in vitro, Biol. Reprod.* **14:**566–571.

Weitlauf, H. M., 1978, Factors in mouse uterine fluid that inhibit the incorporation of [^{3}H]uridine by blastocysts *in vitro, J. Reprod. Fertil.* **52:**321–325.

Weitlauf, H. M., 1982, Comparison of the rates of accumulation of nonpolyadenylated and polyadenylated RNA in normal and delayed implanting mouse embryos, *Dev. Biol.* **93:**266–271.

Weitlauf, H. M., Kiessling, A. A., and Buschman, R., 1979, Comparison of DNA polymerase activity and cell division in normal and delayed implanting mouse embryos, *J. Exp. Zool.* **209:**467–472.

Wimsatt, W. A., 1963, Delayed implantation in the Ursidae, with particular reference to the black bear (*Ursus americanus* Pallus), in: *Delayed Implantation* (A. C. Enders, ed.), University of Chicago Press, Chicago, pp. 49–76.

Wimsatt, W. A., 1974, Morphogenesis of the fetal membranes and placenta of the black bear, *Ursus americanus* (Pallus), *Am. J. Anat.* **140:**471–496.

Wimsatt, W. A., 1975, Some comparative aspects of implantation, *Biol. Reprod.* **12:**1–40.

Wislocki, G. B., and Streeter, G. L., 1938, Development of the macaque embryo, *Contrib. Embryol. Carnegie Inst.* **19:**15–55.

Wong, Y. C., and Dickson, A. D., 1969, A histochemical study of ovoimplantation in the mouse, *J. Anat.* **105:**547–555.

Wright, P. L., 1963, Variations in reproduction cycles in North American mustelids, in: *Delayed Implantation* (A. C. Enders, ed.), University of Chicago Press, Chicago, pp. 77–95.

Wright, P. L., 1966, Observations on the reproductive cycle of the American badger (*Taxidea taxus*), in: *Comparative Biology of Reproduction in Mammals* (I. W. Rowlands, ed.), Academic Press, New York, pp. 27–45.

Wright, P. L., 1981, Commentary. Delayed implantation in the northern fur seal (*Callorhinus ursinus*) and other pinnipeds by J. C. Daniel, Jr., *J. Reprod. Fertil.* *[Suppl.]* **29:**35–50.

Wright, P. L., and Coulter, M. W., 1967, Reproduction and growth in Maine fishers, *J. Wildl. Man.* **31:**70–87.

Yochim, J. M., 1975, Development of the progestational uterus: Metabolic aspect, *Biol. Reprod.* **12:**106–133.

Ziegler, L., 1843, *Beobachtungen über die Brunst und den Embryo der Rehe,* Hannover.

The Implantation Reaction

MARGARET B. PARR and EARL L. PARR

The evolution of the reproductive process has resulted in the development of elaborate adaptive mechanisms to ensure the survival of the offspring. In viviparous animals such adaptations include the development of complex and diverse forms of implantation and placentation in order to support the attachment and development of embryos *in utero*. The implantation process exhibits remarkable diversity among species, most prominently in the extent of trophoblastic invasion into the uterus. Yet the general aim of implantation is accomplished in all species: to attach the embryo to the uterine wall and to establish an intimate union between maternal and fetal tissues so that an exchange of nutrients and waste products can occur. The details of the earliest interactions between the blastocyst and endometrium have been the focus of extensive study. It is our purpose to summarize some of the more important developments in this field since the publication of Finn's fine review of the subject in the second edition of this book (Finn, 1977). In this chapter we have chosen to discuss four aspects of the implantation process: (1) adhesion of the trophoblast to the uterine epithelium; (2) increased vascular permeability at implantation sites; (3) the decidual cell reaction; and (4) loss of epithelial cells surrounding the implanting blastocyst. Our discussion is based primarily on the results of investigations using common laboratory animals, namely, the rat, mouse, and rabbit. In addition, other recent reviews and symposia may be of interest to the reader (Weitlauf, 1979; Glasser and McCormack, 1981; Finn, 1980; Leroy *et al.*, 1980; Glasser and Bullock, 1981; Dey and Johnson, 1980; Kearns and Lala, 1983; Bell, 1983; Kennedy, 1983a; Chávez, 1984; Enders *et al.*, 1983, 1985; Enders and Schlafke, 1986; Yoshinaga *et al.*, 1986).

1. Adhesion

One of the earliest significant events of the implantation process in all species examined is the adhesion of the blastocyst to the uterine epithelium (Enders, 1972). Studies of this process

MARGARET B. PARR and EARL L. PARR ● Department of Anatomy, School of Medicine, Southern Illinois University, Carbondale, Illinois 62901.

have considered the morphology, surface charge, and glycoprotein composition of the apposed cell surfaces. Although the morphological changes in the cell surfaces are now well known, considerably more information will be necessary before we understand the biochemical mechanisms underlying the adhesive process.

1.1. Morphological Changes in the Uterine Epithelial Cell Surface

Morphological changes occur in the apical surface of the uterine epithelium just prior to and during implantation in the rat and mouse. These changes, which are induced by estrogen and progesterone, may be important in leading to the acquisition of adhesiveness and consequently for blastocyst attachment and the initiation of the implantation reaction (Nilsson, 1966a,b). During the early part of the preimplantation period, the luminal surface of the uterine epithelium is characterized by numerous straight, regular microvilli, which are approximately 1 μm in length. Subsequently, the microvilli become less regular (Enders and Schlafke, 1967; Nilsson, 1974), and large surface protrusions appear (Psychoyos and Mandon, 1971a,b; Nilsson, 1972). These protrusions, termed pinopods (Enders and Nelson, 1973), have been shown to mediate endocytosis (Enders and Nelson, 1973; Parr and Parr, 1974, 1977). Closure of the uterine lumen occurs at this time, and microvilli from apposed luminal epithelial cells interdigitate either with one another or, where the embryo is present, with those of the trophoblast. This period of development is called the preattachment phase (Mayer et al., 1967), the apposition stage (Enders and Schlafke, 1969), or the first stage of closure (Pollard and Finn, 1972); it occurs not only during normal pregnancy but also during delayed implantation and in ovariectomized animals treated with progesterone (Martin et al., 1970; Hedlund and Nilsson, 1971). During the next stage, the adhesion stage or the second stage of closure, pinopods disappear (Parr, 1983), and the surface takes on an irregular, undulating configuration. The trophoblast and the uterine epithelium or the opposing epithelial cell surfaces come into intimate contact, leaving a space of approximately 15 nm. The net result of the morphological changes during this period appears to be a flattening of the uterine epithelial cell surface, which may contribute to a closer attachment between the blastocyst and uterine epithelium (Figs. 1 and 2).

In some species the implantation reaction does not proceed much beyond the attachment stage. These species, which include pigs and horses, are said to have epitheliochorial placentation because the fetal trophoblast remains closely apposed to the uterine epithelium throughout pregnancy. In other species, adhesion is followed by trophoblast penetration of the epithelial layer. Schlafke and Enders (1975) have described three types of trophoblast–epithelial interaction. In displacement penetration (rat, mouse), trophoblast processes extend between and beneath the epithelial cells. The cells or their fragments are then phagocytosed, and the trophoblast comes to lie along the basal lamina, which was previously occupied by the displaced uterine cells. In fusion penetration (rabbit), syncytial trophoblast fuses with the uterine epithelial cells. In intrusion penetration (ferret), projections of syncytial trophoblast penetrate between uterine epithelial cells. Despite the differences among species, it appears in all cases that adhesion is a necessary prerequisite to the more intimate form of association that eventually develops as a result of trophoblast penetration.

1.2. Surface Charge on Blastocysts

The possibility that the acquisition of adhesiveness might be correlated with changes in surface charge on the blastocyst and uterine epithelium has prompted considerable investigation. Mouse blastocysts show a loss of negative charge on their surface membrane during the

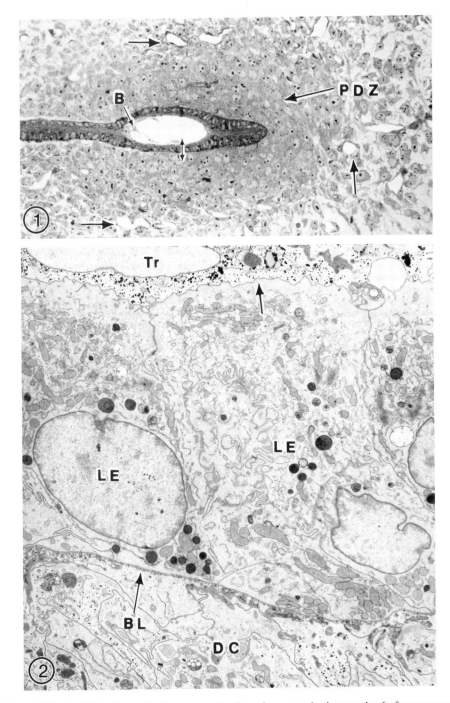

Figure 1. This is a light micrograph of a cross section through a rat uterine horn on day 6 of pregnancy and passing through an implantation site. A blastocyst (B) is present in the uterine lumen and is surrounded by an intact luminal epithelium. The primary decidual zone (PDZ) is a cup-shaped zone of compact cells surrounding the blastocyst. Note the blood capillaries (arrows) at the periphery of the PDZ. A region similar to that at the two-headed arrow is shown in higher magnification in Fig. 2. ×200.

Figure 2. This is an electron micrograph of a region of the uterus similar to that at the two-headed arrow in Fig. 1. The trophoblast (Tr) and the luminal epithelium (LE) are closely apposed at their apical borders (arrow), showing the typical appearance of the adhesion stage of implantation. The epithelial basal lamina (BL) and decidual cells (DC) are seen below the luminal epithelium. ×5300.

implantation period. This has been demonstrated by both electron microscopy (Nilsson *et al.*, 1973; 1975; Jenkinson and Searle, 1977) and free-zone electrophoresis (Nilsson and Njerten, 1982); in the former case one sees reduced binding of positively charged colloidal iron particles to the trophoblast, and in the latter a decrease (30%) in net negative charge densities. In all of these studies pretreatment with neuraminidase markedly reduced the negative charges, suggesting that they are caused by the presence of N-acetylneuraminic or sialic acid in the terminal position of the cell surface carbohydrates. However, enzyme treatment did not completely eliminate the negative charges, which indicates that other molecular groups contribute to surface negativity. The overall negative charge of the blastocyst surface appears to be associated with glycoproteins rather than glycolipids because it is reduced by treatment with two proteolytic enzymes (Jenkinson and Searle, 1977). The decreased negativity of the blastocyst at implantation is apparently independent of maternal influences, since a similar change has been observed in blastocysts implanting *in vitro* (Jenkinson and Searle, 1977; Nilsson *et al.*, 1973, 1975; Nilsson and Njerten, 1982).

1.3. Surface Charge on the Uterine Epithelium

The surface negative charge on uterine epithelial cells at the time of implantation has been characterized using electron microscopy in combination with cytochemical markers such as ruthenium red, polycationic ferritin, and thorium dioxide. In this way, a glycoprotein coat, apparently of negative charge, was observed on the surface membrane of uterine epithelial cells at implantation and during lactational delay (Enders and Schlafke, 1974). The intensity of such labeling was unchanged during early pregnancy in sheep (Guillomot *et al.*, 1982) but was greatly reduced at the time of implantation in mice (Nilsson, 1974) and rabbits (Anderson and Hoffman, 1984) and was completely lost in rats (Hewitt *et al.*, 1979). In rabbits, the labeling was sensitive to neuraminidase and trypsin, suggesting that sialoglycoproteins contribute to surface negativity in that animal. Murphy and Rogers (1981) have shown that binding of ruthenium red is significantly reduced after the administration of estrogen to spayed rats. More recently, using a unique *in vitro* assay system, Morris and Potter (1984) have demonstrated that both mouse blastocysts and uterine epithelial vesicles have negatively charged surfaces and that each can bind to positively charged DEAE-Sephadex beads. This adhesion must involve sialic acid because it was sensitive to neuraminidase. At the time of implantation the epithelial vesicles showed a reduction in negativity consistent with the results of the studies mentioned above.

In addition to a reduction of surface charge on uterine epithelial cells, alterations in the surface coat have also been described. A reduction, loss, or morphological change of the surface coat during implantation has been reported (ferret: Enders and Schlafke, 1972; rat: Salazar-Rubio *et al.*, 1980; mouse: Chavez and Anderson, 1985; rabbit: Anderson and Hoffman, 1984); no change in the surface coat was detected in the bovine uterine epithelium during early pregnancy (Wordinger and Amsler, 1980).

The role of changes in the surface charge or surface coat in causing the blastocyst to adhere to the uterine epithelium remains speculative. Some have suggested that the reduction in the electrostatic repulsion between trophoblast and epithelium may facilitate the juxtaposition of the two surfaces, thereby aiding in the adhesion process (Morris and Potter, 1984). The reduction of surface charge alone is not sufficient for adhesion because surface charge is reduced by estrogen treatment and adhesion does not occur under these conditions (Murphy and Rogers, 1981). One conclusion that can be drawn from the studies of surface charge, especially those using neuraminidase to demonstrate that much of the surface charge resides in sialic acid, is that there are changes in the surface membrane glycoproteins of both the blastocyst and epithelium during the acquisition of adhesiveness.

The possibility that alterations of surface membrane glycoproteins on blastocysts and uterine epithelial cells may be responsible for the acquisition of adhesiveness at implantation has been the focus of considerable attention. Many investigators have tried to characterize these plasma membranes by studying their glycoproteins using lectin binding, autoradiography, and, to a lesser extent, biochemical analysis. Before summarizing the observations made as a result of these various approaches, we consider, very briefly, some of the progress that has been made in studies of cellular adhesion mechanisms in other systems. In particular, many surface proteins isolated from epithelial cells, cells of the nervous system, and other cell types have been shown to be involved in cell-to-cell adhesion. The cell adhesion molecules (CAMs) that have been chemically and functionally characterized are described in detail in recent reviews (Edelman, 1983; Damsky, 1984; Öbrink, 1986; Martz, 1987). It now seems clear that CAMs are involved in cellular adhesion, that several adhesive mechanisms exist involving different CAMs, and that in some cases CAMs may have functions other than simply binding cells together.

One particular group of proteins that may be involved in cell adhesion is the glycosyltransferases. It was originally proposed that this group of enzymes might mediate cell adhesion if they were localized in plasma membranes and bound their specific oligosaccharide substrates in the surface membranes of adjacent cells (Roseman, 1970; Roth *et al.*, 1971). This has been referred to as the Roth hypothesis. Substantial evidence is now available to implicate this mechanism in a variety of cell adhesion or recognition events including cell migration, fertilization, bacterial adhesion, cell differentiation, and immune recognition (Pierce *et al.*, 1980; Shur, 1984). Shur (1982, 1983) has recently demonstrated that embryonal carcinoma cells express in their surface membrane a lactosaminoglycan (LAG) composed of repeating N-acetyllactosamine disaccharides. The surface membrane of the cells also contains a galactosyltransferase that specifically binds the LAGs if UDP-galactose is absent (causing cellular adhesion) or adds galactose to the terminal N-acetylglucosamine of the LAGs if UDP-galactose is added (causing the cells to separate). Cellular adhesion was inhibited by reagents that selectively interfere with galactosyltransferase activity.

1.5. Surface Glycoproteins on Blastocysts

Studies of the possible role of glycosyltransferases in cellular adhesion and in recognition processes generally have prompted further investigation of the relationship between membrane glycoproteins and blastocyst adhesion. In the following sections we describe some of the changes that have been demonstrated in the membrane glycoproteins or glycolipids of blastocysts and the uterine epithelium at implantation. Information about such changes begins to lay a foundation for more detailed work on adhesion between these two cell types.

In 1973, Pinsker and Mintz showed that tritiated glucosamine was incorporated into glycoproteins of high molecular weight on the surface of mouse blastocysts. This result was interpreted as possibly being related to adhesiveness. Since that study, lectins have been used to probe the structure and organization of particular carbohydrate moieties on the surface of blastocysts and their alterations during implantation. Lectins are proteins or glycoproteins that bind specifically to mono- or oligosaccharides—a process that can be inhibited or reversed by the relevant sugars (Goldstein and Hayes, 1979; see Table 1). Investigations of lectin binding have been carried out on blastocysts from the mouse, rat, and hamster. Concanavalin A (Con A), conjugated to a variety of tracers, was shown to bind to the surface of blastocysts, but there is considerable conflict regarding changes in Con A binding during implantation: binding increases (mouse: Wu and Chang, 1978; Wu, 1980a), decreases (mouse: Carollo and Weitlauf,

Table 1. Commonly Used Lectins and Corresponding Carbohydrate Specifications

Lectin	Sugar specificity
Limulus polyagglutinin (LPA)	Sialic acid
Ulex europeus agglutinin I (UEA I)	α-L-Fucose
Concanavalin A (Con A)	β-D-Glucose; α-D-mannose
Succinyl concanavalin A (sCon A)	α-D-Glucose; α-D-mannose
Ricinus communis agglutinin I (RCA I)	β-D-Galactose
Succinyl wheat germ agglutinin (sWGA)	N-Acetyl-β-(1–4)-D-glucosamine
Wheat germ agglutinin (WGA)	N-Acetyl-β-(1–4)-D-glucosamine; sialic acid
Soybean agglutinin (SBA)	N-Acetyl-α-D-galactosamine; D-galactose
Dolichos biflorus agglutinin (DBA)	N-Acetyl-α-D-galactosamine
Peanut agglutinin (PNA)	D-Galactose-β-(1–3)-N-acetylgalactosamine

1981; Rowinski *et al.,* 1976; Magnuson and Stackpole, 1978; hamster: Yanagimachi and Nicolson, 1976), or remains unaltered (mouse: Enders and Schlafke, 1974; Konwinski *et al.,* 1977; rat: Wu, 1980b). The reasons for these conflicting results are uncertain, but they may be related to damage incurred during the collection of the blastocysts (Carollo and Weitlauf, 1981) or to steric interferences with lectin binding, a problem that becomes particularly acute when the lectins are conjugated to relatively large tracers (Chávez and Enders, 1981).

Chávez and his colleagues have studied changes in the binding of lectins to mouse blastocysts during the acquisition of adhesiveness *in vitro* (Chávez and Enders, 1981) and during delayed implantation before and after activation with estrogen (Chávez and Enders, 1981, 1982). Chávez (1986) also has described lectin binding to adhesive and nonadhesive trophectoderm *in situ* using the split-implantation-site technique (Enders and Schlafke, 1979). Taken together, the data indicate that Con A, WGA, UEA-I, and RCA-I bind equally to blastocysts both before and after they become adhesive, but SBA did not bind at either stage. Changes in lectin binding were observed only with PNA, DBA, and sWGA. Changes in the binding of PNA did not appear to be related to the acquisition of adhesiveness but might be involved in the differentiation of the blastocyst (Chávez and Enders, 1981). A loss of DBA binding to the blastocyst surface and of sWGA binding on trophectoderm appeared to be coincident with the acquisition of adhesion (Chávez and Enders, 1982; Chávez, 1986). These results suggest that changes may occur in galactose, N-acetylgalactosamine, and N-acetylglucosamine in glycoproteins on the blastocyst surface at the time of adhesion. The implications of such developments for the adhesive process remain to be elucidated.

As well as describing changes in surface carbohydrates that occur while the blastocyst develops from the preadhesive to the adhesive stage, several investigators have studied the distribution of carbohydrates on the surface of blastocysts. Concanavalin A, when attached to large particulate tracers such as erythrocytes (Sobel and Nebel, 1976) or latex beads (Nilsson *et al.,* 1980), showed a regional pattern of binding to mouse blastocysts at implantation. In both studies there was more binding of particles to the mural trophoblast cells than to the embryonic polar cells, whereas in the binding of Con A erythrocytes to rat blastocysts no regional difference was observed (Enders and Schlafke, 1979). When Con A was attached to smaller tracers such as fluorescein isothiocyanate (FITC) (Sobel and Nebel, 1978), peroxidase

(Enders and Schlafke, 1974; Konwinski *et al.*, 1977), or ferritin (Chávez and Enders, 1982), it bound to the surface of mouse blastocysts at implantation, but no regional differences were observed. On the other hand, when DBA was used, mural trophoblast was found to have about twice as many binding sites as polar cells (Chávez *et al.*, 1984). There was also a greater incorporation of tritiated D-galactose into mural trophoblast cells than into polar cells.

Viewed as a whole, these results suggest that there are differences in the surface carbohydrates of mural and polar trophoblast cells. The technical problems that complicate the interpretation of these experiments have been discussed (Chávez and Enders, 1982; Carollo and Weitlauf, 1981). If there are differences in surface glycoproteins of mouse mural and polar trophoblast cells, they may be related to the fact that it is the mural trophoblast that becomes attached to the uterine epithelium during the adhesion stage. A few days after the adhesion stage, the attached mural trophoblast participates in the formation of the yolk-sac placenta (Welsh and Enders, 1987). This regional differentiation of trophoblastic cell function adds another element of specificity to the study of the biochemical mechanism of blastocyst adhesion. Further research will need to focus on the interaction between the apical membrane of the uterine epithelium and the mural trophoblast, not the whole blastocyst.

Finally, blastocyst attachment to glass or plastic surfaces *in vitro* has been used to study the mechanism of adhesion. Numerous treatments intended to alter surface macromolecules, including neuraminidase, galactose oxidase, trypsin, pronase, hyaluronidase, and tunicamycin, had no effect on blastocyst attachment (Surani, 1979; Sherman and Atienza-Samols, 1978; Atienza-Samols *et al.*, 1980; Webb and Duksin, 1981). However, the use of blastocyst attachment to glass or plastic *in vitro* as a model for adhesion between trophectoderm and uterine epithelium *in vivo* is open to question (Enders *et al.*, 1981). Morris *et al.* (1983) have reported that the attachment of blastocysts to isolated vesicles of uterine epithelium in hanging-drop culture involved an interaction of microvilli from the two surfaces similar to that seen *in vivo*, whereas attachment of blastocysts to inert surfaces, freshly isolated cells, or cultured cell lines differed in several respects.

1.6. Surface Glycoproteins on Uterine Epithelial Cells

Lectins have also been used to probe the surface membrane glycoproteins of uterine epithelial cells. Concanavalin A binding was observed and did not change during early pregnancy in rats (Enders and Schlafke, 1974) and sheep (Guillomot *et al.*, 1982) or in ovariectomized rats treated in several ways with ovarian steroids (Murphy and Rogers, 1981). Enders *et al.* (1980) showed uniform labeling with Con A both inside and outside the imprint site formed in the uterine wall by the rat blastocyst during implantation. As demonstrated by Con A binding, neutral carbohydrates containing glucose and mannose are present in receptive uteri of rat and sheep and do not appear to be altered by the acquisition of adhesiveness or the presence of the blastocyst. It is of interest that the instillation of Con A into the uterine lumen at the time of implantation prevents implantation (mouse: Hicks and Guzman-Gonzalez, 1979; Wu and Gu, 1981; rat: Wu and Gu, 1981).

In rabbits, Anderson *et al.* (1986) have demonstrated binding of WGA, sWGA, SBA, RCA-I, Con A, and UEA-I to the apical membranes of uterine epithelial cells. The extent of lectin binding was essentially the same in estrus and pseudopregnant animals except with RCA-I and sWGA, where greater binding was observed in pseudopregnant animals. Also, the binding of RCA-I, Con A, and sWGA appeared to be less at implantation sites than at nonimplantation sites. These studies were carried out by infusing the labeled lectins into the lumina of fixed uterine horns and then washing and analyzing frozen sections. In fixed cryostat or paraffin-embedded sections of rabbit endometrium, however, Thie *et al.* (1986) could not detect Con A binding to the epithelial apical membranes, although they did detect Con A binding to the basal membranes and WGA binding to the apical membrane.

Proteins have been detergent-extracted from the apical membranes of rabbit epithelial cells in estrus and pseudopregnancy and separated by sodium dodecylsulfate polyacrylamide gel electrophoresis (SDS-PAGE) (Anderson *et al.*, 1986). Western blotting of the isolated proteins showed an increase in the number of RCA-I, sWGA, and Con A binding proteins from uteri of progestational rabbits. The results suggested that pseudopregnancy in rabbits is accompanied by an increase in D-galactose and N-acetylglucosamine on the surface of uterine epithelial cells. Neuraminidase in combination with the aforementioned methods indicated the presence of sialic acid–D-galactose sequences at the nonreducing ends of oligosaccharides in nonreceptive uteri and the reduction of sialic acid in receptive uteri. In addition, a comparison of radioiodinated surface membrane proteins in cultured uterine epithelial cells obtained from estrus and pseudopregnant rabbits indicated that different proteins were present at the two stages (Ricketts *et al.*, 1984). Lampelo *et al.* (1985) have isolated plasma membranes from rabbit endometrial scrapings and found differences in the pattern of membrane proteins from receptive and nonreceptive stages, but their study did not determine whether the specific proteins were derived from the epithelial or stromal cells, nor did it identify specific surface proteins.

In mice, terminal D-galactose groups were present at the apices of uterine epithelial cells on day 5 of pregnancy as determined by RCA-I binding; this localization was accompanied by a reduction in the surface coat as visualized by alkaline bismuth nitrate staining (Chávez and Anderson, 1985). Also relevant to these results are the observations of Murphy and his colleagues. Using freeze–fracture techniques, they showed a marked increase in the number, shape, and aggregation of intramembranous particles (IMPs) in the apical surface membrane of rat uterine epithelial cells during implantation and in spayed rats treated with ovarian hormones (Murphy *et al.*, 1979, 1982). The authors suggest that since IMPs may be attached to membrane carbohydrates, their changes at implantation could indicate that there are changes in the carbohydrate groups exposed at the cell surface and projecting into the uterine lumen. Initial attempts to demonstrate this relationship were negative (Murphy and Swift, 1983), but preliminary evidence now suggests that some sulfated carbohydrate moieties, as demonstrated by colloidal iron hydroxide staining, may be attached to IMPs in the plasma membrane (Murphy and Bradbury, 1984).

Several lines of evidence suggest that mouse uterine epithelial cells *in vitro* synthesize LAGs that can interact with a cell surface galactosyltransferase (Dutt *et al.*, 1987), analogous to the observations made by Shur (1983) on embryonal carcinoma cells. Selective interference with cell surface galactosyltransferase by α-lactalbumin or UDP-galactose interrupted epithelial cell-to-cell adhesion. Whether the cell adhesion studied in this experimental system is most relevant to the adhesion of epithelial cells to one another or to blastocysts is still uncertain. Neither α-lactalbumin nor UDP-galactose interfered with the attachment of blastocysts to the uterine epithelial cells, suggesting that the galactosyltransferase system may not be required for blastocyst adhesion (Dutt *et al.*, 1987). Such an interpretation must be tentative, as indicated by these authors, since epithelial–embryo interaction *in vitro* may not represent blastocyst adhesion *in vivo*. The primary epithelial cell culture used in the *in vitro* studies was evidently not polarized. Because studies using other types of epithelial cells have demonstrated that the absence of tight junctions allows the intermixing of apical and lateral cell surface membrane glycoproteins (Pisam and Ripoche, 1976; Parr and Kirby, 1979), the cultured epithelial cells probably had no true apical membrane.

What can we conclude from the abovementioned studies regarding the mechanisms involved in blastocyst adhesion *in vivo*? There appears to be a reduction in negative charge on the uterine and blastocyst surfaces during early pregnancy that probably results from the masking or removal of terminal sialic acid residues on the surface carbohydrates. There is also a morphological reduction in surface coat, the extent of which varies with the species involved. As suggested by several investigators, the reduction of surface charge and surface coat may facilitate the apposition of the two cell surfaces involved in blastocyst adhesion, but other adhesive mechanisms probably exist as well.

Although many changes in the surface glycoproteins on blastocysts and uterine epithelia have been reported, some of which remain controversial, the available information does not yet provide a sufficient basis for the proposal of any detailed biochemical mechanism for blastocyst adhesion. Changes in D-galactose, acetylgalactosamine, and acetylglucosamine on the blastocyst or uterine epithelium, as well as the synthesis of LAGs by the uterine epithelial cells, are of interest in light of the Roth hypothesis (Roth *et al.*, 1971), but essentially nothing is known of the specific oligosaccharides and glycosyltransferases that might be involved in implantation.

Finally, the cellular mechanisms involved in producing surface changes on the trophectoderm and uterine epithelium are unknown. Reduction of surface charge and surface coat and changes in surface membrane glycoprotein content may arise by internalization of specific old membrane components and/or synthesis and expression of new ones. The relatively active endocytosis of the apical membrane of mouse and rat uterine epithelial cells during the preimplantation period may remove selected glycoproteins from that membrane. The large population of apical vesicles present in these cells during preimplantation (but greatly reduced at the adhesive stage) may fuse with the apical membrane to deliver newly synthesized membrane components needed for adhesion (Parr, 1980).

2. Vascular Permeability

The endometrial response to embryo implantation varies in different species (Mossman, 1937; Finn and Porter, 1975), but one phenomenon appears to be constant: the implantation of blastocysts is preceded by a local increase in uterine vascular permeability leading to stromal edema (Psychoyos, 1973). This was first demonstrated by the intravenous administration of a dye, Pontamine Sky Blue, into pregnant rats at the time of implantation (Psychoyos, 1960). The dye, which binds to albumin in the blood, leaks from the endometrial vessels and forms macroscopically visible blue-colored bands in the uterine horns, each band corresponding to an implantation site. This procedure, referred to as the Pontamine Blue reaction (PBR), is the first macroscopically observable sign of implantation (Finn and McLaren, 1967) and has been reported in many mammalian species (rat: Psychoyos, 1960; hamster: Orsini, 1964; mouse: Finn and McLaren, 1967; sheep: Boshier, 1970; Guillomot *et al.*, 1981; guinea pig: Orsini and Donovan, 1971; rabbit: Hoffman *et al.*, 1978; pig: Keys *et al.*, 1986). The endometrial vascular response is confined to regions of the uterus where blastocysts adhere to the uterine wall and appears to be independent of the extent to which the blastocyst invades the endometrium. The widespread occurrence of increased vascular permeability during implantation suggests that it may be important in serving the early metabolic needs of the developing embryo and endometrium.

2.1. Blood Vessels Responsible for Increased Vascular Permeability

The morphological basis of the increased vascular permeability at implantation has received little attention. Enders and Schlafke (1967) reported the leakage of thorotrast from rat endometrial venules 20 min after intravenous injection, but the morphology of the vessels and the pathway followed by the tracer in leaving the vessels were not studied. More recently, Abrahamsohn *et al.* (1983) have shown that the vascular endothelium in rat implantation sites exhibited fenestrations (0.1 to 0.15 μm) covered by diaphragms and gaps (0.13 to 1.4 μm) between the cells. These features were present in vessels larger than 5 μm in diameter and more than 100 μm away from the uterine epithelium in both mesometrial and antimesometrial regions, but they were not observed in the endothelium at interimplantation sites. To measure the permeability of these vessels, the authors used intravenously administered carbon as a tracer and determined its localization in the endometrium. After 20 min, the tracer was found in the gaps between endothelial cells or between the cells and the basal lamina. A higher frequency of gaps was noted in vessels from carbon-injected rats than in controls, suggesting that the blood vessels at implantation sites were sensitive to the carbon or to some component of the medium in which it was suspended. However, on the basis of these findings and a report that fenestrated capillaries are more permeable to water and small molecules than are continuous capillaries (Bill et al., 1980), the authors suggested that both fenestrations and gaps in the endometrial blood vessels are responsible for the increased vascular permeability and edema during implantation. In a preliminary report, Hoffman and Hoos (1984) examined the morphology of vascular leakage at rabbit implantation sites. They reported the extravasation of carbon from deep endometrial veins at the mesometrial aspect of the implantation chamber. Leakage from these vessels involved gaps between endothelial cells and was inhibited by indomethacin.

Such studies have been understood to indicate that gaps between endothelial cells at implantation sites may be the morphological basis for the PBR (Keys et al., 1986). However, several questions need to be addressed before this view can be accepted. Do blood vessels at implantation sites from rats and rabbits that have not been injected with carbon exhibit gaps between endothelial cells? Are endothelial gaps present at implantation sites in other animals? Does the large size of the carbon particle (30 to 50 nm) make it an inappropriate tracer for studies of the PBR? Would tracers closer in size to the Pontamine Blue–albumin complex cross blood vessels only at gaps between endothelial cells? In partial answer to the last question, Tung et al. (1986) demonstrated a differential permeability of continuous, nonfenestrated capillaries at the periphery of the primary decidual zone (Fig. 1) in rat implantation sites at the time of the PBR. Intravenously administered horseradish peroxidase (HRP, 40 kda) and immunoglobulin G (IgG, 160 kda) conjugated to HRP (IgG–HRP) crossed the capillary endothelium at intercellular junctions. The junctions, which at first glance appeared to be tight junctions, were of the close type in which the outer leaflets of adjacent cell membranes were closely apposed but not fused. The distance between the membranes at the junction was somewhat variable but always less than the width of a cell membrane. Blood vessels with similar morphology were demonstrated in implantation sites from uninjected rats. No gaps were observed between the endothelial cells of any blood vessels in this region. As determined by the density of the HRP reaction product, it appeared that HRP readily penetrated the close junctions of these vessels, whereas the passage of IgG–HRP was impeded (Figs. 3–5). The structure and permeability of blood vessels in other regions of the endometrium at the implantation sites or at interimplantation sites were not studied. Since HRP is similar in size to serum albumin (70 kda), these studies suggest that blood vessels other than those with obvious gaps between endothelial cells may contribute to the PBR.

Also relevant to this discussion is the report of O'Shea et al. (1983), who studied the ultrastructure of the uterine vasculature at the time of increased vascular permeability in rats bearing deciduomata. They reported that fenestrations were present in a few capillaries but that open discontinuities or gaps were rarely observed in the endothelial lining of capillaries and sinusoids and seemed to occur only close to the uterine lumen in association with evidence of vascular degeneration.

Stromal edema in the vicinity of blastocysts 4 hr before the appearance of the PBR has been reported (Lundkvist and Ljungkvist, 1977; Lundkvist, 1979). The edema was most developed in the antimesometrial half of the stroma, half-way between the blastocyst and the myometrium, and did not include the subepithelial stroma surrounding the blastocyst. The

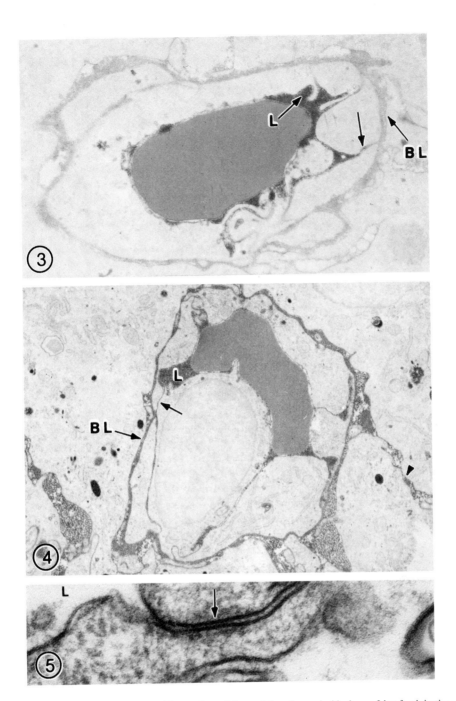

Figure 3. This micrograph shows a capillary at the periphery of the primary decidual zone 2 hr after injection of IgG–HRP on day 7 of pregnancy. Reaction product is dense in the lumen (L) but much less dense in the capillary basal lamina (BL). There is an abrupt change in the density of reaction product at the intercellular cleft between endothelial cells (arrow). This section was not stained. ×12,000.

Figure 4. This micrograph shows a capillary at the periphery of the primary decidual zone at 30 min after injection of HRP on day 7 of pregnancy. The reaction product has the same electron density in the capillary lumen (L), in the intercellular clefts between endothelial cells (arrow), in the capillary basal lamina (BL), and between decidual cells (arrowhead). This section was not stained. ×8200.

Figure 5. This micrograph illustrates the close junctions (arrow) between endothelial cells in the capillaries at the edge of the primary decidual zone on day 7 of pregnancy. L, Capillary lumen. ×119,000.

authors suggested that increased vascular permeability at implantation sites develops gradually and that the PBR is a rather late sign of vascular change. Structural changes in the blood vessels of these animals have not yet been studied. Other data suggest that the PBR and edema are concurrent events (rat: Cecil *et al.*, 1966; rabbit: Hoos and Hoffman, 1980). It appears that edema and increased vascular permeability in the uterus at implantation may be associated with fenestrated endothelium, conspicuous gaps between endothelial cells, or close endothelial cell junctions. Further clarification is needed regarding the distribution of these structures at the implantation site and their permeability to tracers of various molecular weights and charges. It is possible that fenestrated vessels develop in rats and mice in response to ovarian estrogen secretion (Martin *et al.*, 1973), allowing for the early edema described by Lundkvist and Ljungkvist (1977), followed by the formation of gaps or close-type junctions in response to vasoactive mediators, which would result in the extravasation of plasma proteins.

2.2. Role of Prostaglandins in Increased Vascular Permeability

Although it is abundantly clear that there is increased vascular permeability at the site of blastocyst implantation in a wide variety of animals, the cause of this reaction is still under investigation. The fact that the increased permeability is restricted to implantation sites suggests an obligatory role for the blastocyst in this phenomenon. The effect of the blastocyst may be mediated directly through its attachment to the luminal epithelium or by the synthesis and secretion of materials that affect the endometrium. The exact identities of the signals or mediators that pass from the blastocyst to the endometrium are unknown, but prostaglandins (PGs), histamine, and estrogen have been implicated (Dey and Johnson, 1980; Kennedy, 1983a). The nature of the blastocyst signal is currently one of the most interesting questions in implantation biology. In any case, it seems most likely that the blastocyst exerts its effects on the luminal epithelium, which then secretes or releases factors that mediate increased vascular permeability and decidualization. The evidence for this conclusion is the observation that both events can be induced in hormonally sensitized uteri by artificial stimuli in the absence of blastocysts (De Feo, 1967) but that artificial stimuli do not induce decidualization if the luminal epithelium has been previously stripped away (Lejeune *et al.*, 1981).

There is now substantial evidence that PGs are responsible, at least in part, for increased vascular permeability at implantation sites. First, there is a higher concentration of PGs at pontamine blue sites than at other parts of the uterus in several species (rat: Kennedy, 1977; Kennedy and Zamecnik, 1978; hamster: Evans and Kennedy, 1978; rabbit: Sharma, 1979; Pakrasi and Dey, 1982; Hoffman *et al.*, 1984). A second line of evidence comes from the use of antiinflammatory drugs such as indomethacin and aspirin, which decrease PG synthesis by inhibiting the activity of the enzyme prostaglandin synthase. This enzyme catalyzes the conversion of arachidonic acid to PGH_2 (Yamamoto, 1982; Fig. 6). When indomethacin was administered to animals at the time of implantation, it caused a reduction in the amount of endometrial PG (Evans and Kennedy, 1978; Saksena *et al.*, 1976; Hoffman *et al.*, 1984), delayed or reduced the magnitude of the PBR (rat: Kennedy, 1977; Phillips and Poyser, 1981; mouse: Lundkvist and Nilsson, 1980; hamster: Evans and Kennedy, 1978; rabbit: Hoffman *et al.*, 1978; Hoos and Hoffman, 1983), and blocked implantation (rabbit: El-Banna, 1980; mouse: Holmes and Gordashko, 1980; Lau *et al.*, 1973; Saksena *et al.*, 1976). A partial reversal of the antifertility effect of indomethacin was achieved following the administration of $PGF_{2\alpha}$ (Saksena *et al.*, 1976; El-Banna, 1980). Furthermore, PGE_2 and $PGF_{2\alpha}$ induced increased vascular permeability in delayed-implantation animals when used in the place of exogenous estrogen (rat: Oettel *et al.*, 1979; mouse: Holmes and Gordashko, 1980). No single PG has been identified as the exclusive mediator of the PBR, and there appear to be species differences in the predominant type of PG at implantation sites (Kennedy, 1983a).

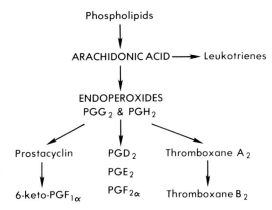

Figure 6. This diagram shows the biosynthetic pathway of prostaglandins and other arachidonic acid metabolites.

2.3. Endometrial Prostaglandins

The studies described above illustrate the involvement of PGs in the PBR, but the source of the PGs was not defined. Additional pieces of evidence have shown that the endometrium synthesizes PGs that mediate increased vascular permeability. Indomethacin inhibited the vascular response to artificial stimuli in uteri of spayed rats sensitized with ovarian hormones (Kennedy, 1979), an effect that was reversed by the administration of PGs into the uterine lumen (Kennedy, 1979, 1980a; Kennedy and Lukash, 1982). The concentration of PGs in the rat endometrium was elevated by artificial stimuli before any change in vascular permeability could be detected (Kennedy, 1979, 1980a; Rankin *et al.*, 1979; Milligan and Lytton, 1983). The concentration of PGs was also elevated at rabbit implantation sites from which the blastocysts and myometrium had been removed (Hoffman *et al.*, 1984). The production of PGs in endometrial homogenates peaked on day 5 of normal pregnancy and pseudopregnancy (Phillips and Poyser, 1981), taking day 1 as the day spermatozoa are detected in the vagina after mating. (Other dating systems have been converted to this one for purposes of comparison in this chapter.) Moreover, recent studies have focused on the identity of the endometrial cells that synthesize PGs. Primary cultures of human glandular epithelial cells and stromal cells produced PGs *in vitro* (Schatz *et al.*, 1987); epithelial cells isolated from rat uteri during pseudopregnancy synthesized PGF and PGE on days 4 to 6, reaching a maximum on day 5 (Moulton, 1984); and PG synthase has been localized in various cell types in the rat endometrium during the periimplantation period (Parr *et al.*, 1988).

The uterine luminal epithelium as a source of PGs in rat implantation sites is of particular interest. Kennedy (1983a) has suggested that these cells may respond to embryonic signals or artificial stimuli by initiating the synthesis of PGs, which would then diffuse into the underlying stroma to bring about increased vascular permeability and decidualization. Although there is no direct evidence that the luminal epithelium synthesizes PGs at implantation, indirect evidence is accumulating (Moulton, 1984; Ohta, 1985; Parr *et al.*, 1988). Several investigators have focused on the important regulatory role of phospholipase A_2 in the mobilization of arachidonic acid from phospholipids (Flower and Blackwell, 1976; Irvine, 1982). The luminal epithelium in rats appears to respond to artificial stimuli by mobilization of arachidonic acid from phospholipids and by phospholipid methylation (Moulton *et al.*, 1987; Moulton and Koenig, 1986). Cox *et al.* (1982) demonstrated a peak of uterine phospholipase A_2 activity just prior to implantation, but no distinction was made between implantation and interimplantation

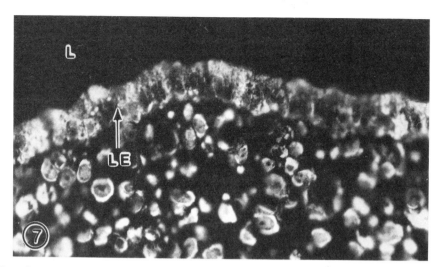

Figure 7. A section through a rat implantation site on the evening of day 5 of pregnancy shows bright fluorescein labeling of prostaglandin synthase in the luminal epithelium (LE) and in adjacent stromal cells that are undergoing decidualization. The primary antibody was a monoclonal mouse IgM antirat PG synthase. L, Uterine lumen. ×425.

sites. Phospholipase activity increased in the endometrium apposed to the blastocyst at the time of implantation in rabbits (Hoffman *et al.,* 1984). A localized depletion of neutral lipids from the luminal epithelium adjacent to blastocysts has been reported and interpreted as a mobilization of precursors for PG synthesis (rat: Boshier, 1976; sheep: Boshier *et al.,* 1987). Also of interest is the observation that PG synthase was detected in the rat luminal epithelium on day 5 by immunohistochemical labeling (Parr *et al.,* 1988; Fig. 7). The labeling of PG synthase in the luminal epithelium declined as implantation proceeded from day 5 to day 7 of pregnancy, a time when the uterus is known to become refractory to implantation (Psychoyos, 1973). The authors thus suggested that PG production by these cells may play a role primarily during the early stages of implantation. The absence of PG receptors in the luminal epithelium (rat: Kennedy *et al.,* 1983a,b; Cao *et al.,* 1984) suggests that although these cells may synthesize PGs, they cannot bind them through receptor-mediated mechanisms.

2.4. *Blastocyst Prostaglandins*

There are numerous studies showing that blastocysts can synthesize PGs, but the role of these PGs in implantation, if any, has not been defined (rabbit: Dey *et al.,* 1980; Harper *et al.,* 1983; Racowsky and Biggers, 1983; sheep: Marcus, 1981; Hyland *et al.,* 1982; Lacroix and Kann, 1982; pig: Watson and Patek, 1979; Lewis and Waterman, 1983; Bazer and First, 1983; cow: Shemesh *et al.,* 1979; Lewis *et al.,* 1982). Prostaglandin synthesis was not detected in rat (Kennedy and Armstrong, 1981) or mouse (Racowsky and Biggers, 1983) blastocysts, but there is indirect evidence that blastocysts may synthesize PGs in these species. Biggers *et al.* (1978) have shown that inhibitors of PG synthesis inhibit hatching of mouse blastocysts *in vitro,* and Racowsky and Biggers (1983) have suggested that the inability to demonstrate PG synthesis in this species may be a result of insensitivity of the methods used thus far. Holmes and Gordashko (1980), using scanning electron microscopy, reported that blastocysts from indomethacin-treated mice were impeded in their morphological activation. Recent evidence shows that preimplantation mouse embryos contain PGE_2 (Nimura and Ishida, 1987), and rat blastocysts at implantation contain PG synthase (Parr *et al.,* 1988; Fig. 8). It is possible that

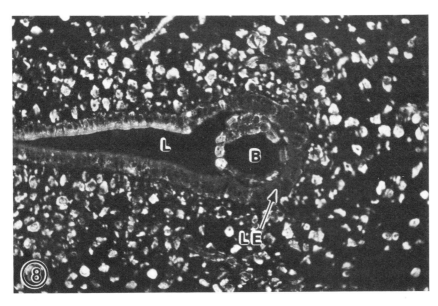

Figure 8. This micrograph shows a rat implantation site on day 5 of pregnancy. Note the specific labeling of PG synthase in the blastocyst (B) and the bright labeling of stromal cells beginning to undergo decidualization. The luminal epithelium (LE) shows patchy labeling. L, Uterine lumen. ×275.

PGs produced by the blastocysts may not have the same physiological functions in all species. Some investigators have suggested that they serve as signals from the blastocyst to the uterus (Marcus, 1981; Lewis *et al.*, 1982; Pakrasi and Dey, 1982), but others have argued that PG synthesis by the blastocyst is required for fluid accumulation and hatching (Biggers *et al.*, 1978, 1981) and for the expansion of the blastocyst in rabbits (Hoffman *et al.*, 1978).

3. The Decidual Cell Reaction

In many mammalian species, the uterus responds to an implanting blastocyst by undergoing extensive modifications that result in the transformation of the endometrium into the decidua. The most conspicuous aspect of this tissue differentiation is the transformation of stromal cells into large, polyploid decidual cells with an epithelioid appearance. The decidual cells are characterized by an accumulation of glycogen and lipid in the cytoplasm, numerous lysosomes, rough endoplasmic reticulum, and extensive cell-to-cell contacts and junctional complexes. The differentiation of the endometrium into decidual tissue is called the decidual cell reaction (DCR) or decidualization, and it involves several changes in the components of the extracellular space less conspicuous than those already mentioned. In the rat and a few other species, decidualization can also be triggered by a variety of artificial stimuli in hormonally prepared uteri. This response results in the formation of a deciduoma, an event that has been studied extensively because it provides a uterine reaction in the absence of embryonic tissue (De Feo, 1967). The deciduoma appears very similar morphologically to the decidua of normal pregnancy (De Feo, 1967).

Early light-microscopic studies established that there were pronounced regional morphological differences in the transformed rat endometrial stroma (decidua) during normal pregnancy. In his now classic paper, Krehbiel (1937) showed that there were two major areas of decidualized tissue: an antimesometrial decidual region consisting of primary and secondary zones and a mesometrial decidual region. These original observations have been confirmed and extended by recent electron-microscopic studies. We summarize the morphological features of the three decidual regions and then discuss the initiation and functions of the DCR.

3.1. The Primary Decidual Zone

The primary decidual zone (PDZ) is a cup-shaped region of transformed fibroblasts surrounding the implanting blastocyst and uterine epithelium at the antimesometrial side of the uterus (Fig. 1). It consists of a narrow band of large cells, three to five cells thick, and is devoid of blood vessels (Enders and Schlafke, 1967; Rogers et al., 1983; Parr and Parr, 1986; Parr et al., 1986; Tung et al., 1986). Rogers et al. (1983), using the combined vascular corrosion casting and scanning electron microscope technique, clearly showed a region comparable to the PDZ free of capillaries at the implantation site. Ultrastructural studies of the PDZ during early pregnancy have shown that its cells contain abundant rough endoplasmic reticulum, lysosomelike bodies, scattered Golgi complexes, microfilaments, numerous microtubules, lipid droplets, and glycogen granules (Enders and Schlafke, 1967; Tachi et al., 1970; Sananes and Le Goascogne, 1976; Schlafke et al., 1985; Parr et al., 1986; Tung et al., 1986; Welsh and Enders, 1987). The cells of the PDZ are tightly packed, and the apposed cell membranes show extensive interdigitations and junctional regions, including gap junctions, desmosome-like junctions, and tight junctions (Parr et al., 1986; Tung et al., 1986). The presence of tight junctions between cells in the PDZ underscores the epithelioid nature of the decidual cells. Gap junctions mediate intercellular communication (Loewenstein, 1966; Gilula et al., 1972) and may facilitate synchronous responses to hormonal signals, coordinate growth of the decidua, and allow the decidua to act as an integrated morphological unit.

The cells of the PDZ exhibit some surprising features. In the rat, flangelike processes from the decidual cells penetrate the basal laminae of the adjacent luminal epithelium and capillary endothelium (Schlafke et al., 1985; Parr et al., 1986; Tung et al., 1986; Welsh and Enders, 1987) (Figs. 9–11). Not only do portions of the decidual cells abut the basal membrane of the endothelial cells without an intervening basal lamina (Parr et al., 1986), but the decidual cells themselves take up positions as part of the wall of the maternal blood vessels and form junctional attachments to the adjacent endothelial cells (Welsh and Enders, 1987). These observations suggest that decidual cells are invasive. Welsh and Enders (1987) have shown that decidual cells lining the maternal vessels eventually degenerate and are replaced by trophoblast cells, allowing the latter to tap the maternal vessels. Thus, the invasive property of the cells of the PDZ in penetrating basal laminae may facilitate the invasion of the trophoblast into the uterine endometrium.

Another characteristic of the rat PDZ is the presence of bundles of collagen fibrils surrounded by plasma membrane in deep invaginations of the decidual cell surface (Parr et al., 1986). Such images suggest that the decidual cells may be involved in a reorganization of the collagen in the PDZ, perhaps including collagen degradation. This cellular activity may be required for the remodeling of the endometrium, including the formation of the PDZ, and for the normal growth and expansion of the developing embryo. Collagen remodeling has been proposed as an important part of the decidualization process in other parts of the uterus (O'Shea et al., 1983; Zorn et al., 1986). In addition, intercellular spaces within the PDZ appear to be filled with a homogeneous electron-dense material that corresponds in position to a mucopolysaccharide substance that has been described at this site in earlier studies (mouse: Finn and Hinchliffe, 1965; rat: Enders and Schlafke, 1979) (Figs. 12–14).

The PDZ is a transient region, developing on day 6 in the rat and showing signs of involution 2–3 days later. Welsh and Enders (1987) have demonstrated that on day 8 of pregnancy the decidual cells next to the trophoblast begin to show morphological features of apoptotic death. Processes of trophoblast cells surround and engulf the dying decidual cells as

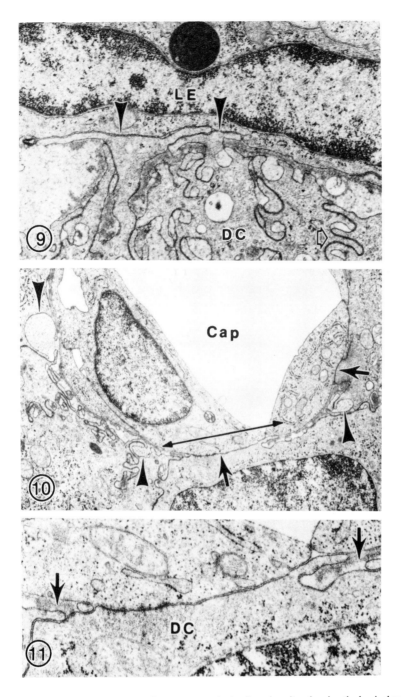

Figure 9. This is an electron micrograph of a rat uterus at the implantation site, showing the luminal epithelium (LE) and the underlying decidual cells (DC). Two flange-like processes of a DC have penetrated the epithelial basal lamina and are seen adjacent to the basal membrane of a luminal epithelial cell (arrowheads). ×17,000.

Figure 10. A blood vessel located at the periphery of the PDZ shows processes from decidual cells (arrows) that have penetrated the basal lamina of the capillary endothelium and lie close to the base of the endothelial cells. Note the clusters of collagen fibrils (arrowheads) at the border of the decidual cells and capillary. The region marked by the two-headed arrow is enlarged in Fig. 11. Cap, Capillary. ×8000.

Figure 11. The decidual cell (DC) has penetrated the basal lamina (arrows) and is seen adjacent to the capillary endothelial cell. ×22,500.

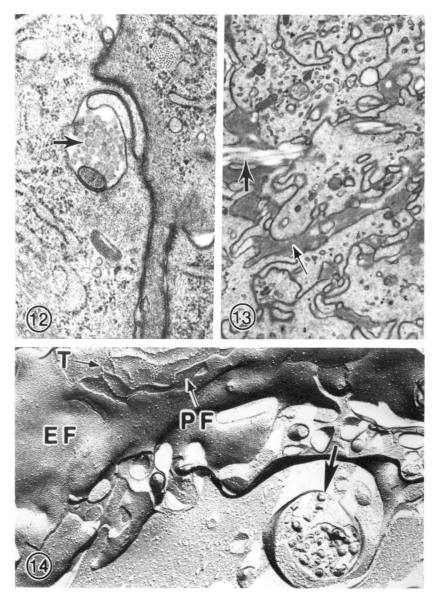

Figure 12. This electron micrograph shows a bundle of collagen fibrils (arrow) seen in transverse section surrounded by the plasma membrane of a decidual cell and invaginated into the cytoplasm of that cell. ×33,000.

Figure 13. This electron micrograph shows pale-staining collagen fibrils cut in longitudinal section (large arrow) and electron-dense material in the extracellular spaces between decidual cells (small arrow). ×15,000.

Figure 14. This is an electron micrograph of a freeze–fracture replica showing decidual cells in the PDZ of rats on day 7 of pregnancy. The micrograph shows tight junctional strands (T) in the P-face (PF) of a decidual cell plasma membrane and a few scattered particles in the E-face (EF). A bundle of collagen fibrils (thick arrow) is seen in a deep invagination of the cell surface membrane. A comparable thin-section image is seen in Fig. 12. ×37,000.

they round up and detach from adjacent cells. After removal of the cells of the PDZ, the trophoblastic cells occupy the space previously occupied by the decidual cells and thus come into contact with the maternal vessels of the secondary decidual zone.

Recent studies have suggested that the PDZ forms a permeability barrier between the blastocyst and the maternal circulation during implantation (Parr and Parr, 1986; Tung *et al.*, 1986). On days 6 and 7 of pregnancy in rats, macromolecules with molecular weights up to and including that of horseradish peroxidase (40 kDa) readily penetrated into the intercellular spaces of the PDZ and thus reached the blastocyst. In contrast, serum albumin (70 kda) and larger macromolecules were largely or completely excluded from the PDZ (Rogers *et al.*, 1983; Parr and Parr, 1986; Tung *et al.*, 1986) (Figs. 15 and 16). An ultrastructural tracer study suggested that there were at least two morphological components to the permeability barrier of the PDZ (Tung *et al.*, 1986). The first barrier component was localized at the intercellular junctions between endothelial cells in the maternal vessels around the periphery of the PDZ. Here, horseradish peroxidase (HRP) readily penetrated through "close" endothelial junctions, while immunoglobulin G conjugated to HRP (IgG–HRP) was impeded but not blocked (Figs. 3–5). Beyond this point, IgG–HRP was effectively excluded from the intercellular spaces of the PDZ, although HRP entered readily. This finding suggests that another selective barrier exists within the PDZ, passing HRP but blocking IgG–HRP. Although the identity of the barrier within the PDZ could not be determined, the fact that discontinuous tight junctions were demonstrated between the cells of the PDZ is of interest. Such junctions could serve as a barrier to macromolecules, and their presence emphasizes the epithelioid nature of the primary decidual cells (Figs. 17–19). Other morphological features of intercellular spaces within the PDZ that could potentially contribute to its barrier function are the extensive interdigitations of the cell surfaces and the amorphous intercellular material.

In the absence of a continuous luminal epithelium at the implantation site from early on day 7 of pregnancy, the PDZ constitutes the only significant barrier between the embryo and maternal blood. By day 9 of pregnancy the PDZ undergoes involution (Welsh and Enders, 1987) and loses its barrier function, but at this time the embryo is surrounded by a continuous and well-developed visceral yolk sac. The tracer studies mentioned above (Parr and Parr, 1986) demonstrated that the yolk sac effectively prevented macromolecules from reaching the underlying embryonic cells on day 9 of pregnancy in rats (Figs. 20 and 21). Parr and Parr (1986) suggested that the PDZ on days 6 to 8 may serve as a temporary barrier preventing immunoglobulins, microorganisms, and immunocompetent cells from reaching the embryo before it develops its own protective layers (Fig. 22). It is noteworthy, however, that this barrier allows the passage of smaller macromolecules between the embryo and the surrounding maternal tissues. That the PDZ may act as a physical barrier to invading trophoblast cells also remains possible (Kirby, 1965). Finally, Tachi *et al.* (1981) have demonstrated that macrophages, which increase in number at rat implantation sites, are absent from the PDZ but are aggregated around its periphery. They suggested that macrophages are unable to cross the PDZ and gain access to paternal antigens, thus resulting in the blockage of the afferent arm of maternal immune recognition.

3.2. Antimesometrial Decidua

Another phase of hyperplasia and hypertrophy occurs on day 6 of pregnancy in the rat, in the stromal cells surrounding the PDZ. This phase results in the formation of the secondary decidual zone (SDZ: Krehbiel, 1937). The SDZ comprises the bulk of antimesometrial decidual tissue and is often referred to, simply, as the antimesometrial decidua. It contributes largely to the formation of the decidua capsularis, which, until the rupture of Reichert's membrane and associated tissues on about day 16 of pregnancy, is associated with the parietal yolk sac.

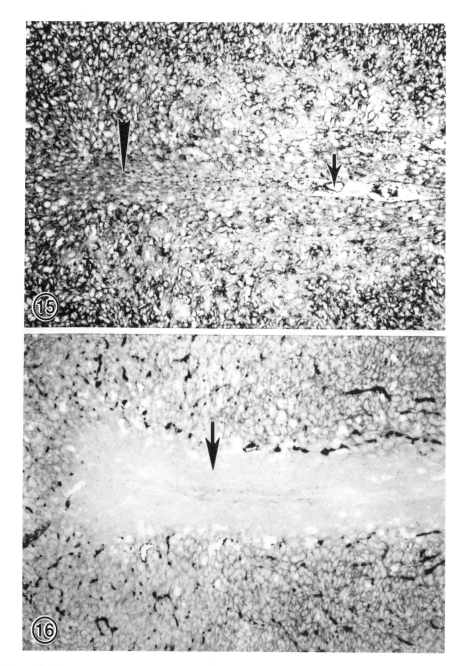

Figure 15. The light micrograph shows the distribution of horseradish peroxidase in a rat implantation site 30 min after i.v. injection on day 7 of pregnancy. Reaction product is present in the interstitial spaces of the endometrium, in the PDZ (arrowhead), and in the blastocyst (arrow). The section was not counterstained. ×110.
Figure 16. This light micrograph shows the distribution of immunoglobulin G conjugated to horseradish perox-idase in an implantation site of a rat uterine horn on day 7 of pregnancy 2 hr after i.v. administration. There is reaction product in the blood vessels and interstitial spaces of the endometrium but not in the PDZ (arrow). The section was not counterstained. ×110.

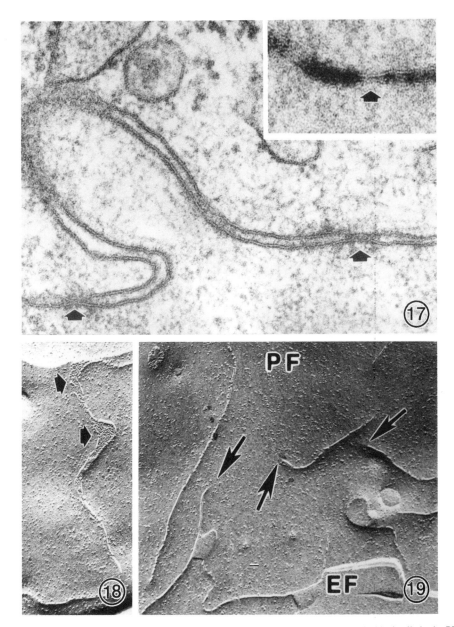

Figure 17. This electron micrograph illustrates two tight junctions (arrows) between decidual cells in the PDZ on day 7 of pregnancy. The external membrane leaflets are fused in the junctions. ×120,000. The inset shows a portion of the PDZ in a day-7 implantation site that was treated with lanthanum. The tracer is present throughout the intercellular spaces between decidual cells except at the tight junction (arrow). ×156,000.

Figures 18 and 19. Electron micrographs of freeze–fracture replicas showing decidual cells in the PDZ of rats on day 7 of pregnancy.

Figure 18. The P-face of a plasma membrane containing a single tight-junctional strand with associated gap-junctional particles (arrows). Each gap-junctional region appears to be enclosed by a tight junctional strand. ×46,000.

Figure 19. Portions of the E- and P-faces of a plasma membrane containing short, discontinuous tight-junctional strands (arrows). ×48,000.

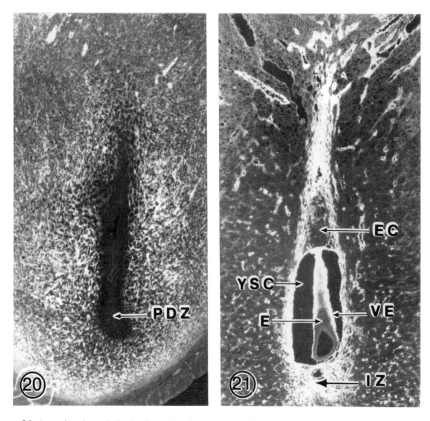

Figure 20. A section through the implantation site in a uterus from a rat injected i.v. with FITC-labeled bovine serum albumin (BSA) on day 7 of pregnancy and killed 1 hr later. Fluorescence is seen in the maternal blood vessels and interstitial spaces of the endometrium but not in the PDZ. ×30.

Figure 21. A section through an implantation site in a uterus from a rat injected i.v. with FITC-labeled BSA on day 9 of pregnancy and killed 1 hr later. There is bright fluorescence in the maternal blood vessels, in and mesometrial to the ectoplacental cone (EC), in the visceral endoderm (VE) of the yolk sac, and in the implantation zone (IZ). VE, Visceral endoderm; YSC, yolk sac cavity. ×30.

The ultrastructural features of cells in the antimesometrial region have been studied extensively in decidua and in deciduomata and appear to be similar in both (rat: Jollie and Bencosme, 1965; Enders and Schlafke, 1967; Tachi *et al.,* 1970; Sananes and Le Goascogne, 1976; Klienfeld *et al.,* 1976; Lundkvist and Ljunkvist, 1977; O'Shea *et al.,* 1983; Welsh and Enders, 1985, 1987; mouse: Finn and Lawn, 1967; Abrahamsohn, 1983; hamster: Orsini *et al.,* 1970; Parkening, 1976).

The glycogen-rich cells are large, polyploid, and often binucleate and contain organelles typical of cells engaged in protein synthesis. The decidualization process is characterized by a reduction of intercellular space and a remodeling of its matrix, as has been shown by a decrease in the number of collagen fibrils (rat: Fainstat, 1963; mouse: Jeffrey, 1981; Martello and Abrahamsohn, 1986; Zorn *et al.,* 1986). Specialized structures that develop on the cell surface include gap junctions, desmosomelike junctions, and extensive areas of lamellar projections, which often interdigitate with those of neighboring cells. Cellular organelles associated with steroidogenesis, such as smooth endoplasmic reticulum and mitochondria with tubular cristae, have been shown to be absent from the cells (O'Shea *et al.,* 1983). The antimesometrial decidua and deciduomata also contain other cell types in small numbers, including lymphocytes, eosinophils, cells of the monocyte–macrophage series, and granulated

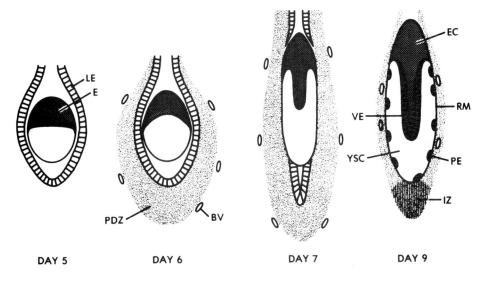

DAY 5   DAY 6   DAY 7   DAY 9

Figure 22. This diagram shows the tissue relationships in the rat implantation site between days 5 and 9 of pregnancy. The PDZ first appears on day 6 as an avascular zone of transformed fibroblasts separating the nearest blood vessels from the uterine luminal epithelium (LE). Early on day 7 the luminal epithelium adjacent to the embryo (E) is lost, and the trophectoderm comes into direct contact with the PDZ. The embryonic yolk sac at this time is not yet well developed, and the PDZ is the only significant barrier between maternal blood vessels (BV) and the embryo. On day 9 the PDZ is thin, and maternal blood spaces are closely adjacent to the parietal endoderm (PE) and Reichert's membrane (RM). The trophoblast has been omitted. On day 9 the visceral endoderm (VE) appears to form an effective barrier between serum macromolecules and embryonic cells. YSC, Yolk sac cavity; EC, ectoplacental cone; IZ, implantation zone.

cells similar to those in the mesometrial decidual region (O'Shea *et al.*, 1983). O'Shea *et al.* (1983) have described a capsule just outside the antimesometrial decidua that consists of a layer of flattened cells that may be the source of appositional growth of the decidua or deciduoma. The basal zone between the capsule and circular muscle was made up of fibrocytelike stromal cells separated by wide bands of collagen fibrils. This zone may contribute to endometrial regeneration following parturition.

3.3. Mesometrial Decidua

Stromal cells in the mesometrial region of the uterus differentiate into decidual cells that form the mesometrial decidua. This region then develops into the decidua basalis, which comes to lie mesometrial to the placenta and persists throughout gestation. O'Shea *et al.* (1983) have described the mesometrial decidua as being composed of cells showing less pronounced differentiation than those on the antimesometrial side. The spiny cells in this zone are referred to as "fixed" cells. They are frequently binucleate and contain large stores of glycogen. The cytoplasmic processes, which give the cells their spiny appearance, form gap junctions and desmosomelike junctions with those of neighboring cells, thus creating a complex meshwork. Here, as in the antimesometrial decidua, there are few collagen fibrils, and the main elements of structural support are provided by spiny cells, their junctions, and microfilaments.

Another population of cells, consisting mainly of granulated cells and often appearing motile, has been observed in the interstices of the meshwork of spiny cell processes. This population was referred to as "free" cells (O'Shea *et al.*, 1983). The appearance of the granulated cells in the decidua was similar to that of granulated cells in the metrial gland, which supports the observation of Stewart and Peel (1981) that the granulated cells within the metrial gland were not restricted to that site. Cells of similar morphological appearance were observed in small numbers at preimplantation stages, spread at random throughout the endometrium. By day 6 in the mouse and day 8 in the rat, however, granulated cells lose their random distribution and begin to appear in increasing numbers in the mesometrial decidua. A short time later they appear in the mesometrial triangle. Strong evidence has accumulated that these granulated metrial gland cells, perhaps in association with decidual tissue and requiring a sufficient and continuing supply of progesterone, are involved in immunologic relationships between maternal and fetal tissues during pregnancy (Bulmer et al., 1987). Another study has suggested that the granulated cells may be natural-killer-like cells (Parr et al., 1987b), but more information will be needed to establish their identity and role in the immunology of pregnancy.

Other cell types with possible immunologic functions have been observed in decidual tissues during the implantation period or throughout pregnancy. These include Fc-receptor-bearing cells (Bernard et al., 1978; Rachman et al., 1981; Kirkwood, 1981; Bell and Searle, 1981; Craggs and Peel, 1983), macrophages (Searle et al., 1983; Tachi et al., 1981; Hunt et al., 1985), dendritic cells (Searle et al., 1983), null lymphocytes (Bernard et al., 1978; Rachman et al., 1981), thy-1-bearing cells (Searle et al., 1983), and T cells lacking IL-1 receptors (Bulmer and Johnson, 1986). It should be pointed out that there is some confusion in the terminology of the various types of cells in the decidua. We suggest that the term "decidual cell" be used only to refer to transformed stromal cells having the morphological features previously described. No other convenient name exists for their identification. Lymphoid cells, resident or transient, such as macrophages and lymphocytes, may be present in the decidualized endometrium and can be referred to by their proper names if their identities are known. Cell preparations obtained by dissociating decidual tissues should not be referred to as decidual cells because a mixture of cell types will generally be present. Such cell preparations could be referred to as "cells of decidual tissue" or "dissociated decidual tissue," which would avoid the implication that the functional activities of the mixed population reside specifically in decidual cells. The roles of decidual cells and their associated lymphoid cells in the immunology of pregnancy have received increased attention in recent years. A review of the relevant literature would be beyond the scope of this chapter, and the reader is referred to several other publications on the subject (Bernard and Rachman, 1980; Bell, 1983; Lala et al., 1986; Clark et al., 1986; Bulmer et al., 1987).

3.4. The Role of Prostaglandins in Initiating Decidualization

There is growing evidence that PGs may be required for the initiation and maintenance of decidualization. The administration of PGs to hormonally primed animals causes the decidual cell response (Tachi and Tachi, 1974; Sananes et al., 1976, 1981; Hoffman et al., 1977; Miller and O'Morchoe, 1982; Kennedy, 1985, 1986; Doktorcik and Kennedy, 1986), indomethacin inhibits its appearance (Sananes et al., 1976, 1980, 1981; Castracane et al., 1974; Tobert, 1976; Rankin et al., 1979), and PGs can override the inhibitory effects of indomethacin (Kennedy and Lukash, 1982; Kennedy, 1985).

The identity of the PGs involved in decidualization is uncertain, however. Both PGE_2 and $PGF_{2\alpha}$ can cause decidualization, but PGE_2 may be more effective than $PGF_{2\alpha}$ in the rabbit (Hoffman et al., 1977) and the rat (Kennedy, 1986). Endometrial binding sites have been detected for PGE_2 (Kennedy et al., 1983a,b) but not for $PGF_{2\alpha}$ (Martel et al., 1985). Concentrations of PGE, PGF, and 6-keto-$PGF_{1\alpha}$ are elevated at implantation sites and in uteri after the application of an artificial deciduogenic stimulus (Kennedy, 1977, 1979, 1980a,b; Kennedy and Zamecnik, 1978; Milligan and Lytton, 1983). Phillips and Poyser (1981) have reported that the PG produced in greatest amount by uterine homogenates from both pregnant and pseudopregnant rats on day 5 is 6-keto-PGF$_{1\alpha}$. In mice, Rankin *et al.* (1979) have suggested that PGI$_2$ (prostacyclin) may mediate decidualization, because tranylcypromine, an inhibitor of PGI$_2$ synthesis, inhibited decidualization. However, PGI$_2$ has not been shown to override the effects of the inhibitor.

Although PGs appear to mediate the DCR, it is not known whether they act directly on endometrial cells or induce decidualization indirectly by some other mechanism. In particular, since PGs are involved with increased vascular permeability that precedes decidualization (Psychoyos, 1973), it is possible that their effects on the DCR may be mediated in part by the increased concentrations of serum components in the endometrium. Attempts have been made to test this possibility. Finn (1965) showed that an increase in vascular permeability induced experimentally in estradiol-sensitized mice was not sufficient to induce decidualization. Milligan and Mirembe (1985) have demonstrated that the intraluminal injection of oil into the uteri of mice treated with progesterone induced a marked increase in vascular permeability that was not followed by a DCR. In addition, Tobert (1976) inhibited decidualization by administering indomethacin 8 hr after the application of a deciduogenic stimulus, a time when the pontamine blue reaction was evident. Still, it is not known in the latter two cases whether the shorter duration of the increased vascular permeability was a factor limiting decidualization. Perhaps the complexities of the *in vivo* condition may be circumvented by studying the effects of PGs on endometrial cells grown *in vitro*. Toward that end, Sananes *et al.* (1980) showed that indomethacin blocked the growth and differentiation of decidual cells *in vitro*, and Daniel and Kennedy (1987) demonstrated that PGE$_2$ stimulated alkaline phosphatase activity in cultured endometrial stromal cells isolated from sensitized rat uteri. This latter observation is relevant to studies of Finn and his colleagues, who demonstrated the presence of alkaline phosphatase in mouse stromal cells following the induction of decidualization in normal pregnancy, and in deciduomata (Finn and Hinchliffe, 1964; Finn and McLaren, 1967). Although the *in vitro* approach may eventually be fruitful, one must be cautious in evaluating such data because there are still numerous problems involved in the establishment of *in vitro* model systems for decidualization (Glasser, 1985; Glasser and McCormack, 1981).

3.5. *Mechanisms of Prostaglandin Effects on Vascular Permeability and Decidualization*

The mechanisms by which PGs cause increased endometrial vascular permeability and decidualization may be similar, and studies of these mechanisms often do not distinguish which end point is affected. We therefore consider in this section how PGs exert their effects on both processes. In general, PGs may exert their influence by altering calcium metabolism, inducing changes in membrane-associated enzymes, interacting with intracellular enzymes, or perhaps by modulating the arrangement of intracellular cytoskeletal elements such as microfilaments and microtubules (Hall and Behrman, 1982). Rankin *et al.* (1977) have suggested that in the uterus cyclic adenosine monophosphate (cAMP) may be a mediator of some of the effects of PGs at implantation. Artificial deciduogenic stimuli bring about a rapid increase in uterine cAMP levels (Leroy *et al.*, 1974; Rankin *et al.* 1977, 1979, 1981; Kennedy, 1983b) that appears to be mediated by PGs because it is inhibited by indomethacin (Rankin *et al.*, 1979). Another study has shown that adenylate cyclase, the enzyme that catalyzes the formation of cAMP, is activated by deciduogenic stimuli (Sanders *et al.*, 1983; Bekairi *et al.*, 1984; Sanders *et al.*, 1986). In addition, cholera toxin, an activator of adenylate cyclase, produces a dose-dependent increase in vascular permeability (Johnston and Kennedy, 1984) and causes decidualization when introduced into the uterine lumen (rat: Kennedy, 1983b; mouse: Rankin *et al.*, 1979). Although cholera toxin led to a tenfold increase in endometrial cAMP in mice (Rankin *et al.*, 1977), it did not increase cAMP levels in rats (Johnston and Kennedy, 1984).

Dey and Hubbard (1981) reported that in rabbits intrauterine administration of an inhibitor of adenylate cyclase decreased the implantation rate. Taken together, these studies suggest a possible role for cAMP in the initiation of implantation, but further studies are needed.

The role of calcium ions in mediating decidualization has been assessed with use of the calcium ionophore A23187. This substance acted as a deciduogenic stimulus when injected into the uterine lumen of pseudopregnant mice (Buxton and Murdoch, 1982) but failed to elicit a response in rats (Feyles and Kennedy, 1987). In the rat, the calcium ionophore had a synergistic effect when used in combination with an activator of protein kinase C, resulting in an inhibition of decidualization. The inhibitory effects did not appear to be mediated by inhibition of PG synthesis in the uterus (Feyles and Kennedy, 1987).

3.6. Decidual Cell Metabolism

There is growing evidence that decidual cells can synthesize PGs throughout pregnancy (Anteby et al., 1975; Huslig et al., 1979; Parr et al., 1988). Decidual cell PGs may participate in the maintenance of increased vascular permeability and differentiation of decidual tissue (Kennedy, 1985). In a recent immunohistochemical study, Parr et al. (1988) demonstrated labeling of PG synthase in differentiating stromal cells surrounding the implanting rat blastocyst on day 5 of pregnancy (Figs. 7 and 8). On days 6 and 7 of pregnancy, cells in the SDZ were strongly labeled, but a marked reduction of labeling was seen in PDZ cells (Fig. 23). These observations suggest that on day 5 differentiating stromal cells synthesize PGs, which might play a role in the initial phases of implantation, but the activity diminishes as the PDZ develops. Cells in the SDZ may then take on the function of PG synthesis so that decidualization and increased vascular permeability are maintained. The changes in PG synthase labeling in the two decidual regions may thus reflect alterations in their functional capacities as implantation proceeds. In addition, PGs synthesized by decidual cells and decidua-associated macrophages may play a role in the immunology of pregnancy (Lala et al., 1986; Searle, 1986; Tawfik et al., 1986).

Carson et al. (1987) have suggested recently that decidual cells may synthesize hyaluronate during the early stages of implantation in the mouse uterus and after the application of artificial stimuli to spayed, hormone-primed animals. In their experiments, a large specific increase in synthesis of hyaluronate occurred in deciduomata and in the uterus on the day of implantation. Increased hyaluronate synthesis may reflect a stromal cell response, since cultured uterine epithelial cells have been shown to synthesize very small amounts of hyaluronate (Dutt et al., 1986). In the in vitro model of implantation, hyaluronate enhanced the attachment and outgrowth of trophoblast cells. Dutt et al. (1986) suggested that hyaluronate synthesis accompanies decidual responses in the endometrium and may promote trophoblastic invasion after penetration of the luminal epithelium. It would be of interest to learn whether the mucopolysaccharidelike substance in the intercellular spaces of the PDZ contains hyaluronate (mouse: Finn and Hinchliffe, 1965; rat: Enders and Schlafke, 1979; Parr et al., 1986).

The synthesis of specific uterine proteins following induction of the decidual reaction has been reported by many investigators (Yoshinaga, 1972, 1974; Denari et al., 1976; Denari and Rosner, 1978; Umapathysivam and Jones, 1978; Bell et al., 1977, 1980; MacDonald et al., 1983; Joshi et al., 1981; Leavitt et al., 1985). Furthermore, the mesometrial and antimesometrial regions of the endometrium show different capacities for protein synthesis (Denari et al., 1976). The functions of specific decidual cell proteins and the reasons for localized differences in the level of synthesis remain to be investigated.

In several species the decidual tissue secretes a prolactinlike substance that possesses luteotropic properties and appears to govern the physiological response of luteal cells to estradiol (Basuray et al., 1983). One investigation indicates that in the rat, decidual prolactin combined with LH from the pituitary acts to sustain ovarian progesterone production from day

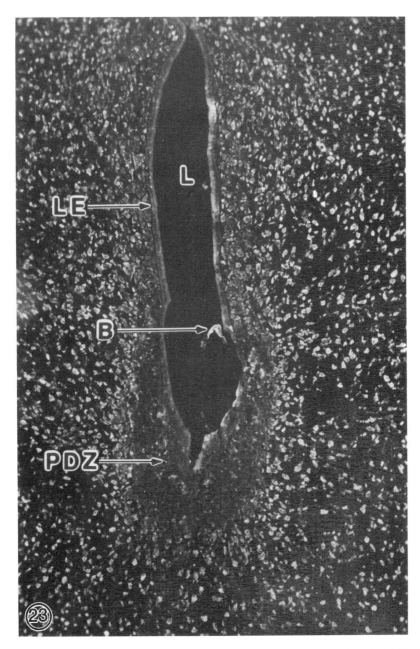

Figure 23. This micrograph shows a rat implantation site on day 6 of pregnancy. Note the labeling of PG synthase in the ectoplacental cone of the blastocyst (B) and in trophoblast cells adherent to the luminal epithelium at the lower right of the blastocyst. The luminal epithelium (LE) and the PDZ exhibit weak or no labeling, but cells in the secondary decidual zone show bright labeling. L, Uterine lumen. ×135.

8 until midpregnancy (Jayatilak *et al.*, 1984). Decidual cells also contain desmin and vimentin (Glasser and Julian, 1986; Glasser *et al.*, 1987), catechol-O-methyltransferase (Inoue *et al.*, 1980), ornithine decarboxylase (Collawn *et al.*, 1981), and alkaline phosphatase (Velardo *et al.*, 1953; Finn and Hinchliffe, 1964), but the significance of these substances is unknown. In some cases, they have been used as markers to distinguish decidual cells from other stromal cells.

3.7. Functions of Decidual Tissue

Although the morphological and endocrinological aspects of decidualization have been extensively studied, the complete significance of the decidual tissue is still a matter for speculation. Many distinct hypotheses have been proposed in regard to its function. It may help nourish the developing embryo (Krehbiel, 1937), protect maternal tissues from excessive trophoblastic invasion (Kirby and Cowell, 1968), isolate each embryo to ensure the development of separate vascular systems and protect each from possible deleterious effects related to the failure of adjacent implantation sites (De Feo, 1967), protect the embryo against immunologic rejection by the mother (Kirby *et al.*, 1966; Beer and Billingham, 1974), act as a barrier between embryonic and maternal circulations (PDZ: Rogers *et al.*, 1983; Parr and Parr, 1986; Tung *et al.*, 1986), provide structural support for the embryo (Welsh and Enders, 1985), secrete a prolactinlike hormone (Kubota *et al.*, 1981; Basuray and Gibori, 1980; Jayatilak *et al.*, 1984), and play a role in the immunology of pregnancy (Bernard and Rachman, 1980; Rachman *et al.*, 1981; Lala *et al.*, 1986; Clark *et al.*, 1986; Bulmer *et al.*, 1987). It is not unreasonable to assume that the decidual tissue, because of its structural complexity, dynamic nature, regional variation, and diverse cell types, may play more than one functional role in the gravid uterus and that each decidual zone may function in a different way. The morphological and (probable) functional heterogeneity of decidual tissues and associated cells emphasizes the importance of using individual, identifiable cell populations in further studies of the biochemical events occurring during pregnancy (Glasser and McCormack, 1981).

4. Epithelial Cell Loss

In common laboratory rodents such as the rat, mouse, and hamster, implantation of the embryo involves the penetration and removal of the adjacent uterine epithelium. Schlafke and Enders (1975) have referred to this process as displacement penetration. The trophoblast sends out cytoplasmic processes that extend to the basal lamina between epithelial cells; the processes continue to grow parallel to this layer and then completely surround and engulf the epithelial cells. The epithelium is thereby removed, and the trophoblast comes to lie next to the epithelial basal lamina. Although it is generally accepted that the epithelial cells die and are phagocytosed by the trophoblast, the cause and mode of cell death are less clear.

4.1. The Uterine Epithelium Adjacent to the Trophoblast

Ultrastructural studies of rat implantation sites have indicated that uterine epithelial cells appear intact and exhibit normal morphological features at the time they are phagocytosed by the trophoblast (Enders and Schlafke, 1967, 1969; Tachi *et al.*, 1970). In hamsters, most epithelial cells in the implantation chamber have normal ultrastructural features until trophoblastic invasion into the epithelium, at which time cell death becomes apparent by the disruption of organelles in a few cells (Parkening, 1976). Poelmann (1975) has reported that in mice the epithelial cells at the time of trophoblast invasion show few signs of degeneration. This is in good agreement with earlier studies in mice (Reinius, 1967; Smith and Wilson, 1974). The common conclusion of these investigators was that the epithelial cells and their organelles were surprisingly well preserved when the trophoblastic cells invaded the epithelial layer. On the other hand, El-Shershaby and Hinchliffe (1975) have described mouse uterine epithelial cells as having numerous large autophagosomes and extensive degeneration of other cellular organelles, an observation that suggests that cell death may be an autolytic process involving autophagosomes and lysosomal enzymes before phagocytosis by trophoblast.

The problem of cell death in general has been studied by Kerr and Wyllie and their associates (Kerr *et al.*, 1972, 1984; Wyllie *et al.*, 1980; Wyllie, 1981), who suggest that cell death occurs by one of two fundamentally different processes, necrosis or apoptosis, and that each mode of cell death presents disparate features. Apoptosis is characterized by shrinkage, blebbing, or fragmentation of the cells, condensation of chromatin and fragmentation of nuclei, and preservation of intact cytoplasmic organelles. Dying cells or their fragments are phagocytosed and degraded by adjacent cells without the accompaniment of cellular inflammation. In addition to these morphological features, the process appears to require energy, macromolecular synthesis involving new gene expression, and the activation of endogenous deoxyribonuclease activity. Inhibitors of RNA and protein synthesis block this form of cell death. In contrast, cell death by necrosis is characterized by surface membrane damage, osmotic swelling of cells and mitochondria, and disintegration of organelles. A cellular inflammatory response occurs in this process. Cells or cell fragments are ingested and degraded by cells of the mononuclear phagocytic system. Necrosis results from disturbances in environmental conditions, such as anoxia, that are inconsistent with continued viability of cells.

There are several lines of evidence suggesting that the death of uterine epithelial cells adjacent to blastocysts at implantation sites is a result of apoptosis or programmed cell death. In an early study in the mouse, Finn and Bredl (1973) suggested that the breakdown of the epithelium was controlled by genetic information that was expressed during implantation. This view has been supported by a study that shows that actinomycin D inhibits the degeneration of the uterine epithelium around the blastocyst and delays decidualization. A recent ultrastructural study of mouse and rat embryo implantation sites has demonstrated that luminal epithelial cells surrounding the blastocysts exhibit the morphological characteristics of apoptosis rather than necrosis: loss of polarity, surface blebbing, shrinkage and fragmentation, intact surface membranes, normal or increased cytoplasmic density, normal cytoplasmic organelles, condensation of chromatin, indentation of the nuclear envelope, and nuclear fragmentation (Parr *et al.*, 1987a). None of the cellular features of necrosis were apparent, suggesting that epithelial cells undergo apoptosis followed by phagocytosis by trophoblast cells (Figs. 24–29).

These morphological studies confirm the suggestion of Smith and Wilson (1974) that cell shrinkage, cytoplasmic condensation, and nuclear indentations in mouse epithelial cells are similar to the features described by Kerr *et al.* (1972), but they do not support some of the observations of El-Shershaby and Hinchliffe (1975) in the mouse. For example, the latter authors have described the presence of numerous swollen organelles and other degenerative changes in the luminal epithelium, whereas Parr *et al.* (1987a) reported that cytoplasmic organelles appeared normal in the epithelium at the time of phagocytosis by trophoblast. It is possible that differences in fixation could account for the disparity in these observations. El-Shershaby and Hinchliffe (1975) also have emphasized the occurrence and increase in size of autophagosomes in the epithelium, which they interpret as signs of autolysis. A few small lysosomelike organelles containing recognizable cell organelles have been observed in mouse and rat epithelial cells (Parr *et al.*, 1987a), but it should be emphasized that autophagosomes are a normal component of many kinds of viable cells. Autophagy is a known cellular mechanism for the degradation of cellular components and redirection of physiological function (Smith and Farquhar, 1966), but its role in cell death is doubtful (Wyllie *et al.*, 1980). The amount of epithelial cell material in trophoblastic heterophagosomes far exceeds that in epithelial cell autophagosomes, and thus, the majority of the digestion of epithelial cells appears to take place in the trophoblast (Parr *et al.*, 1987a). Finally, Parr *et al.* (1987a) have confirmed the description of El-Shershaby and Hinchliffe (1975) regarding loss of epithelial cell polarity, rounding of epithelial cells, peripheral chromatin condensation, and fragmentation of some cells and nuclei. These signs of apoptosis were previously interpreted as indications of cell degeneration (El-Shershaby and Hinchliffe, 1975).

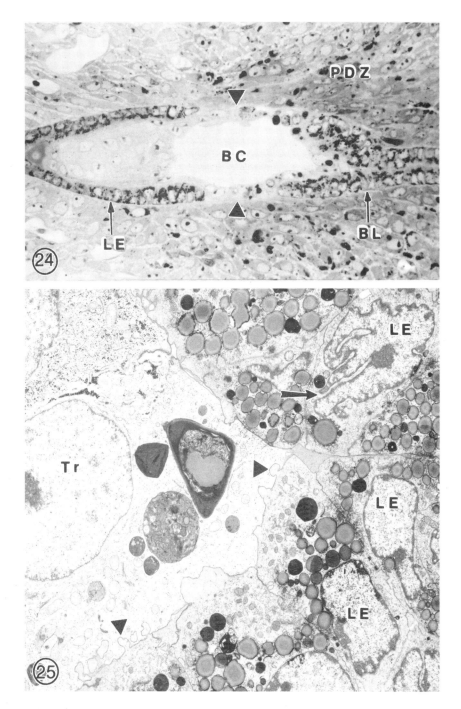

Figure 24. This light micrograph shows a transverse section of a mouse uterus at an implantation site at 8:00 p.m. on day 5 of pregnancy. The embryonic pole of cells is to the left of the blastocyst cavity (BC), while the mural and abembryonic trophoblast cells surround the remainder of the cavity. The uterine luminal epithelium (LE) adjacent to the embryonic pole of the blastocyst retains its polarity, but adjacent to the abembryonic pole the cells are rounded and stratified. Further to the right the luminal epithelium at the antimesometrial side of the uterus again shows normal polarity. At two sites (arrowheads) the epithelial layer is interrupted by the trophoblast, which has invaded to reach the basal lamina (BL). PDZ, Primary decidual zone. ×420.

Figure 25. Trophoblast cells (Tr) in contact with uterine epithelial cells (LE) at the abembryonic pole of a mouse

The proposal that epithelial cell death involves autolysis (El-Shershaby and Hinchliffe, 1975) prompted considerable interest in the possible role of lysosomal enzymes in this process. Several studies reported changes in the activities of lysosomal enzymes in epithelial cells during implantation, but the significance of these changes is uncertain. Biochemical or histochemical determinations of lysosomal enzyme activities at implantation sites show a decrease in cathepsin D in the rat (Moulton, 1974; Moulton et al., 1978), β-glucuronidase in the rat (Roy et al., 1983), and leucylnaphthylamidase in the hamster (Sengupta et al., 1981) and mouse (Paria et al., 1981). On the other hand, acid phosphatase activity has been shown to increase (Sengupta et al., 1979) or remained unchanged (Paria et al., 1981) in the rat and mouse. Acid phosphatase and aryl sulfatase B appear to increase at rat implantation sites, but only 48 hr after the blastocysts make contact with the uterine epithelium (Moulton et al., 1978). It is possible that epithelial cell lysosomal enzymes may participate in the degradation of epithelial cell fragments within trophoblastic heterophagosomes. A possible role for these enzymes in the synthetic or degradative processes required for decidual cell differentiation has also been discussed (Moulton and Elangovan, 1981).

From the evidence, it seems reasonable to conclude that apoptosis, rather than autolysis, is the mode of uterine epithelial cell death in the implantation chamber. Although the causes of cell death remain unknown, the most likely appear to be stimuli coming from either the adjacent trophoblast or the decidual cells or both.

4.3. Effects of Trophoblast on Uterine Epithelium

Trophoblastic cells adhere to the apical surfaces of epithelial cells and could exert a direct cytotoxic effect leading to apoptosis. The killing of target cells by cytotoxic T cells, natural killer cells, and K cells requires adhesion of the lymphocytes to the target cells (Cerottini and Brunner, 1974), and all three kinds of lymphocytotoxicity result in apoptotic death of target cells (Don et al., 1977; Matter, 1979; Carpen et al., 1982; Bishop and Whiting, 1983; Stacey et al., 1985). Target cell killing by K lymphocytes may involve a secretory product, for it has been demonstrated that the Golgi apparatus of the lymphocyte is oriented toward the target cell during killing, and cytotoxic activity can be detected in the medium (Carpen et al., 1982). The cytotoxicity of natural killer and cytotoxic T cells involves cellular contact and the exocytosis of granule contents from the effector cells. The granules contain a protein called perforin, which can be activated by calcium to polymerize on the target cell membrane, forming transmembrane pores that are thought to be involved in target cell death (Podack, 1985; Young and Cohn, 1986).

In the implantation sites of rats and mice, Parr et al. (1987a) have reported occasional trophoblastic Golgi cisternae and associated vesicles near the apposed trophoblast and epithelial cell membranes. The content of the Golgi vesicles had the same staining properties as an amorphous material that was present in the intercellular space. Schlafke and Enders (1975) have described similar morphological features in ferret implantation sites and suggest that the intercellular material is probably secreted by the trophoblast. It has previously been suggested that trophoblast does not exert a direct cytotoxic effect on epithelial cells because epithelial cell membranes, cytoplasm, and organelles remain intact (Enders and Schlafke, 1969). However, recent studies of lymphocytotoxicity have demonstrated that direct cellular cytotoxicity can

---

embryo. The epithelial layer here is stratified, and the cells contain numerous lipid droplets and more darkly stained dense bodies. Their nuclei are more irregular in shape (arrow) and exhibit more peripheral heterochromatin than on the morning of day 5. Projections from the apical surface of epithelial cells indent the surface of trophoblast cells (arrowheads). The latter contain euchromatic nuclei, pale-staining cytoplasm, and large dense bodies with a heterogeneous content. ×4900.

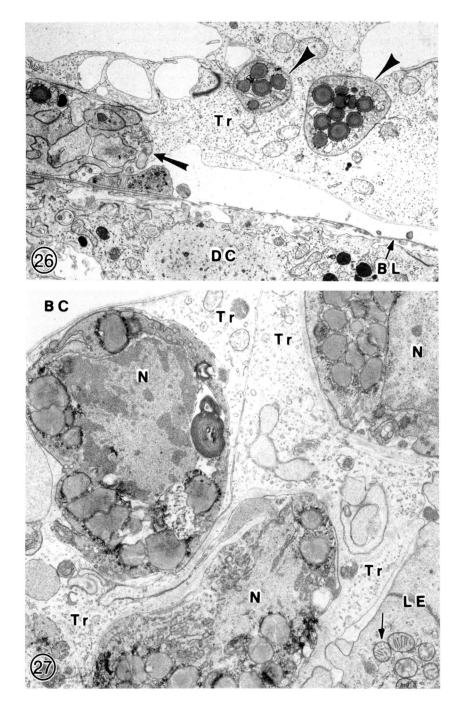

Figure 26. This figure shows a mouse trophoblast cell (Tr) near the epithelial basal lamina (BL) and several decidual cells (DC). At the left side of the micrograph are several small membrane-bound structures containing typical epithelial cell cytoplasm (arrow). The structures may be fragments of epithelial cells. The trophoblast cell contains two large inclusions (arrowheads) that exhibit numerous darkly stained lipid droplets similar to those of epithelial cells. These may be heterophagosomes. ×7300.

Figure 27. Shown are mouse trophoblast cells (Tr) that contain partly or completely phagocytosed uterine epithelial cells the nuclei (N) of which can still be recognized. Note the luminal epithelial cells (LE) that have not yet been phagocytosed; they exhibit apical projections and normal mitochondria. ×10,000.

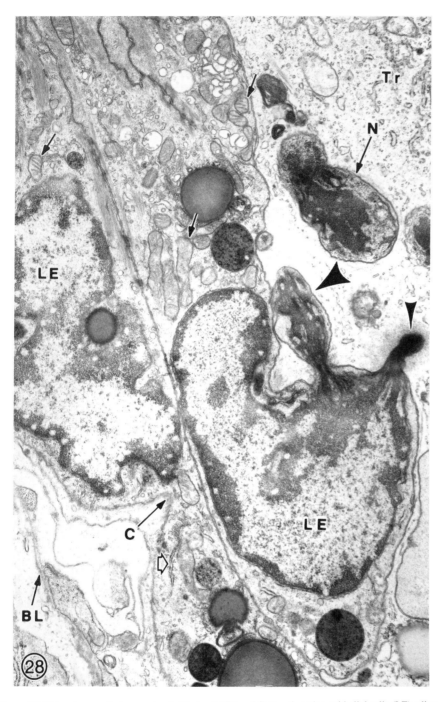

Figure 28. This micrograph shows a trophoblast cell (Tr) and flattened uterine epithelial cells (LE) adjacent to the epithelial basal lamina (BL) in a rat implantation site. The epithelial cell nucleus on the right is fragmenting (arrowheads), and there is a piece of nucleus (N) in the adjacent trophoblast cytoplasm. The epithelial cell on the left shows a narrow constriction (C) below its nucleus. The nucleus is irregular in shape and shows margination of chromatin. Mitochondria in both epithelial cells (arrows) are normal in appearance, as are the rough endoplasmic reticulum cisternae (open arrow). ×13,000.

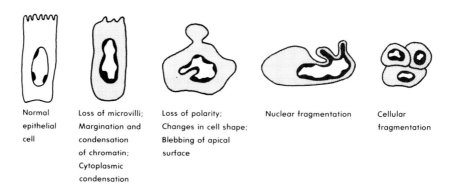

Figure 29. This diagram summarizes the morphological changes characterizing apoptosis in mouse and rat uterine epithelial cells adjacent to trophoblast cells at implantation.

cause apoptotic cell death without any disintegration of cell membranes, organelles, or cytoplasm.

Various investigators have noted the association of proteolytic enzymes with implanting embryos (Denker, 1977, 1980; Kirchner *et al.*, 1971; Pinsker *et al.*, 1974), but none of these studies has characterized the enzyme or demonstrated its involvement in the process of implantation.

4.4. *Effects of Decidual Tissue on Uterine Epithelium*

Some aspect of the decidual reaction may also trigger death of the epithelial cells within the implantation chamber. Epithelial cells might die because they are isolated from their supply of oxygen and nutrients by the closely packed cells of the primary decidual zone (Smith and Wilson, 1974) or because of pH changes in the implantation site (Boving, 1962). Finn and Hinchliffe (1964) and Finn (1977) have argued that the decidual tissue rather than the trophoblast is a likely cause of epithelial cell death because epithelial cells die within an oil-induced deciduoma in the absence of trophoblast. Craig and Jollie (1981) have studied the ultrastructure of rat uterine epithelial cells in an oil-induced deciduoma, but it is not clear from their description whether cell death occurred by apoptosis or necrosis. Differences between normal and oil-induced epithelial cell death have been observed (Hinchliffe and El-Shershaby, 1975), and it appears that oil, but not blastocysts, causes substantial damage to rat uterine epithelial cells (Lundkvist and Nilsson, 1982). Hence, the significance of epithelial cell degeneration in the oil-induced deciduoma remains unclear. At present, the relative importance of trophoblast and decidual cells in causing epithelial cell death in the rodent implantation chamber remains to be elucidated.

ACKNOWLEDGMENTS. Limitations of space prevent us from providing more than a sampling of the extensive recent literature in our bibliography. We thank and apologize to those investigators who have not been cited but who have nonetheless contributed to the development of ideas presented here. Parts of the original research reported in this chapter were supported by grant HD 17480 from the National Institute of Child Health and Human Development. The excellent technical assistance of Kimberly Munaretto, Shonah Hunter, and Shereen Baig and excellent secretarial assistance of Candida Trueblood are gratefully acknowledged. We also thank Matthew Parr (Yale University) for carefully reading and editing the manuscript.

Abrahamsohn, P. A., 1983, Ultrastructural study of the mouse antimesometrial decidua, *Anat. Embryol.* **166**:263–274.

Abrahamsohn, P. A., Lundkvist, O., and Nilsson, O., 1983, Ultrastructure of the endometrial blood vessels during implantation of the rat blastocyst, *Cell Tissue Res.* **229**:269–280.

Anderson, T. L., and Hoffman, L. H., 1984, Alterations in epithelial glycocalyx of rabbit uteri during early pseudopregnancy and pregnancy, and following ovariectomy, *Am. J. Anat.* **171**:321–334.

Anderson, T. L., Olson, G. E., and Hoffman, L. H., 1986, Stage-specific alterations in the apical membrane glycoproteins of endometrial epithelial cells related to implantation in rabbits, *Biol. Reprod.* **34**:701–720.

Anteby, S. O., Bauminger, S., Zor, U., and Lindner, H. R., 1975, Prostaglandin synthesis in decidual tissue of the rat, *Prostaglandins* **10**:991–999.

Atienza-Samols, S. B., Pine, P. P., and Sherman, M. I., 1980, Effects of tunicamycin upon glycoprotein synthesis and development of early mouse embryos, *Dev. Biol.* **79**:19–32.

Basuray, R., and Gibori, G., 1980, Luteotropic action of the decidual tissue of the pregnant rat, *Biol. Reprod.* **23**:507–512.

Basuray, R., Jaffee, R. C., and Gibori, G., 1983, Role of decidual luteotropin and prolactin in the control of luteal cell receptors for estradiol, *Biol. Reprod.* **28**:551–556.

Bazer, F. W., and First, N. L., 1983, Pregnancy and parturition, *J. Anim. Sci.* **57**(Suppl. 2):425–460.

Beer, A. E., and Billingham, R. E., 1974, Host responses to intrauterine tissue, cellular and fetal allografts, *J. Reprod. Fertil. (Suppl.)* **21**:59–88.

Bekairi, A. M., Sanders, R. B., and Yochim, J. M., 1984, Uterine adenylate cyclase activity during the estrous cycle and early progestation in the rat: Responses to fluoride activation and decidual induction, *Biol. Reprod.* **31**:742–751.

Bell, B. C., 1983, Decidualization: Regional differentiation and associated function, *Oxford Rev. Reprod. Biol.* **5**:220–271.

Bell, S. C., and Searle, R. F., 1981, Differentiation of decidual cells in mouse endometrial cell cultures, *J. Reprod. Fertil.* **61**:425–433.

Bell, S. C., Reynolds, S., and Heald, P. J., 1977, Uterine protein synthesis during the early stages of pregnancy in the rat, *J. Reprod. Fertil.* **49**:177–181.

Bell, S. C., Hamer, J., and Heald, P. J., 1980, Induced protein and deciduoma formation in rat uterus, *Biol. Reprod.* **23**:935–940.

Bernard, O., and Rachman, F., 1980, Immunological aspects of the decidual cell reaction, in: *Progress in Reproductive Biology*, Volume 7 (F. Leroy, C. A. Finn, A. Psychoyos, and P. O. Hubinont, eds.), S. Karger, Basel, pp. 135–142.

Bernard, O., Scheid, M., Ripoche, M. A., and Bennett, D., 1978, Immunological studies of mouse decidual cells. I. Membrane markers of decidual cells in the days after implantation, *J. Exp. Med.* **148**:580–591.

Biggers, J. D., Leonov, B. V., Baskar, J. F., and Fried, J., 1978, Inhibition of hatching of mouse blastocysts *in vitro* by prostaglandin antagonists, *Biol. Reprod.* **19**:519–533.

Biggers, J. D., Baskar, J. F., and Torchianan, D. F., 1981, Reduction of fertility of mice by the intrauterine injection of prostaglandin antagonists, *J. Reprod. Fertil.* **63**:365–372.

Bill, A., Tornquist, P., and Alm, A., 1980, Permeability of the intraocular blood vessels, *Trans. Ophthalmol. Soc. U.K.* **100**:332–336.

Bishop, C. J., and Whiting, V. A., 1983, The role of natural killer cells in the intravascular death of intravenously injected murine tumour cells, *Br. J. Cancer* **48**:441–444.

Boshier, D. P., 1970, The Pontamine Blue reaction in pregnant sheep uteri, *J. Reprod. Fertil.* **22**:595–596.

Boshier, D. P., 1976, Effects of the rat blastocyst on neutral lipids and nonspecific esterases in the uterine luminal epithelium at the implantation area, *J. Reprod. Fertil.* **46**:245–247.

Boshier, D. P., Fairclough, R. J., and Holloway, H., 1987, Assessment of sheep blastocyst effects on neutral lipids in the uterine caruncular epithelium, *J. Reprod. Fertil.* **79**:569–573.

Boving, B. G., 1962, Anatomical analysis of rabbit trophoblast invasion, *Contrib. Embryol.* **37**:33–54.

Bulmer, J. N., and Johnson, P. M., 1986, The T-lymphocyte population in first-trimester human decidua does not express the interleukin-2 receptor, *Immunology* **58**:685–687.

Bulmer, D., Peel, S., and Stewart, I., 1987, The metrial gland, *Cell Differ.* **20**:77–86.

Buxton, L. E., and Murdoch, N. R., 1982, Lectins, calcium ionophore A 23187, and peanut oil as deciduogenic agents in the uterus of pseudopregnant mice: Effects of tranylcypromine, indomethacin, iproniazid, and propanol, *Aust. J. Biol. Sci.* **35**:63–72.

Cao, Z.-D., Jones, M. A., and Harper, M. J. K., 1984, Prostaglandin translocation from the lumen of the rabbit uterus *in vitro* in relation to the day of pregnancy or pseudopregnancy, *Biol. Reprod.* **31**:505–519.

Carollo, J. R., and Weitlauf, H. M., 1981, Regional changes in the binding of (^{3}H)concanavalin A to mouse blastocysts at implantation: An autoradiographic study, *J. Exp. Zool.* **218**:247–252.

Carpen, O., Virtanen, I., and Saksela, E., 1982, Ultrastructure of human natural killer cells: Nature of the cytolytic contacts in relation to cellular secretion, *J. Immunol.* **128**:2691–2697.

Carson, D. C., Dutt, A., and Tang, J. P., 1987, Glycoconjugate synthesis during early pregnancy: Hyaluronate synthesis and function, *Dev. Biol.* **120**:228–235.

Castracane, V. D., Saksena, S. K., and Shaikh, A. A., 1974, Effect of IUDs, prostaglandins, and indomethacin on decidual cell reaction in the rat, *Prostaglandins* **6**:397–400.

Cecil, H. C., Hannum, J. A., Jr., and Bitman, J., 1966, Quantitation characterization of uterine vascular permeability changes with estrogen, *Am. J. Physiol.* **211**:1099–1102.

Cerottini, J.-C., and Brunner, K. T., 1974, Cell-mediated cytotoxicity, allograft rejection, and tumor immunity, *Adv. Immunol.* **18**:67–87.

Chávez, D. J., 1984, Cellular aspects of implantation, in: *Ultrastructure of Reproduction* (J. Van Blerkom and P. M. Motta, eds.), Martinus Nijhoff, The Hague, Boston, pp. 247–259.

Chávez, D. J., 1986, Cell surface of mouse blastocysts at the trophectoderm–uterine interface during the adhesive stage of implantation, *Am. J. Anat.* **176**:153–158.

Chávez, D. J., and Anderson, T. L., 1985, The glycocalyx of the mouse uterine luminal epithelium during estrus, early pregnancy, the periimplantation period, and delayed implantation. I. Acquisition of *Ricinus communis* 1 binding sites during pregnancy, *Biol. Reprod.* **32**:1135–1142.

Chávez, D. J., and Enders, A. C., 1981, Temporal changes in lectin binding of peri-implantation mouse blastocysts, *Develop. Biol.* **87**:267–276.

Chávez, D. J., and Enders, A. C., 1982, Lectin binding of mouse blastocysts: Appearance of *Dolichos bifloris* binding sites on the trophoblast during delayed implantation and their subsequent disappearance during implantation, *Biol. Reprod.* **26**:545–552.

Chávez, D. J., Enders, A. C., and Schlafke, S., 1984, Trophectoderm cell subpopulations in the perimplantation mouse blastocyst, *J. Exp. Zool.* **231**:267–271.

Clark, D. A., Brierley, J., Slapsys, R., Daya, S., Damji, N., Chaput, A., and Rosenthal, K., 1986, Trophoblast-dependent and trophoblast independent suppressor cells of maternal origin in murine and human decidua, in: *Reproductive Immunology* (D. A. Clark and B. A. Croy, eds.), Elsevier, New York, pp. 219–226.

Collawn, S. S., Rankin, J. C., Ledford, B. E., and Baggett, B., 1981, Ornithine decarboxylase activity in the artificially stimulated decidual cell reaction in the mouse uterus, *Biol. Reprod.* **24**:528–533.

Cox, C., Cheng, H. C., and Dey, S. K., 1982, Phospholipase A_2 activity in the rat uterus during early pregnancy, *Prostaglandins Leukotrienes Med.* **8**:375–381.

Craggs, R. I., and Peel, S., 1983, Immunological characterization of surface receptors on rat metrial gland cells, *J. Reprod. Immunol.* **5**:27–37.

Craig, S. S., and Jollie, W. P., 1981, Epithelial ultrastructure during decidualization in rats, *Anat. Embryol.* **163**:215–222.

Damsky, C. H., 1984, Integral membrane glycoproteins in cell–cell and cell–substratum adhesion, in: *The Biology of Glycoproteins* (R. J. Ivatt, eds.), Plenum Press, New York, pp. 1–64.

Daniel, S. A. J., and Kennedy, T. G., 1987, Prostaglandin E_2 enhances uterine stromal cell alkaline phosphatase activity *in vitro, Prostaglandins* **33**:241–252.

De Feo, V. J., 1967, Decidualization, in: *Cellular Biology of the Uterus* (R. M. Wynn, ed.), Appleton-Century-Crofts, New York, 191–290.

Denari, J. H., and Rosner, J. M., 1978, Studies on biochemical characteristics of early decidual protein, *Int. J. Fertil.* **23**:123–127.

Denari, J. H., Germino, N. I., and Rosner, J. N., 1976, Early synthesis of uterine proteins after a decidual stimulus in the pseudopregnant rat, *Biol. Reprod.* **15**:1–8.

Denker, H.-W., 1977, Implantation: The role of proteinases and blockage of implantation by proteinase inhibitors, *Adv. Anat. Embryol. Cell Biol.* **53**(5):1–123.

Denker, H.-W., 1980, Role of proteinases in implantation, *Prog. Reprod. Biol.* **7**:28–42.

Dey, S. K., and Hubbard, C. J., 1981, Role of histamine and cyclic nucleotides in implantation in the rabbit, *Cell Tissue Res.* **220**:549–554.

Dey, S. K., and Johnson, D. C., 1980, Reevaluation of histamine in implantation, in: *The Endometrium* (F. A. Kimball, ed.), Spectrum, New York, pp. 269–282.

Dey, S. K., Chien, S. M., Cox, C. L., and Crist, R. D., 1980, Prostaglandin synthesis in the rabbit blastocyst, *Prostaglandins* **19**:449–453.

Doktorcik, P. E., and Kennedy, T. G., 1986, 6-Keto-prostaglandin-E$_1$ and the decidual cell reaction in rats, *Prostaglandins* **32**:679–690.

Don, M. M., Abett, G., Bishop, C. J., Bundeson, P. G., Donald, K. J., Searle, J., and Kerr, J. F. R., 1977, Death of cells by apoptosis following attachment of specifically allergised lymphocytes *in vitro, Aust. J. Exp. Biol. Med. Sci.* **55**:407–417.

Dutt, A., Tang, J.-P., Welply, J. K., and Carson, D. D., 1986, Regulation of N-linked glycoprotein asembly in uteri by steroid hormones, *Endocrinology* **118**:661–673.

Dutt, A., Tang, J.-P., and Carson, D. D., 1987, Lactosaminoglycans are involved in uterine epithelial cell adhesion *in vitro, Dev. Biol.* **119**:27–37.

Edelman, G. M., 1983, Cell adhesion molecules, *Science* **219**:450–457.

El-Banna, A. A., 1980, The degenerative effect on rabbit implantation sites by indomethacin. I. Timing of indomethacin action, possible effect on uterine proteins and the effect of replacement doses of PGF$_{2\alpha}$, *Prostaglandins* **20**:587–599.

El-Shershaby, A. M., and Hinchliffe, J. R., 1975, Epithelial autolysis during implantation of the mouse blastocyst: An ultrastructural study, *J. Embryol. Exp. Morphol.* **33**:1067–1080.

Enders, A. C., 1972, Mechanisms of implantation of the blastocyst, in: *Biology of Reproduction. Basic and Clinical Studies* III (J. T. Velardo and B. A. Kasprow, eds.), Pan American Congress of Anatomy, New Orleans, pp. 313–334.

Enders, A. C., and Nelson, D. M., 1973, Pinocytotic activity of the uterus of the rat, *Am. J. Anat.* **138**:277–300.

Enders, A. C., and Schlafke, S., 1967, A morphological analysis of the early implantation stages in the rat, *Am. J. Anat.* **120**:185–226.

Enders, A. C., and Schlafke, S., 1969, Cytological aspects of trophoblast–uterine interaction in early implantation, *Am. J. Anat.* **125**:1–30.

Enders, A. C., and Schlafke, S., 1972, Implantation in the ferret: Epithelial penetration, *Am. J. Anat.* **133**:291–316.

Enders, A. C., and Schlafke, S., 1974, Surface coats of the mouse blastocyst and uterus during the preimplantation period, *Anat. Rec.* **180**:31–46.

Enders, A. C., and Schlafke, S., 1979, Comparative aspects of blastocyst–endometrial interactions at implantation, in: *Maternal Recognition of Pregnancy, Ciba Foundation Series 64 (New Series)*, Excepta Medica, Amsterdam, pp. 3–32.

Enders, A. C., and Schlafke, S., 1986, Implantation in nonhuman primates and in the human, in: *Comparative Primate Biology*, Volume 3, *Reproduction and Development*, Alan R. Liss, New York, pp. 291–310.

Enders, A. C., Schlafke, S., and Welsh, A. O., 1980, Trophoblastic and uterine luminal epithelial surfaces at the time of blastocyst adhesion in the rat, *Am. J. Anat.* **159**:59–72.

Enders, A. C., Chávez, D. J., and Schlafke, S., 1981, Comparison of implantation *in utero* and *in vitro*, in: *Cellular and Molecular Aspects of Implantation* (S. R. Glasser and D. W. Bullock, eds.), Plenum Press, New York, pp. 365–382.

Enders, A. C., Hendrickx, A. G., and Schlafke, S., 1983, Implantation in the rhesus monkey: Initial penetration of the endometrium, *Am. J. Anat.* **167**:275–298.

Enders, A. C., Welsh, A. O., and Schlafke, S., 1985, Implantation in the rhesus monkey: Endometrial responses, *Am. J. Anat.* **173**:147–169.

Evans, C. A., and Kennedy, T. G., 1978, The importance of prostaglandin synthesis for the initiation of blastocyst implantation in the hamster, *J. Reprod. Fertil.* **54**:255–261.

Fainstat, T., 1963, Extracellular studies of uterus. I. Disappearance of the discrete bundles in endometrial stroma during various reproductive stages in the rat, *Am. J. Anat.* **112**:337–370.

Feyles, V., and Kennedy, T. G., 1987, Inhibitory effect of the intrauterine infusion of phorbol 12-myristate 13-acetate and 1-oleoyl-2-acetylglycerol on the decidual cell reaction in rats, *Biol. Reprod.* **37**:96–104.

Finn, C. A., 1965, Oestrogen and the decidual cell reaction of implantation in mice, *J. Endocrinol.* **32**:223–229.

Finn, C. A., 1977, The implantation reaction, in: *Biology of the Uterus* (R. M. Wynn, ed.), Plenum Press, New York, pp. 245–308.

Finn, C. A., 1980, The endometrium during implantation, in: *The Endometrium*, (F. A. Kimball, ed.), Spectrum, New York, pp. 43–56.

Finn, C. A., and Bredl, J. C. S., 1973, Studies on the development of the implantation reaction in the mouse uterus: Influence of actinomycin D, *J. Reprod. Fertil.* **34**:247–253.

Finn, C. A., and Hinchliffe, J. R., 1964, The reaction of the mouse uterus during implantation and deciduoma formation as demonstrated by changes in the distribution of alkaline phosphatase, *J. Reprod. Fertil.* **8**:331–338.

Finn, C. A., and Hinchliffe, J. R., 1965, Histological and histochemical analysis of the formation of implantation chambers in the mouse uterus, *J. Reprod. Fertil.* **9**:301–309.

Finn, C. A., and Lawn, A. M., 1967, Specialized junctions between decidual cells in the uterus of the pregnant mouse, *J. Ultrastruct. Res.* **20**:321–327.

Finn, C. A., and McLaren, A., 1967, A study of the early stages of implantation in mice, *J. Reprod. Fertil.* **13**:259–267.

Finn, C. A., and Porter, D. G., 1975, *The Uterus,* Publishing Sciences Group, Acton, UK.

Flower, R. J., and Blackwell, G. J., 1976, The importance of phospholipase-A_2 in prostaglandin biosynthesis, *Biochem. Pharmacol.* **25**:285–291.

Gilula, N. B., Reeves, O. R., and Steinback, A., 1972, Metabolic coupling, ionic coupling, and cell contacts, *Nature* **235**:262–265.

Glasser, S. R., 1985, Laboratory models of implantation, in: *Reproductive Toxicology* (R. L. Dixon, ed.), Raven Press, New York, pp. 219–238.

Glasser, S. R., and Bullock, D. W. (eds.), 1981, *Cellular and Molecular Aspects of Implantation,* Plenum Press, New York.

Glasser, S. R., and Julian, J., 1986, Intermediate filament protein as a marker of uterine stromal cell decidualizatioin, *Biol. Reprod.* **35**:463–474.

Glasser, S. R., and McCormack, S. A., 1981, Separated cell types as analytical tools in the study of decidualization and implantation, in: *Cellular and Molecular Aspects of Implantation* (S. R. Glasser and D. W. Bullock, eds.), Plenum Press, New York, pp. 217–239.

Glasser, S. R., Lampelo, S., Munir, M. I., and Julian, J., 1987, Expression of desmin, laminin, and fibronectin during *in situ* differentiation (decidualization) of rat uterine stromal cells, *Differentiation* **35**:132–142.

Goldstein, L. J., and Hayes, C. E., 1979, The lectins: Carbohydrate-containing proteins of plants and animals, *Adv. Carbohyd. Chem. Biochem.* **35**:127–167.

Guillomot, M., Fléchon, J.-E., and Wintenberger-Torres, S., 1981, Conceptus attachment in the ewe: An ultrastructural study, *Placenta* **2**:169–182.

Guillomot, M., Fléchon, J.-E., and Wintenberger-Torres, S., 1982, Cytochemical studies of uterine and trophoblastic surface coats during blastocyst attachment in the ewe, *J. Reprod. Fertil.* **65**:1–8.

Hall, A. K., and Behrman, H. R., 1982, Prostaglandins: Biosynthesis, metabolism, and mechanism of cellular action, in: *Prostaglandins* (J. B. Lee, ed.), Elsevier, New York, pp. 1–38.

Harper, M. J. K., Norris, C. J., and Rajkumar, K., 1983, Prostaglandin release by zygotes and endometria of pregnant rabbits, *Biol. Reprod.* **28**:350–362.

Hedlund, K., and Nilsson, O., 1971, Hormonal requirements for uterine attachment reaction and blastocyst implantation in the mouse, hamster and guinea pig, *J. Reprod. Fertil.* **47**:59–62.

Hewitt, K., Beer, A. E., and Grinnell, F., 1979, Disappearance of anionic sites from the surface of the rat endometrial epithelium at the time of blastocyst implantation, *Biol. Reprod.* **21**:691–707.

Hicks, J. J., and Guzman-Gonzalez, A. M., 1979, Inhibition of implantation by intraluminal administration of concanavalin A in mice, *Contraception* **20**:129–136.

Hoffman, L. H., and Hoos, P. C., 1984, Morphology of vascular leakage at rabbit implantation sites, *Anat. Rec.* **208**:75.

Hoffman, L. H., Strong, G. B., Davenport, G. R., and Frolich, J. C., 1977, Deciduogenic effect of prostaglandins in the pseudopregnant rabbit, *J. Reprod. Fertil.* **50**:231–237.

Hoffman, L. H., DiPietro, D. L., and McKenna, T. J., 1978, Effects of indomethacin on uterine capillary permeability and blastocyst development in rabbits, *Prostaglandins* **15**:823–828.

Hoffman, L. H., Davenport, G. R., and Brash, A. R., 1984, Endometrial prostaglandins and phospholipase activity related to implantation in rabbits: Effects of dexamethasone, *Biol. Reprod.* **30**:544–555.

Holmes, P. V., and Gordashko, B. J., 1980, Evidence of prostaglandin involvement in blastocyst implantation, *J. Embryol. Exp. Morphol.* **55**:109–122.

Hoos, P. C., and Hoffman, L. H., 1980, Temporal aspects of rabbit uterine vascular and decidual responses to blastocyst stimulation, *Biol. Reprod.* **23**:453–459.

Hoos, P. C., and Hoffman, L. H., 1983, Effect of histamine receptor antagonists and indomethacin on implantation in the rabbit, *Biol. Reprod.* **29**:833–840.

Hunt, J. S., Manning, L. S., Mitchell, D., Selanders, J. R., and Wood, G. W., 1985, Localization and characterization of macrophages in murine uterus, *J. Leukocyte Biol.* **38**:255–265.

Huslig, R. L., Fogwell, R. L., and Smith, W. L., 1979, The prostaglandin forming cyclooxygenase of ovine uterus: Relationship to luteal function, *Biol. Reprod.* **21**:589–600.

Hyland, J. H., Manns, J. G., and Humphrey, W. D., 1982, Prostaglandin production by ovine embryos and endometrium *in vitro,* *J. Reprod. Fertil.* **65**:299–304.

Inoue, K., Tice, L. W., and Creveling, C. R., 1980, Immunocytochemical localization of catechol-O-methyltransferase in the pregnant rat uterus, *Endocrinology* **107**:1833–1837.

Irvine, R. F., 1982, How is the level of free arachidonic acid controlled in mammalian cells? *Biochem J.* **204**:3–16.

Jayatilak, R. G., Glaser, L. A., Warshaw, M. L., Herz, Z., Gruber, J. R., and Gibori, G., 1984, Relationship between luteinizing hormone and decidual luteotropin in the maintenance of luteal steroidogenesis, *Biol. Reprod.* **31**:556–564.

Jeffrey, J. J., 1981, Collagen synthesis and degradation in the uterine deciduoma: Regulation of collagenase activity by progesterone, *Coll. Relat. Res.* **1**:257–268.

Jenkinson, E. J., and Searle, R. F., 1977, Cell surface changes on the mouse blastocyst at implantation, *Exp. Cell Res.* **106**:386–390.

Johnston, M. E. A., and Kennedy, T. G., 1984, Estrogen and uterine sensitization for the decidual cell reaction in the rat: Role of prostaglandin E_2 and adenosine $3':5'$-cyclic monophosphate, *Biol. Reprod.* **31**:959–966.

Jollie, W. P., and Bencosme, S. A., 1965, Electron microscopic observations n primary decidua formation in the rat, *Am. J. Anat.* **116**:216–236.

Joshi, S. G., Szarowski, D. H., and Bank, J. F., 1981, Decidua-associated antigens in the baboon, *Biol. Reprod.* **25**:591–598.

Kearns, M., and Lala, P. K., 1983, Life history of decidual cells: A review, *Am. J. Reprod. Immunol.* **3**:78–82.

Kennedy, T. G., 1977, Evidence for a role for prostaglandins in the initiation of blastocyst implantation in the rat, *Biol. Reprod.* **16**:286–291.

Kennedy, T. G., 1979, Prostaglandins and increased endometrial vascular permeability resulting from the application of an artificial stimulus to the uterus of the rat sensitized for the decidual cell reaction, *Biol. Reprod.* **20**:560–566.

Kennedy, T. G., 1980a, Estrogen and uterine sensitization for the decidual cell reaction: Role of prostaglandins, *Biol. Reprod.* **23**:955–962.

Kennedy, T. G., 1980b, Timing of uterine sensitivity for the decidual cell reaction: Role of prostaglandins, *Biol. Reprod.* **22**:519–525.

Kennedy, T. G., 1983a, Embryonic signals and the initiation of blastocyst implantation, *Aust. J. Biol. Sci.* **36**:531–543.

Kennedy, T. G., 1983b, Prostaglandin E_2, adenosine $3':5'$-cyclic monophosphate and changes in endometrial vascular permeability in rat uteri sensitized for the decidual cell reaction, *Biol. Reprod.* **29**:1069–1076.

Kennedy, T. G., 1985, Evidence for the involvement of prostaglandins throughout the decidual cell reaction in the rat, *Biol. Reprod.* **33**:140–16.

Kennedy, T. G., 1986, Intrauterine infusion of prostaglandins and decidualization in rats with uteri differentially sensitized for the decidual cell reaction, *Biol. Reprod.* **34**:327–335.

Kennedy, T. G., and Armstrong, D. T., 1981, The role of prostaglandins in endometrial vascular changes at implantation, in: *Cellular and Molecular Aspects of Implantation* (S. R. Glasser and D. W. Bullock, eds.), Plenum Press, New York, pp. 349–364.

Kennedy, T. G., and Lukash, L. A., 1982, Induction of decidualization in rats by the ultrauterine infusion of prostaglandins, *Biol. Reprod.* **27**:253–260.

Kennedy, T. G., and Zamecnik, J., 1978, The concentration of 6-oxo-$PGF_{1\alpha}$ is markedly elevated at the site of blastocyst implantation in the rat, *Prostaglandins* **16**:599–605.

Kennedy, T. G., Martel, D., and Psychoyos, A., 1983a, Endometrial prostaglandin E_2 binding: Characterization in rats sensitized for the decidual cell reaction and changes during pseudopregnancy, *Biol. Reprod.* **29**:556–564.

Kennedy, T. G., Martel, D., and Psychoyos, A., 1983b, Endometrial prostaglandin E_2 binding during the estrous cycle and its hormonal control in ovariectomized rats, *Biol. Reprod.* **29**:565–571.

Kerr, J. F. R., Wyllie, A. H., and Currie, A. R., 1972, Apoptosis: A basic biological phenomenon with wide-ranging implication in tissue kinetics, *Br. J. Cancer* **26**:239–247.

Kerr, J. F. R., Bishop, C. J., and Searle, J., 1984, Apoptosis, *Recent Adv. Histopathol.* **12**:1–15.

Keys, J. L., King, G. J., and Kennedy, T. G., 1986, Increased uterine vascular permeability at the time of embryonic attachment in the pig, *Biol. Reprod.* **34**:405–411.

Kirby, D. R. S., 1965, The "invasiveness" of the trophoblast, in: *The Early Conceptus, Normal and Abnormal* (W. W. Park, ed.), E. S. Livingstone, Edinburgh, pp. 68–73.

Kirby, D. R. S., and Cowell, T. P., 1968, Trophoblast–host interactions, in: *Epithelial–Mesenchymal Interactions* (R. Fleischmajer and R. E. Billingham, eds.), Williams & Wilkins, Baltimore, pp. 64–77.

Kirby, D. R. S., Billington, W. D., and James, D. A., 1966, Transplantation of eggs to the kidney and uterus of immunised mice, *Transplantation* **4**:713–718.

Kirchner, C., Hirchlauser, C., and Kionke, M., 1971, Protease activity in rabbit uterine secretion 24 hr before implantation, *J. Reprod. Fertil.* **27**:259–260.

Kirkwood, K. J., 1981, Immunoglobulin and complement receptor-bearing cells in cultures of mouse decidual tissue, *J. Reprod. Fertil.* **62**:345–352.

Kleinfeld, R. G., Morrow, H. A., and De Feo, V. J., 1976, Intercellular junctions between decidual cells in the growing deciduoma of the pseudopregnant rat uterus, *Biol. Reprod.* **15**:593–603.

Konwinski, M., Vorbrodt, A., Solter, D., and Koprowski, H., 1977, Ultrastructural study of concanavalin A binding to the surface of preimplantation mouse embryos, *J. Exp. Zool.* **200**:311–324.

Krehbiel, R. H., 1937, Cytological studies of the decidual reaction in the rat during early pregnancy and the production of deciduomata, *Physiol. Zool.* **10**:212–234.

Kubota, T., Kumasaka, T., Yaoi, Y., Suzuki, A., and Saito, M., 1981, Study on immunoreactive prolactin of decidua in early pregnancy, *Acta Endocrinol.* **96**:258–264.

Lacroix, M. C., and Kann, G., 1982, Comparative studies of prostaglandins $F_{2\alpha}$ and E_2 in late cyclic and early pregnant sheep: *In vitro* synthesis by endometrium and conceptus effects of *in vivo* indomethacin treatment on establishment of pregnancy, *Prostaglandins* **23**: 507–526.

Lala, P. K., Parhar, P. S., Kearns, M., Johnson, S., and Scodras, J. M., 1986, Immunologic aspects of the decidual response, in: *Reproductive Immunology* (D. A. Clark and B. A. Croy, eds.), Elsevier, New York, pp. 190–198.

Lampelo, S. A., Ricketts, A. D., and Bullock, D. W., 1985, Purification of rabbit endometrial plasma membranes from receptive and non-receptive uteri, *J. Reprod. Fertil.* **75**:475–484.

Lau, I. F., Saksena, S. K., and Chang, M. C., 1973, Pregnancy blockage by indomethacin, an inhibitor of prostaglandin synthesis: Its reversal by prostaglandins and progesterone in mice, *Prostaglandins* **4**:795–803.

Leavitt, W. W., MacDonald, R. G., and Shwaery, G. T., 1985, Characterization of deciduoma marker proteins in hamster uterus: Detection in decidual cell cultures, *Biol. Reprod.* **32**:631–643.

Lejeune, B., Van Hoeck, J., and Leroy, F., 1981, Transmitter role of the luminal uterine epithelium in the induction of decidualization in rats, *J. Reprod. Fertil.* **61**:235–240.

Leroy, F., Vansande, J., Shetgen, G., and Brasseur, D., 1974, Cyclic AMP and the triggering of the decidual reaction, *J. Reprod. Fertil.* **39**:207–211.

Leroy, F., Finn, C. A., Psychoyos, A., and Hubinont, P. O. (eds.), 1980, *Progress in Reproductive Biology,* Volume 7, S. Karger, Basel.

Lewis, G. S., and Waterman, R. A., 1983, Metabolism of arachidonic acid *in vitro* by porcine blastocysts and endometrium, *Prostaglandins* **25**:871–880.

Lewis, G. S., Thatcher, W. W., Bazer, F. W., and Curl, J. S., 1982, Metabolism of arachidonic acid *in vitro* by bovine blastocysts and endometrium, *Biol. Reprod.* **27**:431–439.

Loewenstein, W. R., 1966, Permeability of membrane junctions, *Ann. N.Y. Acad. Sci.* **137**:441–472.

Lundkvist, O., 1979, Morphometric estimation of stromal edema during delayed implantation in the rat, *Cell Tissue Res.* **199**:339–348.

Lundkvist, O., and Ljungkvist, I., 1977, Morphology of the rat endometrial stroma at the appearance of the pontamine blue reaction during implantation after an experimental delay, *Cell Tissue Res.* **184**:453–466.

Lundkvist, O., and Nilsson, B. O., 1980, Ultrastructural changes of the trophoblast–epithelial complex in mice subjected to implantation blocking treatment with indomethacin, *Biol. Reprod.* **22**:719–726.

Lundkvist, O., and Nilsson, B. O., 1982, Endometrial ultrastructure in the early uterine response to blastocysts and artificial deciduogenic stimuli in rats, *Cell Tissue Res.* **225**:355–364.

MacDonald, R. G., Morency, K. O., and Leavitt, W. W., 1983, Progesterone modulation of specific protein synthesis in the decidualized hamster uterus, *Biol. Reprod.* **28**:753–766.

Magnuson, T., and Stackpole, C. W., 1978, Lectin-mediated agglutination of preimplantation mouse embryos, *Exp. Cell Res.* **116**:466–469.

Marcus, G. J., 1981, Prostaglandin formation by the sheep embryo and endometrium as an indication of maternal recognition of pregnancy, *Biol. Reprod.* **25**:56–64.

Martel, D., Kennedy, T. G., Monier, M. N., and Psychoyos, A., 1985, Failure to detect specific binding sites for prostaglandin $F_{2\alpha}$ in membrane preparations from rat endometrium, *J. Reprod. Fertil.* **75**:265–274.

Martello, E. M. V. G., and Abrahamsohn, P. A., 1986, Collagen distribution in the mouse endometrium during decidualization, *Acta Anat.* **127**:146–150.

Martin, L., Finn, C. A., and Carter, J., 1970, Effects of progesterone and oestradiol-17β on the luminal epithelium of the mouse uterus, *J. Reprod. Fertil.* **21**:461–469.

Martin, L., Hallowes, R. C., Finn, C. A., and West, D. G., 1973, Involvement of the uterine blood vessels in the refractory state of the uterine stroma which follows oestrogen stimulation in progesterone-treated mice, *J. Endocrinol.* **56**:309–314.

Martz, E., 1987, LFA-1 and other accessory molecules functioning in adhesion of T and B lymphocytes, *Hum. Immunol.* **18**:3–37.

Matter, A., 1979, Microcinematographic and electron microscopic analysis of target cell lysis induced by cytotoxic T lymphocytes, *Immunology* **36**:179–190.

Mayer, G., Nilsson, O., and Reinius, S., 1967, Cell membrane changes of uterine epithelium and trophoblast during blastocyst attachment in the rat, *Z. Anat. Entwickl. Gesch.* **126**:43–48.

Miller, M. M., and O'Morchoe, C. C. C., 1982, Decidual cell reaction induced by prostaglandin $F_{2\alpha}$ in the mature oophorectomized rat, *Cell Tissue Res.* **225**:189–200.

Milligan, S. R., and Lytton, F. D. C., 1983, Changes in prostaglandin levels in the sensitized and non-sensitized uterus of the mouse after the intrauterine instillation of oil or saline, *J. Reprod. Fertil.* **67**:373–377.

Milligan, S. R., ar.d Mirembe, F. M., 1985, Intraluminally injected oil induces changes in vascular permeability in the "sensitized" and "nonsensitized" uterus of the mouse, *J. Reprod. Fertil.* **74**:95–104.

Morris, J. E., and Potter, S. W., 1984, A comparison of developmental changes in surface charge in mouse blastocysts and uterine epithelium using DEAE beads and dextran sulfate *in vitro, Dev. Biol.* **103**:190–199.

Morris, J. E., Potter, S. W., Rynd, L. S., and Buckley, P. M., 1983, Adhesion of mouse blastocysts to uterine epithelium in culture: A requirement for mutual surface interactions, *J. Exp. Zool.* **225**:467–479.

Mossman, H. W., 1937, Comparative morphogenesis of the fetal membranes and accessory uterine structures, *Contrib. Embryol. Carnegie Inst.* **26**:129–246.

Moulton, B. C., 1974, Ovum implantation and uterine lysosomal enzyme activity, *Biol. Reprod.* **10**:543–548.

Moulton, B. C., 1984, Epithelial cell function during blastocyst implantation, *J. Biosci.* **6**(Suppl. 2):11–21.

Moulton, B. C., and Elangovan, S., 1981, Lysosomal mechanisms in blastocyst implantation and early decidualization, in: *Cellular and Molecular Aspects of Implantation* (S. R. Glasser and D. W. Bullock, eds.), Plenum Press, New York, pp. 335–344.

Moulton, B. C., and Koenig, B. B., 1986, Hormonal control of phospholipid methylation in uterine epithelial cells during sensitivity to deciduogenic stimuli, *Endocrinology* **118**:244–249.

Moulton, B. C., Koenig, B. B., and Borkan, S. C., 1978, Uterine lysosomal enzyme activity during ovum implantation and early decidualization, *Biol. Reprod.* **19**:167–170.

Moulton, B. C., Schuler, J. A., and Leftwich, J. B., 1987, Effect of a deciduogenic stimulus on arachidonic acid turnover in uterine phospholipids, *Biol. Reprod.* **36**(Suppl. 1): 66.

Murphy, C. R., and Bradbury, S., 1984, Colloidal iron hydroxide staining of surface carbohydrates after glycerol treatment of uterine epithelial cells, *Histochemistry* **80**:45–48.

Murphy, C. R., and Rogers, A. W., 1981, Effects of ovarian hormones on cell membranes in the rat uterus: III. The surface carbohydrates at the apex of the luminal epithelium, *Cell Biophys.* **3**:305–320.

Murphy, C. R., and Swift, J. G., 1983, Relationships between intramembranous particles and surface coat carbohydrates in cells of a compact tissue, *J. Cell Sci.* **64**:123–136.

Murphy, C. R., Swift, J. G., Mukherjee, T. M., and Rogers, A. W., 1979, Effects of ovarian hormones on cell membranes in the rat uterus. I. Freeze–fracture studies of the apical membrane of the luminal epithelium, *Cell Biophys.* **1**:181–193.

Murphy, C. R., Swift, J. G., Mukherjee, T. M., and Rogers, A. W., 1982, Changes in the fine structure of the apical plasma membrane of endometrial epithelial cells during implantation in the rat, *J. Cell. Sci.* **55**:1–12.

Nilsson, B. O., and Njerten, S., 1982, Electrophoretic quantification of the changes in the average net negative surface charge density of mouse blastocysts implanting *in vivo* and *in vitro, Biol. Reprod.* **27**:485–493.

Nilsson, O., 1966a, Estrogen-induced increase of adhesiveness in uterine epithelium of mouse and rat, *Exp. Cell Res.* **43**:239–241.

Nilsson, O., 1966b, Structural differentiation of luminal membrane in rat uterus during normal and experimental implantations, *Z. Anat. Entwickl.* **125**:152–159.

Nilsson, O., 1972, Ultrastructure of the process of secretion in the rat uterine epithelium at preimplantation, *J. Ultrastruct. Res.* **40**:572–580.

Nilsson, O., 1974, Changes of the luminal surface of the rat uterus of blastocyst implantation, *Z. Anat. Entwickl.* **144**:337–342.

Nilsson, O., Lindqvist, I., and Ronquist, G., 1973, Decreased surface charge of mouse blastocysts at implantation, *Exp. Cell Res.* **83**:421–423.

Nilsson, O., Lindqvist, I., and Ronquist, G., 1975, Blastocyst surface charge and implantation in the mouse, *Contraception* **11**:441–450.

Nilsson, O., Naeslund, G., and Curman, B., 1980, Polar differences of delayed and implanting mouse blastocysts in binding of alcian blue and concanavalin A, *J. Exp. Zool.* **214**:177–180.

Nimura, S., and Ishida, K., 1987, Immunohistochemical demonstration of prostaglandin E_2 in preimplantation mouse embryos, *J. Reprod. Fertil.* **80**:505–508.

Öbrink, B., 1986, Epithelial cell adhesion molecules, *Exp. Cell Res.* **163**:1–21.

Oettel, M., Koch, M., Kurischko, A., and Schubert, K., 1979, A direct evidence for the involvement of prostaglandin $F_{2\alpha}$ in the first step of estrone-induced blastocyst implantation in the spayed rat, *Steroids* **33**:1–8.

Ohta, Y., 1985, Histochemical localization of prostaglandin synthetase in the rat endometrium with reference to decidual cell reaction, *Proc. Jpn. Acad. [B]* **61**:467–470.

Orsini, M. W., 1964, Implantation: A comparison of conditions in the pregnant and pseudopregnant hamster, in: *5th International Congress on Animal Reproduction and Artificial Insemination,* Volume 7, Trento, 309–319.

Orsini, M. W., and Donovan, B. T., 1971, Implantation and induced decidualization of the uterus in the guinea pig, as indicated by Pontamine Blue, *Biol. Reprod.* **5**:270–2811.

Orsini, M. W., Wynn, R. M., Harris, J. A., and Bulmash, J. M., 1970, Comparative ultrastructure of the decidua in pregnancy and pseudopregnancy, *Am. J. Obstet. Gynecol.* **106**:14–25.

O'Shea, J. D., Kleinfeld, R. G., and Morrow, H. A., 1983, Ultrastructure of decidualization in the pseudopregnant rat, *Am. J. Anat.* **166**:271–298.

Pakrasi, P. L., and Dey, S. K., 1982, Blastocyst is the source of prostaglandins in the implantation site in the rabbit, *Prostaglandins* **24**:73–77.

Paria, B. C., Sengupta, J., and Manchanda, S. K., 1981, Involvement of lysosomal enzymes in mouse embryo implantation: Effect of the antioestrogen, CI-628 citrate, *J. Endocrinol.* **90**:83–88.

Parkening, T., 1976, An ultrastructural study of implantation in the golden hamster. III. Initial formation and differentiation of decidual cells, *J. Anat.* **122**:485–498.

Parr, E. L., and Kirby, W. M., 1979, An immunoferritin labeling study of H-2 antigens on dissociated epithelial cells, *J. Histochem. Cytochem.* **27**:1327–1336.

Parr, E. L., Tung, H. N., and Parr, M. B., 1987a, Apoptosis as the mode of uterine epithelial cell death embryo implantation in mice and rats, *Biol. Reprod.* **36**:211–225.

Parr, E. L., Parr, M. B., and Young, J. D.-E., 1987b, Localization of a pore-forming protein (perforin) in granulated metrial gland cells, *Biol. Reprod.* **37**:1327–1335.

Parr, M. B., 1980, Endocytosis in the uterine epithelium during early pregnancy, *Prog. Reprod. Biol.* **7**:81–91.

Parr, M. B., 1983, Relationship of uterine closure to ovarian hormones and endocytosis in the rat, *J. Reprod. Fertil.* **68**:185–188.

Parr, M. B., and Parr, E. L., 1974, Uterine luminal epithelium: Protrusions mediate endocytosis not apocrine secretion in the rat, *Biol. Reprod.* **11**:220–233.

Parr, M. B., and Parr, E. L., 1977, Endocytosis in the uterine epithelium of the mouse, *J. Reprod. Fertil.* **50**:151–153.

Parr, M. B., and Parr, E. L., 1986, Permeability of the primary decidual zone in the rat uterus: Studies using fluorescein-labeled proteins and dextrans, *Biol. Reprod.* **34**:393–403.

Parr, M. B., Tung, H. N., and Parr, E. L., 1986, The ultrastructure of the rat primary decidual zone, *Am. J. Anat.* **176**:423–436.

Parr, M. B., Parr, E. L., Munaretto, K., Clark, M. R., and Dey, S. K., 1988, Immunohistochemical localization of prostaglandin synthase in the rat uterus and embryo during the peri-implantation period, *Biol. Reprod.* **38**:333–343.

Phillips, C. A., and Poyser, N. L., 1981, Studies on the involvement of prostaglandins in implantation in the rat, *J. Reprod. Fertil.* **62**:73–81.

Pierce, M., Turley, E. A., and Roth, S., 1980, Cell surface glycosyltransferase activities, *Int. Rev. Cytol.* **65**:1–47.

Pinsker, M. C., and Mintz, B., 1973, Change in cell-surface glycoproteins of mouse embryos before implantation, *Proc. Nat. Acad. Sci. USA* **70**:1645–1648.

Pinsker, M. C., Sacco, A. G., and Mintz, B., 1974, Implantation-associated proteinase in mouse uterine fluid, *Dev. Biol.* **38**:285–290.

Pisam, M., and Ripoche, P., 1976, Redistribution of surface macromolecules in dissociated epithelial cells, *J. Cell Biol.* **71**:907–920.

Podack, E. R., 1985, The molecular mechanism of lymphocyte mediated tumor cell lysis, *Immunol. Today* **6**:21–27.

Poelmann, R. E., 1975, An ultrastructural study of implanting mouse blastocysts: Coated vesicles and epithelium formation, *J. Anat.* **119**:421–434.

Pollard, R. M., and Finn, C. A., 1972, Ultrastructure of the uterine epithelium during hormonal induction of sensitivity and insensitivity to a decidual stimulus in the mouse, *J. Endocrinol.* **55**:293–298.

Psychoyos, A., 1960, La réaction déciduale est précédée de modifications précoces de la perméabilité capillaire de l'utérus, *C. R. Seances Soc. Biol.* **154**:1384.

Psychoyos, A., 1973, Endocrine control of egg implantation, in: *Handbook of Physiology*, Section 7, Volume 2, Part 2, (R. O. Greep, E. B. Astwood, and S. R. Geiger, eds.), Williams & Wilkins, Baltimore, MD, pp. 187–215.

Psychoyos, A., and Mandon, P., 1971a, Etude de la surface de l'épithélium utérin au microscope électronique à balayage. Observations chez la ratte au 4e et au 5e jour de la gestation, *C.R. Hebd. Seances Acad. Sci. (Paris)* **272:**2723–2725.

Psychoyos, A., and Mandon, P., 1971b, Scanning electron microscopy of the surface of the rat uterine epithelium during delayed implantation, *J. Reprod. Fertil.* **26:**137–138.

Rachman, F., Bernard, O., Scheid, M. P., and Bennett, D., 1981, Immunological studies of mouse decidual cells. II. Studies of cells in artificialy induced decidua, *J. Reprod. Immunol.* **3:**41–48.

Racowsky, C., and Biggers, J. D., 1983, Are blastocyst prostaglandins produced endogenously? *Biol. Reprod.* **29:**379–388.

Rankin, J. C., Ledford, B. E., and Baggett, B., 1977, Early involvement of cyclic nucleotides in the artificially stimulated decidual cell reaction in the mouse uterus, *Biol. Reprod.* **17:**549–554.

Rankin, J. C., Ledford, B. E., Jansson, H. T., and Baggett, B., 1979, Prostaglandins, indomethacin and the decidual cell reaction in the mouse uterus, *Biol. Reprod.* **20:**399–404.

Rankin, J. C., Ledford, B. E., and Baggett, B., 1981, The role of prostaglandins and cyclic nucleotides in artificially stimulated decidual cell reaction in the mouse uterus, in: *Cellular and Molecular Aspects of Implantation* (S. R. Glasser and D. W. Bullock, eds.), Plenum Press, New York, pp. 428–430.

Reinius, S., 1967, Ultrastructure of blastocyst attachment in the mouse, *Z. Zellforsch. Mikrosk. Anat.* **77:**257–266.

Ricketts, A. P., Scott, D. W., and Bullock, D. W., 1984, Radioiodinated surface proteins of separated cell types from rabbit endometrium in relation to the time of implantation, *Cell Tissue Res.* **236:**421–429.

Rogers, P. A. W., Murphy, C. R., Rogers, A. W., and Gannon, B. J., 1983, Capillary patency and permeability in the endometrium surrounding the implanting rat blastocyst, *Int. J. Microcirc. Clin. Exp.* **2:**241–249.

Roseman, S., 1970, The synthesis of complex carbohydrates by multiglycosyltransferase systems and the potential function in intercellular adhesion, *Chem. Phys. Lipids* **5:**270–299.

Roth, S., McGuire, J. E., and Roseman, S., 1971, Evidence for cell-surface glycosyltransferases—potential role in cellular recognition, *J. Cell Biol.* **51:**536–547.

Rowinski, J., Solter, D., and Kaprowski, H., 1976, Changes of concanavalin A induced agglutinability during preimplantation mouse development, *Exp. Cell Res.* **100:**404–408.

Roy, S. K., Sengupta, J., and Manchanda, S. K., 1983, Histochemical study of beta-glucuronidase in the rat uterus during implantation and pseudopregnancy, *J. Reprod. Fertil.* **68:**161–164.

Saksena, S. K., Lau, I. F., and Chang, M. C., 1976, Relationship between oestrogen, prostaglandin $F_{2\alpha}$, and histamine in delayed implantation in the mouse, *Acta Endocrinol.* **91:**801–807.

Salazar-Rubio, M., Gil-Recasens, M. E., Hicks, J. J., and Gonzalez-Angulo, Y. A., 1980, High resolution cytochemical study of uterine epithelial cell surface of the rat at identified sites previous to blastocyst–endometrial contact, *Arch. Invest. Méd. (Méx.)* **11:**117–127.

Sananes, N., and Le Goascogne, C., 1976, Decidualization in prepuberal rat uterus, *Differentiation* **5:**133–144.

Sananes, N., Baulieu, E.-E., and Le Goascogne, C., 1976, Prostaglandin(s) as inductive factor of decidualization in the rat uterus, *Mol. Cell. Endocrinol.* **6:**153–158.

Sananes, N., Weiller, S., Baulieu, E.-E., and Le Goascogne, C., 1980, Decidualization *in vitro, Prog. Reprod. Biol.* **7:** 125–134.

Sananes, N., Baulieu, E.-E., and Le Goascogne, C., 1981, A role for prostaglandins in decidualization of the rat uterus, *J. Endocrinol.* **89:**25–33.

Sanders, R. B., Bekairi, A. M., and Yochim, J. M., 1983, Estrogen sensitive uterine adenylate cyclase in the rat, *Fed. Proc.* **42:**1852.

Sanders, R. B., Bekairi, A. M., Abulaban, F. S., and Yochim, J. M., 1986, Uterine adenylate cyclase in the rat: Responses to a decidual-inducing stimulus, *Biol. Reprod.* **35:**100–105.

Schatz, F., Markiewicz, L., and Gurpide, E., 1987, Differential effects of estradiol, arachidonic acid, and A 23187 on prostaglandin $F_{2\alpha}$ output by epithelial and stromal cells of human endometrium, *Endocrinology* **120:**1465–1471.

Schlafke, S., and Enders, A. C., 1975, Cellular basis of interaction between trophoblast and uterus at implantation, *Biol. Reprod.* **12:**41–65.

Schlafke, S., Welsh, A. O., and Enders, A. C., 1985, Penetration of the basal lamina of the uterine luminal epithelium during implantation in the rat, *Anat. Rec.* **212:**47–56.

Searle, R. F., 1986, Intrauterine immunization, in: *Reproductive Immunology* (D. A. Clark and B. A. Croy, eds.), Elsevier, New York, pp. 211–218.

Searle, R. F., Bell, S. C., and Billington, W. D., 1983, Ia antigen-bearing decidual cells and macrophages in cultures of mouse decidual tissue, *Placenta* **4**:139–148.

Sengupta, J., Roy, S. K., and Manchanda, S. K., 1979, Hormonal control of implantation: A possible role of lysosomal function in th embryo–uterus interaction, *J. Steroid Biochem.* **11**:729–744.

Sengupta, J., Paria, B. C., and Manchanda, S. K., 1981, Effect of an oestrogen antagonist on implantation and uterine leucylnaphylamidase activity in the ovariectomized hamster, *J. Reprod. Fertil.* **62**:437–440.

Sharma, S. C., 1979, Temporal changes in PGE, PGF$_\alpha$, oestradiol-17β and progesterone in uterine venous plasma and endometrium of rabbits during early pregnancy, *INSERM Symp.* **91**:243–264.

Shemesh, M., Milaguir, F., Ayalon, N., and Hansel, W., 1979, Steroidogenesis and prostaglandin synthesis by cultured bovine blastocysts, *J. Reprod. Fertil.* **56**:181–185.

Sherman, M. I., and Atienza-Samols, S. B., 1978, *In vitro* studies on the surface adhesiveness of mouse blastocysts, in: *Human Fertilization* (H. Ludwig and P. F. Tauber, eds.), Georg Thieme, Stuttgart, pp. 179–180.

Shur, B. D., 1982, Evidence that galactosyltransferase is a surface receptor for poly(N)-acetyl lactosamine glycoconjugates on embryonal carcinoma cells, *J. Biol. Chem.* **257**:6871–6878.

Shur, B. D., 1983, Embryonal carcinoma cell adhesion: The role of surface galactosyltransferase and its 90K lactosaminoglycan substrate, *Dev. Biol.* **99**:360–372.

Shur, B. D., 1984, The receptor function of galactosyltransferases during cellular interactions, *Mol. Cell. Biochem.* **61**:143–158.

Smith, A. F., and Wilson, I. B., 1974, Cell interaction at the maternal–embryonic interface during implantation in the mouse, *Cell Tissue Res.* **152**:525–542.

Smith, R. E., and Farquhar, M. G., 1966, Lysosome function in the regulation of the secretory process in cells of the anterior pituitary glands, *J. Cell Biol.* **31**:319–347.

Sobel, J. S., and Nebel, L., 1976, Concanavalin A agglutinability of developing mouse trophoblast, *J. Reprod. Fertil.* **47**:399–402.

Sobel, J. S., and Nebel, L., 1978, Changes in concanavalin A agglutinability during development of the inner cell mass and trophoblast of mouse blastocysts *in vitro*, *J. Reprod. Fertil.* **52**:239–248.

Stacey, N. H., Bishop, C. J., Halliday, J. W., Halliday, W. J., Cooksley, W. G. E., Powell, L. W., and Kerr, J. F. R., 1985, Apoptosis as the mode of cell death in antibody-dependent lymphocytotoxicity, *J. Cell Sci.* **74**:169–179.

Stewart, I., and Peel, S., 1981, Granulated metrial gland cells in the virgin and early pregnant mouse uterus, *J. Anat.* **133**:535–541.

Surani, M. A. H., 1979, Glycoprotein synthesis and inhibition of glycosylation by tunicamycin in preimplantation mouse embryos: Compaction and trophoblast adhesion, *Cell* **18**:217–227.

Tachi, C., and Tachi, S., 1974, Cellular aspects of ovum implantation and decidualization in the rat, in: *Physiology and Genetics of Reproduction,* Part B (E. M. Coutinho and F. Fuchs, eds.), Plenum Press, New York, pp. 263–286.

Tachi, C., Tachi, S., Knyszynski, A., and Lindner, H. R., 1981, Possible involvement of macrophages in embryo–maternal relationships during ovum implantation in the rat, *J. Exp. Zool.* **217**:81–92.

Tachi, S., Tachi, C., and Lindner, H. R., 1970, Ultrastructural features of blastocyst attachment and trophoblastic invasion in rat, *J. Reprod. Fertil.* **21**:37–56.

Tawfik, O. W., Hunt, J. S., and Wood, G. W., 1986, Implication of prostaglandin E$_2$ in soluble factor-mediated immune suppression by murine decidual cells, *Am. J. Reprod. Immunol. Microbiol.* **12**:111–117.

Thie, M., Bochskanl, R., and Kirchner, C., 1986, Glycoproteins in rabbit uterus during implantation. Differential localization visualized using ^{3}H-N-acetyl-glucosamine labeling and FITC-conjugated lectins, *Histochemistry* **84**:73–79.

Tobert, J. A., 1976, A study of the possible role of prostaglandins in decidualization using a nonsurgical method for the instillation of fluids into the uterine lumen, *J. Reprod. Fertil.* **47**:391–393.

Tung, H. N., Parr, M. B., and Parr, E. L., 1986, The permeability of the primary decidual zone in the rat uterus: An ultrastructural tracer and freeze–fracture study, *Biol. Reprod.* **35**:1045–1058.

Umapathysivam, K., and Jones, W. R., 1978, An investigation of decidual specific proteins in the rat, *Int. J. Fertil.* **23**:138–142.

Velardo, J. T., Dawson, A. B., Olsen, A. G., and Hisaw, F. L., 1953, Sequence of histological changes in the uterus and vagina of the rat during prolongation of pseudopregnancy associated with the presence of deciduomata, *Am. J. Anat.* **93**:273–305.

Watson, J., and Patek, E. E., 1979, Steroid and prostaglandin secretion by the corpus luteum, endometrium and embryos of cyclic and pregnant pigs, *J. Endocrinol.* **82**:425–428.

Webb, C. G., and Duskin, D., 1981, Involvement of glycoproteins in the development of early mouse embryos: Effect of tunicamycin and a, a'-dipyridyl *in vitro*, *Differentiation* **20**:81–86.

Weitlauf, H., 1979, Implantation, in: *Animal Models for Research on Conception and Fertility* (N. J. Alexander, ed.), PARFR Series on Fertility Regulation, Harper & Row, Hagerstown, MD, pp. 238–252.

Welsh, A. O., and Enders, A. C., 1985, Light and electron microscopic examination of the mature decidual cells of the rat with emphasis on the antimesometrial decidua and its degeneration, *Am. J. Anat.* **172**:1–29.

Welsh, A. O., and Enders, A. C., 1987, Trophoblast–decidual cell interactions and establishment of maternal blood circulation in the parietal yolk sac placenta of the rat, *Anat. Rec.* **217**:203–219.

Wordinger, R. J., and Amsler, K. R., 1980, Histochemical identification of the glycocalyx layer in the bovine oviduct and endometrium, *Anim. Reprod. Sci.* **3**:189–193.

Wu, J. T., 1980a, Concanavalin A binding capacity of preimplantation mouse embryos, *J. Reprod. Fertil.* **58**:455–461.

Wu, J. T., 1980b, Concanavalin A binding capacity of preimplanation rat embryos, *J. Exp. Zool.* **213**:377–382.

Wu, J. T., and Chang, M. C., 1978, Increase in concanavalin A binding sites in mouse blastocysts during implantation, *J. Exp. Zool.* **105**:447–453.

Wu, J. T., and Gu, Z., 1981, The effect of intrauterine injection of concanavalin A on implantation in mice and rats, *Contraception* **23**:667–676.

Wyllie, A. H., 1981, Cell death: A new classification separating apoptosis from necrosis, in: *Cell Death in Biology and Pathology* (I. D. Bowen and R. A. Lockshin, eds.), Chapman and Hall, London, pp. 9–34.

Wyllie, A. H., Kerr, J. F. R., and Currie, A. R., 1980, Cell death: The significance of apoptosis, *Int. Rev. Cytol.* **68**:251–306.

Yamamoto, A., 1982, Purification and assay of PGH synthase from bovine seminal vesicles, *Methods Enzymol.* **86**:55–60.

Yanagimachi, R., and Nicolson, G. L., 1976, Lectin-binding properties of hamster egg zona pellucida and plasma membrane during maturation, *Exp. Cell Res.* **100**:249–257.

Yoshinaga, K., 1972, Rabbit antiserum to rat deciduoma, *Biol. Reprod.* **6**:51–57.

Yoshinaga, K., 1974, Interspecific cross-reactivity of deciduoma antiserum: Interaction between mouse deciduoma and antiserum to rat deciduoma, *Biol. Reprod.* **11**:50–55.

Yoshinaga, K. (ed.), 1986, *Annals of the New York Academy of Sciences,* Volume 476, *Nidation,* New York Academy of Sciences, New York.

Young, J. D.-E., and Cohn, Z. A., 1986, Cell-mediated killing: A common mechanism, *Cell* **46**:641–642.

Zorn, T. M. T., Bevilacqua, E. M. A. F., and Abrahamsohn, P. A., 1986, Collagen remodeling during decidualization in the mouse, *Cell Tissue Res.* **244**:443–448.

Regeneration in the Primate Uterus

The Role of Stem Cells

HELEN A. PADYKULA

Artificial programming of the menstrual cycle in rhesus monkeys is a remarkable advance in primate uterine biology (Hodgen, 1983). Ovariectomized mature monkeys receive sub-cutaneous silastic implants of estradiol and progesterone that mimic the serum steroidal hormonal profile of a natural 28-day menstrual cycle. Transfer of surrogate preimplantation embryos into the ampulla of the fallopian tube during artificial cycles has resulted in successful pregnancies and birth of normal offspring. This achievement was followed by production of fertile cycles in women who had been ovariectomized or had primary ovarian failure (Lutjen *et al.*, 1984; Navot *et al.*, 1986). These fundamental demonstrations established that primate uterine cyclic growth depends primarily on an appropriate pattern of systemic estradiol and progesterone secretion.

These basic experiments united the primate uterus with the uteri of subprimates in mutual dependence on ovarian steroids for cyclicity. They have also provided an important primate model in the rhesus monkey for experimentation that will ultimately lead to better understanding of the control mechanisms that guide cyclic endometrial growth and differentiation in women and other menstruating primates. Recently, another important factor related to the control of endometrial mitotic activity has been identified in the rat endometrium. Although cell proliferation is under the control of serum and tissue estradiol, its mitogenic action is effected through the mediation of epidermal growth factor (EGF) binding to endometrial tissue EGF receptors (Mukku and Stancel, 1985). This observation provides an avenue for identifying control mechanisms that produce differential mitotic patterns within tissues. A new era is upon us that will center on localization of tissue growth factors such as angiogenic factor (AGF), fibroblastic growth factor (FGF), and others.

HELEN A. PADYKULA • Department of Cell Biology, University of Massachusetts Medical School, Worcester, Massachusetts 01655.

In addition to the systemic ovarian steroidal secretion, an essential intrinsic endometrial tissue mechanism consists of an omnipresent small pool of multipotential stem cells that divide slowly. It is assumed that, at the outset of puberty or of a new menstrual cycle, stem cells give rise to progenitor cells that divide more rapidly and become committed to specific pathways of differentiation to give rise to characteristic endogenous endometrial cell types. That is, initial estrogen-stimulated cell growth involves mitotic recruitment and differentiation of luminal and glandular epithelial cells, stromal fibroblasts, endometrial granular cells, and the cellular components of the endometrial microvasculature. The synthesis of the endometrial extracellular matrix is also under steroidal control through cellular activity.

1. Endometriectomy and the Location of the Endometrial Stem Cells

From primate reproductive biology and human clinical practice, it has long been known that removal of all visible endometrial tissue by curettage in women and monkeys is followed, after a short delay, by rapid reconstruction of a new endometrium that can support pregnancy. Since the basal portions of the endometrial glands interdigitate with myometrial stroma and smooth muscle at the endometrial–myometrial junction, it may be inferred that endometrial stem cells for epithelial, stromal, and vascular components are located near or within the endometrial–myometrial junction.

Carl Hartman (1944) provided graphic evidence of the effects of repeated regeneration of the rhesus monkey uterus after endometriectomy (Fig. 1), as expressed in the following excerpts selected by Dr. John McCracken from Hartman's fundamental publication:

> Endometriectomy, as I practiced it, consisted of removal of most of the endometrium, including the basalis. In six experiments, the endometrium was wiped out as clean as possible with a cotton sponge, so that no vestige of mucosa was visible to the naked eye—yet perfect regeneration occurred.
>
> More than 200 endometriectomies were performed on intact rhesus monkeys, both cycling and in early pregnancy. The greatest number of hysterotomies in one animal was four. However, five animals had endometriectomies performed three times at intervals of two to four months. Twenty-eight animals were operated upon twice. The purpose of this approach was to obtain implanting embryos and also to conserve the animals for further use and to obtain additional specimens from the same animal. Coincidentally using the endometriectomy technique, an unsurpassed opportunity was provided to study the regenerative powers of the endometrium.

Quantitative analyses of estrogen and progesterone receptors in the monkey endometrium were performed during the luteal phase between days 17 and 22 to obtain enough tissue for analysis (Kreitman-Gimbal et al., 1979). Repeated endometriectomies were performed on several monkeys to obtain adequate endometrial tissue without negative consequences. After curettage of the rabbit endometrium, regeneration of the luminal epithelium was rapidly initiated at 3 hr; at 72 hr, regeneration of the endometrium was complete, and the endometrium resembled that of the control (Schenker et al., 1971).

Thus, the regenerative capacity of the mammalian endometrium is impressive. It resembles that of the epidermis in that a relatively small number of the stem cells can reconstruct the original structure quite effectively. Human epidermal stem cells have been identified within the basal and immediately suprabasal cells (Sun and Lavker, 1982). Moreover, isolated human epidermal stem cells of an individual will proliferate and form sheets in culture that can be transferred to sites of severe burns in the same individual to promote healing without immunologic rejection. As for the endometrium, it remains to be determined whether or not the most basal endometrial region is the only site of multipotential stem cells.

Cyclic endometrial renewal consists of a small pool of multipotential stem cells that

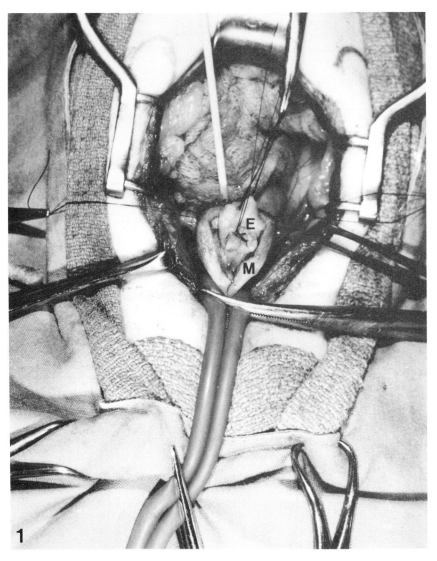

Figure 1. Surgical endometriectomy, mature rhesus monkey. The endometrium is removed by cutting along the endometrial–myometrial junction with a scalpel. A suture through the endometrial tissue (E) serves to lift it as it is being separated from the myometrium (M). Dr. John A. McCracken of the Worcester Foundation for Experimental Biology derived this technique from C. G. Hartman's (1944) original description of endometriectomy.

divide slowly (Fig. 2). Under systemic hormonal changes, such as the cyclic increase in the serum level of estradiol, it can be postulated that stem cells migrate and give rise to a group of progenitor cells that become committed to specific types of cell differentiation, e.g., epithelial, stromal, and vascular, within certain microenvironments (Hall, 1983). Progenitor cells have higher mitotic rates than do stem cells, and thus the result is progressive endometrial growth. The "options" for progenitor cells are (1) to continue mitotic activity with concomitant differentiation or (2) to become postmitotic and thus transient. In relation to primate endometrial regeneration, the destination of migrating stem–progenitor cells may be the four zones or microenvironments of the primate endometrium.

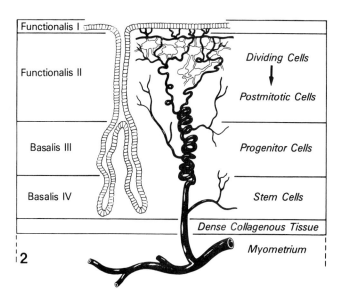

Figure 2. Endometrial zonation of the rhesus monkey adapted from Bartelmez (1951). The primate endometrium consists of four structurally distinct zones. The germinal basalis consists of two zones, basalis III and basalis IV. The functionalis is composed of two zones, functionalis I and functionalis II. Endometrial regeneration after endometriectomy proceeds from the remnants of basalis IV, and that after the menses from basalis III and IV.

2. Compartmentalization of the Primate Endometrium

The uterine endometrium of mammals possesses a germinal compartment that persists from cycle to cycle during reproductive life (Figs. 2 and 3). The germinal compartment gives rise to a transient compartment for the purpose of accommodating implantation of the blastocyst as well as providing for the maternal component of the placenta if pregnancy should occur. Thus, after a menstrual cycle or the close of pregnancy, the transient component is eliminated, only to be recreated.

In subprimate mammals, it is difficult to distinguish between the germinal and transient endometrial compartments because cell death and regression of the transient tissue occur *in situ* (Padykula, 1981). However, in menstruating primates the endometrial functionalis, the transient compartment, is shed by tissue sloughing accompanied by bleeding. At the close of menses, the germinal basalis remains and enters into the hormonal environment of the next cycle to produce a new functionalis.

Thus, the rhesus monkey provides a natural system for analysis of the germinal and transient endometrial compartments because of the clearcut separation of the transient cells at the close of menses. Then, during the subsequent menstrual cycle, it is possible to trace the origin of the transient compartment from the germinal compartment during estrogen and progesterone dominance.

The neuroendocrine features of the rhesus hypothalamic–ovarian circuit have been carefully defined and are comparable to those of women (Knobil, 1980). In women and monkeys, the menstrual cycles are approximately 28 days in length, with ovulation occurring approximately 38 hr after the LH surge. Thus, the rhesus monkey is an appropriate model for identifying intraendometrial control mechanisms that make provision for the possibility of pregnancy during a cycle by preparing a transient ''home'' for an embryo within the functionalis. In addition, the control mechanisms should insure that the germinal basalis will persist from cycle to cycle. These control mechanisms remain to be defined.

zone I   **zone II**

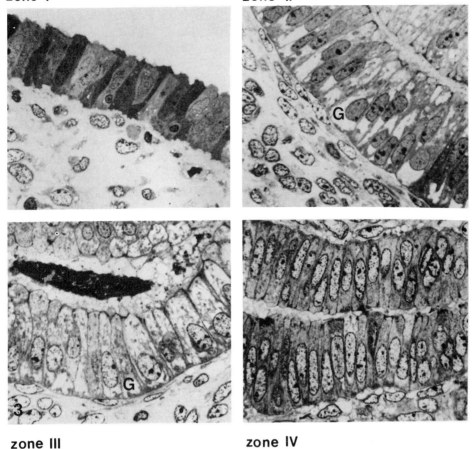

zone III   **zone IV**

Figure 3. Histological zonation of the human endometrium, day 19 of the menstrual cycle. The epithelia of the four zones were photographed at the same magnification. Note the zonal variation in epithelial cell height, shape, and degree of glycogen storage (G).

Our recent studies on [³H]thymidine ([³H]-TdR) incorporation during the natural menstrual cycle have provided data that may lead to definition of the cyclic origin of the functionalis as well as the germinal mechanisms within the basalis. To interpret the pattern of [³H]-TdR incorporation into endometrial tissue, it is necessary to consider the zonal subcompartmentalization of the functionalis and basalis of the rhesus and human endometria, as defined histologically (Bartelmez, 1951, 1957) and ultrastructurally (Kaiserman-Abramof and Padykula, 1987).

3.   Zonation of the Primate Endometrium

Compartmentalization extends beyond the major subdivision of germinal basalis and transient functionalis. Bartelmez (1951, 1957) identified four histologically different horizontal zones in the rhesus and human endometria as follows (Figs. 2 and 3):

Functionalis	Zone I:	Luminal epithelium and subjacent stroma
	Zone II:	Upper endometrium in which the straight region of the glands course and are widely separated by stroma
Basalis	Zone III:	Midregions of the glands that are widely separated by stroma
	Zone IV:	Basal regions of the glands in a fibrous stroma adjacent to the endometrial–myometrial junction

This endometrial quadripartite zonation had been largely ignored until functional differences were identified among the four zones by autoradiography (Padykula *et al.*, 1984a). A single intravenous injection of [^{3}H]thymidine was made on a specific day of the menstrual cycle. One hour later endometrial biopsies were obtained by hysterotomy. Plastic sections (2 μm) were used to prepare autoradiographs from which the zonal labeling indices for the luminal and glandular epithelia were determined (Table 1). At that time, other laboratories were localizing estrogen receptors through immunocytochemistry in the cynomolgus monkey (West and Brenner, 1983; McClellan *et al.*, 1986). Zonal differences were also observed in the distribution of these receptors in human endometria during the menstrual cycle (Press *et al.*, 1984, 1985, 1986).

Table 1. Zonal Distribution of Mitotic Activity
in Rhesus Endometrium: Epithelial
Labeling Index[a]

Day of cycle	Zone			
	I	II	III	IV
9[b]	7%	13%	9%	3%
−2	11%	10%	6%	1%
−1	10%	10%	5%	2%
−1	—	14%	7%	3%
0	11%	7%	5%	4%
+1	11%	11%	5%	5%
+2	12%	13%	7%	4%
+3	9%	11%	6%	7%
+5	3%	0%	3%	9%
+6	9%	1%	1%	9%
+10	2%	2%	1%	11%
+14	0%	0%	0%	0%

[a]Zonal variation in [^{3}H]thymidine incorporation 1 hr following a single i.v. injection on each of ten days of the menstrual cycle. During the periovulatory period (−2 to +3 days), the labeling index of functionalis I and II is approximately 10%, whereas basalis III has an index of 5–6%. Between days +5 and +14, progesterone action inhibits epithelial mitosis and thus decreases the labeling indices in functionalis I and II and basalis III. In contrast, mitotic activity in basalis IV epithelium rises steadily from 1% to 11% between days −2 and +10. A minimum of 2000 cells/zone per specimen were used to determine LI. From Padykula *et al.* (1984b).
[b]On biological day 9, the serum estradiol concentration was less than 50 pg/ml.

Although current understanding of cyclic renewal of the primate endometrium is fragmentary, it is possible to construct an hypothesis for cyclic endometrial growth derived from the data on [³H]thymidine incorporation during the natural menstrual cycle. The pioneer effort in this approach was made by Ferenczy *et al.* (1979), who incubated slices of human endometrium *in vitro* with [³H]-TdR. Labeling of nuclei occurred only at the surface of the slices; thus, the data were limited and did not permit functional interpretation.

It was therefore necessary to use an appropriate animal model, such as the mature female rhesus monkey, to effect *in vivo* labeling on specific days during the 28-day rhesus menstrual cycle (Padykula *et al.*, 1984a,b). Initial [³H]-TdR labeling centered around the estradiol peak on the premise that estrogen is a mitogen for epithelial, stromal, and vascular cells during the proliferative phase, i.e., estrogen dominance. A single intravenous injection of [³H]-TdR was made, and an endometrial biopsy was taken 1 hr later and prepared for plastic sections (2 μm) for light microscopy and ultrathin sections for electron microscopy. Autoradiographs were prepared in an effort to obtain a plane of section that ran parallel to the endometrial glands and coiled arterioles to provide accurate recognition of the four zones.

4.1. Epithelial Mitotic Activity in the Transient Compartment during Estrogen Dominance

Zonal variation in the [³H]-TdR labeling indices was visually evident in the autoradiographs. As the data in Table 1 indicate, high epithelial proliferative activity in the functionalis was evident from −2 to +3 days of estrogen dominance. In contrast, epithelial cells of the basalis had lower labeling indices (LI). Overall, the epithelial LI of the functionalis was approximately 10%, whereas that of the basalis III was 5–6%, and that of basalis IV progressively increased from 1 to 6%. Thus, during estrogen dominance, the epithelial [³H]-TdR LI of the functionalis is approximately twice that of the basalis.

4.2. Germinal Mechanisms in the Endometrial Basalis

During the postovulatory period of progesterone dominance, the zonal pattern of [³H]-TdR uptake was identifiable on day +5 by the antiestrogenic action of progesterone as an inhibitor of epithelial proliferation in the functionalis I and II and basalis III (Table 1) (Padykula *et al.*, 1984b). In contrast, basalis IV escapes progesterone inhibition, as the [³H]-TdR labeling index from −2 to +10 days continues to increase to 11% (Fig. 4). Here it is possible to make an important correlation between the autoradiographic data and the immunocytochemical distribution of the estrogen receptor in the cyclic human and monkey (artificial menstrual cycles) (Press *et al.*, 1984; McClellan *et al.*, 1986). During the preovulatory (proliferative) phase, nuclear estrogen receptor is localized in all four zones of the glandular and luminal epithelia. However, this reactivity decreased steadily in zones I, II, and III during the postovulatory period of progesterone dominance, but not in the deep basalis (zone IV). Hence, this persistence of estrogen receptor correlates with the steadily increasing mitotic activity of epithelial cells in zone IV.

Thus, in the most basal regions of the preovulatory endometrium, high epithelial activity persists along with nuclear binding of the estrogen receptor. In other words, zone IV epithelial cells "escape progesterone mitotic inhibition." The deep endometrium contains unique germinal cells that differentiate under the control of a distinctly different mechanism from that of

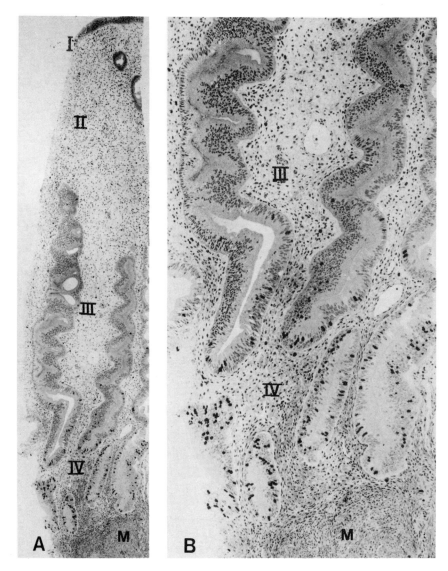

Figure 4. Autoradiograph, day +10, rhesus endometrium. These low- and high-power figures demonstrate [³H]thymidine incorporation by the glandular epithelium of basalis IV during progesterone dominance. Note the lack of reactivity in basalis III.

the functionalis and basalis III. Histologists have long recognized increasing epithelial pseudostratification in the basalis during the late luteal phase. Pseudostratification reflects the crowding of columnar glandular cells that are being rapidly produced.

Continued high epithelial proliferation in the basalis IV during progesterone dominance requires special comment. Progesterone is used clinically in human endometrial cancer to suppress abnormal mitotic activity. It is likely that basalis IV of the human endometrium may also "escape progesterone inhibition," and thus clinicians should be aware of this possibility until the mitotic control mechanisms for germinal basalis IV have been identified.

1. The basalis is a bifunctional germinal compartment that will reconstruct a new functionalis.

2. The transient functionalis expands rapidly during the mitogenic stimulus of estrogen dominance. A fundamental functional and structural dichotomy exists within the basalis. During postovulatory rising serum progesterone, epithelial proliferation is inhibited in basalis III and functionalis I and II. In contrast, proliferation in basalis IV continues to increase at least to day 10 or 12.

3. The basalis expands primarily by heightened epithelial cell proliferation in basalis IV, which "escapes inhibition by progesterone." Simultaneously, the nuclear estrogen receptor persists in high concentration only in basalis IV during progesterone dominance.

4. The heightened postovulatory rate of production of basalis IV epithelial cells contributes to intracyclic growth for the possibility of pregnancy as well as for intercycle stem cell continuity.

5. After menses, the program of basalis III includes rapid covering of the menstrual wound and reinitiation of mitotic activity to recreate the zonal microenvironments in the new functionalis.

6. The program for postmenstrual reconstruction or pregnancy is most likely prepared during the cellular expansion that occurs during progesterone dominance of the preceding menstrual cycle.

7. By day +14, epithelial proliferation is inhibited in all zones of the premenstrual endometrium (Bartelmez, 1951; Noyes *et al.,* 1950) (Table 1). Intercycle mitotic quiescence persists until day 4–5 of the next cycle as a new group of stem-progenitor cells is activated (McClellan *et al.,* 1986).

6. References

Bartelmez, G. W., 1951, Cyclic changes in the endometrium of the rhesus monkey (Macaca mulatta), *Contrib. Embryol. Carnegie Inst.* **34**:99–146.

Bartelmez, G. W., 1957, The phases of the menstrual cycle and their interpretation in terms of the pregnancy cycle. *Am. J. Obstet. Gynecol.* **74**:931–955.

Bensley, C. M., 1951, Cyclic fluctuations in the rate of epithelial mitosis in the endometrium of the rhesus monkey, *Contrib. Embryol. Carnegie Inst.* **34**:87–98.

Brenner, R. M., McClellan, M. C., and West, N. B., 1984, Immunocytochemistry of estrogen receptors in stroma and epithelium during menstruation and repair, *J. Cell Biol.* **99**:215A.

Ferenczy, A., 1980, Regeneration of the human endometrium, in: *Progress in Surgical Pathology,* Volume 1 (C. M. Genoglio and L. M. Wolff, eds.), Masson, Paris.

Ferenczy, A., Bertrand, G., and Gelfand, M. M., 1979, Proliferation kinetics of human endometrium during the normal menstrual cycle, *Am. J. Obstet. Gynecol.* **133**:859–867.

Hall, A. K., 1983, Stem cell is a stem cell is a stem cell, *Cell* **33**:11–12.

Hartman, C. G., 1944, Regeneration of the monkey uterus after surgical removal of the endometrium and accidental endometriosis, *West. J. Surg. Obstet. Gynecol.* **52**:87–102.

Hodgen, G. D., 1983, Surrogate embryo transfer combined with estrogen–progesterone therapy in monkeys, *J.A.M.A.,* **250**:2167–2171.

Kaiserman-Abramof, I. R., and Padykula, H. A., 1987, Ultrastructural zonation of the primate endometrium (rhesus monkey), *Anat. Rec.* **218**:70A.

Knobil, E., 1980, The neuroendocrine control of the menstrual cycle, *Recent Prog. Horm. Res.* **36**:53–88.

Kreitmann-Gimbal, B., Bayard, F., Nixon, W. E., and Hodgen, G. D., 1980, Patterns of estrogen and progesterone receptors in monkey endometrium during the normal menstrual cycle, *Steroids* **35**:471–475.

Lavker, R. M., and Sun, T. T., 1983, Epidermal stem cells, *J. Invest. Dermatol. [Suppl.]*:1215–1275.

Lutjen, P., Trounson, A., Leeton, J., Findlay, J., Wood, C., and Renou, P., 1984, The establishment and maintenance of pregnancy using *in vitro* fertilization and embryo donation in a patient with primary ovarian failure, *Nature* **307**:174–175.

McClellan, M., West, N. B., and Brenner, R. M., 1986, Immunocytochemical localization of estrogen receptors in the macaque endometrium during the luteal–follicular transition, *Endocrinology* **19**:2467–2475.

Mukku, V. R., and Stancel, G. M., 1985, Regulation of epidermal growth factor receptor by estrogen, *J. Biol. Chem.* **260**:9820–9824.

Navot, D., Laufer, N., Kopolovic, J., Rabinowitz, R., Birkenfeld, A., Lewin, A., Granat, M., Margalioth, E. J., and Schenker, J. G., 1986, Artificially induced endometrial cycles and establishment of pregnancies in the absence of ovaries, *N. Engl. J. Med.* **315**:806–811.

Noyes, R. W., 1973, Normal phases of the endometrium, in: *The Uterus*, Chapter 7 (H. J. Norris and A. T. Hertig, eds.), Williams & Wilkins, Baltimore.

Noyes, R. W., Hertig, A. T., and Rock, J., 1950, Dating the endometrial biopsy, *Fertil. Steril.* **1**:3–25.

Padykula, H. A., 1981, Shifts in uterine stromal cell populations during pregnancy and regression, in: *Cellular and Molecular Aspects of Implantation* (S. R. Glasser and D. W. Bullock, eds.), Plenum Press, New York, pp. 197–216.

Padykula, H. A., Coles, L. G., McCracken, J. A., King, N. W., Longcope, C., and Kaiserman-Abramof, I. R., 1984a, A zonal pattern of cell proliferation and differentiation in the rhesus endometrium during the estrogen surge, *Biol. Reprod.* **31**:1103–1118.

Padykula, H. A., Coles, L. G., McCracken, J. A., King, N. W., Jr., Longcope, C., and Kaiserman-Abramof, I. R., 1984b, Production of progenitor cells for postmenstrual endometrial reconstruction in the cyclic rhesus monkey, *Biol. Reprod.* **30**(Suppl. 1):92.

Padykula, H. A., Coles, L. G., Okulicz, W. C., Rapaport, S. I., McCracken, J. A., King, Jr., N. W., Longcope, C., and Kaiserman-Abramof, I. R., 1989, The basalis of the primate endometrium: A bifunctional germinal compartment, *Biol. Reprod.* (in press).

Press, M. F., Nousek-Goebel, N., Herbst, A. L., and Greene, G. F., 1984, Immunocytochemical assessment of estrogen receptor distribution in the human endometrium throughout the menstrual cycle, *Lab. Invest.* **51**:495–503.

Press, M. F., Nousek-Goebel, N., Herbst, A. L., and Greene, G., 1985, Immunocytochemical microscopic localization of estrogen receptor with monoclonal estrophilin antibodies, *J. Histochem. Cytochem.* **33**:915–924.

Press, M. F., Nousek-Goebel, N., Bur, M., and Greene, G., 1986, Estrogen receptor localization in the female genital tract, *Am. J. Pathol.* **123**:280–292.

Schenker, J. G., Sacks, M. I., and Plishuk, W. Z., 1971, I. Regeneration of rabbit endometrium following curettage, *Am. J. Obstet. Gynecol.* **111**:970–978.

Suzuki, M., Goawa, M., Tamada, T., Nagura, H., and Watanabe, K., 1984, Immunocytochemical localization of secretory component and IgA in the human endometrium in relation to the menstrual cycle, *Acta Histochem. Cytochem.* **17**:223.

West, N. B., and Brenner, R. M., 1983, Estrogen receptor levels in the oviduct and endometria of cynomolgus macaques during the menstrual cycle, *Biol. Reprod.* **29**:1303–1312.

The Human Endometrium
Cyclic and Gestational Changes

RALPH M. WYNN

The endometrium is an ideal tissue for study of the interrelated effects of ovarian hormones, enzymes, and prostaglandins. Advances in the biochemistry and physiology of the uterus have stimulated reinterpretation of the cyclic morphological changes in the endometrium. Concomitantly, ultrastructural studies have bridged the gap between the large body of cytochemical information and the conventional histological studies of endometrial development and disease.

This chapter deals with the histological and submicroscopic structure of the normal human endometrium as well as the vascular changes in normal and hypertensive pregnancies. Regeneration is discussed in detail in Chapter 10, and pathological changes are described in Chapter 12. Relevant clinical topics include the anatomic events of menstruation, preparation for decidualization, and the ultrastructural effects of steroidal and intrauterine contraceptive agents.

1. Histology

The normal cyclic changes in the endometrium are closely correlated with those in the ovary. The proliferative, or preovulatory, phase of endometrial development corresponds temporally to the follicular phase of the ovarian cycle. The postovulatory, or secretory, phase of the endometrium corresponds to the ovarian luteal phase. Teleologically, these cyclic alterations may be considered preparation of the endometrium for nidation of the ovum. In a cycle in which fertilization does not occur, the endometrium sloughs; that is, menstruation ensues.

The earliest major description of the cyclic histological changes in the human endo-

RALPH M. WYNN ● Departments of Obstetrics and Gynecology and Anatomy and Cell Biology, Wayne State University School of Medicine, Detroit, Michigan 48201.

289

metrium appeared in the first decade of this century (Hitschmann and Adler, 1908). The paper to which most modern studies refer was published over 40 years later (Noyes *et al.*, 1950). These histological descriptions refer to the most advanced consistent change in the functional zone of the normal endometrium. The location of the endometrium within the corpus, furthermore, determines to a considerable extent the response of that tissue to the hormones of the menstrual cycle. Elucidating this well-known observation, Tsibris *et al.* (1981) reported an uneven distribution of estradiol and progesterone receptors in human endometrium. They showed that the concentration of cytoplasmic receptors for these steroids is highest at the fundus and lower toward the cervix, whereas the corresponding nuclear receptors are distributed inversely.

The highest concentrations of estrogen and progesterone receptors are found during the midproliferative phase of the cycle, at a time when estradiol in the plasma is rising and mitotic activity in the endometrial cells is maximal. Estradiol promotes the synthesis of both estradiol and progesterone receptors, whereas progesterone inhibits the synthesis of estradiol receptors. The sex hormones appear to function in intranuclear activation of receptors that initiate alterations in functions of target cells. Details of receptor biology are found in Chapter 7.

Dating of the endometrium refers to the classic 28-day cycle, in which ovulation is assumed to occur on day 14. Because the postovulatory phase is constant (14 days ± 36 hr), it is appropriate to designate the third postovulatory day, for example, as day 17. The day immediately preceding menstruation is day 28, and the first day of bleeding is day 1. Because the range of the normal menstrual cycle is from 21 to 35 days, the preovulatory phase may vary in length from 7 to 21 days. Because of this variation, it is inappropriate to designate the days of the preovulatory phase of the cycle by numbers. Instead, the terms "early," "mid," and "late," proliferative are used. For example, in a 28-day cycle with a 14-day preovulatory phase, days 1–4 would coincide with the menstrual period; days 5–7 would be early proliferative; days 8–10 would be midproliferative; and days 11–14 would be late proliferative, ovulation occurring on or very near day 14.

The first half of the endometrial cycle, before ovulation, is concerned with growth or proliferation; the second half is concerned with epithelial and stromal differentiation. During the first half of the postovulatory phase, or the third week of a typical 28-day cycle, specific synchronized changes occur in the endometrial epithelium, particularly the glands of the zona spongiosa. During the second half of the endometrial cycle, or the fourth week of a 28-day cycle, the histological changes affect primarily the stroma, leading to a predecidual reaction. If fertilization fails to occur, the stromal reaction regresses and menstruation ensues. If pregnancy occurs, the endometrial changes progress to formation of true decidua. The major histological changes during the endometrial cycle are summarized in Table 1.

The early preovulatory (proliferative) endometrium measures only 1–2 mm in thickness. The superficial epithelium, composed of cuboidal cells, appears to be regenerating. The glands are short, straight, narrow, and partially collapsed (Fig. 1). Mitotic figures frequently are seen in both epithelium and compact stroma, which consists of stellate cells with scanty cytoplasm. During the midproliferative phase, the epithelial cells become columnar. The glands elongate and become more tortuous. Stromal edema may appear at this stage, although it is inconstant and soon regresses. Mitotic figures are most obvious at this time. During the late proliferative phase, the glands continue to increase in length and tortuosity. Individual columnar epithelial cells achieve their greatest height, and pseudostratification of nuclei is maximal (Fig. 2).

The first distinct histological change in the postovulatory (secretory) phase occurs about 48 hr after ovulation (day 16), when subnuclear vacuolation of the glandular epithelium becomes prominent. Initially, these large, regularly distributed vacuoles displace the nuclei upward to create a pattern of pseudostratification. After all the vacuoles have passed the nuclei, pseudostratification disappears, with nuclei returning to the bases of their cells. Increases in diameter and tortuosity of the glands accompany these changes.

On day 17, the glandular epithelium shows an orderly row of nuclei with homogeneous

Table 1. Major Histological Features of the Human Endometrium during an Ideal 28-Day Cycle

Phase of the cycle	Day	Glands	Stroma
Early proliferative	5–7	Straight with small circular cross section; low epithelium; basal nuclei; occasional mitoses	Spindly cells with relatively large nuclei; occasional mitoses
Midproliferative	8–10	Longer with slight tortuosity; nuclei pseudostratified; numerous mitoses	Variable edema; numerous mitoses
Late proliferative	11–14	Marked tortuosity; wide lumen; maximal pseudostratification of nuclei	Less edema; many mitoses
Early secretory	15–18	Lumina wide; nuclei basal on day 16; the subnuclear vacuole passes nucleus on day 18; mitoses disappearing	Relatively compact; rare mitoses
Midsecretory	19–23	Sawtooth; nuclei returned to basal position; intraluminal secretion maximal; no mitotic figures	Edema maximal on day 22; first appearance of pseudodecidual cuff of cells around small arteries on day 23
Late secretory	24–28	Regression, with fraying of luminal epithelial surface	Maximal predecidual reaction; infiltration by leukocytes and later erythrocytes
Menses	1–4	Breakdown of epithelium with menstrual slough	Hemorrhage into stroma and endometrial slough

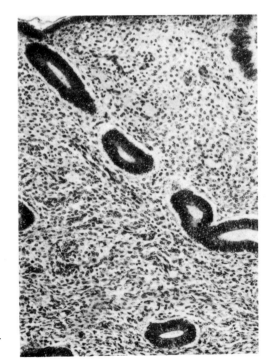

Figure 1. Early proliferative endometrium showing short, narrow, straight glands.

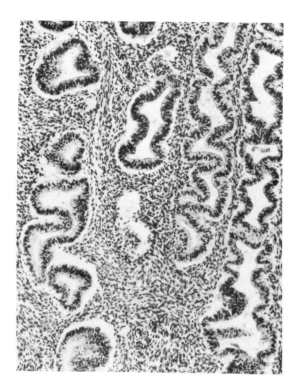

Figure 2. Late proliferative endometrium showing long, dilated, tortuous glands.

cytoplasm above them and large vacuoles below (Fig. 3). By day 18, the vacuoles push past the nuclei, decreasing in size and entering the cytoplasm nearer to the glandular lumen. By day 19, most of the nuclei have returned to the bases of the cells, and most of the vacuoles have discharged their contents. Day 19 may resemble day 16 with its early vacuolation or may even resemble the late proliferative phase, but it is distinguished from the earlier phases by intraluminal secretion and absence of pseudostratification and mitotic figures. By day 20, acidophilic intraluminal secretion reaches its peak. Thereafter, it becomes inspissated and more darkly stained (Fig. 4).

Dating of the second half of the postovulatory phase (days 21–28) depends largely on stromal characteristics. Edema is rather constant in the midsecretory period, abruptly increasing on day 21 and reaching its peak on day 22. The stromal cells at this stage appear as small, dense, nearly naked nuclei with only a rim of cytoplasm.

On day 23, endometrial spiral arterioles become more prominent because of enlargement of the nuclei and increase in the cytoplasm of the periarteriolar stromal cells. This cuff of stromal cells around the arterioles of the zona compacta is the earliest predecidual change. By day 24, distinct collections of periarteriolar predecidual cells may be identified.

Similar predecidual cells begin to differentiate beneath the epithelium of the surface on or about day 25. During the next 48 hr, patches of these cells begin to coalesce, forming solid sheets of well-developed decidua-like cells by day 27.

Around day 24 of a cycle in which pregnancy does not occur, glandular epithelial involution begins. The epithelium of the dilated and tortuous glands is thrown into tufts, creating the serration that is characteristic of the last week of the cycle. The previously tall columnar epithelium diminishes in height. Its nuclei appear shrunken, and its cytoplasmic borders become ragged and indistinct (Fig. 5).

A few lymphocytes may be scattered throughout the stroma in the proliferative and early secretory phases, but the differentiation of predecidua is accompanied by a sharp increase in

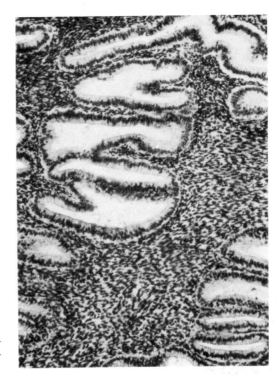

Figure 3. Early secretory (day-17) endometrium showing regularly aligned subnuclear vacuoles.

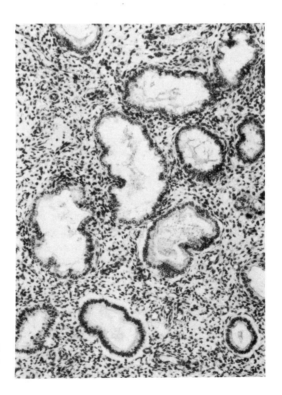

Figure 4. Midsecretory (day-21) endometrium showing low glandular epithelium and inspissated intraluminal secretion.

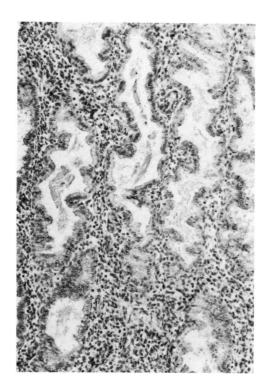

Figure 5. Late secretory (day-25) endometrium showing serrated glands with ragged cytoplasmic borders (secretory exhaustion) and sparse intervening connective tissue.

lymphocytic infiltration. Polymorphonuclear leukocytes, which first appear in large numbers on day 26, are obvious by day 27. According to Bardawil (1987), many of these alleged leukocytes may be distinct predecidual cells, in the shrunken cytoplasm of which granules (*Körnchenzellen*) are found. These granules may contain relaxin and lytic enzymes that play a role in the onset of menstruation. Microscopic areas of focal necrosis and hemorrhage appear a few hours before the onset of menstruation.

In the second half of the secretory phase, three strata, or zones, of endometrium can be distinguished. The zona compacta is the uppermost layer, so named because it consists of broad fields of compact hypertrophied stromal cells between the rather narrow necks of glands. The zona spongiosa is the middle zone, so called because of the lacy, labyrinthine appearance caused by the large numbers of dilated, tortuous glands with little intervening stroma. The zona basalis, the deepest layer, is in contact with the myometrium, because there is no uterine submucosa. The basalis is composed of bases of glands surrounded by dense stroma. The compacta and spongiosa form the zona functionalis. Part of the endometrium regenerates from the basal layer; by the time bleeding ceases, the endometrial surface is normally restored. During pregnancy, the zona compacta and the zona spongiosa are converted into decidua compacta and decidua spongiosa, respectively (Fig. 6).

2. Ultrastructure

2.1. The Normal Menstrual Cycle

Because the endometrium is a highly sensitive target tissue for the ovarian hormones, and because its morphological changes are critical in the investigation of infertility, it has been

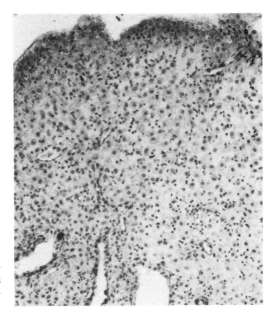

Figure 6. Decidua parietalis of early pregnancy showing transformation of stromal cells in the compact zone into large rounded and polygonal elements.

studied extensively by electron microscopy for 30 years. The following description is based on studies published from my laboratory and elsewhere (Borell *et al.,* 1959; Cavazos *et al.,* 1967; Colville, 1968; Gompel, 1962; Nilsson, 1962a,b; Sengel and Stoebner, 1970a,b; Themann and Schünke, 1963; Wessel, 1960; Wetzstein and Wagner, 1960; Wienke *et al.,* 1968; Wynn and Harris, 1967b; Wynn and Woolley, 1967).

Examination of endometrial ultrastructure reveals cytoplasmic secretion into the glandular lumina throughout the cycle. The terms ''secretory'' and ''proliferative'' therefore do not accurately reflect the histological pattern. Since various degrees of differentiation may occur in the same endometrium from area to area and even from cell to cell, ultrastructural dating is based on the most advanced consistent pattern in the specimen, as with histological classification. The basal endometrium remains essentially unchanged throughout the proliferative phase, whereas cyclic changes affect primarily the glands in the zona spongiosa. The superficial epithelium undergoes less obvious cyclic alteration. The pseudostratification noted with the light microscope is not seen in thin sections if tangential cuts are avoided. Endometrial nuclei during the preovulatory period are large, regular, and oval, with prominent nucleoli (Fig. 7). Mitotic figures are seen throughout the proliferative phase, most prominently in glandular epithelium and most frequently in midproliferative nuclei. The epithelial cytoplasm is poorly differentiated, containing numerous ribosomes but relatively few extensive channels of endoplasmic reticulum or elaborate Golgi complexes.

Mitochondria are scattered randomly throughout the cytoplasm in the early proliferative phase. Around the time of ovulation they are located primarily near the base of the cell. They then enlarge, forming prominent cristae and developing in relation to polyribosomes and perinuclear patches of glycogen. Shortly before ovulation the small accumulations of glycogen coalesce to form large deposits between the nucleus and the basal plasma membranes, resulting in well-defined structures that may be detected with the electron microscope about 2 days before the appearance of the typical ''subnuclear vacuole'' noted with the light microscope.

The Golgi apparatus increases in size during the midproliferative period, with the addition of flattened saccules and microvesicles. Microvilli are found on all well-preserved epithelial cells. Endometrial cells with typical cilia are found throughout the cycle, but they are much more common in the lower uterine segment and endocervix. Extensive pinocytosis is not

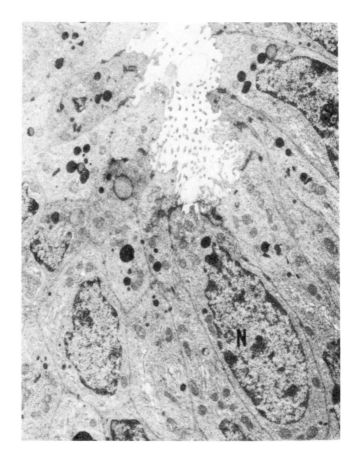

Figure 7. Low-power electron micrograph of early proliferative endometrium (tangential section) showing large, dense nuclei (N).

evident. Typical terminal bars and desmosomes occur between epithelial cells (Fig. 8). No annulate lamellae or myelin figures are seen in well-preserved normal endometrium.

The stromal changes in the preovulatory phase vary temporally and topically. Endometrial stroma is essentially ordinary moderately dense connective tissue, varying greatly in proportions of collagen, ground substance, and cells. The late proliferative stroma resembles that of the early secretory phase, which also is variable. The stromal nuclei are relatively large and usually denser than those of the epithelial cells. Mitotic figures are found throughout the proliferative phase, most regularly in the midproliferative. The usually scant cytoplasm may be reduced to a mere rim, surrounding the "naked nuclei" seen with the light microscope. Large numbers of endometrial granulocytes are uncommon, and plasma cells are rarely seen except around the time of the menses.

The changes in endometrial organelles during the proliferative phase thus reflect a pattern consistent with growth and endogenous metabolism rather than elaboration of proteins for export. The end of the proliferative phase is characterized by cessation of development of these organelles, possibly a "braking" effect of progesterone.

Ultrastructural features confined to the secretory phase have been identified. Confluent subnuclear patches of glycogen and large mitochondria can first be detected by electron microscopy on or about day 14, or approximately 36–48 hr before subnuclear vacuolation can be recognized by light microscopy (Fig. 9). The mitochondria that first appear about the time

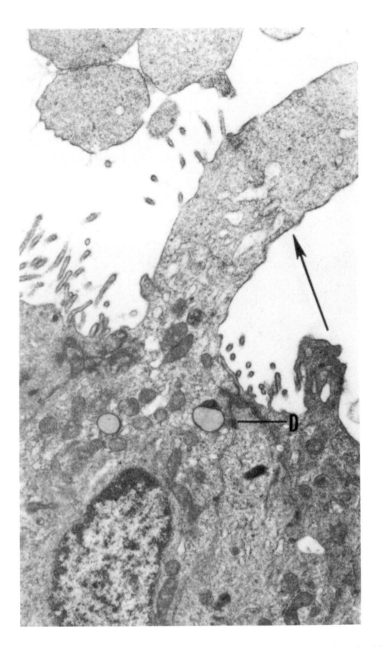

Figure 8. Midproliferative endometrium showing large cytoplasmic projection (arrow) into glandular lumen. Desmosome (D) joins adjacent epithelial cells.

of ovulation are several times larger than the typical organelles of the proliferative phase, and they have prominent cristae (Fig. 10). Not more than a few of these giant mitochondria are found in any individual cell. These giant mitochondria may be related to the increased energy required for the metabolism of glycogen. By day 17, deposits of glycogen are scattered diffusely through the cytoplasm, and supranuclear Golgi complexes are dense and well developed. Smaller mitochondria are distributed prominently between convolutions of the plasma membranes.

Between days 17 and 20, a characteristic nucleolar channel system is maximally conspic-

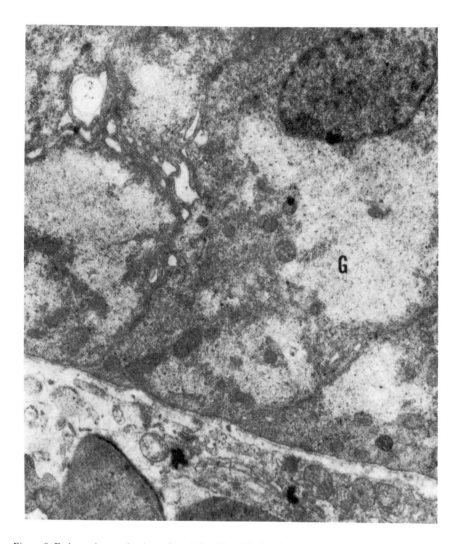

Figure 9. Endometrium at the time of ovulation (day 14) showing a subnuclear patch of glycogen (G).

uous (Fig. 11). This structure is described in detail in Section 2.2. Endoplasmic reticulum is not prominent, but mitochondria continue to enlarge and elongate, and convolutions of the plasma membranes continue to increase. By day 19 or 20, large projections from the surfaces of the glandular epithelial cells are found in association with extensive intraluminal secretion (Fig. 12). Organelles are sparse within the cytoplasmic promontories, although ribosomes, glycogen, and occasionally mitochondria and isolated reduced cisterns of endoplasmic reticulum may be seen.

The irregular protrusions from the apical surfaces of the luminal epithelial cells have been reinterpreted by Parr and Parr (1974). Because they observed these structures with all fixatives that they employed, they concluded that they were not artifacts of fixation. Reabsorption of ferritin from the uterine lumen of the rat on the fifth day of pregnancy suggested that these apical protrusions were involved in the formation of endocytotic vacuoles. Parr and Parr (1974) found no evidence that these apical protrusions were pinched off to form apocrine secretion. We have described secretory protrusions in the luteal phase of the human endo-

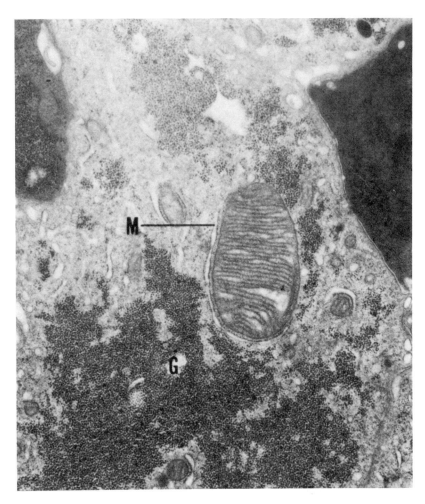

Figure 10. Early postovulatory endometrium showing a giant mitochondrion (M) and a subnuclear deposit of glycogen (G). (This patient had an intrauterine device *in situ* when the specimen was obtained.)

metrial cycle that resemble apocrine secretion (Wynn and Woolley, 1967), and similar structures have been described in other species.

Bulges from the apical surfaces of luminal or glandular epithelial cells in the luteal phase of the human endometrium were seen by Borell *et al.* (1959), Wessel (1960), Wynn and Woolley (1967), Colville (1968), and Armstrong *et al.* (1973). These authors suggested that the protrusions, after being pinched off, degenerate to form nutritive material for the embryo before implantation. Several studies, however, did not report the pinching off of these apical protrusions (Gompel, 1962; Cavazos *et al.,* 1967; Sengel and Stoebner, 1970b).

By about day 19 or 20, the cytoplasm has ceased to differentiate further. The Golgi apparatus, however, remains fairly complex, and the nuclei have returned from luminal to basal positions. Free cytoplasmic lipid and annulate lamellae are rarely seen in well-preserved tissues.

By day 22, intraluminal secretion is prominent, and the cells contain fewer intracytoplasmic secretory granules. There is little suggestion of pseudostratification. Apical microvilli are somewhat shorter, and epithelial cells themselves are lower. Basal laminae are thicker, and plasma membranes are maximally folded.

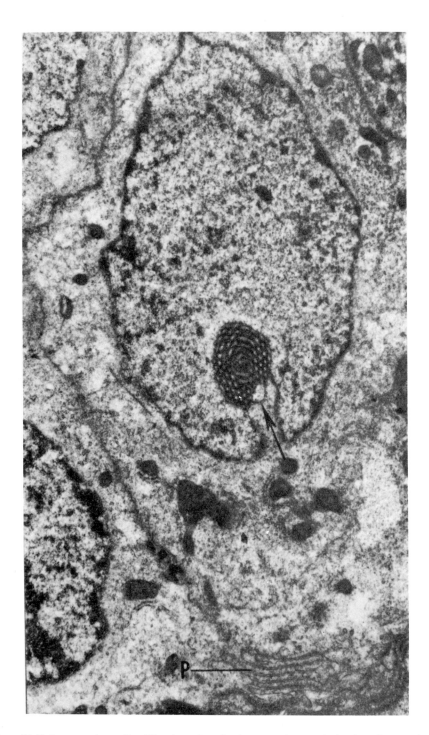

Figure 11. Early postovulatory (day-17) endometrium showing a prominent nucleolar channel system (arrow) and convoluted plasma membranes (P).

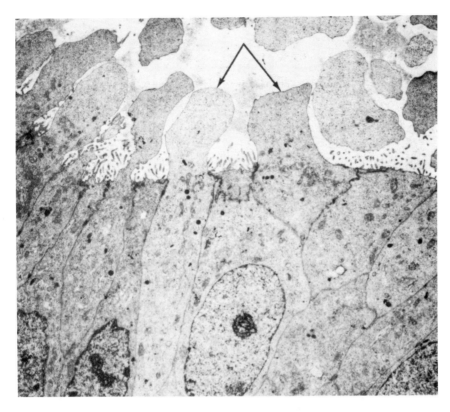

Figure 12. Midsecretory (day 20) endometrium showing apical secretion (arrows) into the glandular lumen.

By day 23, the granular endoplasmic reticulum has become less prominent, and the number of nucleolar channel systems has decreased greatly. Occasionally Golgi complexes still appear well developed, and deposits of glycogen and lipid are scattered throughout the epithelial cells. The slender, elongated mitochondria resemble those of decidual cells, and the plasma membranes are highly convoluted. Mitochondria are distributed basally and peripherally and small patches of glycogen are seen apically.

On day 24, isolated deposits of glycogen, large Golgi complexes, fragments of endoplasmic reticulum, and numerous small mitochondria are seen. The plasma membranes remain maximally convoluted, and complex intercellular spaces develop. Basal laminae of capillaries and epithelium may be separated by only wisps of connective tissue.

During the last few days of the cycle, the epithelial nuclei are basal; the apical surfaces are irregular; and the convolutions of the plasma membranes remain extensive. There are no consistent changes in size or number of microvilli. Nucleolar channel systems and giant mitochondria are not found.

In a cycle in which pregnancy does not occur, signs of cytoplasmic degeneration (stromal hemorrhage, increased numbers of lysosomes and lipid granules, and clumping of nuclear chromatin) appear by day 25. The morphological events of menstruation are discussed in Section 3.2. The decidual cell of pregnancy does not regress but maintains its numerous characteristic slender mitochondria and short cisterns of endoplasmic reticulum. The fibrillar connective tissue is condensed to form a "capsule" around the cell, and a characteristic epithelioid pattern is established (Fig. 13). Ultrastructural details of decidualization are found in Section 2.3.

Epithelial ultrastructural changes during the first half of the secretory phase of the cycle

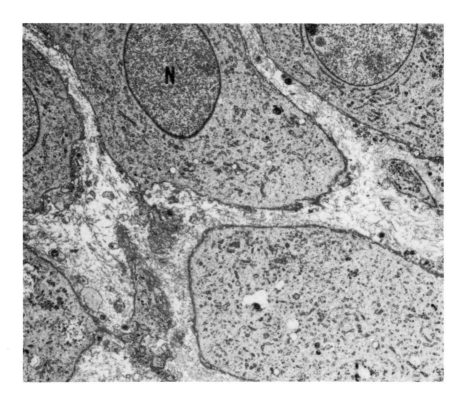

Figure 13. Parietal decidua from early (6 weeks) gestation showing rather poorly differentiated cytoplasm with numerous slender mitochondria, extensive intercellular matrix, and typical small, ovoid nuclei (N).

are well defined. The phase of maximal secretory activity is characterized by elaboration of glycoprotein granules associated with large mitochondria, polyribosomes, rough endoplasmic reticulum, and well-developed Golgi complexes. During the second postovulatory week, ultrastructural differentiation of the epithelium diminishes; the subsequent cyclic changes affect primarily the stroma.

Fine-structural development of the endometrial epithelium does not progress notably beyond the late preovulatory stages. The first half of the postovulatory phase is concerned with elaboration and secretion of cytoplasmic products into the glandular lumina. The second postovulatory week is concerned with development of the stroma into predecidual tissue.

2.2. *The Nucleolar Channel System*

The structure now commonly designated a nucleolar channel system (NCS) was first described by Dubrauszky and Pohlmann (1960), although its discovery is often credited to other investigators who reported it in the English literature several years later. Both the morphogenesis and the functional significance of this structure have generated considerable controversy. Two studies (Armstrong *et al.,* 1973; More *et al.,* 1974) have done much to explain this structure. Because it is found most commonly between days 17 and 20 of the normal cycle, it is easy to miss in specimens that are collected at other times of the cycle. Cavazos *et al.* (1967) and Cavazos and Lucas (1973), in their extensive studies of the endometrium, obtained samples at 5-day intervals (days 5, 10, 15, 20, and 25 of the normal human cycle). They therefore were unable to detect these structures, which are most prominent around day 19.

More *et al.* (1975) described a three-dimensional reconstruction of the NCS (Fig. 14). From the inner nuclear membrane arise two tubules, which form a nine-turn spiral to terminate bluntly at the apex. The NCS develops at the apex of an invagination of both inner and outer nuclear membranes. It is an ordered, hollow, spherical stack of interdigitating membrane-bound tubules, 60–100 nm in diameter, embedded in a dense matrix surrounding a core of lightly granular material. Toward the end of the cycle the NCS appears more commonly as a dense disordered mass of tubules lacking a central core, often occurring as a protrusion of the nucleus (More *et al.*, 1974).

More *et al.* (1974) suggest that the NCS may be extruded and possibly incorporated into giant lysosomes. They conclude that the NCS may be contiguous with the true nucleolus or separate from it. In assessing the function of the nucleolar channel system, they postulate that progesterone causes derepression of the genome, with the production of new varieties of messenger ribonucleic acid (mRNA). Several enzymes (Section 2.6) such as acid phosphatase and phosphorylase, which increase during the secretory phase, require the mediation of mRNA. Thus the NCS is thought to provide the pathway for rapid transport of new mRNA into the cytoplasm to act as a template for new protein. More *et al.* (1974) conclude that the NCS may not always be of nucleolar origin and suggest the term "nuclear channel system" as more appropriate.

Since the early 1960s it has been known that ovulation is followed shortly by three ultrastructural changes in the human endometrial epithelium: subnuclear accumulation of large deposits of glycogen in the glandular cells, appearance of giant mitochondria (Fig. 15), and formation of nucleolar channel systems (Fig. 16). In an attempt to separate the effects of

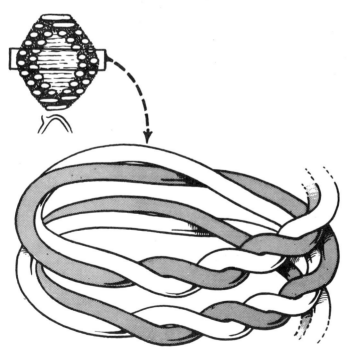

Figure 14. Schematic representation of a portion of the nucleolar channel system. Courtesy of Dr. Ian A. R. More.

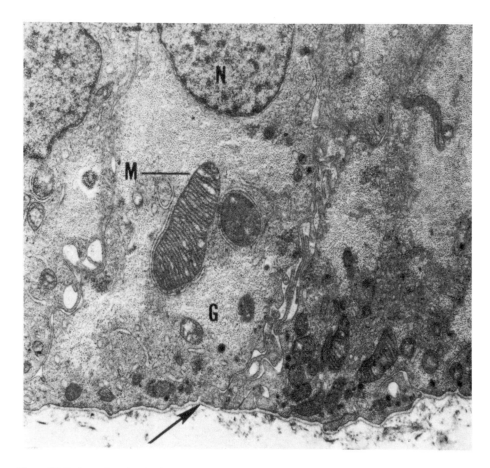

Figure 15. Endometrium shortly after ovulation (day 15 of a 28-day cycle), showing a giant mitochondrion (M) and glycogen (G) between the nucleus (N) and the basal lamina (arrow).

ovulation from those of the accompanying hormonal milieu, MacLennan *et al.* (1971) studied endometrial ultrastructure of the normally cycling baboon. The experimental plan was to castrate the baboon, replace steroidal hormones, and observe the effects on the development of the NCS. During the secretory phase of the cycle, glandular epithelial nuclei of the baboon develop a prominent nucleolonema that stands out from the pars amorpha. This structure is most pronounced the day after ovulation, but nothing comparable to the NCS of the human endometrium is found. The baboon thus proved to be an unsuitable model for study of the human NCS.

More recently, Pryse-Davies *et al.* (1979) have shown that the NCS could be produced *in vivo* by progesterone in postmenopausal endometrium; *in vitro* production also has been demonstrated. Thus, the appearance of the NCS does not necessarily indicate ovulation.

2.3. The Decidua

Formation of decidua is a unique example of rapid histogenesis in a normal adult mammal. Nevertheless, until the study by Wynn (1974), on which the following description is based, electron microscopy of the decidua had dealt almost exclusively with experimental animals, mainly rodents, and had provided only isolated fine-structural details of the human

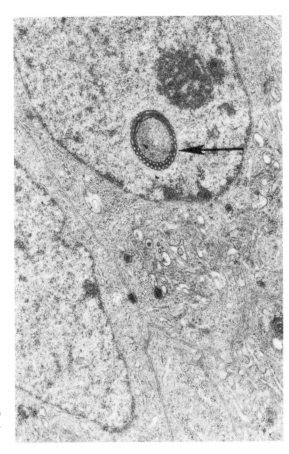

Figure 16. Early postovulatory (day-17) endometrium showing the nucleolar channel system (arrow).

decidua (Lawn *et al.,* 1971), often incidental to a discussion of the trophoblast. Although comparative studies may suggest biological principles, the great diversity in structure and function of the decidua among even closely related species requires knowledge of the human decidua to draw valid conclusions about such phenomena as implantation and its inhibition in man.

In this discussion, "decidua" refers to the pregnant endometrium (epithelium and stroma), some of which is shed at parturition, and a "decidual cell" refers specifically to the transformed polygonal glycogen-containing stromal cell. According to these definitions, even the closely related macaque, which forms an epithelial plaque rather than an extensive stromal reaction, is a poor model for the study of human decidual development.

To eliminate problems of histogenetic identification, the description that follows is confined to the parietal and capsular deciduas. The basal decidua and the complex elements that are often confused with trophoblast have been considered elsewhere (Wynn, 1967a, 1972).

The ultrastructural features of the human decidua are foreshadowed in the stromal cells of the endometrium during the second postovulatory week. The epithelial cells have convoluted plasma membranes, small slender mitochondria, large Golgi complexes, and relatively sparse microvilli. The major changes in endometrial development affect the stroma. Many of the cells are typical fusiform fibrocytic elements with moderately well-differentiated cytoplasm. The laminae externae of these stromal elements are well developed. Between stromal cells, tight junctions (maculae, zonae, and fasciae occludentes) but not true desmosomes are found. In addition, gap junctions may form between processes of the same cell. Unusual features of predecidual cells that are shared by the early true decidua are deep projections of one cell into

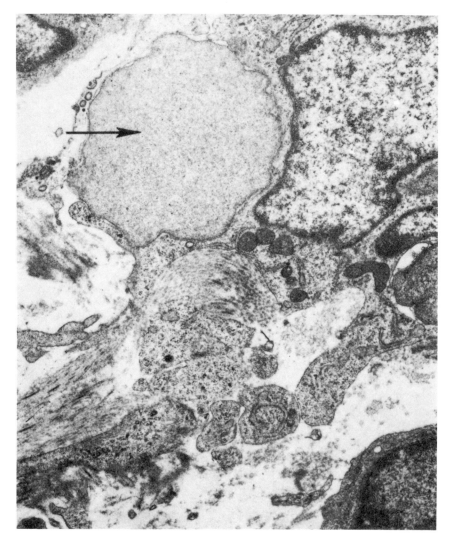

Figure 17. Predecidual cells of endometrial stroma on day 25 of the menstrual cycle. A cytoplasmic process of one cell (arrow) indents the cytoplasm of another.

the cytoplasm of another (Fig. 17). These invaginations of homogeneous cytoplasm resemble inclusions at low magnification, but intercellular membranes are seen with high resolution. Abundant collagen and fibrinoid, some of which appears to be intracellular, surround the stromal cells. Phagocytic activity in the decidual cells may facilitate the decidual reaction through removal of collagen from the endometrial stroma. Ciliated stromal elements are found in the secretory phase of the menstrual cycle as well as in true decidua.

The decidual reaction in human endometrium is accompanied by synthesis of prolactin. Maslar *et al.* (1986) reported that progesterone can induce and maintain decidualization and synthesis of prolactin in organ culture. They found, furthermore, that long-term production of prolactin is not maintained without progesterone. Paradoxically, progesterone exerts a transient inhibitory effect on production of prolactin. The interrelated phenomena of stromal differentiation and synthesis of decidual prolactin require further elucidation. A current study by Sakbun *et al.* (1987) reports, furthermore, that parietal decidual cells and the "decidua-like" cells of the basal plate of the placenta may produce relaxin in addition to prolactin.

During the first few months of gestation, the decidua parietalis and the decidua capsularis resemble each other in detail. Apparent secretory activity is maximal during the first 10 weeks. A transitional phase occurs during the tenth to 12th weeks, and ultrastructural evidence of diminution in activity follows during the 12th to 14th weeks. The capsularis usually disappears by the 14th week.

The decidual cell of early pregnancy is surrounded by fine reticular fibers and occasionally by fibrinoid. Its cytoplasm is generally homogeneous and moderately well developed. Some of the smaller cells appear better differentiated. The typical stromal cell has a large pale nucleus. The epithelium contains sparsely granular endoplasmic reticulum, most of it in vesicular form. Fine filaments course throughout the epithelium, occasionally forming a terminal web beneath the microvillous border, but they do not form bundles as they do in the connective tissue. Epithelial Golgi complexes are moderately well developed, and mitochondria are slender and dense. True desmosomes are found between adjacent epithelial cells.

By 6 weeks, the endoplasmic reticulum of the stromal cell has become maximally differentiated. The nuclear envelope remains smooth, and the collagenous extracellular material is compact. Unusual cytoplasmic features at this stage are projections of the plasma membrane containing extremely osmiophilic bodies (Fig. 18), many of which look like lysosomes and appear to be associated with the formation of extracellular coats. The delicate mitochondria remain small and numerous. A few of the better-differentiated elements resemble fibroblasts. The low ratio of nuclear to cytoplasmic size explains the apparent absence of nuclei from many sections of decidual cells.

By 8 weeks, the granular endoplasmic reticulum of the epithelial cell is maximally developed. Mitochondria are small and most abundant above the nucleus, which appears to be invaginated by numerous lipoprotein granules. The microvilli are low and scanty. Golgi complexes are moderately well developed and distended. The basal plasma membrane is highly convoluted. True desmosomes and tight junctions are prominent. At 8 weeks, many of the stromal cells lie very close to the basal lamina, and some seem to share certain ultrastructural features with the epithelium. The stromal cells near the capillaries are best developed. A few of the cells form extracellular spaces between the decidua and basal lamina that contain granules, some of which are consistent morphologically with procollagen (Fig. 19).

Tekelioğlu-Uysal *et al.* (1975) described coated and uncoated vesicles at the sites of frequent thickenings of the cell membrane. They interpreted these findings as evidence that the decidual cells are capable of extruding protein or proteinlike substances into the intercellular spaces. As described earlier by Wynn (1967a, 1972), the decidual cells of the trophoblastic junctional zone with their large Golgi complexes and well-developed endoplasmic reticulum appeared more active than did those of the parietal decidua.

At 10 weeks, the capsular decidua, which still resembles the parietal decidua, begins to regress (Fig. 20). The epithelium is laden with lipid and glycogen but contains relatively few organelles. Microvilli are found in reduced numbers. The stroma is still rich in granular endoplasmic reticulum, much of it in vesicular form, but more free ribosomes are noted at this stage. A few stromal cells are ultrastructurally complex, resembling basal decidual cells, but larger numbers are degenerate. Some of the fusiform decidual cells have cytoplasmic streamers.

By 12 weeks, even in the parietal decidua, degeneration of the epithelium is extensive. There is no further ultrastructural differentiation of the stroma beyond this stage. Processes of decidual cytoplasm make very close contact with capillary endothelium.

By 22 weeks, degeneration of the fusiform parietal stromal cells as well is noted, along with deposition of considerable basement-membrane-like material. Some of this deposit appears to be intracellular but more likely represents indentation of the cytoplasm from without.

At 28 weeks, the decidual cell contains short fragments of endoplasmic reticulum and

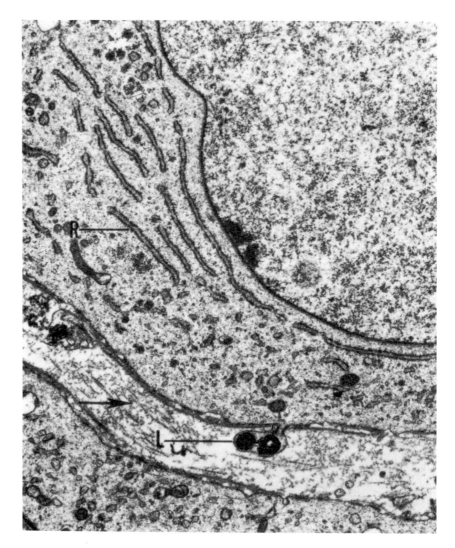

Figure 18. Decidua parietalis of early (6 weeks) gestation showing parallel channels of rough-surfaced endoplasmic reticulum (R). Lysosomelike bodies (L) are contained in projections from the decidual surface. Fibrillar material (arrow) forms an extracellular coat around the stromal cell.

Golgi complexes with prominent condensed tubules. Mitochondria remain small and delicate. Lamina externa, collagen, and fibrinoid are prominent. Fine fibrillar material appears to be discharged into the extracellular space from the stromal cytoplasm. A terminal web forms near the surface, as in epithelium.

At term, a thin layer of epithelium may be distinguished in certain portions of the decidua parietalis. The epithelial cells have low microvilli and prominent deposits of glycogen. Many of the stromal cells that lie close to the epithelium are surrounded by a lamina externa that closely resembles the basal lamina of the epithelium. The cytoplasm of the parietal decidual cell is homogeneous and not highly differentiated. Such an element cannot easily be confused with trophoblast, as can a complex basal decidual cell.

Wynn and Woolley (1967) found that after the first few postovulatory days there was no further increase in Golgi complexes or granular endoplasmic reticulum in the human endometrial epithelium. Only in the third week of the menstrual cycle do the stromal changes that

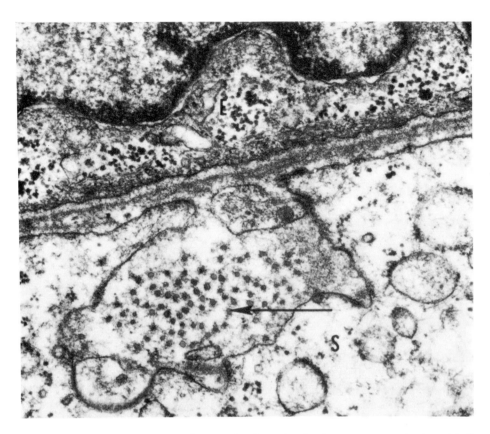

Figure 19. Detail of parietal decidual cell at 8 weeks of gestation showing numerous granules (arrow) in the space between epithelium (E) and stroma (S).

culminate in the decidual reaction appear. Specifically, on day 22, broader contacts between the decidual cells are found. On day 23, the individual stromal cells enlarge, and the cytoplasm is packed with glycoprotein. On day 25, the ground substance is more compact, and the first signs of regression occur if the patient is not pregnant. If pregnancy occurs, endometrial development progresses to form true decidua. In their study of the stromal cells during the second half of the cycle, Wienke *et al.* (1968) noted a "margin of condensation," which we interpret to be similar to a lamina externa. Tropocollagen, the precursor of collagen, is secreted into the extracellular space, where polymerization occurs. Collagen very likely functions to support the decidua, and the accumulated glycogen and glycoprotein nourish the early conceptus.

Lawn *et al.* (1971) studied the junctions between human decidual cells and concluded that they connected processes of the same cell rather than those between adjacent cells. Because these gap junctions in the human decidua could not form a significant barrier, Lawn *et al.* (1971) reasoned that the extracellular matrix was a more important mechanical barrier in human placentation. The dense extracellular material surrounding the mature human decidual cell is ultrastructurally similar to the basal lamina of the epithelium. Osmiophilic membrane-bound inclusions associated with well-developed endoplasmic reticulum and intracellular fibrils suggest intracellular secretion of this material, intracellular digestion, or a combination of these two processes.

Kearns and Lala (1983) have ascribed an immunologic role to the decidua. Among the relevant manifestations are suppression of the mixed lymphocyte reaction and the proliferative response of lymphocytes to cells of allogeneic grafts and T-cell mitogens.

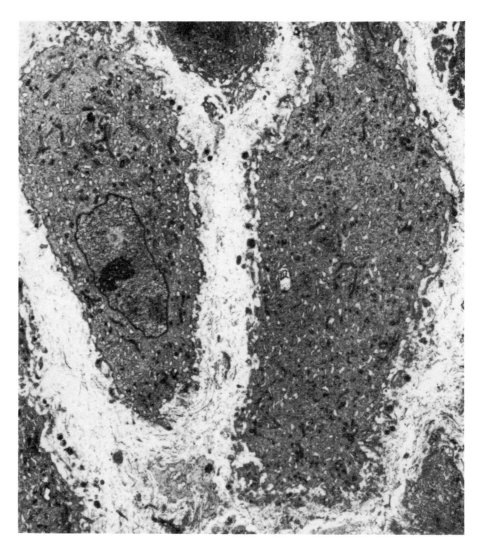

Figure 20. Decidua capsularis at 10 weeks of gestation showing slender mitochondria and small vesicles of endoplasmic reticulum. This tissue closely resembles the decidua parietalis at the same stage of gestation.

2.4. *The Arias–Stella Reaction*

The history of the endometrial morphological changes commonly associated with the name of Arias–Stella has been discussed by Wynn and Harris (1967a). These changes, associated with the proximity of chorionic tissue, are often described in connection with ectopic pregnancy, but they also have been identified in normal intrauterine pregnancy, abortion (De Brux and Ancla, 1964), and hydatidiform mole (Wynn and Harris, 1967a). The nuclear hypertrophy and abundant cytoplasmic secretion in the endometrial epithelium have been considered either a direct reponse to chorionic gonadotropin or an indirect effect mediated through hypersecretion of estrogen and progesterone. Thrasher and Richart (1972) pointed out that the Arias–Stella reaction differs ultrastructurally from carcinoma of the endometrium in that the distribution of chromatin is more homogeneous in the Arias–Stella endometrium. They concluded also that polyploidy, which presumably results from endomitosis and subsequent nuclear fusion, explains the abnormal appearance of the nuclei. In contrast, the nuclear DNA in endometrial carcinoma is usually nearly diploid or aneuploid. The excess secretion of hormones beyond that of the normal menstrual cycle was offered as an explanation of the increased size of the nucleus, the hyperchromatism, the polymorphism, and the loss of polarity.

According to Wynn (1974), the ultrastructural features of the epithelium are consistent with a hypersecretory interpretation of the Arias–Stella reaction (Fig. 21). The nuclei are large and irregular, but the chromatin is rather evenly distributed. Microvilli are low, and zonae adhaerentes are prominent. Parallel channels of granular endoplasmic reticulum, large mitochondria, and microtubules are abundant, particularly in supranuclear regions. The cytoplasm is crowded with many small oval mitochondria and lipoprotein granules. Some of the mitochondria lack cristae entirely; others have prominent transverse cristae. The Golgi complexes have numerous stacked saccules, and the plasma membranes are complexly interdigitated.

In his study of the endometrium associated with hydatidiform mole, Wynn (1974) found within the epithelium electron-rare intranuclear bodies with a fine filamentous structure and intramitochondrial crystalloids. The nuclear membrane was tortuous, and the prominent nucleolus was skeinlike. Near the nucleolus were electron-rare fields about 2 μm in diameter. Within these fields were round or oval structures containing numerous fine filaments (Fig. 22). Within the mitochondria, crystalloids about 0.5 μm in largest diameter appeared to lie between the cristae (Fig. 23). These findings probably reflect the high concentrations of steroidal and protein hormones that are associated with trophoblastic growths and very likely other gestational states as well.

2.5. Scanning Electron Microscopy

Scanning electron microscopy of the endometrium, notably by Ferenczy et al. (1972), Ferenczy and Richart (1974), and Johannisson and Nilsson (1972), has confirmed the findings of transmission electron microscopy and added important details about the luminal epithelial

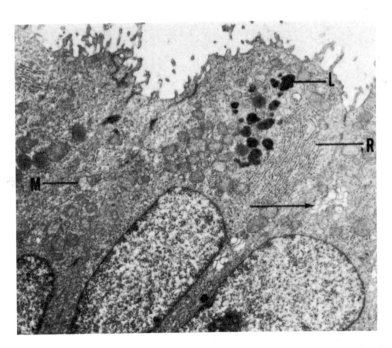

Figure 21. Endometrial epithelium associated with invasive hydatidiform mole showing the Arias–Stella reaction with numerous mitochondria (M), endoplasmic reticulum (R), osmiophilic droplets (L), and dilated Golgi complexes (arrow).

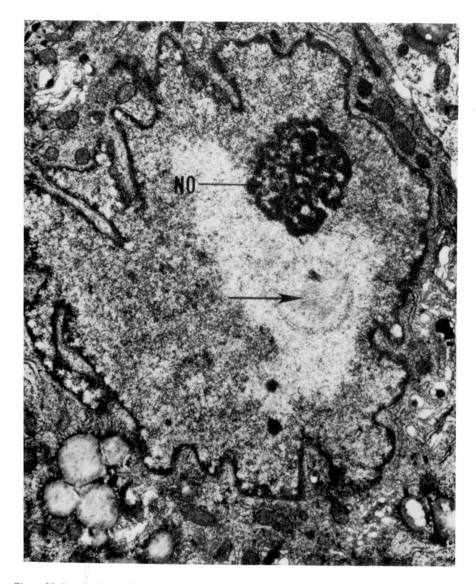

Figure 22. Detail of an endometrial epithelial nucleus associated with benign hydatidiform mole showing skeinlike nucleolus (NO) and an electron-lucent field containing an oval area with fine filaments (arrow).

surface and its cilia. In general, during the normal proliferative phase, the epithelium is composed of ciliated cells and low, nonciliated cells with small microvilli. Under the influence of estrogen, the number of ciliated cells and the size and abundance of the microvilli of the nonciliated cells increase. According to Johannisson and Nilsson (1972), during the secretory phase, the size and number of the microvilli decrease, and the protrusions of apical cytoplasm into the uterine lumen become more prominent. They stated that the cilia decrease during the secretory phase and degenerate during pregnancy and that cilia are more abundant near the cervix and around glandular orifices.

Ferenczy *et al.* (1972) also found changing proportions of dome-shaped, nonciliated to ciliated cells during the endometrial cycle. In the early proliferative phase (Fig. 24), the ratio of nonciliated to ciliated cells was about 30:1, whereas in the late proliferative phase (Fig.

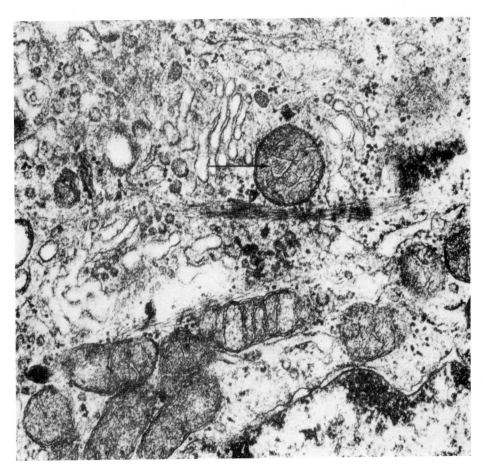

Figure 23. Detail of endometrial epithelial cytoplasm associated with benign hydatidiform mole showing a crystalloid structure (arrow) within a mitochondrion.

25), the ratio fell to 15:1. From day 21 on, the proportion of ciliated cells decreased to about 40 or 50 nonciliated cells to one ciliated cell, but ciliated cells were always readily identified throughout the postovulatory phase. Apocrine secretion is most readily identified by scanning electron microscopy between the 20th and 24th days of the cycle (Fig. 26).

Ferenczy *et al.* (1972) and most other workers agree that withdrawal of estrogen leads to deciliation. Masterson *et al.* (1975) concluded that the proportion of ciliated cells increases during the proliferative phase to reach a maximum of 20%, which is maintained during the ovulatory phase and then declines. This study also suggests that the precursors of ciliated cells are sensitive to estrogen and that the fall in their numbers during the secretory phase reflects negative influence of progesterone. Another study by More and Masterson (1975) suggests that the previously reported reduction in numbers of ciliated cells in the secretory phase may be only an apparent loss, resulting from heretofore unrecognized secretory activity of those cells.

Scanning electron microscopy confirms that the epithelium of the endometrial surface undergoes less cyclic change than does that of the glands. Perhaps the steadier rate of synthesis of ribonucleoprotein results in the greater number of ciliated cells and the earlier and more sustained appearance of cytoplasmic glycogen. With respect to the morphological response to the changing hormonal milieu, as exemplified by ciliogenesis, the epithelium of the superficial endometrium resembles that of the oviduct more than that of the endometrial glands.

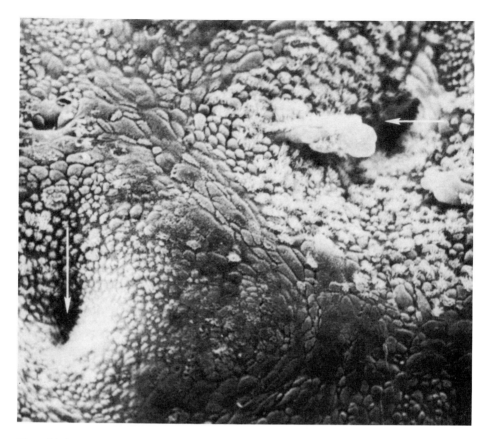

Figure 24. Scanning electron micrograph of an early proliferative endometrium showing glandular orifices (arrows) surrounded by ciliated cells. Courtesy of Dr. Alex Ferenczy.

Martel *et al.* (1981) provided a detailed scanning electron microscopic study of the surface of the luminal endometrial epithelium during the human menstrual cycle. They claimed that cyclic alterations in the luminal epithelial cells, particularly the nonciliated microvillous elements, permit dating of the endometrial biopsy to within 2 to 3 days and elucidated ultrastructurally many hormonally determined dysfunctional states.

Studies by both scanning and transmission electron microscopy demonstrate similar effects of the ovarian hormones on cyclic endometrial structure, as summarized by Ferenczy and Richart (1974). Estrogen stimulates rapid growth of cells by accelerating DNA-dependent synthesis of RNA. Estrogen also influences the metabolism of glycogen and phospholipid, the synthesis of alkaline and acid phosphatases, and the rate of mitosis. Progesterone causes further accumulation and secretion of glycogen, mucopolysaccharides, lipid, and hydrolytic enzymes. The principal morphological manifestations of secretory activity include the endoplasmic reticulum (protein), glycogen granules, mitochondria (phosphorylation), and Golgi complexes, which are involved in the formation of secretory vesicles containing mucopolysaccharides.

2.6. Ultrastructural Localization of Enzymes

Ultracytochemical studies of the human endometrial cycle have provided another means of correlating morphological changes with metabolic functions. According to Sawaragi and

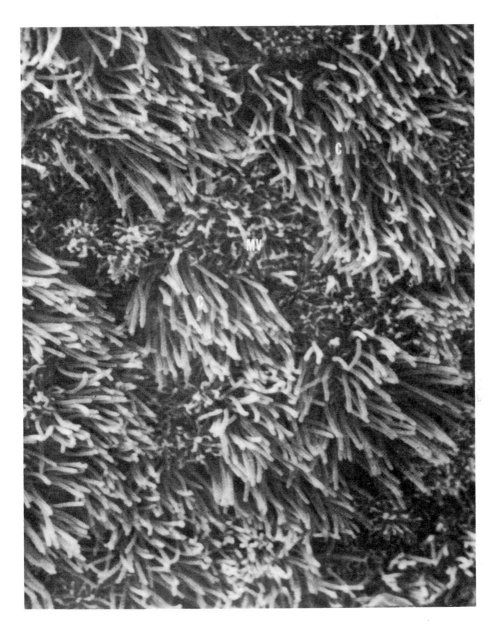

Figure 25. Scanning electron micrograph of a late proliferative endometrium showing clusters of ciliated (C) and microvillous, nonciliated (MV) cells. Courtesy of Dr. Alex Ferenczy.

Wynn (1969), alkaline phosphatase is found on epithelial plasma membranes throughout the proliferative phase and into the midsecretory phase (Fig. 27). Acid phosphatase is observed in lysosomes of glandular epithelium after day 21. The release of lysozyme from these structures may be an immediate precursor of menstruation (Section 3.2). Glucose-6-phosphatase is most evident around the time of ovulation and in the early secretory phase, localized mainly within cisternae of endoplasmic reticulum (Fig. 28). Adenosine triphosphatase was studied by Colville (1968), who found it on the cell membranes and microvilli in the proliferative but not the secretory phase.

Bardawil (1987) summarized the enzymatic changes throughout the menstrual cycle.

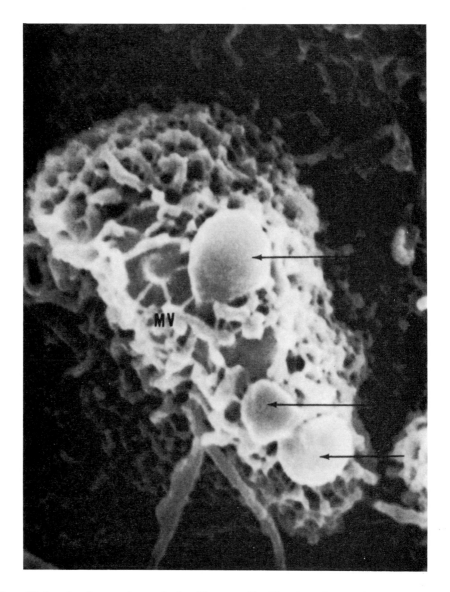

Figure 26. Scanning electron micrograph of a midsecretory (day-22) endometrium showing apical cytoplasmic projections (arrows) that resemble apocrine secretion. Microvilli (MV) are shorter and less abundant than those of the proliferative endometrium. Courtesy of Dr. Alex Ferenczy.

During the proliferative phase are found increases in alkaline phosphatase, β-glucuronidase, glucose-6-phosphatase, and reduced nicotinamide-adenine dinucleotide phosphate (NADPH) in addition to increases in RNA. During the secretory phase glycogen, glycoprotein, other proteins, and lipid are produced in association with increases in acid phosphatase, glucose-6-phosphate dehydrogenase, lactic dehydrogenase, succinic dehydrogenase, cytochrome oxidase, malic dehydrogenase, and isocitric dehydrogenase. The timed appearances of these enzymes during the endometrial cycle suggest that they are biochemical determinants of the events leading to menstruation, on the one hand, or implantation, on the other.

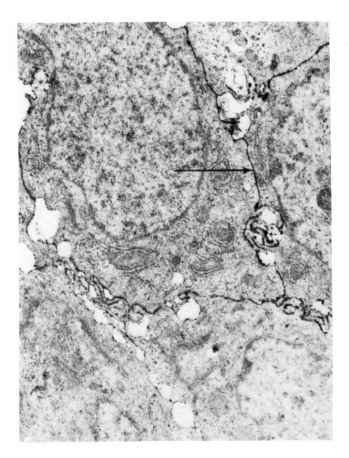

Figure 27. Midsecretory (day-21 to -22) endometrium showing persistence of the reaction product for alkaline phosphatase along plasma membranes (arrow).

3. Clinical Correlations

3.1. Effects of Contraceptive Agents

Studies of the effects of oral contraceptives on endometrial ultrastructure (Friedrich, 1967; Wynn and Sawaragi, 1969; Cavazos and Lucas, 1973) have in general been able to relate morphological alterations to the ratios and types of the estrogens and progestins and to the duration of administration of the drugs. As predicted by histological observations, the contraceptive steroids cause glandular atrophy and premature differentiation of the stroma into predecidua. Under cyclic therapy the cytoplasmic organelles in the glands are poorly developed, and protein synthesis appears minimal. The stromal elements in the secretory phase, however, have abundant glycogen and well-developed endoplasmic reticulum and Golgi complexes. With all conventional agents that presumably inhibit ovulation the nucleolar channel systems fail to develop. Maruffo *et al.* (1974) showed that both combined and sequential agents prevented morphological changes associated with ovulation (giant mitochondria and nucleolar channel systems). The now unavailable sequential agents, however, were associated with an endometrium that was more nearly normal histologically. These authors reported,

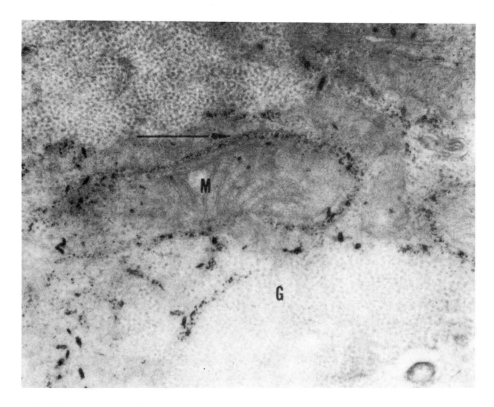

Figure 28. Early secretory (day-18) endometrium showing the reaction product for glucose-6-phosphatase in the endoplasmic reticulum (arrow) in proximity to a mitochondrion (M) and a deposit of glycogen (G).

furthermore, that well-developed rough-surfaced endoplasmic reticulum, giant mitochondria, and nucleolar channel systems were all present in the endometrium affected by megestrol acetate (17α-acetoxy-6-methyl-6-dehydroprogesterone), a low-dose progestin that presumably does not inhibit ovulation. This result might be expected if the nucleolar channel system is related to a specific range of ratios of estrogen to progestin, but unfortunately these authors did not illustrate the NCS in their paper.

Caution is required in the interpretation of the ultrastructural effects of steroidal contraceptive drugs. For example, the suggestion that pills containing only a progestin could cause progestational development of an endometrium unprimed by estrogen must be questioned in light of the knowledge that progestinic compounds such as quingestanol, a 3-enol ether of a δ4-3-ketosteroid, have potent intrinsic estrogenic properties. Detailed knowledge of the metabolic pathways of the synthetic progestins is thus requisite to an interpretation of their morphological effects.

Gudmundsson *et al.* (1987) studied the appearance of the endometrium subjected to 6 months of continuous treatment with nafarelin acetate, a GnRH superagonist, in daily doses of 125 or 250 μg. Using light and transmission electron microscopy they detected no endometrial hyperplasia but only signs of low metabolic activity and weak synthesis of protein.

Studies of the ultrastructural effects of the intrauterine device (IUD) have met with only limited success, largely because of the sampling errors inherent in the application of the electron microscope to histopathology. With the light microscope, Wynn (1968) was able to show no consistent histopathological effect of the IUD on the endometrium except for the inflammation in the vicinity of the device. Wynn (1967b) and Wynn and Sawaragi (1969), in ultrastructural studies, reported asynchronous development of the endometrium in proximity to the IUD. In a later study, Czernobilsky *et al.* (1975) concluded that the IUD exerts its effect through several mechanisms. They found asynchronous development of the endometrium in about one-third of their patients. Most of the asynchrony resulted from a delay in endometrial development, although in a few cases an advance was described, as previously reported by Wynn (1967b, 1968). Czernobilsky *et al.* (1975) unfortunately used patients with infertility as the controls, but their study nevertheless produced two significant findings. First, there was no correlation between the incidence of asynchrony and the duration of usage of the IUD. Second, the early secretory endometrium was often mixed with late proliferative in the patients with IUDs. Thus our earlier finding of nucleolar channel systems in "proliferative" endometrium (an indication of advanced ultrastructural development) might instead be interpreted to show late proliferative endometrium in the secretory phase (histological delay).

Nilsson *et al.* (1974) have used the electron microscope to elucidate the mode of action of the copper-coated IUD. They reported that "light areas" were less extensive in the endometria in contact with the Copper-T. The authors suggest that the Copper-T causes a decrease in endometrial α-amylase, with a resulting increase in content of glycogen in the secretory phase. The decrease in light areas in the endometrium associated with the IUD might indicate interference with the degradation of glycogen, perhaps as a result of enzymatic inhibition. Because these effects were seen only after long-term use of the copper IUD, there is still no explanation for the immediate contraceptive effectiveness of the device on the basis of an interference with endometrial metabolism of carbohydrates.

3.2. Menstruation

Morphological studies of the cyclic loss and regeneration of endometrial tissue have not yet provided an explanation for all the clinical phenomena of menstruation. McLennan and Rydell (1965) suggested that the loss of endometrial tissue was less extensive than earlier investigators had thought. In their opinion, regeneration of the uterine mucosa could occur from residual spongiosa rather than from the deepest elements of the basalis. If parts of the compact and spongy layers remain, some of the superficial portion of the endometrium during the so-called early proliferative phase would best be considered reorganization of tissue under a new epithelial cover rather than new growth.

Ferenczy (1976), in a study using scanning electron microscopy, concluded that the period of endometrial repair lasts about 48 hr, from about day 2–3 to about day 4–5. According to him, endometrial repair involves new formation of superficial epithelium and is initiated when the zona basalis is denuded of its overlying zona spongiosa. He believes that the epithelium of the endometrial surface is regenerated by simultaneous proliferation from two sources. The more important is the exposed ends of the basal glands, and the other is the persistent, intact superficial covering of the lower uterine and cornual segments. Ferenczy (1976) concluded that a lack of estrogen-dependent morphological phenomena such as mitosis and ciliogenesis suggests that the initial processes operating in endometrial reconstruction simply reflect repair of tissues and are independent of cyclic hormonal stimuli. Ferenczy (1976), moreover, noted no transformation of stromal cells into superficial epithelial cells. Baggish *et al.* (1967), however, earlier concluded that cells at the stromoepithelial border have a tendency to form metaplastic (squamoid) elements, which are later replaced by mature columnar cells.

In a more recent study, Ferenczy (1980) has provided further details of the processes of menstruation and endometrial regeneration. He believes that during repair of the endometrial surface migration of epithelial cells is followed by replication. The first epithelial cells involved in resurfacing are flattened, with abundant microvilli, intracellular intermediate filaments, microtubules, and pseudopodial projections. These features are thought to reflect ameboid motility that is promoted by cyclic adenosine monophosphate and the interaction of actin-containing filaments with myosin-containing plasma membranes. Ferenczy (1980) also suggested that kinetic and ultrastructural data do not support the view that new endometrium is regenerated directly from persistent spongiosa or stromal fibroblasts. He has suggested, furthermore, that fibroblasts contribute to endometrial epithelial repair indirectly, through their influence on growth factors and their provision of cellular support to the newly resurfacing epithelial cells.

Ultrastructural studies do not support the contention of McLennan and Rydell (1965) that endometrial healing involves rapid metamorphosis of residual secretory elements to proliferative tissue. Ferenczy (1976) has suggested, however, that prolonged menses might result from delayed separation of the functionalis from the underlying basalis and that anovulatory bleeding might result from superficial loss of mucosa not extending to the basalis. In both of these common clinical disorders, the basal zone must be freed from the overlying tissue, as can be accomplished by curettage, which then allows regeneration of the epithelium, thereby terminating the abnormal bleeding.

Henzl *et al.* (1972), among others, have attempted to formulate a lysosomal concept of menstruation. They noted an increase in acid phosphatase in the second half of the menstrual cycle and postulated that progesterone causes an accelerated development of lysosomes in the stroma. Downie *et al.* (1974) showed an increase in prostaglandin $F_{2\alpha}$ ($PGF_{2\alpha}$) up to the time of menses and a rise in PGE_2 during the luteal phase. If PG causes venous constriction, the resulting stasis could effect disruption of endothelial cells. With disintegration of the lysosomal membranes acid hydrolases would be liberated, thus further disrupting cell membranes and breaking down the endometrium. It may thus be possible to relate the cyclic variations in levels of estrogen and progesterone to prostaglandins, acid phosphatase, lysosomes, and, ultimately, menses.

4. Structural Vascular Changes in Normal and Hypertensive Pregnancies

Perhaps the most significant vascular lesion in the gravid endometrium is that described by Robertson *et al.* (1967). These investigators originally held that certain highly specific

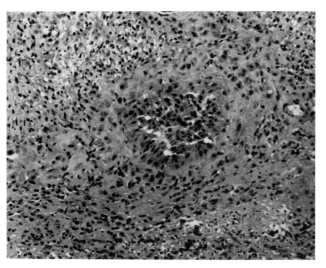

Figure 29. Basal decidua (placental bed) in the first trimester of pregnancy, heavily infiltrated with extravillous migratory trophoblast. A plug of endovascular trophoblast in a spiral (uteroplacental) artery initiates "physiological changes" in the maternal vessel. Courtesy of Professor W. B. Robertson.

changes could be identified in preeclampsia. The history of placental pathology in preeclampsia, including the lesion described by Robertson's group, was summarized by Wynn (1978). The major thesis of Robertson and co-workers is as follows. In normal pregnancy the ''physiological'' changes in the uterine vessels extend from the decidual terminations of the spiral arteries as far as the radial arteries deep in the myometrium. In all pregnancies, furthermore, the trophoblast produces extensive structural alterations in the maternal spiral arteries (Fig. 29). Brosens *et al.* (1972) reported that in preeclampsia these physiological changes are restricted to the decidual branches of the spiral arteries and fail to reach the myometrial trunks or radial arteries. In essential hypertension the myometrial arterial segments show hyperplastic

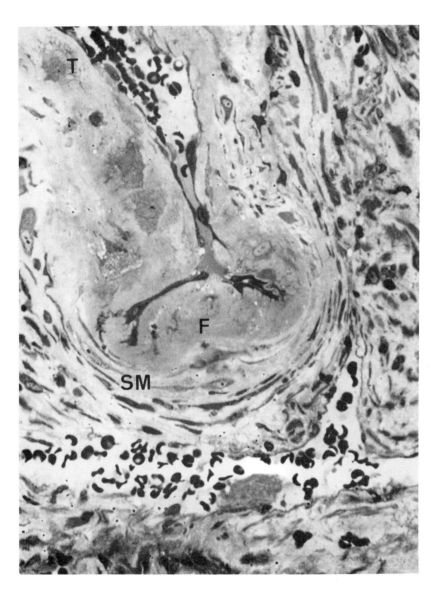

Figure 30. Thick section of a decidual spiral artery in the placental bed in normal pregnancy at term. The musculoelastic elements of the arterial wall are replaced by fibrinoid (F), in which large cells are embedded. Many of these cells appear to be trophoblastic (T). The vascular lumen is lined by an uninterrupted layer of endothelium. Focally, some smooth muscle cells (SM) in the outer layers of the media are preserved. Courtesy of Dr. Frank De Wolf.

arteriosclerosis. When preeclampsia is superimposed on essential hypertension, the physiological changes are still restricted to the decidual segments of the spiral arteries, but there is hyperplastic arteriosclerosis in the myometrial segments. These morphological features imply a reduced blood supply to the placenta from the start of a preeclamptic pregnancy. The onset of clinical manifestations in preeclampsia is accompanied by acute atherosis in the spiral arteries. This acute lesion is characterized by fibrinoid necrosis associated with an infiltration of foam cells. The basal arteries remain unaffected by these physiological changes. In the uteroplacental arteries in normal pregnancy, a convoluted layer of fibrinoid beneath the cellular intimal cushion replaces the internal elastic laminae, and externally cellular fibrous connective tissue replaces the muscular tunica media. In preeclampsia, the spiral artery at the myometriodecidual junction has a normal structure, and the myometrial arteries retain normal elastic tissue. The atherotic change comprises fibrinoid necrosis and the infiltration of

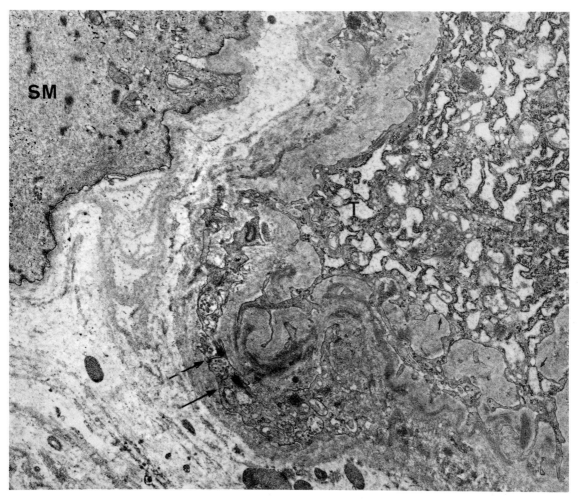

Figure 31. Electron micrograph of a spiral artery in normal pregnancy at term showing a smooth muscle cell (SM) and a trophoblastic cell (T) surrounded by amorphous material of moderate electron density. Long, narrow cytoplasmic processes are connected by desmosomes (long arrows). The endoplasmic reticulum is well developed, and its distended cisternae are filled with amorphous material. In places the membranes of the cisternae fuse with the plasma membranes of the cells (short arrows), suggesting that some of the peritrophoblastic fibrinoid is produced by these cells. Courtesy of Dr. Frank De Wolf.

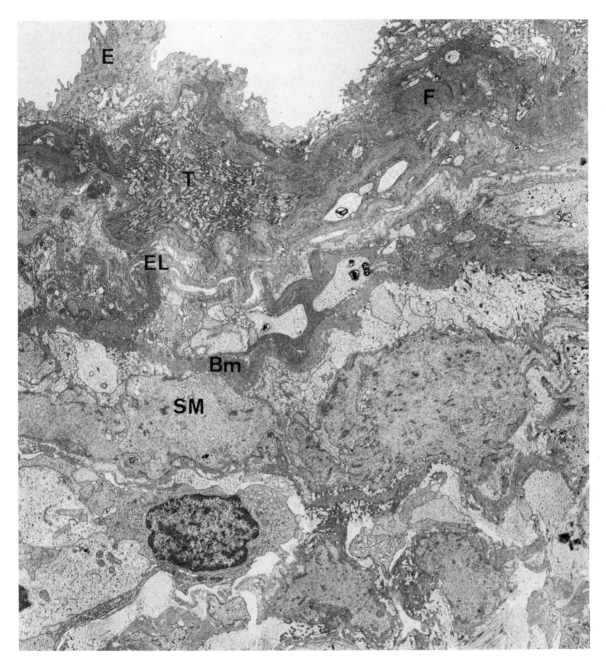

Figure 32. Spiral artery from the placental bed within the myometrium at about 14 weeks of gestation. The intima is lined by an uninterrupted hypertrophic endothelium (E) with villous projections from its surface. Beneath the endothelium is trophoblast (T) and closely related fibrinoid (F). Between the intima and the media, an elastic lamella (EL) may still be recognized. The smooth muscle (SM) of the media is somewhat disorganized, with an increase in interstitial fluid and ground substance and a thickening of the basement membrane (Bm). Courtesy of Dr. Frank De Wolf.

lipophages into the damaged vascular wall. In essential hypertension the hyperplastic changes involve all layers of the myometrial spiral artery.

In the first detailed electron microscopic studies of the spiral arteries in normal and hypertensive pregnancies, De Wolf *et al.* (1973, 1975) illustrated the atherotic lesion of preeclampsia (Figs. 30–37). They described endothelial damage, insudation of constituents of the plasma into the vascular wall, proliferation of myointimal cells, and medial necrosis. They stated that the fat accumulates first in myointimal cells; later, macrophages engulf lipid-rich debris from disintegrating myogenic foam cells. De Wolf *et al.* (1975) believe that the first evidence of arterial damage is fibrinoid necrosis and that the lipid changes are secondary. It is

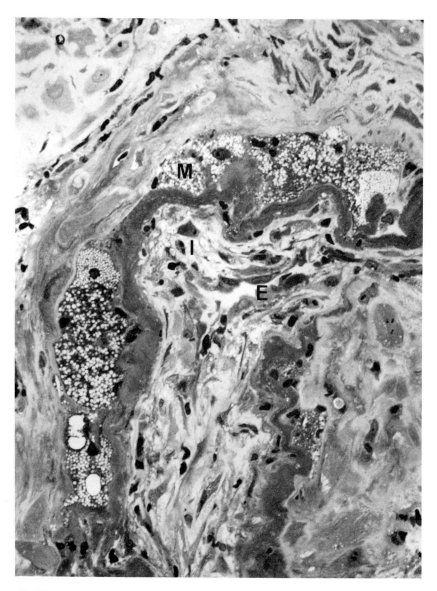

Figure 33. Thick section of decidual spiral artery in the placental bed in pregnancy complicated by severe preeclampsia. The vascular lumen is lined by endothelial cells (E). The intima (I) is thickened as a result of proliferation of myointimal cells, some of which show early accumulation of lipid. The smooth muscle of the media (M) is in an advanced stage of accumulation of lipid. Courtesy of Dr. Frank De Wolf.

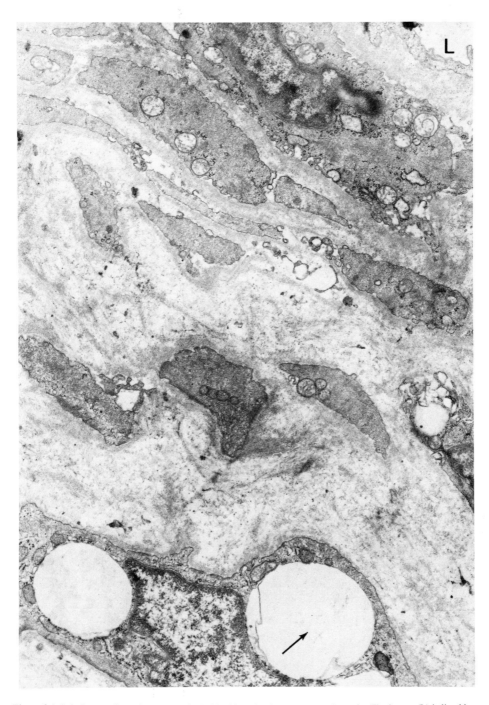

Figure 34. Spiral artery from the myometriodecidual junction in severe preeclampsia. The lumen (L) is lined by endothelium. The intima is thickened as a result of haphazard proliferation of myointimal cells, one of which shows extensive accumulation of lipid (arrow). Courtesy of Dr. Frank De Wolf.

important to be certain that the vessels are not altered by trophoblast before their structure is assessed. That is, atherosis may be diagnosed only in vessels that have been unaffected by physiological change. Thus, it is necessary to examine myometrial arterial segments, because physiological changes occur in both normal and preeclamptic pregnancies in the distal decidual segments. Robertson's (1967) definition of atherosis requires necrosis in the wall of a formerly normal vessel.

Sheppard and Bonnar (1976), in an ultrastructural study of the spiral arteries in pregnancy complicated by fetal growth retardation, reported occlusive lesions similar to those described by the Robertson group, irrespective of the presence or absence of hypertension. Brosens *et al.* (1977) countered that although there may be some restriction of physiological changes in fetal growth retardation without hypertension, the atherotic lesion was specifically associated with proteinuric preeclampsia.

In a more recent ultrastructural study, Sheppard and Bonnar (1981) again investigated the spiral arteries in hypertensive and normotensive pregnancies and in cases of fetal growth retardation. They reaffirmed their conclusion that identical lesions could be found in hypertensive and normotensive pregnancies complicated by fetal growth retardation, and they found no arteriopathy that was specific for preeclampsia. At the present writing, W. B. Robertson (personal communication, 1987) believes that in preeclampsia there is a defect in placentation in that only about 50 to 60% of the spiral arteries (100 to 150 in normal pregnancy) are converted to uteroplacental arteries by the action of migratory cytotrophoblast. In those arteries that are found in preeclampsia the physiological changes are restricted to the decidual seg-

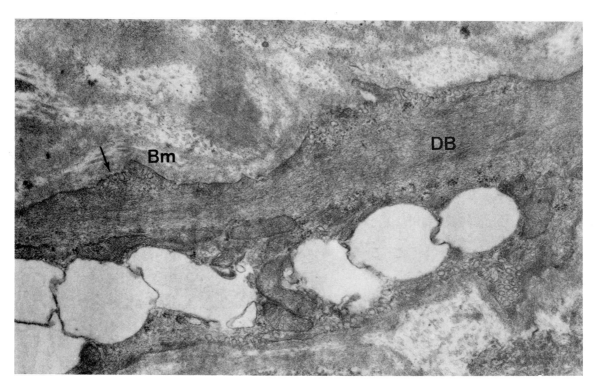

Figure 35. High-magnification electron micrograph showing detail of the vessel in Fig. 34. The myointimal cell has a basement membrane (Bm) and contains cytoplasmic filaments, dense bodies (DB), micropinocytotic vesicles (arrow), and an advanced degree of accumulation of lipid. Courtesy of Dr. Frank De Wolf.

ments, about 50% of which are so affected. In full-blown preeclampsia acute atherosis is found in myometrial segments of uteroplacental arteries, basal arteries, spiral arteries in the decidua parietalis, and spiral arteries in the basal decidua and basal plate that were missed by migratory trophoblast and hence did not undergo physiological changes. W. B. Robertson (personal communication, 1987) agrees that the atherotic lesion may be found in the basal plate and basal decidua in certain cases of fetal growth retardation in both normotensive and hypertensive pregnancies but not so constantly as in preeclampsia. He believes, furthermore, that the incidence of acute atherosis in preeclampsia is about 50% and that the extent of atherosis does not necessarily parallel the degree of hypertension. He suggests that the maternal vessels that are attached to the chorioamnion be examined more carefully to ascertain possible differences in the various complications of pregnancy. Robertson summarizes his thinking, correctly I believe, with the opinion that the arteriopathy of preeclampsia, although perhaps not pathognomonic, is at least highly characteristic of the disorder.

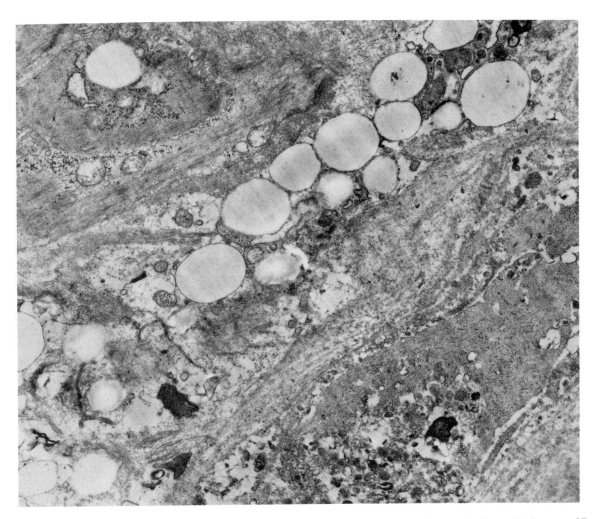

Figure 36. Intima of a spiral artery within the myometrium in severe preeclampsia showing a degenerative foam cell. Courtesy of Dr. Frank De Wolf.

ACKNOWLEDGMENTS. I am indebted to Professor Alex Ferenczy for the scanning electron micrographs and for helpful review of the manuscript; to Professor William B. Robertson for valuable discussions of the vascular lesions described in this chapter; to Dr. Frank De Wolf for the photomicrographs and electron micrographs of the vessels in normal and preeclamptic pregnancies; and to Dr. Raul M. Quillamor for his diligent editorial assistance.

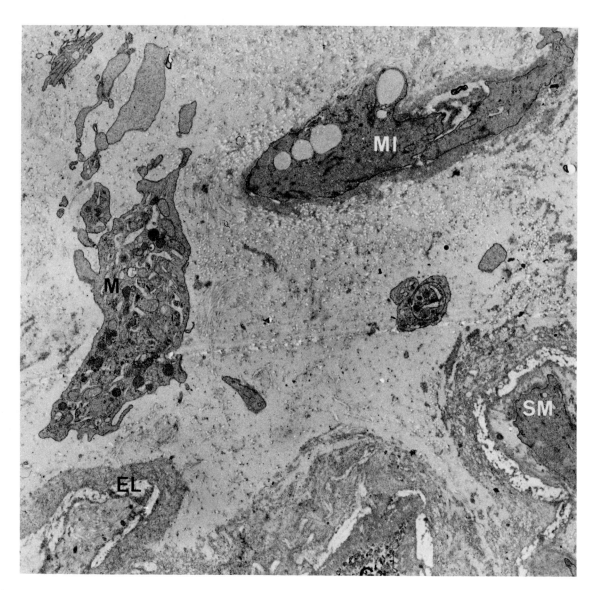

Figure 37. Myometrial segment of a spiral artery in severe preeclampsia. The intima (top) is separated from the media (bottom) by an elastic lamella (EL), the intimal side of which is associated with a band of fine granular and fibrillar material. Also shown are an intimal macrophage (M), a myointimal cell with early lipid vacuolation (MI), a medial smooth muscle cell (SM), and a degenerated medial ghost cell (G). Courtesy of Dr. Frank De Wolf.

Armstrong, E. M., More, I. A. R., McSeveney, D., and Chatfield, W. R., 1973, Reappraisal of the ultrastructure of the human endometrial glandular cell, *J. Obstet. Gynaecol. Br. Commonw.* **80:**446–460.

Baggish, M. S., Pauerstein, C. J., and Woodruff, J. D., 1967, Role of stroma in regeneration of endometrial epithelium, *Am. J. Obstet. Gynecol.* **99:**459–466.

Bardawil, W. A., 1987, Endometrium, in: *Gynecologic Endocrinology,* 4th ed. (J. J. Gold and J. B. Josimovich, eds.), Plenum Press, New York, pp. 185–245.

Borell, U., Nilsson, O., and Westman, A., 1959, The cyclical changes occurring in the epithelium lining the endometrial glands. An electron-microscopical study in the human being, *Acta Obstet. Gynecol. Scand.* **38:**364–377.

Brosens, I. A., Robertson, W. B., and Dixon, H. G., 1972, The role of the spiral arteries in the pathogenesis of preeclampsia, in: *Obstetrics and Gynecology Annual,* Volume 1 (R. M. Wynn, ed.), Appleton-Century-Crofts, New York, pp. 177–191.

Brosens, I., Dixon, H. G., and Robertson, W. B., 1977, Fetal growth retardation and the arteries of the placental bed, *Br. J. Obstet. Gynaecol.* **84:**656–664.

Cavazos, F., and Lucas, F. V., 1973, Ultrastructure of the endometrium, in: *The Uterus* (H. J. Norris, A. T. Hertig, and M. R. Abell, eds.), Williams & Wilkins, Baltimore, pp. 136–174.

Cavazos, F., Green, J. A., Hall, D. G., and Lucas, F. V., 1967, Ultrastructure of the human endometrial glandular cell during the menstrual cycle, *Am. J. Obstet. Gynecol.* **99:**833–854.

Colville, E. A., 1968, The ultrastructure of the human endometrium, *J. Obstet. Gynaecol. Br. Commonw.* **75:**342–350.

Czernobilsky, B., Rotenstreich, L., Mass, N., and Lancet, M., 1975, Effect of intrauterine device on histology of endometrium, *Obstet. Gynecol.* **45:**64–66.

De Brux, J., and Ancla, M., 1964, Arias–Stella endometrial atypias. Case study with the electron microscope, *Am. J. Obstet. Gynecol.* **89:**661–669.

De Wolf, F., De Wolf-Peeters, C., and Brosens, I., 1973, Ultrastructure of spiral arteries in the human placental bed at the end of normal pregnancy, *Am. J. Obstet. Gynecol.* **117:**833–848.

De Wolf, F., Robertson, W. B., and Brosens, I., 1975, The ultrastructure of acute atherosis in hypertensive pregnancy, *Am. J. Obstet. Gynecol.* **123:**164–174.

Downie, J., Poyser, N. L., and Wunderlich, M., 1974, Levels of prostaglandins in human endometrium during the normal menstrual cycle, *J. Physiol. (Lond.)* **236:**465–472.

Dubrauszky, V., and Pohlmann, G., 1960, Strukturveränderungen am Nukeolus von Korpusendometriumzellen während der Sekretionsphase, *Naturwissenschaften* **47:**523–524.

Ferenczy, A., 1976, Studies on the cytodynamics of human endometrial regeneration. I. Scanning electron microscopy, *Am. J. Obstet. Gynecol.* **124:**64–74.

Ferenczy, A., 1980, Regeneration of the human endometrium, in: *Progress in Surgical Pathology,* Volume 1 (C. M. Fenoglio and M. Wolff, eds.), Masson, USA, New York, pp. 157–173.

Ferenczy, A., and Richart, R. M., 1974, *Female Reproductive System: Dynamics of Scan and Transmission Electron Microscopy,* John Wiley & Sons, New York.

Ferenczy, A., Richart, R. M., Agate, F. J., Jr., Purkerson, M. L., and Dempsey, E. W., 1972, Scanning electron microscopy of the human endometrial surface epithelium, *Fertil. Steril.* **23:**515–521.

Friedrich, E. R., 1967, Effects of contraceptive hormone preparations on the fine structure of the endometrium, *Obstet. Gynecol.* **30:**201–219.

Gompel, C., 1962, The ultrastructure of the human endometrial cell studied by electron microscopy, *Am. J. Obstet. Gynecol.* **84:**1000–1009.

Gudmundsson, J. A., Lindgren, A., Lundkvist, Ö., Nillius, S. J., and Bergquist, C., 1987, Endometrial morphology after 6 months of continuous treatment with a new gonadotropin-releasing hormone superagonist for contraception, *Fertil. Steril.* **48:**52–56.

Henzl, M. R., Smith, R. E., Boost, G., and Tyler, E. T., 1972, Lysosomal concept of menstrual bleeding in humans, *J. Clin. Endocrinol. Metab.* **34:**860–875.

Hitschmann, F., and Adler, L., 1908, Der Bau der Uterusschleimhaut des geschlechtsreifen Weibes mit besonderer Berücksichtigung der Menstruation, *Monatsschr. Geburtshilfe Gynaekol.* **27:**1–82.

Johannisson, E., and Nilsson, L., 1972, Scanning electron microscopic study of the human endometrium, *Fertil. Steril.* **23:**613–625.

Kearns, M., and Lala, P. K., 1983, Life history of decidual cells: A review, *Am. J. Reprod. Immunol.* **3:**78–82.

Lawn, A. M., Wilson, E. W., and Finn, C. A., 1971, The ultrastructure of human decidual and predecidual cells, *J. Reprod. Fertil.* **26**:85–90.

MacLennan, A. H., Harris, J. A., and Wynn, R. M., 1971, Menstrual cycle of the baboon. II. Endometrial ultrastructure, *Obstet. Gynecol.* **38**:359–374.

Martel, D., Malet, C., Gautray, J. P., and Psychoyos, A., 1981, Surface changes of the luminal uterine epithelium during the human menstrual cycle: A scanning electron microscopic study, in: *The Endometrium: Hormonal Impacts* (J. de Brux, R. Mortel and J. P. Gautray, eds.), Plenum Press, New York, pp. 15–29.

Maruffo, C. A., Casavilla, F., Van Nynatten, B., and Perez, V., 1974, Modifications of the human endometrial fine structure induced by low-dose progestogen therapy, *Fertil. Steril.* **25**:778–787.

Maslar, I. A., Powers-Craddock, P., and Ansbacher, R., 1986, Decidual prolactin production by organ cultures of human endometrium: Effects of continuous and intermittent progesterone treatment, *Biol. Reprod.* **34**:741–750.

Masterson, R., Armstrong, E. M., and More, I. A. R., 1975, The cyclical variation in the percentage of ciliated cells in the normal human endometrium, *J. Reprod. Fertil.* **42**:537–540.

McLennan, C. E., and Rydell, A. H., 1965, Extent of endometrial shedding during normal menstruation, *Obstet. Gynecol.* **26**:605–621.

More, I. A. R., and Masterson, R. G., 1975, The fine structure of the human endometrial ciliated cell, *J. Reprod. Fertil.* **45**:343–348.

More, I. A. R., Armstrong, E. M., McSeveney, D., and Chatfield, W. R., 1974, The morphogenesis and fate of the nucleolar channel system in the human endometrial glandular cell, *J. Ultrastruct. Res.* **47**:74–85.

More, I. A. R., Armstrong, E. M., and McSeveney, D., 1975, Observations on the three-dimensional structure of the nucleolar channel system of the human endometrial glandular cell, *J. Anat.* **119**:163–167.

Nilsson, O., 1962a, Electron microscopy of the glandular epithelium in the human uterus. I. Follicular phase, *J. Ultrastruct. Res.* **6**:413–421.

Nilsson, O., 1962b, Electron microscopy of the glandular epithelium in the human uterus. II. Early and late luteal phase, *J. Ultrastruct. Res.* **6**:422–431.

Nilsson, O., Hagenfeldt, K., and Johannisson, E., 1974, Ultrastructural signs of an interference in the carbohydrate metabolism of human endometrium produced by the intrauterine copper-T device, *Acta Obstet. Gynecol. Scand.* **53**:139–149.

Noyes, R. W., Hertig, A. T., and Rock, J., 1950, Dating the endometrial biopsy, *Fertil. Steril.* **1**:3–25.

Parr, M. B., and Parr, E. L., 1974, Uterine luminal epithelium: Protrusions mediate endocytosis, not apocrine secretion, in the rat, *Biol. Reprod.* **11**:220–233.

Pryse-Davies, J., Ryder, T. A., and MacKenzie, M. L., 1979, *In vivo* production of the nucleolar channel system in postmenopausal endometrium, *Cell Tissue Res.* **203**:493–498.

Robertson, W. B., Brosens, I., and Dixon, H. G., 1967, The pathological response of the vessels of the placental bed to hypertensive pregnancy, *J. Pathol. Bacteriol.* **93**:581–592.

Sakbun, V., Koay, E. S. C., and Bryant-Greenwood, G. D., 1987, Immunocytochemical localization of prolactin and relaxin C-peptide in human decidua and placenta, *J. Clin. Endocrinol. Metab.* **65**:339–343.

Sawaragi, I., and Wynn, R. M., 1969, Ultrastructural localization of metabolic enzymes during the human endometrial cycle, *Obstet. Gynecol.* **34**:50–61.

Sengel, A., and Stoebner, P., 1970a, Ultrastructure de l'endomètre humain normal. I. Le chorion cytogène, *Z. Zellforsch.* **109**:245–259.

Sengel, A., and Stoebner, P., 1970b, Ultrastructure de l'endomètre humain normal. II. Les glandes, *Z. Zellforsch.* **109**:260–278.

Sheppard, B. L., and Bonnar, J., 1976, The ultrastructure of the arterial supply of the human placenta in pregnancy complicated by fetal growth retardation, *Br. J. Obstet. Gynaecol.* **83**:948–959.

Sheppard, B. L., and Bonnar, J., 1981, An ultrastructural study of utero-placental spiral arteries in hypertensive and normotensive pregnancy and fetal growth retardation, *Br. J. Obstet. Gynaecol.* **88**:695–705.

Tekelioğlu-Uysal, M., Edwards, R. G., and Kişnişçi, H. A., 1975, Ultrastructural relationships between decidua, trophoblast and lymphocytes at the beginning of human pregnancy, *J. Reprod. Fertil.* **42**:431–438.

Themann, H., and Schünke, W., 1963, The fine structure of the glandular epithelium of the human endometrium, electron microscopic morphology, in: *The Normal Human Endometrium* (H. Schmidt-Matthiesen, ed.), McGraw-Hill, New York, pp. 99–134.

Thrasher, T. V., and Richart, R. M., 1972, Ultrastructure of the Arias–Stella reaction, *Am. J. Obstet. Gynecol.* **112**:113–120.

Tsibris, J. C., Fort, F. L., Cazenave, C. R., Cantor, B., Bardawil, W. A., Notelovitz, M., and Spellacy, W.

N., 1981, The uneven distribution of estrogen and progesterone receptors in human endometrium, *J. Steroid Biochem.* **14**:997–1003.

Wessel, W., 1960, Das elektronenmikroskopische Bild menschlicher endometrialer Drüsenzellen während das menstruellen Zyklus, *Z. Zellforsch.* **51**:633–657.

Wetzstein, R. H., and Wagner, H., 1960, Elektronenmikroskopische Untersuchungen am menschlichen Endometrium, *Anat. Anz.* **108**:362–375.

Wienke, E. C., Cavazos, F., Hall, D. G., and Lucas, F. V., 1968, Ultrastructure of the human endometrial stroma cell during the menstrual cycle, *Am. J. Obstet. Gynecol.* **102**:65–77.

Wynn, R. M., 1967a, Fetomaternal cellular relations in the human basal plate. An ultrastructural study of the placenta, *Am. J. Obstet. Gynecol.* **97**:832–850.

Wynn, R. M., 1967b, IUDs: Effects on ultrastructure of human endometrium, *Science* **156**:1508–1510.

Wynn, R. M., 1968, Fine structural effects of intrauterine contraceptives on the human endometrium, *Fertil. Steril.* **19**:867–882.

Wynn, R. M., 1972, Cytotrophoblastic specializations: An ultrastructural study of the human placenta, *Am. J. Obstet. Gynecol.* **114**:339–355.

Wynn, R. M., 1974, Ultrastructural development of the human decidua, *Am. J. Obstet. Gynecol.* **118**:652–670.

Wynn, R. M., 1978, The placenta in preeclampsia, in: *Hypertensive Disorders in Pregnancy* (F. K. Beller and I. MacGillivray, eds.), Georg Thieme, Stuttgart, pp. 45–49.

Wynn, R. M., and Harris, J. A., 1967a, Ultrastructure of trophoblast and endometrium in invasive hydatidiform mole (chorioadenoma destruens), *Am. J. Obstet. Gynecol.* **99**:1125–1135.

Wynn, R. M., and Harris, J. A., 1967b, Ultrastructural cyclic changes in the human endometrium. I. Normal preovulatory phase, *Fertil. Steril.* **18**:632–648.

Wynn, R. M., and Sawaragi, I., 1969, Effects of intra-uterine and oral contraceptives on the ultrastructure of the human endometrium, *J. Reprod. Fertil. Suppl.* **8**:45–57.

Wynn, R. M., and Woolley, R. S., 1967, Ultrastructural cyclic changes in the human endometrium. II. Normal postovulatory phase, *Fertil. Steril.* **18**:721–738.

Endometrial Hyperplasia and Neoplasia

ALEX FERENCZY and
CHRISTINE BERGERON

The pathogenesis of endometrial hyperplasia and its relationship to carcinoma have long been issues of concern to students of endometrial pathology (Hertig and Sommers, 1949; Hertig *et al.*, 1949; Beutler *et al.*, 1963; Gusberg and Kaplan, 1963; Vellios, 1972; Gusberg *et al.*, 1974; Welch and Scully, 1977; Tavassoli and Kraus, 1978; Fox and Buckley, 1982; Ferenczy *et al.*, 1983; Kurman *et al.*, 1985; Ferenczy, 1988). More specifically, the morphological diagnosis, the potential for invasive carcinoma, and the appropriate treatment of hyperplastic endometria remain hotly debated and controversial subjects. Difficulties in obtaining consensus have resulted from several complex factors, both morphological and clinical. For example, histologically benign endometrial glands may present with worrisome architecture, mimicking malignancy, whereas glandular cells with a benign appearance or very subtle cytological modifications may demonstrate extensive invasive growth patterns of well-differentiated carcinoma.

An even more important reason for our fragmentary knowledge and poor understanding of the natural history of endometrial hyperplasia has been the inability to construct and carry out statistically meaningful long-term prospective follow-up studies on patients with endometrial hyperplasia without interfering with its biological behavior (Gusberg *et al.*, 1974). Indeed, in most patients presenting with abnormal uterine bleeding, the initial diagnostic ascertainment was made by endometrial curettage. This procedure may remove the entire abnormal endometrium, thus being therapeutic as well as diagnostic. Conversely, the curettage may not sample the entire endometrial lining, and the areas of greater histological or cytological severity may escape microscopic identification. In such cases, the initially obtained endometrial sample is histologically underdiagnosed and incorrectly interpreted as a "progressive

---

ALEX FERENCZY and CHRISTINE BERGERON ● Departments of Pathology and Obstetrics and Gynecology, McGill University and The Sir Mortimer B. Davis Jewish General Hospital, Montreal, Quebec H3T 1E2, Canada.

lesion," and the undetected disease is eventually discovered on follow-up. Other limitations of most of the earlier prospective studies included small numbers of patients followed for only a relatively short period of time and the use of pelvic radiotherapy to control uterine bleeding associated with a hyperplastic endometrium with or without presumed potential for carcinoma (Gusberg *et al.*, 1974). Ionizing radiation even at relatively small doses may be potentially carcinogenic to the endometrium. This in turn may result in an artificially high rate of neoplasia in lesions not otherwise at risk for carcinoma.

All these pitfalls and drawbacks in studying the human endometrium in pathological states have led to a confusing, nonreproducible, and therapeutically irrelevant terminology (Winkler *et al.*, 1984) and to a poor understanding of their precise natural history. Nevertheless, the general and traditional concept that has developed over the years is that women with endometrial hyperplasia are at increased risk of developing carcinoma (Hertig *et al.*, 1949; Beutler *et al.*, 1963; Vellios, 1972; Gusberg *et al.*, 1963, 1974; Welch and Scully, 1977; Tavassoli and Kraus, 1978; Fox and Buckley, 1982; Ferenczy *et al.*, 1983; Kurman *et al.*, 1985; Ferenczy, 1988). Endometrial hyperplasias were thought, furthermore, to form a histological and presumably biological spectrum that begins with a simple exaggeration of the normal proliferative state and ends with a highly atypical form representing the most significant state prior to invasive carcinoma (Hertig and Sommers, 1949; Hertig *et al.*, 1949; Beutler *et al.*, 1963; Gusberg *et al.*, 1963, 1974; Welch and Scully, 1977; Tavassoli and Kraus, 1978). Supporting further the concept of a continuum is the relatively frequent finding of coexistent hyperplasia and adenocarcinoma in the same endometrium (Beutler *et al.*, 1963; Welch and Scully, 1977; Tavassoli and Kraus, 1978).

In recent years several attempts have been made to subdivide this spectrum by both clinical and laboratory means into more homogeneous and therapeutically as well as prognostically relevant categories (Fox and Buckley, 1982; Colgan *et al.*, 1983; Aausems *et al.*, 1985; Kurman *et al.*, 1985; Ferenczy, 1988). The results of these studies have challenged the existing concept and suggest that the risk of endometrial carcinoma is not uniform in women with so-called hyperplasia but is concentrated in those with cytological atypia. This chapter reviews both the laboratory and clinical evidence that has led to a reinterpretation of the traditional data and the development of a two-disease, hyperplasia and neoplasia, concept as opposed to that of a continuum.

1. Laboratory Evidence

1.1. Histology

Endometrial proliferations without cytological atypia constitute a group of lesions displaying a variety of architectural alterations ranging from simple (Fig. 1A,B) to complex (Fig. 1C,D). In the former, the most common form of hyperplasia, the architecture deviates little from the normal proliferative endometrium. The glands vary in size; many are voluminous, others are dilated, and still others are normal or even small. The lining epithelium is usually formed of pseudostratified tall and columnar cells (Fig. 1A,B) or, in cystic dilated glands, flat cuboidal cells. The ratio of stroma to glands is normal because the stroma is also hypercellular. The gland cells lack cytological atypia, and numerous normal mitoses may be present in both epithelial and stromal cells. These lesions are traditionally named anovulatory, persistent proliferative endometrium, cystic glandular hyperplasia, or simple or mild hyperplasia (Hertig and Sommers, 1949; Hertig *et al.*, 1949; Beutler *et al.*, 1963; Gusberg *et al.*, 1974; Vellios, 1974; Welch and Scully, 1977; Tavassoli and Kraus, 1978; Fox *et al.*, 1982; Ferenczy *et al.*,

1983). The terms adenomatous hyperplasia, moderate hyperplasia, or complex hyperplasia refer to voluminous glands with complex convolutions and epithelial buddings into the adjacent and reduced stroma (Fig. 1C,D). The lining epithelium of these glands, however, is formed of regular tall columnar cells with no nuclear atypia.

In contrast to the aforementioned lesions, endometrial proliferations with cytological atypia are characterized by glandular cells with enlargement, rounding, and pleomorphism of the nucleus, loss of polarity, and clumped or coarse nuclear chromatin with macronucleoli (Fig. 2A,B). The cytoplasm may be reduced or relatively abundant, with a clear or granular appearance, and is sometimes eosinophilic. These cytological alterations are usually accompanied by glandular alterations, including crowding with a "back-to-back" pattern and intraluminal tufting (Fig. 2B), which produces a cribriform or "gland-in-gland" pattern. The stroma/gland ratio is usually in favor of the glands. These lesions are referred to variously as atypical adenomatous hyperplasia, severe hyperplasia, hyperplasia with cytological atypia, atypical complex hyperplasia, or carcinoma *in situ* (Hertig *et al.*, 1949; Beutler *et al.*, 1963; Vellios, 1974; Gusberg *et al.*, 1974; Welch and Scully, 1977; Tavassoli and Kraus, 1978; Fox and Buckley, 1982; Ferenczy *et al.*, 1983; Kurman *et al.*, 1985).

Epithelial proliferations with cytological atypia that are no longer confined to the glands include well-differentiated adenocarcinoma. By definition, such lesions invade either the stroma (intramucosal carcinoma) or the myometrium. Intramucosal carcinomas usually replace large portions of preexisting stroma, or the glands have ragged contours or an extensive papillary pattern and are associated with a desmoplastic, inflammatory, or necrotic reaction of the invaded stromal tissue (Fig. 3) (Kurman *et al.*, 1982). These histological criteria delineate biologically significant lesions with a greater likelihood of metastasis than those in which invasion is absent.

1.2. Electron Microscopy

Viewed with the transmission electron microscope, endometrial proliferations without cytological atypia have ultrastructural features that correspond to hyperestrogenic states (Ferenczy and Richart, 1974; Ferenczy *et al.*, 1979, 1983; Fenoglio *et al.*, 1982). The glands are rich in mitochondria, Golgi apparatus, free and bound ribosomes, primary lysosomes, and intermediate filaments (Fig. 4A). Scanning electron microscopy demonstrates increased numbers of cilia and alkaline-phosphatase-rich surface microvilli compared with cyclic proliferative endometrium (Fig. 4B) (Table 1). The spindle-shaped fibroblasts resemble those of middle or late proliferative endometrium except for extracellular collagen synthesis, evidence for which is minimal. These ultrastructural alterations suggest that nuclear DNA synthesis, a prerequisite for the mitotic phase of the cell cycle, prevails rather than production of extracellular collagen fibers. The stroma in hyperplasia frequently contains lipid-laden foam cells in close contact with the adjacent spindle-shaped stromal fibroblasts (Ferenczy and Richart, 1974). Lipid bodies contain cholesterol, a precursor of sex steroids. It is not clear whether endometrial foam cells in hyperplasia are merely a reflection of estrogenic stimulation or are also related to intraendometrial steroid metabolism (Dallenbach and Rudolph, 1974).

Endometrial proliferations with cytological atypia display significant qualitative and quantitative modifications in the organization of intracellular organelles (Ferenczy and Richart, 1974; Fenoglio *et al.*, 1982; Ferenczy *et al.*, 1983), which are pleomorphic and disorganized (Fig. 5A). Because of cellular crowding, the cytoplasmic membranes are irregular and complexly convoluted. Estrogen-dependent ciliogenesis, microvilli (Fig. 5B), and primary lysosomal activity are decreased, and the nuclear membrane is distended.

The abovementioned changes are similar to those seen in well-differentiated invasive carcinoma (Ferenczy and Richart, 1974; Ferenczy *et al.*, 1983). However, the number of

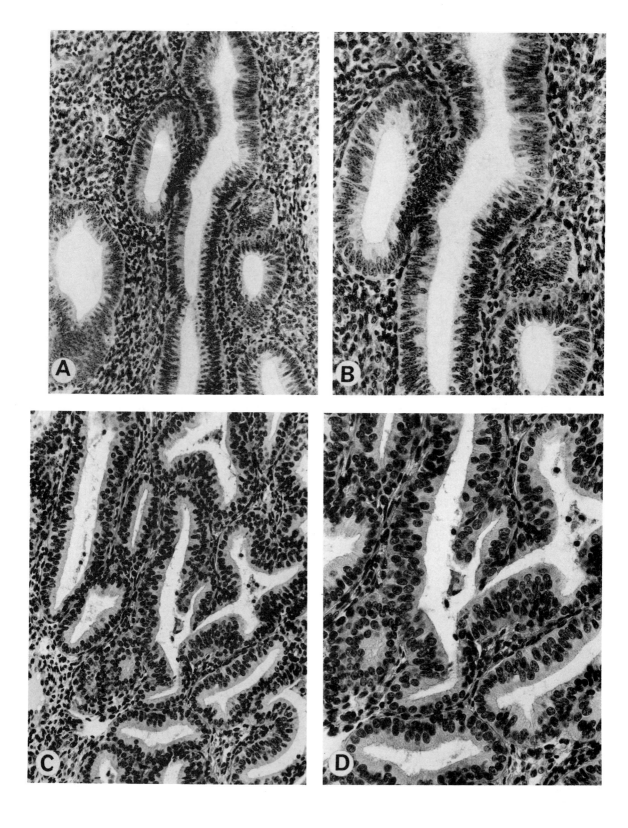

ciliated cells is further reduced, as is the length of surface microvilli, and cytonuclear pleomorphism is more pronounced (Fig. 6A,B). Specialized estrogen-related cellular changes are rare or absent in poorly differentiated grade 3 endometrial carcinomas, probably as a reflection of neoplastic dedifferentiation rather than of reduced estrogenic stimulation. Indeed, neoplastic dedifferentiation of endometrial epithelial cells results in loss or impairment of the cellular mechanisms that are necessary to respond to estrogens.

1.3. Morphometry, DNA–Feulgen Microspectrophotometry, and Flow Cytometry

With quantitative cytomorphology, morphometry allows objective assessment of a variety of morphological features and has recently been applied to diagnostic pathology (Baak and Oort, 1983). Stereological features and nuclear characteristics have been measured so that one lesion can be compared with another. The most constant stereological discriminators in the endometrium are the volume percentages of the epithelium and glands and the inner surface density of the glands (Baak et al., 1981). The best nuclear discriminators are the standard deviation of nuclear area and nuclear perimeter (Colgan et al., 1983; Aausems et al., 1985; Oud et al., 1986; Roberts et al., 1986; Fu et al., 1988). These criteria express best the degree of dispersion that corresponds to an increase in nuclear atypia and pleomorphism.

Hyperplasias without cytological atypia contain morphometric discriminators closer to normal than to invasive carcinoma, whereas those with cytological atypia resemble carcinomas (Table 1). In one study (Colgan et al., 1983), nuclear features predicted progression of hyperplasia with cytological atypia to carcinoma with 80% accuracy.

Unfortunately, measurements of DNA content by Feulgen microspectrophotometry and flow cytometry, used to distinguish between cellular proliferations with and without invasive potential as well as between normal and invasive carcinoma, are not useful for study of the endometrium (Wagner et al., 1967; Sachs et al., 1974; Feichter et al., 1982; Iversen, 1986). Unlike the situation in precancerous and cancerous conditions in general (Atkin, 1976), in which nuclear aneuploidy corresponds to significant chromosomal alterations with numerous markers, most well-differentiated endometrial adenocarcinoma cells and their precursors have diploid or near diploid nuclear DNA content indistinguishable from that of either normal or hyperplastic glandular cells (Sachs et al., 1974; Feichter, 1982; Iversen, 1986). The reason for the ''normal'' DNA content in invasive and noninvasive endometrial neoplasia is not clear, but it is also found frequently in other sex-steroid target organs such as the breast (Trent, 1985) and prostate (Stephenson et al., 1987). The high proportion of diploid carcinomas may reflect the generally better prognosis of endometrial compared to ovarian (Friedlander et al., 1983) and cervical carcinomas (Jakobsen, 1984).

Cytogenetic studies of endometrial and breast carcinomas (Katayama and Jones, 1967; Trent and Davis, 1979; Trent, 1985; Couturier et al., 1986; Gibas and Rubin, 1987) demonstrate only subtle numerical (trisomy $1q$ or 10) rather than structural aberrations of the chromo-

---

Figure 1. Endometrial proliferations without cytological atypia. (A) Endometrial hyperplasia (also referred to as mild or simple hyperplasia or anovulatory persistent proliferative endometrium). The glands are voluminous with lateral epithelial buddings (arrow) but overall resemble glands seen in late proliferative endometrium (H&E, ×250). (B) At higher magnification, the glands are lined by regular columnar cells with pseudostratified pencil-shaped nuclei. The chromatin is finely granular and evenly distributed. Nucleoli are visible (H&E, ×450). (C) Endometrial hyperplasia (also referred to as moderate or complex hyperplasia or adenomatous hyperplasia). The glands are voluminous, and their architecture is complex. They are in tight apposition and have epithelial buddings into the stroma. The glands occasionally have a Y-shaped configuration (middle). (D) At still higher magnification, there is slight rounding of the nuclei, which lack cytological atypia (H&E, ×450). From Ferenczy and Gelfand (1986), with permission.

somes, in keeping with the diploid to near-diploid DNA values found by DNA–Feulgen microspectrophotometry in these lesions. Moreover, one study (Trent and Davis, 1979) found similar alterations in D-group chromosomes in both endometrial carcinoma and "hyperplasia." Unfortunately, the authors provided no information about the presence or absence of cytological atypia in their hyperplastic lesions. The lack of nuclear aneuploidy produces normochromasia and often hypochromasia of nuclei on routine H&E sections, making the distinction between exuberant hyperplasia and early well-differentiated adenocarcinoma difficult on the basis of the appearance of nuclear chromatin alone.

1.4. In Vitro DNA Histoautoradiography

With use of a labeled nucleoprotein precursor such as tritiated thymidine, the cytokinetics, including duration of the S phase of DNA synthesis and cell-doubling time of endometrial tissues, can be evaluated on a semiobjective basis. The S phase coupled with the cell-doubling time of hyperplasia without cytological atypia is similar to that of proliferative endometrium (Table 1). In contrast, the duration of the S phase and the cell-doubling time in cytologically atypical lesions, including invasive carcinoma, are significantly longer than in hyperplasia without such atypia (Ferenczy, 1983) (Table 1). Prolongation of the DNA S phase of the cell cycle is a frequent feature of both intraepithelial and invasive neoplasia.

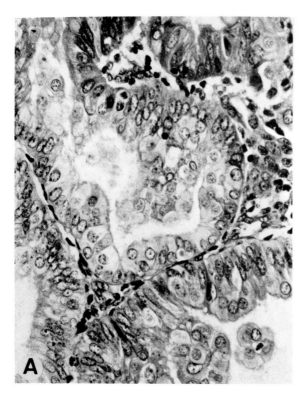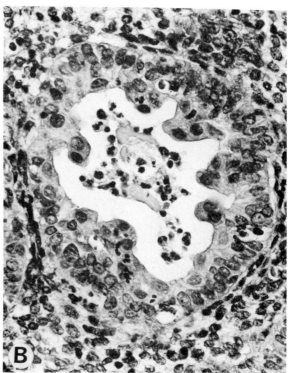

Figure 2. Endometrial proliferations with cytological atypia or endometrial intraepithelial neoplasia (EIN) (also referred to as atypical adenomatous or severe hyperplasia). (A) The glands contain intraluminal tufting and budding but are surrounded by stroma. The gland cells have abundant eosinophilic cytoplasm and "irregular" nuclear pseudostratification with prominent nucleoli. Cellular cohesion is lost (H&E, ×250). (B) A large gland is lined by cells with tiny papillary intraluminal projections. The nuclei are rounded and pleomorphic with coarse, aggregated chromatin. The stromal cells resemble those of proliferative endometrium, and there is no evidence of invasion (H&E, ×250). From Ferenczy and Gelfand (1986), with permission.

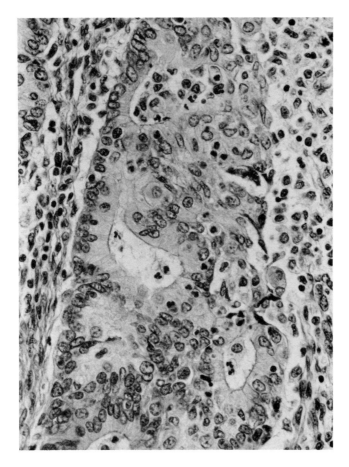

Figure 3. Well-differentiated invasive adenocarcinoma of the endometrium. Invasion of the stroma is evidenced by the ragged outline of the neoplastic gland and an inflammatory stromal response (H&E, ×250).

1.5. Immunohistochemistry

Sex steroid hormones regulate the growth of the endometrium. Normal endometrial growth is estradiol (E_2) dependent, and progesterone (Pg) inhibits E_2-mediated endometrial cell proliferation. The presence of estrogen receptors (ER) and progesterone receptors (PgR) is a prerequisite for the expression of E_2 and Pg actions, respectively (Clark *et al.*, 1985). Synthesis of PgR is regulated mainly by E_2, and its presence reflects the E_2 sensitivity of a target tissue (Leavitt *et al.*, 1977). Earlier studies using tissue homogenates (charcoal-coated receptor binding assays) found both ER and PgR elevated in hyperplasias and reduced in neoplasia (Janne *et al.*, 1979; Shyamala and Ferenczy, 1981). These methods, however, fail to provide data on the precise localization of receptors within the various components of human endometrium. The recently developed monoclonal antibodies to ER and PgR (King and Greene, 1984; Sullivan *et al.*, 1986) can trace sex steroid receptors by immunocytochemistry, and their relative distributions in epithelium and stroma can be evaluated. Both normal and hyperplastic endometria without cytological atypia display a high content of ER and PgR in both the epithelium and the stroma (Fig. 7A,B) (Bergeron *et al.*, 1988a,b). These results confirm the E_2 sensitivity of these tissues and suggest an intact ER mechanism. Their potential to respond to progesterone or progestagens is evidenced by their high PgR concentrations.

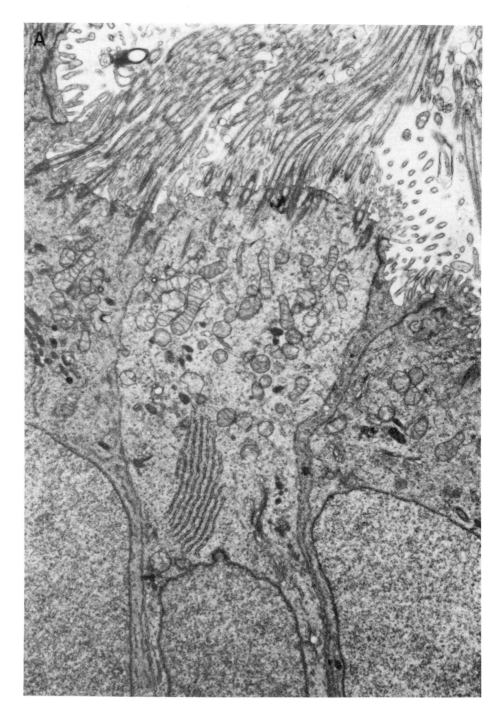

Figure 4. Endometrial hyperplasia. (A) Mature ciliated cells have abundant mitochondria, free and bound ribosomes, and Golgi apparatuses. Ciliary shafts alternate with slender microvilli (×5800). (B) The endometrial surface is composed predominantly of ciliated cells (×5640). Insert: The nonciliated cells have more numerous microvilli and microvillous promontories than do those of cystic glandular hyperplasia (×21,600).

In contrast, hyperplastic endometria with cytological atypia contain lower concentrations of ER and PgR in the epithelium (Fig. 8A,B), and the levels are comparable to those of invasive carcinoma (Fig. 9A,B) (Bergeron *et al.,* 1988a,b). This finding suggests a relative epithelial insensitivity to E_2 in these abnormal endometria and a low potential to respond to progesterone or progestagens (see Section 2). Interestingly, the ER and PgR contents in the stroma of cytologically atypical endometrial tissues, including invasive carcinoma, remain high. It has been suggested that in various tissue systems, particularly in targets of steroid hormones, epithelial growth is dependent on a mesenchymal support, which in turn is controlled by sex steroid hormones (Cunha *et al.,* 1983; Kratochwil, 1986). Whether ER and PgR play a role in mediating an E_2-dependent paracrine (extracellular) regulation of the epithelium as previously suggested is unknown (Cunha *et al.,* 1983).

On the basis of the available pertinent laboratory evidence it appears that hyperplasias with and without cytological atypia are made of different epithelial cell populations. Those without atypia are an exaggeration of normal, cyclic proliferative endometrium, whereas those with atypias are precursors of invasive carcinoma. If cytological atypia makes it possible to distinguish precursors of carcinoma (intraepithelial neoplasia) from nonprecursors (hyperplasia), then lesions with and without atypia should be named differently to emphasize their different morphology and natural history (Table 2). Endometrial lesions with cytological atypia may be referred to by a unifying generic term *endometrial intraepithelial neoplasia* (EIN) rather than by confusing and clinically meaningless names such as atypical adenomatous

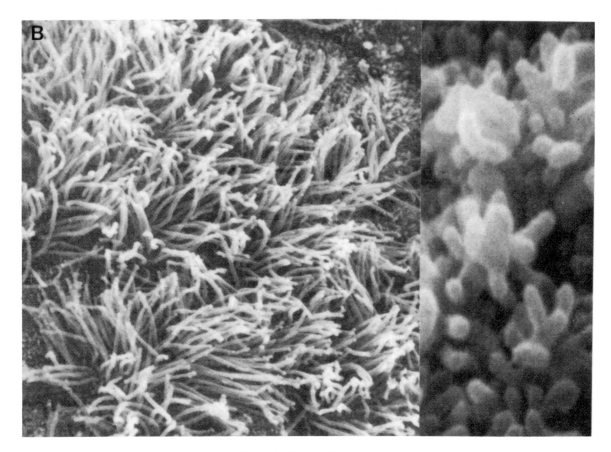

Figure 4. (Continued)

hyperplasia, severe hyperplasia, or carcinoma *in situ*. Such nomenclature should, in time, lead to easier and more appropriate therapeutic decisions. It is important to emphasize that the term "neoplasia" is not synonymous with invasive carcinoma. Rather, it refers to a lesion that, in contrast to hyperplasia, rarely regresses, tends to persist or recur after conservative treatment, and may progress to carcinoma.

2. Clinical Evidence

Most cases of asymptomatic endometrial hyperplasias are found incidentally in a regressed form in elderly, estrogen-deprived women in whom the uterus is removed for prolapse or at autopsy. Histologically, the endometrium is thickened and polypoid and retains the

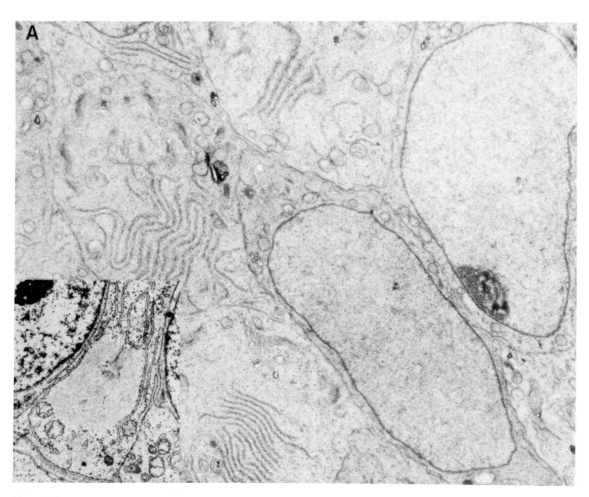

Figure 5. Endometrial intraepithelial neoplasia. (A) Nuclei are enlarged and pleomorphic. The GER–Golgi element–mitochondria complex is well developed, but primary lysozomes and glycogen particles are rare (×7900). Insert: Microfilaments tend to aggregate in the basal portion of neoplastic cells, and membranes of GER often appear in a complex, convoluted pattern (×8450). (B) There is a sharp decrease in the number of ciliated cells compared with hyperplastic endometrium. The nonciliated cells have short microvilli and exhibit variation in shape and size. Individual cell degeneration, suggested by ruptured and wrinkled surface plasma membranes, is a commonly encountered feature (×4550).

exaggerated height of a hyperplastic mucosa (Ferenczy, 1987). However, the glandular cells are definitely atrophic, as is the stroma, which is fibrotic. Similarly, most lesions associated with bleeding are reversible to normal proliferative, to secretory, or to persistent atrophic endometrium by one or more curettages or by progestagenic suppressive therapy (Wentz, 1966; Eichner and Abellera, 1971; Gal, 1986; Kurman et al., 1985; Ferenczy and Gelfand, 1988).

In a prospective study of 65 postmenopausal women with histologically proven endometrial hyperplasia followed for a mean period of 7 years, an 80% complete response rate has been obtained with cyclic progestagen therapy consisting of 10 mg medroxyprogesterone acetate (Provera) daily for 14 days a month (Ferenczy and Gelfand, 1988). Similar experience has been published by others (Kurman et al., 1982; Gal, 1986). Of greater significance, none of the lesions in these 65 patients, including the 20% with persistent and recurrent hyperplasia, progressed to carcinoma during the 7-year follow-up period. The low or negligible risk of carcinoma in women with endometrial hyperplasia seems to be supported by an earlier long-term longitudinal study by McBride (1959). He failed to find higher rates of carcinoma (4/1000) than in the general population (6–9/1000) (Koss et al., 1981) in his series of 500 postmenopausal women with endometrial hyperplasia whom he followed from their premenopausal years. Although occasional progression of endometrial hyperplasia to carcinoma has been reported (Chamlian and Taylor, 1970; Kurman et al., 1985), such cases are almost exclusively confined to premenopausal women with polycystic ovary syndrome. These women are presumed to be genetically and metabolically predisposed to chronic anovulation and are at

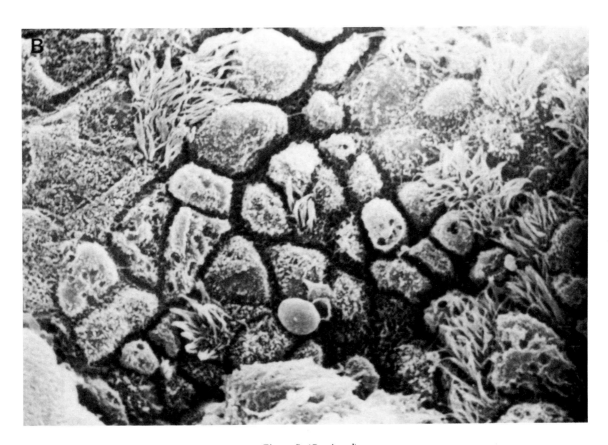

Figure 5. (Continued)

significantly higher risk of corpus carcinoma than are their postmenopausal counterparts (without polycystic ovary syndrome) (Fechner, 1974). Furthermore, careful review of illustrations and descriptions of hyperplasia that presumably progressed to carcinoma revealed significant cytological atypia in most cases (Chamlian and Taylor, 1970; Kurman *et al.*, 1985). In a prospective study, Koss *et al.* (1981) found the same number of cases of endometrial hyperplasia (9/1000) as of carcinoma (9/1000) in over 1000 asymptomatic postmenopausal women. This finding is in great contrast to other carcinoma precursor lesions, which consistently are found significantly more often than their invasive counterparts, the arguing against the "precursor" nature of endometrial hyperplasia. Indeed, according to the prevalence and incidence of corpus carcinoma, if hyperplasia were its precursor, it should be found at least nine to ten times more often than carcinoma (Koss *et al.*, 1981).

In contrast to endometrial hyperplasia without atypia, the majority of patients (15/20, 75%) with cytologically atypical lesions failed to respond to daily relatively high doses of oral medroxyprogesterone therapy (Ferenczy and Gelfand, 1988). Similar experience has been reported by others (Eichner and Abellera, 1971; Gusberg *et al.*, 1974; Kurman *et al.*, 1985). Although a certain proportion of endometria with cytological atypia responded to progestational agents, the lesions tended to recur after therapy had been discontinued (Eichner and

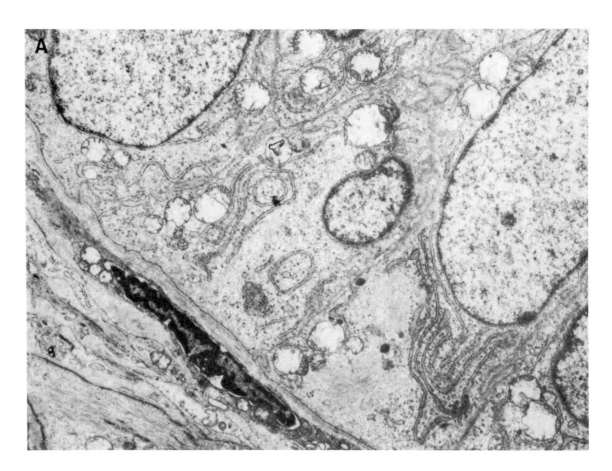

Figure 6. Well-differentiated invasive adenocarcinoma of endometrium. (A) There is a more pronounced variation in nuclear and mitochondrial sizes as well as in the convolution of the GER system than in noninvasive adenocarcinoma cells. Microfilaments are concentrated in a supranuclear location (×4400). (B) There is cellular pleomorphism throughout the surface. Ciliated cells are decreased in number. Microvilli covering the nonciliated cells are short, and the surface plasma membranes are poorly preserved (×2500).

Abellera, 1971; Ferenczy and Gelfand, 1984). The general experience with cytologically atypical endometria showed, furthermore, that persistent or recurrent disease was associated with high risks of carcinoma (Chamlian and Taylor, 1970; Gusberg et al., 1974; Ferenczy and Gelfand, 1988). For example, in our study progression rates of patients with persistent and recurrent disease were as high as 5/15 (33%) (Ferenczy and Gelfand, 1988). According to several earlier prospective and retrospective studies of women with cytologically atypical glandular proliferations, endometrial adenocarcinoma developed in as many as 75% of the cases (Hertig et al., 1949; Beutler et al., 1963; Gusberg et al., 1974; Welch and Scully, 1977; Tavassoli and Kraus, 1978; Fox and Buckley, 1982; Kurman et al., 1985). The clinical pertinence of cytological atypia as the most important single indicator for the subsequent development of carcinoma has also been observed in other reproductive organs including the breast (Dupont and Page, 1985) and prostate (Gleason, 1985).

Why some cases of hyperplasia and many of EIN fail to respond to progestagens (Eichner and Abellera, 1971; Gal, 1986; Kurman et al., 1985) is not clear. It is possible that pro-gestagen-resistant hyperplastic and carcinoma-precursor endometria are relatively poor in or devoid of progestagen receptors (PgR). Charcoal-coated binding assays invariably found higher PgR concentrations in hyperplastic endometria than in either their proliferative or neoplastic counterparts, whereas in cytologically atypical lesions PgR levels were lower than those in normal but higher than those in invasive carcinoma (Janne et al., 1979; Shyamala and Fer-

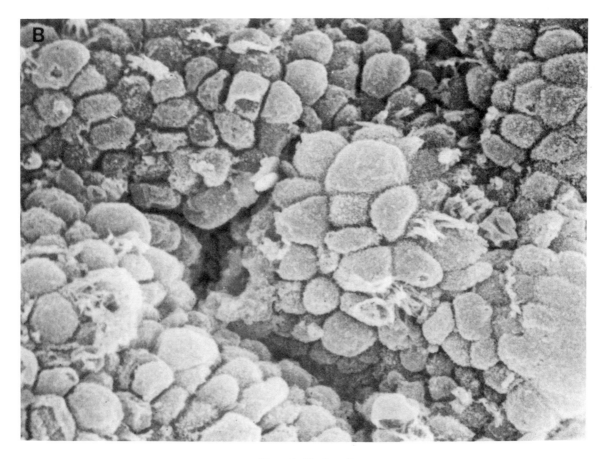

Figure 6. (Continued)

Table 1.   Morphological and Biochemical Characteristics of Endometrial Hyperplasia and Neoplasia[a]

	Proliferative	EH	EIN	Ca grade I
Cytological atypia	No	No	Yes	Yes
Cilia	3+	6+	1–2+	1–2+
Intracellular organelles[b]	Uniform and regular arrangement		Pleomorphic and disorganized	
Volume percentage epithelium	10	20	50–60	50–60
SD nuclear area	10	10	15	20
SD nuclear perimeter	2	3	4	5
DNA S-phase duration	Short		Prolonged	
Estrogen and progesterone receptors	High in nuclei of epithelial and stromal cells		Low, concentrated mainly in nuclei of stromal cells	

[a]EH, endometrial hyperplasia; EIN, endometrial intraepithelial neoplasia; Ca, carcinoma; SD, standard deviation.
[b]Including intermediate filaments, mitochondria, Golgi, and primary lysosomes.

enczy, 1981). Immunohistochemical studies detailed earlier showed relatively high albeit heterogeneously distributed intranuclear PgRs in both the glands and stroma of hyperplastic endometrium, but mainly in the stroma of carcinoma precursors (Bergeron *et al.,* 1988b).

It is interesting that endometrial hyperplasia in nonresponders was associated with a complex, adenomatous growth pattern (77%) more often than in the responder group (13%)

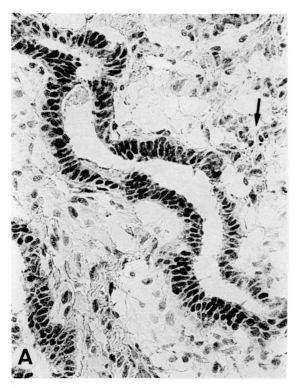 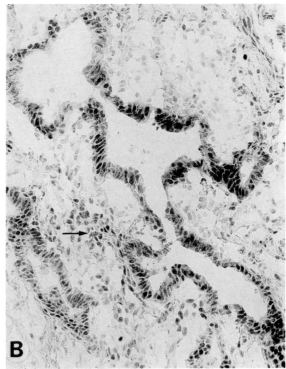

Figure 7. Immunohistochemical localization of ER (A) and PgR (B) in hyperplasia. (A) Strong nuclear staining is observed in the epithelial and stromal (arrow) nuclei (no counterstain, ×250). (B) Lining of a complex voluminous gland with intense nuclear staining. Some stromal nuclei stain strongly as well (arrow) (no counterstain, ×250).

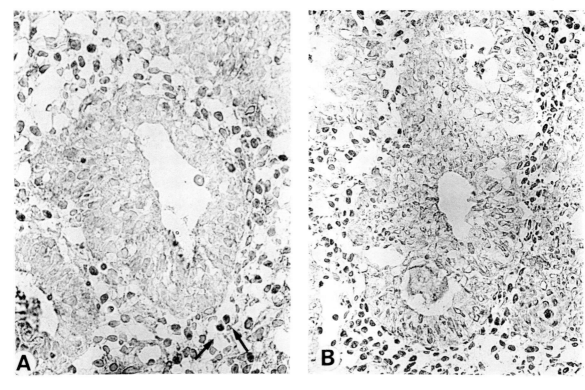

Figure 8. Immunohistochemical localization of ER (A) and PgR (B) in endometrial intraepithelial neoplasia. (A) The glandular cells are devoid of receptors in contrast to the strong nuclear staining reaction of stromal cells (arrow) (no counterstain, ×250). (B) The stromal nuclei stain strongly, but the epithelial cells contain weak or no staining reaction (no counterstain, ×450).

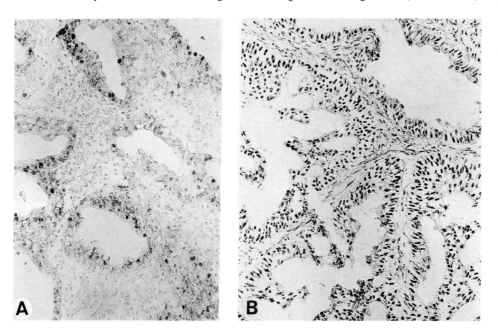

Figure 9. Immunohistochemical localization of ER (A) and PgR (B) in well-differentiated carcinoma. (A) Both epithelial and stromal cells have heterogeneous nuclear ER content (no counterstain, ×250). (B) The epithelial cells demonstrate intense nuclear staining for PgR (no counterstain, ×250).

Table 2. Nomenclature of Endometrial
Hyperplasia and Neoplasia

Endometrial hyperplasia (EH)
Endometrial intraepithelial neoplasia (EIN)
Invasive carcinoma[a]

[a]Invasion of the endometrial stroma (intramucosal) or myometrium.

(Ferenczy and Gelfand, 1988). It is possible, although unproved, that PgRs in medroxyprogesterone-resistant endometria are not functional or that only a small proportion of endometrial tissue contains high concentrations of PgRs or that PgRs are concentrated in the stroma rather than the glandular epithelium. The fact that secretory differentiation in most glands and stroma is partial or abortive supports these speculations. The observation that stromal decidualization often occurs without significant secretory changes in the neighboring endometrial glands of progestagen-resistant endometrial tissues (Fig. 10) lends further support.

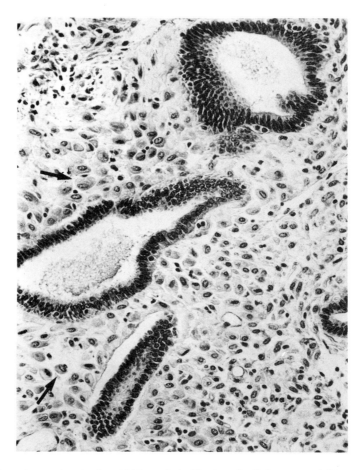

Figure 10. Progestagen-resistant endometrial hyperplasia. The stromal cells have responded to progestagens as evidenced by their complete decidual transformation (arrows), but the lining epithelium of the glands has undergone comparatively less secretory differentiation (H&E, ×250).

Invasive carcinoma and/or EIN may coexist with hyperplasia in the same endometrium, suggesting a pathogenic continuum (Hertig *et al.,* 1949; Beutler *et al.,* 1963; Gusberg and Kaplan, 1963; Welch and Scully, 1977; Tavassoli and Kraus, 1978). However, coexistence does not necessarily imply a cause–effect relationship and therefore does not contradict the two-disease concept. Indeed, in such cases, endometrial hyperplasia and intraepithelial invasive neoplasia form distinct histological (Fig. 11) and immunocytochemical entities (Bergeron *et al.,* 1988a,b) and fail to demonstrate continuity.

The mechanisms responsible for the pathogenic development of both hyperplasia and EIN/carcinoma in the same endometrium are not clear. Carcinogenesis in general involves initiation and promotion (potentiation) of oncogenes in target cells. The initiators induce genetic alterations in the cells, which, if stimulated by a promoter, may develop into clinical cancer (Becker, 1981). Initiators of human endometrial carcinogenesis have not yet been identified (Lucas, 1981; Satyaswaroop and Mortel, 1981). Estradiol (E$_2$) and its receptors, however, are potent promoters of endometrial growth (Meissner *et al.,* 1957; Smith *et al.,* 1975; Clark *et al.,* 1985). It may be speculated that both "cancer-initiated" and "noninitiated" cells are present in the same endometrium in many women. In such patients the growth-promoting effect of E$_2$ in the absence of or failure to respond to progestagenic suppression may

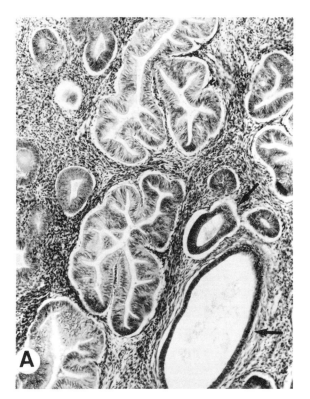

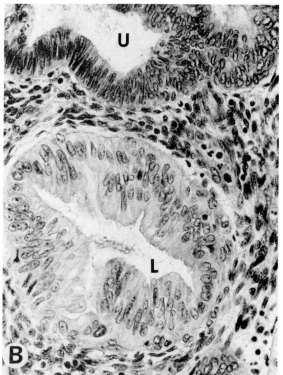

Figure 11. Endometrial intraepithelial neoplasia associated with endometrial hyperplasia. (A) Endometrial glands typical of EIN are close to but separated from hyperplastic glands (arrows) H&E, ×125). (B) Detailed view of EIN (L) and EH (U) separated from each other by fibrocellular stroma. The clear staining charac-teristics of EIN cells including their nuclei contrast with the hyper-chromatic but regularly arranged pencil-shaped nuclei of the adjacent EH (H&E, ×450). From Ferenczy and Gelfand (1986), with permission.

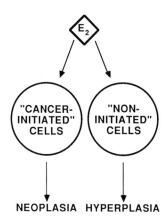

Figure 12. Possible pathogenic mechanism of coexistent endometrial hyperplasia and neoplasia. Estradiol (E$_2$), a potent growth promoter of endometrial epithelial cells, potentiates "carcinoma-initiated" cells to develop into neoplasia, whereas "noninitiated" cells develop into hyperplasia. In such an endometrium, neoplasia coexists with hyperplasia.

lead to the development of "cancer-initiated" cells into neoplasia. The "noninitiated" cells in the same endometrium develop into hyperplasia (Fig. 12).

It appears that in tissues that are targets of steroid hormones, epithelial growth is dependent on mesenchymal support, which in turn is controlled by sex steroid hormones (Cunha *et al.*, 1983; Hunter, 1985; Kratochwil, 1986). Conversely, the epithelium seems to control the response of the mesenchyme to these hormones by stimulating the function of appropriate receptors. As outlined earlier in this chapter, our immunoperoxidase studies of steroid receptors showed impairment in intensity and distribution of estrogen receptor content in EIN and invasive carcinoma compared with the epithelium and stroma of normal and hyperplastic endometria (Figs. 7–9) (Bergeron *et al.*, 1988a). These findings may suggest a disturbance in the mutual dependence of epithelium and mesenchyme in the normal control of growth and function by steroid hormones. This disturbance in turn may be related to endometrial carcinogenesis.

Typically, the carcinomas that are associated with endometrial hyperplasia are seen in relatively young patients (under 55 years of age) with a hyperestrogenic background as evidenced by obesity and long-term replacement therapy with estrogen alone (Horwitz and Feinstein, 1986). Typically, these women have FIGO stage I, well-differentiated, focal carcinomas with high estrogen and progesterone receptor concentrations and nearly 100% 5-year survival rates (Budwit-Novotny *et al.*, 1986; Geisinger *et al.*, 1986; Bergeron *et al.*, 1988a). Such "good-prognosis" carcinomas contrast with their "bad-prognosis" counterparts, which are diagnosed in elderly (60 years or older) hypoestrogenic women who are underweight rather than overweight and have seldom received estrogen replacement therapy. They have atrophic rather than hyperplastic endometrium adjacent to poorly differentiated, progesterone-receptor-poor carcinoma that demonstrates deep myometrial and vascular invasion (Budwit-Novotny *et al.*, 1986; Geisinger *et al.*, 1986; Bergeron *et al.*, 1988a). The 5-year survival rates in such women are a dismal 25% (Boronow *et al.*, 1984). These observations support the present concept of two distinct pathogenic types of corpus carcinoma (Ober, 1971; Bokhman, 1983; Boronow *et al.*, 1984; Deligdisch and Cohen, 1985).

4. Clinical Implications of the Two-Disease Concept

A classification, either clinical or pathological, is meaningful provided it is reproducible and can be related to appropriate management (Table 2). The revised concept of endometrial hyperplasia and neoplasia holds that hyperplasia is morphologically and clinically benign and has negligible or no potential to become carcinoma. In contrast, EIN closely resembles well-differentiated, invasive adenocarcinoma of the endometrium and is a significant precursor lesion. The single most important morphological feature that distinguishes hyperplasia from EIN is cytological atypia. The morphological and clinical implications of this classification include improved diagnostic accuracy and therapeutic decisions. Hyperplasia may be managed by conservative, suppressive progestational therapy, whereas EIN is best treated by hysterectomy unless the patient desires to conceive or is at high risk for surgical complications.

5. References

Aausems, E. W. M. A., Van der Kamp, J. K., and Baak, J. P. A., 1985, Nuclear morphometry in the determination of the prognosis of marked atypical endometrial hyperplasia, *Int. J. Gynecol. Pathol.* **4**:180–185.

Atkin, N. B., 1976, *Cytogenetic Aspects of Malignant Transformation,* S. Karger, New York.

Baak, J. P. A., and Oort, J., 1983, *A Manual of Morphometry in Diagnostic Pathology,* Springer-Verlag, Berlin, Heidelberg, New York.

Baak, J. P. A., Kurver, P. H. J., Diegenbach, P. C., Delemarre, J. F. M., Brekelmans, E. C. M., and Nieuwlaat, J. E., 1981, Discrimination of hyperplasia and carcinoma of the endometrium by quantitative microscopy—a feasibility study, *Histopathology* **5**:61–68.

Becker, F. F., 1981, Recent concepts of initiation and promotion in carcinogenesis, *Am. J. Pathol.* **105**:3–9.

Bergeron, C., Ferenczy, A., and Shyamala, G., 1988a, Distribution of estrogen receptors in various cell types of normal, hyperplastic and neoplastic human endometrial tissues, *Lab. Invest.* **58**:338–344.

Bergeron, C., Ferenczy, A., Toft, D. O., and Shyamala, G., 1988b, Immunocytochemical study of progesterone receptors in hyperplastic and neoplastic endometrial tissues, *Cancer. Res.* (in press).

Beutler, H. K., Dockerty, M. B., and Randall, L. M., 1963, Precancerous lesions of the endometrium, *Am. J. Obstet. Gynecol.* **86**:433–443.

Bokhman, J. V., 1981, Two pathogenic types of endometrial carcinoma, *Gynecol. Oncol.* **15**:10–17.

Boronow, R. C., Morrow, C. P., and Creasman, W. T., 1984, Surgical staging in endometrial cancer: Clinical-pathologic findings of a prospective study, *Obstet. Gynecol.* **63**:825–832.

Budwit-Novotny, D. A., McCarty, K. S., Cox, E. B., Soper, J. T., Mutch, D. G., Creasman, W. T., Flowers, J. T., and McCarty, J. S., Jr., 1986, Immunohistochemical analyses of estrogen receptor in endometrial adenocarcinoma using a monoclonal antibody, *Cancer Res.* **46**:5419–5425.

Chamlian, D. L., and Taylor, H. B., 1970, Endometrial hyperplasia in young women, *Obstet. Gynecol.* **36**:659–665.

Clark, J. H., Schrader, W. T., and O'Malley, B. W., 1985, Mechanisms of steroid hormone action, in: *Textbook of Endocrinology* (J. D. Wilson, and D. W. Foster, eds.), W. B. Saunders, Philadelphia.

Colgan, T. J., Norris, H. J., Foster, W., Kurman, R. J., and Fox, C. H., 1983, Predicting the outcome of endometrial hyperplasia by quantitative analysis of nuclear features using a linear discriminant function, *Int. J. Gynecol. Pathol.* **1**:347–352.

Couturier, J., Vielh, P., Salmon, R., and Dutrillaux, B., 1986, Trisomy and tetrasomy for long arm of chromosome 1 in near diploid human endometrial adenocarcinomas, *Int. J. Cancer* **38**:17–19.

Cunha, G. R., Chung, L. W. K., Shannon, J. M., Taguchi, O., and Fujii, H., 1983, Hormone-induced morphogenesis and growth: Role of mesenchymal–epithelial interactions, *Recent Prog. Horm. Res.* **39**:559–598.

Dallenbach, F. D., and Rudolph, H. E., 1974, Foam cells and estrogen activity of the human endometrium, *Arch. Gynäkol.* **217**:335–347.

Deligdisch, L., and Cohen, C. J., 1985, Histologic correlates and virulence implications of endometrial carcinoma associated with adenomatous hyperplasia, *Cancer* **56**:1452–1455.

Dupont, W. D., and Page, D. L., 1985, Risk factors for breast cancer in women with proliferative breast disease, *N. Engl. J. Med.* **312**:146–151.

Eichner, E., and Abellera, M., 1971, Endometrial hyperplasia treated by progestagens, *Obstet. Gynecol.* **38**:739–741.

Fechner, R. E., and Kaufman, R., 1974, Endometrial adenocarcinoma in Stein–Leventhal syndrome, *Cancer* **34**:444–452.

Feichter, G. E., Hoffken, H., Heep, J., Haag, D., Heberling, D., Brandt, H., Rummel, H., and Goerttler, K.,

1982, DNA-flow-cytometric measurements on the normal, atrophic, hyperplastic, and neoplastic human endometrium, *Virchows Arch.* [*Pathol. Anat.*] **398**:53–65.

Fenoglio, C. M., Crum, C. P., and Ferenczy, A., 1982, Endometrial hyperplasia and carcinoma. Are ultrastructural, biochemical and immunocytochemical studies useful in distinguishing between them? *Pathol. Res. Pract.* **174**:257–284.

Ferenczy, A., 1983, Cytodynamics of endometrial hyperplasia and neoplasia, part II: *In vitro* DNA histoautoradiography, *Hum. Pathol.* **14**:77–82.

Ferenczy, A., 1987, Anatomy and histology of the uterine corpus, in: *Blaustein's Pathology of the Female Genital Tract*, (R. J. Kurman, ed.), Springer-Verlag, New York, pp. 141–157.

Ferenczy, A., 1988, Endometrial hyperplasia and neoplasia: A two disease concept, in: *Contemporary Issues in Obstetrics and Gynecology*, Vol 3: *Gynecology Oncology* (R. L. Berkowitz, C. Cohen, and N. G. Kale, eds.), Churchill Livingston, New York, pp. 197–213.

Ferenczy, A., and Gelfand, M. M., 1984, Outpatient endometrial sampling with endocyte: Comparative study of its effectiveness with endometrial biopsy, *Obstet. Gynecol.* **63**:295–302.

Ferenczy, A., and Gelfand, M. M., 1986, Hyperplasia vs. neoplasia: Two tracks for the endometrium? *Contemp. Ob/Gyn.* **28**:79–96.

Ferenczy, A., and Gelfand, M. M., 1988, The biologic significance of cytologic atypia in progestagen treated endometrial hyperplasia, *Am. J. Obstet. Gynecol.* (in press).

Ferenczy, A., and Richart, R. M., 1974, *Female Reproductive System: Dynamics of Scan and Transmission Electron Microscopy*, John Wiley & Sons, New York.

Ferenczy, A., Bertrand, G., and Gelfand, M. M., 1979, Proliferation kinetics of human endometrium during the normal menstrual cycle, *Am. J. Obstet. Gynecol.* **133**:859–867.

Ferenczy, A., Gelfand, M. M., and Tzipris, F., 1983, The cytodynamics of endometrial hyperplasia and carcinoma. A review, *Ann. Pathol.* **3**:189–202.

Fox, H., and Buckley, C. H., 1982, The endometrial hyperplasias and their relationship to endometrial neoplasia, *Histopathology* **6**:493–510.

Freidlander, M. L., Taylor, I. W., Russell, P., Musgrove, E. A., Hedley, D. W., and Tattersall, M. H. N., 1983, Ploidy as a prognostic factor in ovarian cancer, *Int. J. Gynecol. Pathol.* **2**:55–63.

Fu, Y. S., Ferenczy, A., Huang, I., and Gelfand, M. M., 1988, Digital imaging analysis of normal, hyperplastic and malignant endometrial cells, *Anal. Quant. Cytol. Histol.* **10**:139–149.

Gal, D., 1986, Hormonal therapy for lesions of the endometrium, *Semin. Oncol.* **13**:33–36.

Geisinger, K. R., Homesley, H. D., Morgan, T. M., Kute, T. E., and Marshall, R. B., 1986, Endometrial adenocarcinoma. A multiparameter clinicopathologic analysis including the DNA profile and the sex steroid hormone receptors, *Cancer* **58**:1518–1525.

Gibas, Z., and Rubin, S. C., 1987, Well-differentiated adenocarcinoma of endometrium with simple karyotypic changes: A case report, *Cancer Genet. Cytogenet.* **25**:21–26.

Gleason, D. F., 1985, Atypical hyperplasia, benign hyperplasia and well-differentiated adenocarcinoma of the prostate, *Am. J. Surg. Pathol.* **9**:53–69.

Gusberg, S. B., and Kaplan, A. L., 1963, Precursors of corpus cancer IV: Adenomatous hyperplasia or stage 0 carcinoma of the endometrium, *Am. J. Obstet. Gynecol.* **87**:662–678.

Gusberg, S. B., Chen, S. J., and Cohen, C. J., 1974, Endometrial cancer: Factors influencing the choice of treatment, *Gynecol. Oncol.* **2**:308–313.

Hertig, A. T., and Sommers, S. C., 1949, Genesis of endometrial carcinoma. I. Study of prior biopsies, *Cancer* **2**:946–956.

Hertig, A. T., Sommers, S. C., and Bengloff, H., 1949, Genesis of endometrial carcinoma. III. Carcinoma *in situ*, *Cancer* **2**:964–971.

Horwitz, R. I., and Feinstein, A. R., 1986, Estrogens and endometrial cancer. Responses to arguments and current status of an epidemiologic controversy, *Am. J. Med.* **81**:503–507.

Hunter, T., 1985, Oncogenes and growth control, *Trends Biochem. Sci.* **10**:275–280.

Iversen, O. E., 1986, Flow cytometric deoxyribonucleic acid index: A prognostic factor in endometrial carcinoma, *Am. J. Obstet. Gynecol.* **155**:770–776.

Jakobsen, A., 1984, Prognostic impact of ploidy level in carcinoma of the cervix, *Am. J. Clin. Oncol.* **7**:475–480.

Janne, O., Kauppila, A., Kontula, K., Syrjala, P., and Vihko, R., 1979, Female sex steroid receptors in normal, hyperplastic and carcinomatous endometrium. The relationship to serum steroid hormones and gonadotropins and changes during medroxyprogesterone acetate administration, *Int. J. Cancer* **24**:545–554.

Katayama, K. P., and Jones, H. W., 1967, Chromosomes of atypical (adenomatous) hyperplasia and carcinoma of the endometrium, *Am. J. Obstet. Gynecol.* **97**:978–983.

King, W. J., and Greene, G. L., 1984, Monoclonal antibodies localize oestrogen receptor in the nuclei of target cells, *Nature* **307**:745–747.

Koss, L. G., Schreiber, K., Oberlander, S. G., Moukhtar, M., Levine, H. S., and Moussouris, H. F., 1981, Screening of asymptomatic women for endometrial cancer, *Obstet. Gynecol.* **57**:681–691.

Kratochwil, K., 1986, The stroma and the control of cell growth, *J. Pathol.* **149**:23–24.

Kurman, R. J., and Norris, H. J., 1982, Evaluation of criteria for distinguishing atypical endometrial hyperplasia from well-differentiated carcinoma, *Cancer* **49**:2547–2559.

Kurman, R. J., Kaminski, P. T., and Norris, H. J., 1985, The behavior of endometrial hyperplasia. A long-term study of ''untreated'' hyperplasia in 170 patients, *Cancer* **56**:403–412.

Leavitt, W. W., Chen, T. J., and Allen, T. C., 1977, Regulation of progesterone receptor formation by estrogen action, *Ann. N.Y. Acad. Sci.* **286**:210–225.

Lucas, W. E., 1981, Estrogen—a cause of gynecologic cancer? *Cancer* **48**:451–454.

McBride, J. M., 1959, Pre-menopausal cystic hyperplasia and endometrial carcinoma, *J. Obstet. Gynaecol. Br. Emp.* **66**:288–296.

Meissner, W. A., Sommers, S. C., and Sherman, G., 1957, Endometrial hyperplasia, endometrial carcinoma, and endometriosis produced experimentally by estrogen, *Cancer* **10**:500–509.

Ober, W. B., 1971, Adenocarcinoma of the endometrium: A pathologist's view, in: *Symposium on Endometrial Cancer* (M. G. Brush, R. W. Taylor, and D. C. Williams, eds.), William Heinemann, London, pp. 73–81.

Oud, P. S., Reubsaet-Veldhuizen, J. A. M., Henderik, J. B. J., Pahlplatz, M. M. M., Hermkens, H. G., Tas, J., James, J., and Vooijs, G. P., 1986, DNA and nuclear protein measurement in isolated nuclei of human endometrium, *Cytometry* **7**:318–324.

Roberts, D. K., Lavia, L. A., Freedman, R. S., Horbelt, D. V., and Busby-Walker, N., 1986, Nuclear and nucleolar areas: A quantitative assessment of endometrial neoplasia, *Obstet. Gynecol.* **68**:705–708.

Sachs, H., Wamtach, E. V., and Wurthner, K., 1974, DNA content of normal, hyperplastic and malignant endometrium, determined cytophotometrically, *Arch. Gynecol.* **217**:349–365.

Satyaswaroop, P. G., and Mortel, R., 1981, Endometrial carcinoma: An aberration of endometrial cell differentiation, *Am. J. Obstet. Gynecol.* **140**:620–623.

Shyamala, G., and Ferenczy, A., 1981, The effect of sodium molybdate on the cytoplasmic estrogen and progesterone receptors in human endometrial tissues, *Diag. Obstet. Gynecol.* **3**:277–282.

Smith, D. C., Prentice, R., Thompson, D. J., and Herrmann, W. L., 1975, Association of exogenous estrogen and endometrial carcinoma, *N. Engl. J. Med.* **293**:1164–1167.

Stephenson, R. A., James, B. C., Gay, H., Fair, W. R., Whitmore, W. F., Jr., and Melamed, M. R., 1987, Flow cytometry of prostate cancer: Relationship of DNA content to survival, *Cancer Res.* **47**:2504–2509.

Sullivan, W. P., Beito, R. G., Proper, J., Krco, C. J., and Toft, D. O., 1986, Preparation of monoclonal antibodies to the avian progesterone receptor, *Endocrinology* **119**:1549–1557.

Tavassoli, F., and Kraus, F. T., 1978, Endometrial lesions in uteri resected for atypical endometrial hyperplasia, *Am. J. Clin. Pathol.* **70**:770–779.

Trent, J. M., 1985, Cytogenetic and molecular biologic alterations in human breast cancer: A review, *Breast Cancer Res. Treat.* **5**:221–229.

Trent, J. M., and Davis, J. R., 1979, D-group chromosome abnormalities in endometrial cancer and hyperplasia, *Lancet* **2**:361.

Vellios, F., 1972, Endometrial hyperplasias, precursors of endometrial carcinoma, in: *Pathology Annual* (S. C. Sommers, ed.), Appleton–Century–Crofts, New York, pp. 201–229.

Wagner, D., Richart, R. M., and Turner, J. Y., 1967, Deoxribonucleic acid content of presumed precursors of endometrial carcinoma, *Cancer* **20**:2067–2077.

Welch, W. R., and Scully, R. E., 1977, Precancerous lesions of the endometrium, *Hum. Pathol.* **8**:503–512.

Wentz, W. B., 1966, Treatment of persistent endometrial hyperplasia with progestagen, *Am. J. Obstet. Gynecol.* **96**:999–1004.

Winkler, B., Alvarez, S., Richart, R. M., and Crum, C. P., 1984, Pitfalls in the diagnosis of endometrial neoplasia, *Obstet. Gynecol.* **64**:185–194.

13

Biochemistry of the Myometrium and Cervix

GABOR HUSZAR and MICHAEL P. WALSH

The uterus comprises the corpus (endometrium and myometrium) and the cervix. Although the functions of each are important, the events related to myometrial contractility, because they are the most visible, have received the most attention. Our understanding of smooth muscle contractility has advanced a great deal in the past decade. Most important in this respect has been the recognition that the interaction of actin and myosin is regulated by myosin light chain phosphorylation in contrast to skeletal muscles in which regulation occurs through troponin/tropomyosin associated with the actin filament. In the case of the myometrium, regulation is more complex, because the cellular events of myometrial contractility are modulated by the endocrine events of the menstrual cycle and gestation. Another key development in the understanding of uterine function was the recognition that myometrium and cervix are functionally interrelated and act in concert to bring about the cervical and myometrial events of labor (Huszar, 1979, 1980, 1983, 1986; Huszar *et al.*, 1986).

During pregnancy, the myometrium relaxes to accommodate the developing fetus and products of conception, whereas at the end of pregnancy it provides the rhythmic tonic contractions of labor that lead to the expulsion of the uterine contents. In the first part of gestation the cervix is hard and firmly holds the uterine contents. The biochemical process of ''cervical maturation'' commences at about the 34th week of pregnancy, together with other prelabor myometrial events, until the cervical os is fully dilated at delivery. The close coordination between the myometrium and cervix is essential for normal uterine function, and defects in this relationship cause maternal and fetal morbidity.

Much of our understanding of the regulation of smooth muscle contraction comes from studies of nonuterine smooth muscles, particularly avian gizzard and mammalian vascular smooth muscles. Although there are clear differences between uterine and other smooth muscles with respect to morphological, electrophysiological, and pharmacological properties,

GABOR HUSZAR • Department of Obstetrics and Gynecology, Yale University School of Medicine, New Haven, Connecticut 06510.   MICHAEL P. WALSH • Department of Medical Biochemistry, University of Calgary, Calgary, Alberta T2N 4N1, Canada.

it has become increasingly clear that the elements and regulation of the contractile process are common to all types of smooth muscle. It is reasonable, therefore, to discuss the fundamentals of transmembrane Ca^{2+} fluxes and the roles of various muscle cell organelles and contractile proteins as well as the contractile regulation of smooth muscles in general terms, with the cautionary note that many of the details remain to be verified in the myometrium.

1. The Structure of the Myometrium

1.1. Cellular Organization

The myometrium is not a homogeneous muscle tissue as is skeletal muscle. It is composed of muscle cells that are embedded in connective tissue, an arrangement that facilitates the transmission of contractile forces generated by individual muscle cells. The muscle cells communicate with each other by means of gap junctions. These cell-to-cell contacts are believed to synchronize myometrial function by conducting electrophysiological stimuli during labor. In the final weeks of pregnancy, when the so-called Braxton–Hicks irregular contractions and cervical maturation occur, the myometrial gap junctions gradually increase in number and size until the commencement of labor (Garfield *et al.*, 1982). The formation of myometrial gap junctions has been studied in *in vitro* organ cultures, and regulatory roles for estrogen, progesterone, and prostaglandins have been established (Garfield *et al.*, 1980). In parturient rats, it was demonstrated that the frequency of myometrial gap junctions more closely corresponds to the concentrations of estrogen receptors (increased gap junctions) and progesterone receptors (decreased gap junctions) than to the levels of circulating steroids (Saito *et al.*, 1985). More recent experiments with the antiprogesterone RU 486 indicated that progesterone suppresses myometrial contractility by inhibiting gap junction formation, perhaps at the level of protein biosynthesis (Garfield *et al.*, 1987). The modulation of gap junction synthesis by various hormones and pharmacological agents appears to be essential for the coordination of labor.

Beyond the hormonal milieu of pregnancy, the stretch effect of the growing conceptus on the uterine wall also affects the formation of gap junctions. In studies on three groups of postpartum rats (Wathes and Porter, 1982), gap junctions were stimulated by administration of estrogen, by inflation of the uterine horn with a balloon, and by the simultaneous administration of both of these stimuli. Gap junction densities high enough to be comparable to those at parturition were obtained only in animals that received a combination of the two treatments. In other experiments a relationship was established among the electrical activity and the conductivity properties of the rat myometrium and the density of gap junctions (Verhoeff *et al.*, 1984). This finding indicates that the various related components of myometrial cellular regulation, including the formation of gap junctions, enhanced electrical activity, and the response to estrogen, oxytocin, and other hormones, are simultaneous events that collectively contribute to the increased myometrial activity of labor. However, at least in primates, progesterone receptor blockade did not change the events of prostaglandin biosynthesis and cervical maturation in parturition (Haluska *et al.*, 1987).

1.2. Filament Structure and Function

The need for a functional link such as gap junctions among the individual myometrial cells is essential, since smooth muscles are not organized into fibers, fibrils, and filaments as are skeletal muscles. The intracellular organization is also different; the thick myosin and thin actin filaments occur in long, random bundles throughout the smooth muscle cells, and the continuity of these filaments is not interrupted by Z-lines. Because of this organization, smooth muscles can exert pulling force in any direction, whereas in skeletal muscle, the direction of contraction/force generation is always aligned with the axis of the muscle fibers and the constituent actin and myosin filaments (Huxley, 1971) (Fig. 1).

Other differences are related to the structure of the actin and myosin filaments (Fig. 2). In smooth muscle cells there are three distinct types of filaments (A. V. Somlyo, 1980): thin filaments (6–8 nm in diameter) composed mainly of actin monomers polymerized into a double-helical strand; intermediate filaments (10 nm in diameter) composed mainly of desmin, vimentin, or both; and thick filaments (15–18 nm in diameter) composed of aggregated myosin molecules. In skeletal muscle actin filaments originate in each Z-line and point toward the center of the sarcomere. Myosin filaments are also bidirectional: myosin molecules are laid down from the center of the sarcomere toward the Z-lines. Thus, in skeletal muscle the thick and thin filaments are interrupted, and the bidirectional configuration repeats itself in each sarcomere. In smooth muscle myosin molecules are aligned in the same direction and form long, uninterrupted filaments. This unidirectional polarity enables actin to interact with myosin along the entire length of the thick filament, which explains the severalfold greater shortening ability of smooth muscle compared to skeletal muscle.

The intermediate filaments and dense bodies are not active participants in the contractile process; rather, they form a flexible structural network that links actin and myosin filaments into integrated mechanical units. The dense bodies act as "functional" Z-lines by providing attachment sites for actin. Dense bodies and Z-lines both contain α-actinin as their major protein. Electron micrographs of saponin-treated smooth muscle indicate that the free ends of

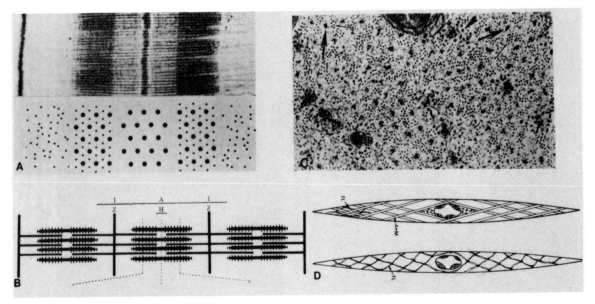

Figure 1. (A,B) Electron microscopic and diagrammatic representation of the structure of striated muscle, showing overlapping arrays of actin- and myosin-containing filaments, the latter with projecting cross bridges (Huxley, 1971). (C) Cross section of a smooth muscle cell. Thick filaments (large arrows) have a diameter of about 160 Å, and the center-to-center spacing is approximately 600 to 700 Å. Thin filaments (small arrows) have a mean diameter of about 70 Å. Intermediate filaments (arrowhead) are about 100 Å in diameter (A. P. Somlyo and Somlyo, 1974). (D) Schematic diagram of the contractile apparatus and proposed arrangement of "contractile units." Each unit consists of a bundle of actin and myosin filaments (A+M) connecting opposing sites on the cell surface. The 100-Å filaments (FL) form a network between the actin–myosin filament groups (Small, 1977). From Huszar (1980), with permission.

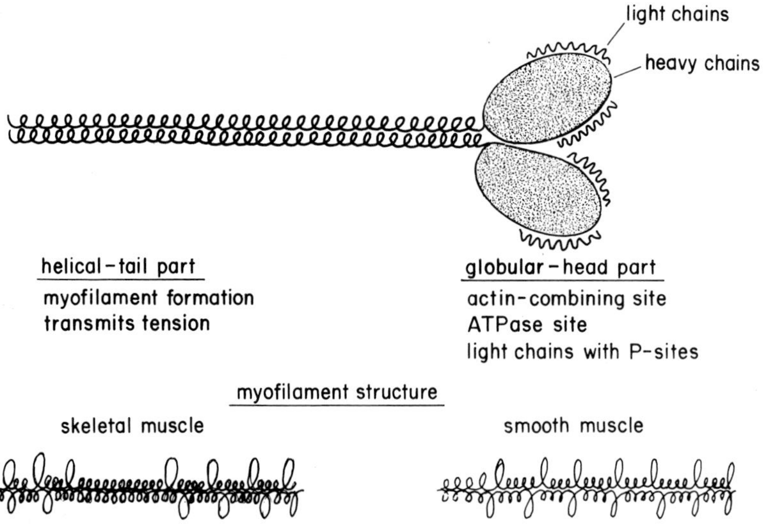

light chains

heavy chains

helical–tail part
myofilament formation
transmits tension

globular–head part
actin-combining site
ATPase site
light chains with P-sites

myofilament structure

skeletal muscle

smooth muscle

Figure 2. Schematic structures of myosin and myofilaments. Myosin is a 140-nm molecule composed of a helical tail (myofilament formation) and a globular head (actin-combining and ATPase sites and the associated myosin light chains). The myofilaments are bidirectional in skeletal muscle but unidirectional and uninterrupted in smooth muscle. From Huszar (1983), with permission.

actin filaments interdigitate with myosin filaments, an arrangement that suggests that a sarcomerelike structure connects adjacent dense bodies by actin and overlapping myosin filaments (A. V. Somlyo, 1980). In fact, when the dense bodies and associated actin filaments in smooth muscle of vas deferens were decorated with myosin heads (Bond and Somlyo, 1982), the resulting "arrowheads" always pointed away from the dense bodies (Fig. 3), similar to the direction of the actin filaments originating in the Z-bands of skeletal muscles. The precise filament structure is not clear (Bagby, 1983), but this organized yet highly flexible arrangement enables the uterus to generate forces in any axis necessary and to assume virtually any shape to accommodate fetuses in various positions and of various sizes during labor.

It is well established in both smooth and skeletal muscle that contraction is based on a relative sliding of actin and myosin filaments without an internal change in the length of either filament (Huxley, 1971). The sliding action is caused by the cyclic formation of cross bridges (myosin heads interacting with actin monomers), conformational changes in the myosin heads that effectively move the myosin filament along the actin filament, and dissociation (detachment) of the myosin head at the end of each cycle. Cross-bridge cycling occurs at the expense of ATP hydrolysis, which provides the driving force for contraction.

2. Calcium and Contractile Regulation

2.1. The Importance of Ca^{2+} Ions

Calcium ions play a central role in the regulation of a wide variety of cellular processes, including smooth muscle contraction. An enormous ($\sim 10^4$-fold) Ca^{2+} concentration gradient exists between the extracellular milieu ($\sim 10^{-3}$ M) and intracellular cytosol ($\sim 10^{-7}$ M). This gradient across the plasma membrane, which in smooth muscle is called the sarcolemma, is

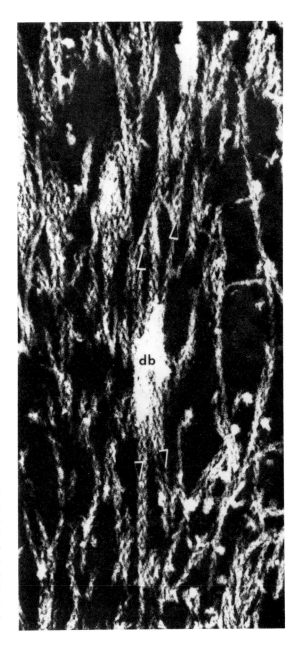

Figure 3. Longitudinally sectioned cytoplasmic dense body from a saponin-treated
vas deferens smooth muscle cell. Myosin-
subfragment-1-decorated thin filaments
(applied arrowhead markers) insert into
each end of the dense body (db); the direction of the arrowheads is away from the
dense body at each end. The micrograph is
reproduced with reverse contrast.
×84,000. From Bond and Somlyo (1982),
with permission.

maintained by a variety of mechanisms. Calcium-dependent activation of contraction involves
an elevation of cytosolic free Ca^{2+} concentration from a resting level of $\sim 10^{-7}$ M to $0.5-1 \times 10^{-6}$ M. The Ca^{2+} may originate from the extracellular space, the intracellular Ca^{2+}-storing
organelle, the sarcoplasmic reticulum (SR), or both. Because the diffusional distance between
the extracellular space and the contractile elements in smooth muscle is short, extracellular
Ca^{2+} may be as important as Ca^{2+} stored within the SR, unlike the situation for striated
muscles in which SR Ca^{2+} is of major importance. The increase in cytosolic free Ca^{2+}
concentration is detected by intracellular high-affinity Ca^{2+}-binding proteins, which convert
the Ca^{2+} signal to specific cellular responses.

2.2. The Source of Activating Calcium

The role of intracellular calcium in smooth muscle contractility is supported by experiments with electron probe analysis, in which the SR was identified as the major intracellular store for calcium (A. P. Somlyo et al., 1982). Smooth muscles contain a well-developed SR (1.5–7.5% of cell volume), which sequesters enough Ca^{2+} to fulfill the contractile needs of the smooth muscle cell, e.g., large elastic arteries, estrogen-treated or pregnant uterus (A. P. Somlyo, 1985). The potential role of mitochondria as a source of activating Ca^{2+} was also seriously considered for many years. However, it is now generally recognized that mitochondria, despite their high capacity to accumulate Ca^{2+} ions, do not function as sinks of Ca^{2+} for contractile regulation because of their low affinity for Ca^{2+} ($K_d \sim 10$ μM). However, because cells cannot survive cytosolic free Ca^{2+} concentrations of >10 μM, the mitochondria play an important role in buffering Ca^{2+} in the high concentration ranges, thus offering protection against Ca^{2+}-induced cell death (A. P. Somlyo, 1985).

The Ca^{2+} concentration within the nucleus of a smooth muscle cell appears to be regulated independently of cytosolic Ca^{2+}, which is desirable because many nuclear events, including the transcriptional events of protein biosynthesis, are dependent on specific Ca^{2+} concentrations. The independent regulation of nuclear Ca^{2+} in smooth muscles was demonstrated in single cells by Fay and co-workers (Williams et al., 1987), who found, using fura-2 (a calcium-sensor dye), that intranuclear Ca^{2+} concentration rose from 200 nM to not more than 300 nM following depolarizing stimuli that induced a rise of cytosolic Ca^{2+} >700 nM.

2.3. Measurements of Cellular Ca^{2+} Transients

More than 20 years ago, Filo et al. (1965) observed a strong Ca^{2+} dependence of contraction in glycerinated vascular smooth muscle: tension development did not occur below 1.8×10^{-7} M free Ca^{2+} and was maximal at 10^{-6} M. Direct evidence for Ca^{2+} transients (changes in calcium concentrations) in response to contraction-inducing stimuli has become available with the development of the Ca^{2+} indicators. Morgan and Morgan (1982) used the photoprotein aequorin, either microinjected or loaded by reversible permeabilization of smooth muscle cells, to demonstrate Ca^{2+} transients in response to electrical stimulation or to the pharmacological agents angiotensin and phenylephrine. The observed peak of free Ca^{2+} concentration preceded the development of tension. Recently, a class of Ca^{2+} indicator dyes, including quin-2 and fura-2 developed by Roger Tsien (Grynkiewicz et al., 1985), has received wide application in the study of Ca^{2+} transients. These dyes bind Ca^{2+} selectively [their structures are based on Ca^{2+} chelator compounds ethyleneglycolbis-(β-aminoethylether)-N,N,N',N'-tetraacetic acid (EGTA) and 1,2-bis-(2-aminophenoxy)ethane-N,N,N',N'-tetraacetic acid (BAPTA)], and changes occur in their fluorescence properties that are proportional to the cytosolic free Ca^{2+} concentration. Loading isolated toad stomach smooth muscle cells with quin-2 and fura-2 enabled Fay and co-workers to determine the resting free cytosolic Ca^{2+} concentration to be ~ 130 nM (Williams et al., 1987; Williams and Fay, 1986). Using aequorin, DeFeo and Morgan (1985) reported a resting cytosolic free Ca^{2+} concentration of 180 nM in the portal vein and 270 nM in the aorta of ferrets. The distribution of Ca^{2+} within a single toad stomach smooth muscle cell was also observed using a combination of fura-2 and digital imaging microscopy (Williams et al., 1985): Free Ca^{2+} concentration in the nucleus and SR of the resting cell was greater than that in the cytosol. These Ca^{2+} gradients were abolished by Ca^{2+} ionophores, compounds that eliminate the physiological Ca^{2+}-barrier properties of membranes.

The relevance of extracellular calcium versus intracellular calcium in the regulation of smooth muscle contraction is not yet a settled issue. The importance of extracellular calcium has been demonstrated in various experiments (Batra, 1982; Van Breemen *et al.*, 1982). In one study, contraction was initiated by potassium or by norepinephrine in the presence of diltiazem, a drug that blocks the membrane calcium channels that allow the influx of calcium. In the case of potassium activation, the rate of calcium influx and the development of muscle tone showed a parallel pattern, indicating that the potassium-induced contractility was caused by the influx of extracellular calcium. On the other hand, with norepinephrine the inhibition was delayed, which suggests that during norepinephrine-induced contraction the initial calcium is released from intracellular calcium stores. Stimulation of dye-loaded smooth muscle cells by K^+ depolarization, electrical stimulation, or variety of agonists (e.g., carbachol) in the presence or absence of extracellular Ca^{2+} revealed that the importance of extracellular versus intracellular Ca^{2+} in the increase of the cytosolic free Ca^{2+} concentration varies depending on the stimulus and the particular smooth muscle (Sumimoto and Kuriyama, 1986; Bitar *et al.*, 1986a).

3. Regulation of Transmembrane Ca^{2+} Fluxes

A variety of mechanisms exist that maintain the intracellular low Ca^{2+} concentrations in the resting state and, on contractile activation, facilitate the rise in cytosolic free Ca^{2+} concentration. Since the cytoplasmic calcium may originate from the extracellular milieu and the SR, systems regulating Ca^{2+} fluxes are present in both the sarcolemma and sarcoplasmic reticulum membranes. Some allow or induce Ca^{2+} movement into the cytosol, and others facilitate calcium extrusion. The prevailing cytosolic free Ca^{2+} concentrations therefore reflect the balance of these mechanisms that regulate Ca^{2+} movement among the various compartments (Fig. 4).

3.1. Mechanisms of Ca^{2+} Efflux

In the sarcolemma, two important systems exist that maintain the low resting cytosolic free Ca^{2+} concentration by transporting Ca^{2+} from the cytosol to the extracellular milieu: the Ca^{2+}-transport ATPase or (Ca^{2+}, Mg^{2+})-ATPase (Fig. 4, 7) and the Na^+/Ca^{2+} exchanger (Fig. 4, 8).

3.1.1. Ca^{2+}-Transport ATPase

The Ca^{2+}-transport ATPase, or Ca^{2+} pump, has been isolated from smooth muscle sarcolemma, and the Ca^{2+} transport function of the enzyme was confirmed in artificial lipid vesicles (Furukawa and Nakamura, 1984; Wuytack *et al.*, 1984, 1985). The enzyme has a subunit mass of 130 kda and is activated by the Ca^{2+}-dependent regulatory protein calmodulin in a Ca^{2+}-dependent manner. A similar enzyme has been reported in the human myometrium (Popescu and Ignat, 1983). The (Ca^{2+}, Mg^{2+})-ATPase appears to be the principal mechanism of Ca^{2+} transport to the extracellular space. It retains a basal level of activity in the absence of Ca^{2+}/calmodulin, i.e., at resting cytosolic free Ca^{2+}, whereas elevation of the cytosolic Ca^{2+} concentration leads to activation of the system and restoration of the resting cytosolic free Ca^{2+} level. In myometrial membrane preparations from both nonpregnant and pregnant uterus, oxytocin inhibits the sarcolemmal (Ca^{2+}, Mg^{2+})-ATPase. This effect, which is proportional to the density of oxytocin receptors (Soloff and Sweet, 1982), may explain the relationship between oxytocin binding and increased myometrial contractility (Sakamoto and Huszar, 1984a).

3.1.2. Na^+/Ca^{2+} Exchanger

As in all other excitable cells, a Na^+ concentration gradient exists across the sarcolemma of a smooth muscle cell with external and internal sodium concentrations of 145 mM and 12 mM, respectively. Similarly, there is a K^+ concentration gradient in the opposite direction (4 mM outside and 139 mM inside). These ion gradients are maintained by a (Na^+, K^+)-ATPase (Fig. 4). Under normal physiological conditions, the Na^+/Ca^{2+} exchanger, which can expel Ca^{2+} at the expense of Na^+ influx, allows three Na^+ ions to flow into the cell in exchange for a single Ca^{2+} ion. The Na^+ is then extruded by the (Na^+, K^+)-ATPase. This situation can be verified in preparations of right-side-out membrane vesicles with a high Na^+ concentration inside and a low Na^+ concentration outside. In such an experimental system the membrane-bound Na^+/Ca^{2+} exchanger will move Na^+ to the outside and Ca^{2+} to the inside (Casteels *et al.*, 1986).

The Na^+/Ca^{2+} exchangers have a high K_m (2–20 μM) and velocity, whereas the Ca^{2+}-transport ATPase has a low velocity and high affinity (K_m ~0.4 μM) (Baker, 1975). However, Na^+/Ca^{2+} exchange across the smooth muscle sarcolemma appears to be of minor importance compared to the (Ca^{2+}, Mg^{2+})-ATPase in accomplishing Ca^{2+} extrusion (Casteels *et al.*, 1986).

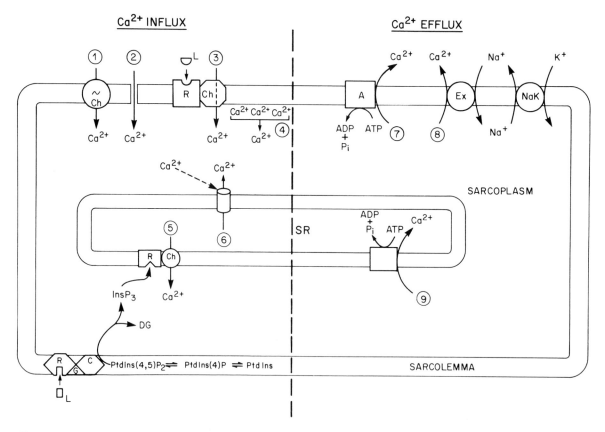

Figure 4. Conceptual overview of Ca^{2+} regulation in smooth muscle cells. Ch, channel; C, phospholipase C; R, receptor; G, guanine nucleotide-binding protein; A, Ca^{2+}-transport ATPase; Ex, Na^+/Ca^{2+} exchanger; NaK, (Na^+/K^+)-ATPase; L, ligand; DG, diacyl glycerol. 1, voltage-operated Ca^{2+} channels; 2, passive influx of Ca^{2+} ("Ca^{2+} leak"); 3, receptor-operated Ca^{2+} channels; 4, Ca^{2+} release from association with the sarcolemma; 5, InsP$_3$-mediated Ca^{2+} release from SR; 6, Ca^{2+}-induced Ca^{2+} release; 7, sarcolemmal Ca^{2+}-transport ATPase; 8, Na^+/Ca^{2+} exchange; 9, SR Ca^{2+}-transport ATPase.

The SR membranes of smooth muscles, including the myometrium, contain an intracellular ATP-dependent Ca^{2+}-transport pump (Fig. 4, 9), which is an important regulator of cytoplasmic calcium level and thus of the contractile state of the muscle. The SR Ca^{2+} pump has a mass of 100 kda and is immunologically distinct from the sarcolemmal Ca^{2+} pump and the Ca^{2+} pump of skeletal muscle SR (Casteels *et al.*, 1986). Antibodies against the cardiac muscle SR Ca^{2+} pump, however, do recognize the smooth muscle SR Ca^{2+} pump (Casteels *et al.*, 1986).

The SR Ca^{2+}-transport ATPase is regulated by an associated multisubunit protein, phospholamban, which has been isolated and thoroughly characterized in cardiac SR (Kirchberger *et al.*, 1974). It copurifies with the SR Ca^{2+}-transport ATPase, suggesting an association. Antibody to phospholamban stains SR of cardiac, smooth, and slow-twitch (red) skeletal muscles but not SR in fast-twitch (white) skeletal muscles (Jorgensen and Jones, 1986; Raeymaekers and Jones, 1986). To suggest further a regulatory role, phospholamban in the heart is a substrate of cAMP-dependent protein kinase (Tada and Katz, 1982), a Ca^{2+}/calmodulin-dependent protein kinase (LePeuch *et al.*, 1979), and protein kinase C (Movsesian *et al.*, 1984). Phosphorylation of phospholamban enhances the activity of the Ca^{2+}-transport ATPase. Similar regulation is likely in smooth muscle but remains to be established.

In cardiac and skeletal SR, Ca^{2+} is stored bound to calsequestrin (MacLennan *et al.*, 1983), a highly acidic protein that contains a single asparagine-linked carbohydrate unit. This protein of 42 kda (Fliegel *et al.*, 1987) binds Ca^{2+} with high capacity (~40–50 Ca^{2+} ions/molecule) and low affinity ($K_d \sim 1$ mM), clearly an ideal situation for a Ca^{2+} storage sink that readily surrenders its Ca^{2+} to the cytosol on demand. In skeletal muscle, calsequestrin is localized in the terminal cisternae at a concentration of ~100 mg/ml so that, at saturation, it can bind up to ~100 mM Ca^{2+}. Recent work from Casteels' group indicates the presence of calsequestrin in smooth muscle SR (Wuytack *et al.*, 1987). This finding had been suggested earlier on the basis of electron microscopic and electron microprobe analysis studies (A. P. Somlyo, 1985).

3.3. Mechanisms of Ca²⁺ Influx

3.3.1. Sarcolemmal Mechanisms

Cytoplasmic free Ca^{2+} may enter from the extracellular milieu on appropriate stimulation. Two main routes exist for Ca^{2+} entry into the cytosol: voltage-operated Ca^{2+} channels (Fig. 4, 1) and receptor-operated Ca^{2+} channels (Fig. 4, 3) (Hurwitz, 1986). Prostaglandins allow entry of Ca^{2+} into the cell, perhaps via specific Ca^{2+} channels.

Calcium channeling is based on a complex of membrane-bound glycoproteins with a roughly cylindrical configuration and an aqueous pore at the center. The Ca^{2+} channels are thought to exist in three possible states, the open conformation (activated state) and two closed conformations (deactivated and inactivated states). Ca^{2+} entry via a single sarcolemmal Ca^{2+} channel has been estimated to be $\sim3 \times 10^6$ ions/sec (Holz *et al.*, 1986), much faster than the flux of Ca^{2+} through a single Ca^{2+} pump site of the cardiac SR (~30 ions/sec) (Armstrong and Eckert, 1987).

When the membrane is depolarized to an appropriate level, voltage-operated Ca^{2+} channels convert to the activated state, allowing a substantial Ca^{2+} influx into the cell. Receptor-operated Ca^{2+} channels are opened in response to activating ligands (e.g., neurotransmitters or hormones) that bind to specific receptors associated with the channel. Guanine nucleotide-binding proteins regulate Ca^{2+} channels and may couple channels and receptors directly

(Brum *et al.*, 1984). The Ca^{2+} channel activity may also be modulated by phosphorylation (e.g. Shigekawa *et al.*, 1976; Tsien, 1983; Kaczmarek, 1986; Galizzi *et al.*, 1987).

Voltage-operated Ca^{2+} channels have been divided into three types (long, transient, and neuronal) on the basis of their conductance properties. The long- and transient-type Ca^{2+} channels are important in smooth muscle activation. The long-type Ca^{2+} channels are blocked by a variety of so-called Ca^{2+} channel blockers, including 1,4-dihydropyridines such as nifedipine and nitrendipine, and are activated by structural analogues such as Bay K8644, a Ca^{2+} channel agonist (Triggle and Janis, 1987). The dihydropyridine-sensitive Ca^{2+} channel is particularly abundant in the transverse-tubule membranes of skeletal muscle and has been isolated from this source in several laboratories (e.g., Curtis and Catterall, 1986). The isolated voltage-operated Ca^{2+} channel protein has five distinct subunits: α_1 (175 kda), α_2 (143 kda), β (54 kda), γ (30 kda), and δ (24–27 kda) (Leung *et al.*, 1987; Takahashi *et al.*, 1987). The complete amino acid sequence of the α_1 subunit of the dihydropyridine receptor of skeletal muscle has been predicted from its cDNA structure (Tanabe *et al.*, 1987). Dihydropyridine, nitrendipine, and similar agents bind to myometrial strips, inhibit spontaneous or oxytocin-mediated contractility in a dose-related manner, and significantly delay labor in the rat model (Sakamoto and Huszar, 1984b; Janis and Triggle, 1986; Holbrook *et al.*, 1987).

To date we have no structural information on the receptor-operated Ca^{2+} channels. The relative contributions of voltage-dependent and receptor-operated channels to Ca^{2+} influx are likely to vary from one smooth muscle type to another. Recent evidence from studies with sea urchin eggs (Irvine and Moor, 1986) also suggests the possibility that inositol 1,3,4,5-tetrakisphosphate may open the receptor-operated Ca^{2+} channels in the plasma membrane to allow extracellular Ca^{2+} to enter the cytosol.

As an alternative Ca^{2+}-entry mechanism, Van Breemen and his colleagues have postulated a "Ca^{2+} leak" (passive influx of Ca^{2+}) (Fig. 4, 2) whereby Ca^{2+} consistently enters the smooth muscle cell at a slow rate (Van Breemen *et al.*, 1986). In addition, it has been suggested that a pool of Ca^{2+} may be associated with the inner surface of the plasmalemma (possibly associated with phospholipids) in the resting cell (Fig. 4, 4). Membrane depolarization would disrupt this interaction, releasing Ca^{2+} into the cytosol. The presence of such a discrete Ca^{2+} pool is experimentally difficult to prove and will require high-resolution electron microprobe analysis.

3.3.2. *Release of Ca^{2+} from the SR by Inositol 1,4,5-Trisphosphate*

Recent advances toward an understanding of Ca^{2+} release from the SR into the cytosol are based on a series of elegant studies in nonmuscle cells. After the discovery by Hokin and Hokin (1953) that pancreatic inositide metabolism was stimulated in response to acetylcholine, Michell (1975) proposed that inositide metabolism is involved in the modulation of intracellular Ca^{2+} concentration. It is now evident that the important link between inositides and Ca^{2+}-regulation is inositol 1,4,5-trisphosphate [$Ins(1,4,5)P_3$]. Plasma membranes commonly contain small amounts of phosphatidylinositol (PtdIns), phosphatidylinositol 4-phosphate [PtdIns(4)P], and phosphatidylinositol 4,5-bisphosphate [$PtdIns(4,5)P_2$]. Ligand binding induces activation of a specific phospholipase C, which hydrolyzes $PtdIns(4,5)P_2$ to form $Ins(1,4,5)P_3$ and 1,2-diacylglycerol (Fig. 5). A GTP-binding protein, homologous to the guanine nucleotide-binding regulatory proteins of the adenylate cyclase system, is believed to couple the receptor to phospholipase C (Berridge and Irvine, 1984). The products of $PtdIns(4,5)P_2$ hydrolysis have now been recognized as second messengers, i.e., intracellular molecules that transmit the extracellular signals to bring about the desired physiological response (Nishizuka, 1984; Berridge and Irvine, 1984).

Studies with smooth muscle tissues suggest an important role for $Ins(1,4,5)P_3$ in release of Ca^{2+} from the SR. Stimulation of rabbit arterial strips with norepinephrine led to an increase in PtdIns turnover (Hashimoto *et al.*, 1986). Furthermore, following incubation of the tissue with radiolabeled inositol, norepinephrine transiently increased the quantities of radioactive Ins(1,4,5)P$_3$ metabolites. Ins(1,4,5)P$_3$ is a water-soluble compound that diffuses in the cytosol and apparently interacts with a specific receptor in the SR membrane (Spät *et al.*, 1986). This interaction opens a Ca^{2+} channel [which is either the Ins(1,4,5)P$_3$ receptor itself or may be coupled to the Ins(1,4,5)P$_3$ receptor] in the SR membrane, causing the release of Ca^{2+} from the SR into the cytosol (Fig. 4, 5).

Administration of Ins(1,4,5)P$_3$ to skinned smooth muscle fibers in micromolar concentrations (similar to that known to occur in agonist-induced intact nonmuscle cells) can release sufficient Ca^{2+} from the SR to elicit development of maximal force (A. V. Somlyo *et al.*, 1985; Bitar *et al.*, 1986b; Hashimoto *et al.*, 1986). Also, smooth muscles contain substantially higher (~35-fold) levels of Ins(1,4,5)P$_3$ phosphatase than does skeletal muscle (Walker *et al.*, 1987). That Ins(1,4,5)P$_3$-induced Ca^{2+} release plays a role *in vivo* was supported by studies using "caged Ins(1,4,5)P$_3$" (Walker *et al.*, 1987). The caged compound, a photolabile precursor of Ins(1,4,5)P$_3$, is ineffective in releasing SR Ca^{2+} and is not a substrate of the endogenous Ins(1,4,5)P$_3$ phosphatase. Laser pulse photolysis of rabbit main pulmonary arterial fibers loaded with the caged compound released active Ins(1,4,5)P$_3$ and induced a full contraction at 0.5 μM with activation rates ($t_{1/2}$ to peak tension ~3 sec) compatible with *in vivo* contractions (Walker *et al.*, 1987).

Ins(1,4,5)P$_3$, like other second messengers, must be generated rapidly but also removed rapidly to allow the timely restoration of resting cellular conditions. This action is accomplished in two ways (Fig. 5). Ins(1,4,5)P$_3$ can be hydrolyzed by a 5-phosphatase (5-phosphomonoesterase) to Ins(1,4)P$_2$, which is in turn hydrolyzed by a distinct phosphatase to Ins1P (and probably Ins4P) and finally to inositol, which is recycled back into membrane polyphosphoinositides. As an alternative to hydrolysis, Ins(1,4,5)P$_3$ can be phosphorylated to inositol 1,3,4,5-tetrakisphosphate [Ins(1,3,4,5)P$_4$], which may in turn be further phosphorylated to InsP$_5$ and InsP$_6$. The Ins(1,4,5)P$_3$ kinase is Ca^{2+} and calmodulin dependent (Rossier

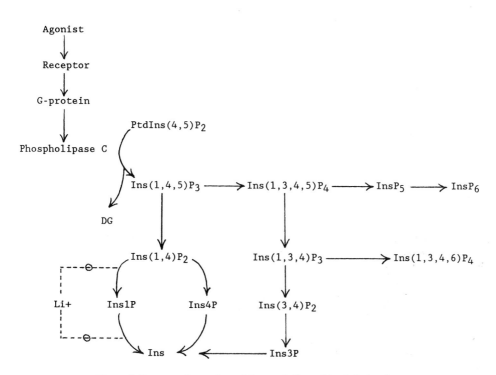

Figure 5. Current understanding of the metabolism of inositol phosphates.

et al., 1987; Yamaguchi *et al.*, 1987). In addition, Ins(1,3,4,5)P$_4$ can be hydrolyzed to Ins(1,3,4)P$_3$, an inactive isomer of Ins(1,4,5)P$_3$. It is likely that the relative importance of alternative pathways of inositol phosphate metabolism will vary from one smooth muscle to another.

3.3.3. Ca^{2+}-Induced Ca^{2+} Release

The phenomenon of Ca^{2+}-induced Ca^{2+} release has been extensively studied in skeletal and cardiac muscles (Endo, 1977), and its occurrence and importance in smooth muscle have been suggested (Itoh *et al.*, 1985). In this process, a small influx of extracellular Ca^{2+}, or release of Ca^{2+} bound to the inner surface of the sarcolemma, triggers the release of Ca^{2+} from the SR by a presently undefined mechanism.

4. Contractile Proteins of the Myometrium

4.1. Myosin

Myosin is the principal protein of muscle contraction. It is laid down in myofilaments, which optimizes the interaction with the other major contractile protein, actin. Myosin is also an enzyme that facilitates conversion of the chemical energy of ATP into motion/force generation during contraction. In smooth muscles, such as the myometrium, the myosin molecule is composed of two heavy chains of 200 kda and two pairs of light chains of 17 and 20 kda (Fig. 2). The globular head of myosin carries three important sties: (1) the actin-combining site, where myosin and actin interact; (2) the ATPase site, where ATP is hydrolyzed; and (3) the 20-kda light chains, which provide the key element of contractile regulation through reversible phosphorylation. The mechanism of contraction at the molecular level is identical in all muscles and is based on the interaction of actin and myosin. It is well established that the common signal for contractile regulation of skeletal and smooth muscles is calcium. However, the mechanism of calcium regulation is different in the two muscles (Fig. 6). In skeletal muscles, regulation is associated with the actin filament: Ca^{2+} binds to the troponin C subunit of the troponin–tropomyosin complex, inducing conformational changes in the proteins and allowing actin–myosin interaction and contraction. In smooth muscles, however, there is now overwhelming evidence that the actin–myosin interaction is regulated by phosphorylation of the 20-kda light chains of myosin catalyzed by the enzyme myosin light chain kinase (MLCK), which is calcium dependent. The actin–myosin interaction can take place only if myosin light chains (MLC) have been phosphorylated. That the activation of actomyosin ATPase activity and contraction are both dependent on MLC phosphorylation is supported by various data *in vivo* and *in vitro*. The activation of contraction by increasing calcium concentrations parallels the increase in levels of P$_i$ incorporation into myosin. Also, a correlation has been shown between the phosphorylation of MLCs and actomyosin ATPase activity in smooth muscles, including the uterus (Chacko *et al.*, 1977; Sherry *et al.*, 1978; Lebowitz and Cooke, 1979; Janis *et al.*, 1981; Kerrick and Hoar, 1981). An example of such a regulatory system in a human reproductive organ is the smooth muscle of the human placenta. When the MLCs were phosphorylated, placental actomyosin ATPase activity simultaneously increased about fourfold in comparison with the activity of unphosphorylated myosin (Huszar and Bailey, 1979a).

Fragmentation of smooth muscle myosin with a variety of proteases has provided useful information about the domain structure of the molecule. The globular head is the N-terminal end of the heavy chain (Fig. 7). Myosin can be cleaved by chymotrypsin into light meromyosin (composed of the last two-thirds of the tail) and heavy meromyosin (composed of the

SKELETAL MUSCLE

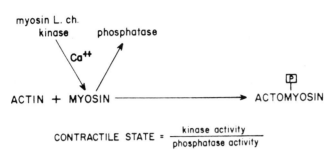

SMOOTH MUSCLE

$$\text{CONTRACTILE STATE} = \frac{\text{kinase activity}}{\text{phosphatase activity}}$$

Figure 6. The common role of calcium in the regulation of actin–myosin interaction in skeletal and smooth muscles. TN, troponin; TM, tropomyosin. From Huszar (1981), with permission.

two globular heads and one-third of the tail) (Seidel, 1980). Heavy meromyosin can be cleaved with papain to subfragment-1 (free myosin heads), which retains the actin binding and the ATPase site (Seidel, 1980). *Staphylococcus aureus* V8 protease is very useful for generating heavy meromyosin and subfragment-1 (the globular head) with intact light chains (Ikebe and Hartshorne, 1985a). These fragments are widely used in studies of myosin enzymatic properties.

4.1.1. Conformational Transitions in Smooth Muscle Myosin

Light-chain phosphorylation induces a substantial conformational change in monomeric myosin *in vitro* (Suzuki *et al.*, 1982; Trybus *et al.*, 1982; Craig *et al.*, 1983). The non-phosphorylated myosin exhibits a sedimentation coefficient of 10 S, whereas the phosphory-lated protein sediments at 6 S. Electron microscopy has revealed that the tail in 10 S myosin is bent in two places (about one-third and two-thirds of the way down the tail from the head–tail junction) and is folded so that the distal bend comes in close proximity to the neck region. On

Figure 7. Proteolytic fragments of smooth muscle myosin. Each heavy chain consists of a long α-helical tail and a globular head. The two tails are wound around each other to form an α-helical coiled coil. Two light chains with masses of about 15 and 20 kda are associated noncovalently with each globular head. ''P'' denotes the site of phosphorylation (serine-19) on each of the 20-kda light chains. The major fragments of light meromyosin (LMM)

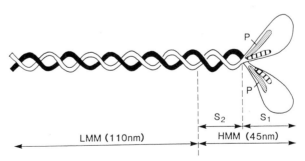

and heavy meromyosin (HMM) and the further degradation products of HMM subfragment-1 (S_1) and HMM subfragment-2 (S_2) can be generated by a variety of proteases (see text).

the other hand, the tail in 6 S myosin is elongated, resembling skeletal muscle myosin (Onishi and Wakabayashi, 1982; Trybus *et al.*, 1982; Craig *et al.*, 1983). Ikebe *et al.* (1983) demonstrated an important correlation between transition from 10 S to 6 S myosin and conversion of myosin from an inactive to an active state. Studies with proteolytic fragments of smooth muscle myosin indicate that the functionally important effect of light chain phosphorylation is a conformational change in the neck region of the myosin molecule (the head–tail junction) (Ikebe and Hartshorne, 1984). A similar conformational change is thought to occur in filamentous myosin (Ikebe and Hartshorne, 1984, 1985a), the state in which myosin occurs in both contracted and relaxed smooth muscles (A. V. Somlyo *et al.*, 1981). In physiological terms, phosphorylation induces a functionally important conformational change in the neck region of myosin, which leads to a state in which the myosin Mg^{2+}-ATPase may be activated by actin.

4.1.2. Myosin Isoforms

Isoforms of skeletal and cardiac muscle myosin heavy chains have been demonstrated by isolation and sequencing of homologous peptides and by electrophoresis of the native proteins in various gel systems. With respect to smooth muscles, two myosin heavy-chain isoforms, which differ by about 4 kda in molecular mass, were demonstrated (Rovner *et al.*, 1986; Kawamoto and Adelstein, 1987). At present, it is not clear whether native myosin exists as heavy chain homodimers or heterodimers. Isoforms of myosin were also demonstrated in human thoracic aorta and lower saphenous vein and in rabbit aorta and uterus by pyrophosphate gel electrophoresis (Lema *et al.*, 1986). However, Kawamoto and Adelstein (1987), using cultured cells, detected no major differences in two-dimensional tryptic peptide maps between the two rat aortic heavy chains, nor did these peptide maps differ from those of vas deferens or uterine heavy chains.

The question of tissue-specific isoforms of smooth muscle myosin heavy chain was studied in detail by comparison of two-dimensional cyanogen bromide peptide maps of myosin heavy chains isolated from chicken and turkey gizzards, dog aorta, and human esophagus, stomach, urinary bladder, uterus, and placenta (Huszar and Vigue, 1986). The gizzard heavy chains were found to be identical, but differences in the various human myosin heavy chains indicated tissue-specific isoforms. Species differences also were apparent among the heavy chains of human, cow, and rabbit myometrial smooth muscle. However, uterine heavy chains from nonpregnant and pregnant cows were not different. Skeletal and cardiac myosin isoforms are known to differ in their actin-activated myosin Mg^{2+}-ATPase activities (Pope *et al.*, 1980), raising the possibility that the contractile properties of smooth muscles may be influenced by their myosin isoform types.

4.2. Thin Filament Proteins

Actin is structurally highly conserved, consistent with its involvement in diverse contractile and motile processes and its ability to interact with a large number of proteins. Actin has three important properties: (1) it polymerizes to form long filaments in a reversible manner (G-actin $\rightleftharpoons$ F-actin transition); (2) it combines with myosin and activates its Mg^{2+}-ATPase activity; and (3) it binds to tropomyosin and other regulatory proteins, e.g., troponin in striated muscles and MLCK in smooth muscles. The actin monomer is 42 kda (374 or 375 amino acids) and exists in several isoforms. In smooth muscle two actins were found: the α and γ types, which differ by only three amino acids, all at the N terminus (Vanderkerckhove and Weber, 1979). The α variant is predominant in vascular smooth muscles, and the γ variant in the gastrointestinal system. In other smooth muscles, e.g., uterus (Vandekerckhove and Weber, 1979; Fatigati and Murphy, 1984), there are approximately equal amounts of smooth α

and γ actins. Most smooth muscles also contain cytoplasmic α and β actins (Fatigati and Murphy, 1984).

Tropomyosin is present in smooth muscle, such as the myometrium, at a molar ratio to actin monomers of 1:6 to 1:7. It is composed of two elongated, α-helical polypeptides of 33 kda coiled around each other and is located in the grooves of the actin strands. Each tropomyosin molecule spans seven actin monomers, consistent with the *in vivo* stoichiometry. Smooth muscle tropomyosin exists in two isoforms, α and β (α having a higher mobility on SDS-polyacrylamide gel electrophoresis). In chicken gizzard, the protein exists predominantly as the heterodimer (Sanders *et al.*, 1986). Rabbit and pig uterine smooth muscles, however, contain only the β-tropomyosin species (Cummins and Perry, 1974). The function of tropomyosin in smooth muscles has not yet been clearly defined, although it has a significant potentiating effect on the actin-activated myosin Mg^{2+}-ATPase *in vitro* (Sobieszek and Small, 1977; Miyata and Chacko, 1986).

5. Regulation of Myometrial Contractility

5.1. Calmodulin

As discussed earlier, the major regulator of contraction in smooth muscles is Ca^{2+}. In the resting cell, the cytoplasmic free Ca^{2+} level is 130 nM. Physiological stimuli such as membrane depolarization or contractile agents (acetylcholine, norepinephrine, etc.) may cause a transient increase in sarcoplasmic free Ca^{2+} to about 500–700 nM, which is detected by the "Ca^{2+} sensor protein" calmodulin. Calmodulin can bind 4 moles Ca^{2+}/mole with high affinity (K_ds in the micromolar range) (Potter *et al.*, 1983). The Ca^{2+} binding induces a dramatic change in calmodulin conformation (Klee, 1980), which exposes a hydrophobic domain(s) of interaction with target enzymes. On binding to calmodulin, these enzymes are usually converted from the inactive apoenzyme to the active holoenzyme of Ca^{2+}_4·calmodulin·enzyme.

5.2. Calmodulin-Dependent Myosin Light Chain Kinase

The most important calmodulin-dependent enzyme in the regulation of smooth muscle contractility is MLCK (Stull *et al.*, 1986). Myosin light chain kinase, a single polypeptide, binds with a very high affinity to the Ca^{2+}/calmodulin complex [e.g., K_d of the bovine stomach enzyme is 1.3 nM (Walsh *et al.*, 1982a)] in a 1:1 molar ratio. The MLCK of smooth muscles has a molecular mass in the range of 130–160 kda (Stull *et al.*, 1986); in porcine myometrium it is 130 kda (Higashi *et al.*, 1983). About 60% of the smooth muscle (chicken gizzard) MLCK sequence has been deduced from the cloned cDNA corresponding to the C-terminal region of the kinase (Fig. 8; Guerriero *et al.*, 1986). The N-terminal 40% of the molecule remains to be sequenced.

Myosin light chain kinase also occurs in skeletal muscles, e.g., in the rabbit (65 kda), although its role in striated muscles is unclear. The rabbit skeletal muscle enzyme consists of 603 amino acids of known sequence (Fig. 8; Takio *et al.*, 1985, 1986). The calmodulin-binding site is located at the C terminus; a 27-residue synthetic peptide corresponding to this region (residues 577–603) binds calmodulin very tightly (Blumental h *et al.*, 1985). The homologous binding region in the chicken gizzard enzyme (residues 473–501 in Fig. 8) is quite distant from the C-terminus. However, synthetic peptides similar to this sequence of the

RS 1 Ac-A T E N G A V E L G I Q S L S T D E A S K G A A S E E S L A

RS 31 A E K D P A P P D P E K G P G P S D T K Q D P D P S T P K K

RS 61 D A N T P A P E K G D V V P A Q P S A G G S Q G P A G E G G

RS 91 Q V E A P A E G S A G K P A A L P Q Q T A T A E A S E K K P
CG 1   W M K F R K Q I Q E N E Y I K I E N A E N

RS 121 E A E K G P S G H Q D P G E P T V G K K V A E G Q A A A R R
CG 22 S S K L T I S S T K Q E H C G C Y T L V V E N K L G S R Q A

RS 151 G S P A F L H S P S C P A I I A S T E K L P A Q K P L - S E A
CG 52 Q V N L T V V D K P D P P A G T P C A S D I R S S S L T L S W

RS 181 S E L I F E G V P A T P G P T E P G P A K A E G G V D L L A
CG 83 Y G S S Y D G G S A V Q S Y T V E I W N S V D N K W T D L T

RS 211 E S Q K E A G E K A P G Q A D Q A K V Q G D T S R G I E F Q
CG 113 T C R S T S F N V Q D L Q A D R E Y K F R V R A A N V Y G I

RS 241 A V P S E R P R P E V G Q A L C L P A R E E D C F Q I L D D
CG 143 S E P S Q E S E V V K V G E K Q E E E L K E E E A E L S D D

RS 271 C P P P P A P F P H R I V E L R T G N V S S E F S M N S K E
CG 173 E G K E T E V N Y Q T V T I N T E Q K V S - D V Y - N I E E

RS 301 A L G G G K F G A V C T C T E K S T G L K L A A Q V I K K Q
CG 201 R L G S G K F G Q V F R L V E K K T G K V W A G Q F F K A Y

RS 331 T P K D K E M V M L E I E V M N Q L N H R N L I Q L Y A A I
CG 231 S A K E K E N I R D E I S I M N C L H H P K L V Q C V D A F

RS 361 E T P H E I V L F M E Y I E G G E L F E R I V D E D Y H L T
CG 261 E E K A N I V M V L E M V S G G E L F E R I I D E D F E L T

RS 391 E V D T M V F V R Q I C D G I L F M H K M R V L H L D L K P
CG 291 E R E C I K Y M R Q I S E G V E Y I H K Q G I V H L D L K P

RS 421 E N I L C V N T T G H L V K I I D F G L A R R Y N P N E K L
CG 321 E N I M C V N K T G T S I K L I D F G L A R R L E S A G S L

RS 451 K V N F G T P E F L S P E V V N Y D Q I S D K T D M W S L G
CG 351 K V L F G T P E F V A P E V I N Y E P I G Y E T D M W S I G

RS 481 V I T Y M L L S G L S P F L G D D D T E T L N N V L S G N W
CG 381 V I C Y I L V S G L S P F M G D N D N E T L A N V T S A T W

Figure 8. Comparison of the partial amino acid sequence of chicken gizzard (CG) MLCK with the complete sequence of the rabbit skeletal muscle (RS) enzyme. The sequences are aligned to give maximal homology with deletions indicated by dashes. Boxed residues are identical in the two kinases. The catalytic domain is in the region 302–508, and the calmodulin-binding domain residues are 577–595 (using the numbering for the skeletal muscle enzyme). The serine residues in the smooth muscle enzyme (491 or 492 and 505) that are phosphorylated by the cAMP-dependent protein kinase are circled. The ATP-binding lysine residue (325) is circled, and the consensus sequence (residues 303–308 on the N-terminal side, -GLY-X-GLY-X-X-GLY-) is underlined.

```
RS  511  Y F D E E T F E A V S D E A K D F V S N L I V K E Q G A R M
CG  411  D F D D E A F D E I S D D A K D F I S N L L K K D M K S R L

RS  541  S A A Q C L A H P W L N N L A E K A K R C N R R L K S Q R L
CG  441  N C T Q C L Q H P W - - - L Q K D T K N M E A K K L S K D R

RS  571  L K K Y L M K R R - W K K N F I A V S A A N R - F K K I S S S G
CG  468  M K K Y - M A R R K W Q K T G H A V R A I G R L S S M A M I S G

RS  601  A L M
CG  499  M S G R K A S G S S P T S P I N A D K V E N E D A F L E E V

CG  529  A E E K P H V K P Y F T K T I L D M E V V E G S A A R F D C

CG  559  K I E G Y P D P E V M W Y K D D Q P V K E S R H F Q I D Y D

CG  589  E E G N C S L T I S E V C G D D D A K Y T C K A V N S L G E

CG  619  A T C T A E L L V E T M G K E G E G E G E G E E D E E E E E

CG  649  E
```

Figure 8. (Continued)

smooth muscle enzyme also bind calmodulin in a Ca^{2+}-dependent manner and inhibit the calmodulin-induced activation of MLCK (Lukas *et al.*, 1986; Kemp *et al.*, 1987).

Limited proteolysis of MLCK has been extremely useful in studies of the structure–function relationship (Walsh, 1985; Foyt *et al.*, 1985). Several distinct domains can be recognized: a catalytic active site, a calmodulin-binding site, and two sites of phosphorylation by cAMP-dependent protein kinase (Fig. 9). A 70-kda peptide fragment of chicken gizzard MLCK generated by *Staphylococcus aureus* V8 protease digestion retains all these sites. It has been suggested, but not proved, that the remainder of the molecule may serve to bind the kinase to the actin filament (Walsh, 1985; Dabrowska *et al.*, 1982). Other enzymatic fragments also have indicated the mechanism whereby calmodulin binding induces activation of MLCK. An 80-kda chymotryptic fragment is fully active in the absence of Ca^{2+} and calmodulin (Walsh *et al.*, 1982b). On tryptic digestion of MLCK (Foster *et al.*, 1986; Ikebe *et al.*, 1987b), a 64-kda fragment is produced that is completely inactive and has lost the ability to bind calmodulin (Fig. 9). Further digestion generates a 61-kda MLCK peptide that is constitutively active.

It therefore appears that the apoenzyme form of MLCK is inactive because an inhibitory peptide domain is folded in a way that masks the active site. Binding of Ca^{2+}/calmodulin induces a conformational change leading to the exposure of the active site. In analogous fashion, chymotryptic digestion of the kinase removes the inhibitory peptide domain of MLCK, unmasking the active site. The inhibitory peptide region is part of the calmodulin-binding domain, and removal of a portion of this sequence results in loss of calmodulin binding but not substrate interaction with the MLCK active site. Kemp *et al.* (1987) found that a calmodulin-binding 22-residue peptide corresponding to residues 460–481 of smooth muscle MLCK (Fig. 8) resembles the sequence around the phosphorylated serine of the 20-kda myosin light chain. This finding suggests that, in the apoenzyme of MLCK, this domain of the kinase would be bound at the substrate binding site. Binding of Ca^{2+}/calmodulin would unfold the active site and allow access for the myosin light chains.

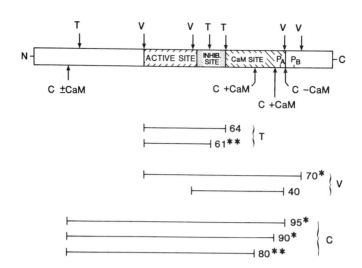

Figure 9. The domain structure of smooth muscle MLCK from the N- to the C-terminal end. Sites of proteolysis are indicated by arrows. T, trypsin; V, *S. aureus* V8 protease; C, α-chymotrypsin; CaM, calmodulin. The presence of bound calmodulin affects chymotryptic digestion as shown. The bars below the kinase depict the important fragments generated by the three proteases. Their M_r values (in kilodaltons) are indicated at the right. P_A and P_B represent sites A (ser 491 or 492) and B (ser 505) phosphorylated by cAMP-dependent protein kinase. Asterisks denote active fragments that require Ca^{2+} for activity; double asterisks denote Ca^{2+}-independent active fragments. The 64-kda tryptic peptide and the 40-kda *Staphylococcus aureus* protease peptide lack enzymatic activity.

The catalytic domain of MLCK (residues 200–450; Fig. 8) is homologous with cAMP-dependent protein kinase and the catalytic subunit of phosphorylase *b* kinase (Guerriero *et al.*, 1986). The protein kinases contain a consensus sequence, -GLY-X-GLY-X-X-GLY-, located 16–28 residues towards the N terminus from the lysine, which is involved in ATP binding (Kamps *et al.*, 1984). These are residues 203–208 (-GLY-SER-GLY-LYS-PHE-GLY-) and 225 (LYS) in Fig. 8. Two sites of phosphorylation by cAMP-dependent protein kinase were identified as serines 491 (or 492) and 505 (Lukas *et al.*, 1986; Payne *et al.*, 1986). The former is phosphorylated only in the absence of bound calmodulin, whereas the latter is phosphory-lated in either the presence or absence of bound calmodulin.

5.3. *The Mechanism of MLCK Action*

Myosin light chain kinase catalyzes phosphorylation of a serine residue (SER-19) near the N terminus of the 20-kda light chain (Pearson *et al.*, 1984). The primary structure around this phosphorylation site is remarkably similar to the calmodulin-binding domains of chicken gizzard and rabbit skeletal muscle MLCK (Fig. 10), causing the pseudosubstrate behavior of the MLCK peptide previously discussed. The basic residues located toward the N terminus from SER-19 and the hydrophobic residues PHE-22 and VAL-21 at the C-terminal side have a particularly important influence on the V_{max} of phosphorylation (Kemp *et al.*, 1982, 1983; Kemp and Pearson, 1985; Pearson *et al.*, 1986).

Turkey gizzard MLCK phosphorylates gizzard myosin with apparent K_m and V_{max} values of approximately 15 μM and 15 μmole/min per mg, respectively (Persechini and Hartshorne, 1981). The activities of smooth muscle MLCKs, including the porcine myometrial enzyme, are highly dependent on Ca^{2+} and calmodulin. *In vitro* studies of the kinetics of light chain phosphorylation have led to two schools of thought: those investigators who believe that the

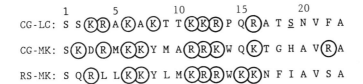

Figure 10. The distribution of basic amino acids near the phosphorylated serine in the 20-kda light chain of chicken gizzard myosin (CG-LC) and in the calmodulin-binding domains of chicken gizzard (CG-MK) and rabbit skeletal muscle (RS-MK) MLCKs. The N-terminal 23 residues of the light chain are shown with the homologous regions of the two MLCKs, which, on the numbering of Fig. 8, are residues 464–486 for the chicken gizzard enzyme and 567–589 for the rabbit skeletal muscle enzyme. Basic residues are circled, and the phosphorylated serine (residue 19) in the light chain is underlined.

two heads of a myosin are randomly phosphorylated (Chacko, 1981; Chacko and Rosenfeld, 1982; Trybus and Lowey, 1985) and others who maintain that phosphorylation is negatively cooperative and therefore occurs by an ordered mechanism (Persechini and Hartshorne, 1981; Ikebe *et al.*, 1982; Sellers *et al.*, 1983). Similarly, controversy exists as to whether both heads of myosin need to be phosphorylated before actin activation of the myosin Mg^{2+}-ATPase can occur (see Trybus and Lowey, 1985, for discussion). The direct correlation between the level of myosin phosphorylation and the velocity of shortening [cross-bridge cycling rate (Aksoy *et al.*, 1982)] in vascular smooth muscle does not support a negatively cooperative phosphorylation mechanism in which only doubly phosphorylated myosin is activated by actin. Furthermore, Persechini *et al.* (1986) provided evidence supportive of a random phosphorylation mechanism in intact bovine tracheal smooth muscle strips.

5.4. *Modulation of Smooth Muscle Contractility by MLCK*

There appears to be a positive correlation between the level of myosin phosphorylation and the velocity of shortening in skinned and intact smooth muscle fibers (Dillon *et al.*, 1981; Persechini *et al.*, 1986). The ATP analogue adenosine 5′-O-(3-thiotriphosphate), abbreviated ATPγS, is a good substrate for MLCK, but thiophosphorylated myosin is not dephosphorylated by myosin light chain phosphatase. Permanently thiophosphorylated gizzard myosin does not require Ca^{2+} for actin activation of the Mg^{2+}-ATPase (Sherry *et al.*, 1978). Furthermore, incubation of skinned smooth muscle fibers with ATPγS also induces a Ca^{2+}-insensitive activation of tension (Cassidy *et al.*, 1979; Hoar *et al.*, 1979).

The reversibility of the effect of myosin phosphorylation on actin activation of the Mg^{2+}-ATPase was demonstrated using MLCK and myosin light chain phosphatase *in vitro* (Sellers *et al.*, 1981). The actin-activated ATPase rate of unphosphorylated myosin (4 nmole P_i/mg myosin per min) rose to 51 nmole/mg per min when myosin was phosphorylated to the extent of 2 moles P_i/mole myosin. Subsequent dephosphorylation with myosin light chain phosphatase decreased the ATPase rate to 5 nmole/mg myosin per min. Rephosphorylation with MLCK increased the rate again to 46 nmole/mg myosin per min. Similar results on the phosphorylation-dependent actin–myosin interaction were obtained with actomyosin preparations from the human placenta (Huszar and Bailey, 1979a,b). Myosin phosphatases also have been used to induce relaxation in skinned fibers of hog carotid artery (Rüegg *et al.*, 1982), chicken gizzard (Hoar *et al.*, 1985), and rat uterine smooth muscle (Haeberle *et al.*, 1985).

Further experiments probing the regulation of smooth muscle contractility were based on pharmacological agents, including phenothiazines, e.g., trifluoperazine (Levin and Weiss, 1979), and naphthalenesulfonamides (Hidaka *et al.*, 1981), which bind to calmodulin in a Ca^{2+}-dependent manner and inhibit its interaction with MLCK. These compounds inhibited both phosphorylation of the myosin light chain and actin-activated Mg^{2+}-ATPase of gizzard myosin (Hidaka *et al.*, 1980). The calmodulin antagonists also inhibited tension development or induced relaxation of skinned (e.g., Kanamori *et al.*, 1981; Silver and Stull, 1983) and intact (e.g., Hidaka *et al.*, 1978) smooth muscle fibers.

The Ca^{2+}-independent MLCK chymotrypic fragment described above was used in smooth muscle actomyosin (Walsh *et al.*, 1982b, 1983) and skinned fiber preparations (Walsh *et al.*, 1982c, 1983; Mrwa *et al.*, 1985) to study the effects of myosin phosphorylation on the actin-activated myosin Mg^{2+}-ATPase and tension development. A gizzard actomyosin preparation that contained MLCK and calmodulin exhibited Ca^{2+}-sensitive actomyosin ATPase activity (75.9% Ca^{2+} sensitivity) as expected. With the Ca^{2+}-independent MLCK preparation, the Ca^{2+} sensitivity of the ATPase was essentially abolished (5.2% Ca^{2+} sensitivity). In skinned-fiber experiments, incubation with Ca^{2+}-independent MLCK and ATP in the absence of Ca^{2+} elicited phosphorylation of the 20-kda light chain and development of tension comparable to that observed in the presence of Ca^{2+}-dependent MLCK. Maximal tension development could, therefore, be accounted for solely on the basis of myosin phosphorylation.

Such studies strongly support the idea that myosin phosphorylation and dephosphorylation are key events in the "on–off" switch in actin activation of the myosin Mg^{2+}-ATPase. Initiation of tension development in smooth muscles may occur in response to electrical impulse, K^+ ions, and pharmacological agonists, all of which cause phosphorylation of myosin light chains during isometric contraction (reviewed by Kamm and Stull, 1985, and Hartshorne, 1987).

5.5. *Myosin Light Chain Phosphatase*

The notion that myosin phosphorylation plays a central role in smooth muscle contraction led to the isolation and characterization of myosin light chain phosphatase from diverse smooth muscle tissues. Two phosphatases were isolated from turkey gizzard by Pato and Adelstein (1980): one contains three subunits of 60, 55, and 38 kda (the catalytic subunit) in equal molar ratios and is relatively nonspecific; the other contains a single polypeptide chain of 43 kda, requires Mg^{2+} for activity, and appears to be specific for the 20-kda light chain. However, neither of these phosphatases can dephosphorylate intact myosin; therefore, they are unlikely to dephosphorylate myosin *in vivo*. Similar enzymes have been isolated from bovine aorta and chicken gizzard (Werth *et al.*, 1982; Pato and Kerc, 1986). Two other phosphatases that can dephosphorylate intact myosin were identified in turkey gizzard (Pato and Kerc, 1985). At present it is unclear whether myosin phosphatases are subject to some form of regulation. It seems likely that the phosphatase activity is unregulated *in vivo* and that the level of myosin phosphorylation in the muscle at a given time is dependent exclusively on the MLCK activity.

5.6. *Phosphorylation of Myosin Light Chain and Heavy Chains by Other Kinases*

In addition to MLCK, various other protein kinases are able to phosphorylate the isolated 20-kda light chain of smooth muscle myosin: cAMP-dependent protein kinase (Noiman, 1980), casein kinase II (Singh *et al.*, 1983), the epidermal growth factor (EGF) receptor tryosine kinase (Gallis *et al.*, 1983), phosphorylase kinase (Singh *et al.*, 1983), glycogen synthase kinase I (Singh *et al.*, 1983), and a Ca^{2+}/calmodulin-dependent protein kinase (Fukunaga *et al.*, 1982). These enzymes, however, do not phosphorylate light chains of intact myosin and therefore are unlikely to be of physiological significance. However, intact myosin is phosphorylated *in vitro* by *Acanthamoeba* myosin I heavy chain kinase (on SER-19 of the 20-kda light chains) (Hammer *et al.*, 1984), protease-activated kinase I (also on SER-19)

(Tuazon and Traugh, 1984), and the Ca^{2+}- and phospholipid-dependent protein kinase (protein kinase C) (Nishikawa *et al.*, 1983).

Protein kinase C is a widely distributed enzyme with a relatively broad substrate specificity (Nishizuka, 1984). It is activated by an increase in cytosolic Ca^{2+} concentration, by phorbol esters (tumor promoters), and by the second messenger 1,2-diacylglycerol, which is generated by membrane polyphosphoinositide turnover in response to a variety of extracellular messengers (peptide hormones, growth factors, muscarinic cholinergic and α-adrenergic agents). The enzyme also requires acidic phospholipids, e.g., phosphatidylserine, for activity; these are supplied by the plasma membrane. Ikebe *et al.* (1987a) observed phosphorylation of gizzard heavy meromyosin by protein kinase C at three sites, all on the 20-kda light chains: SER-1, SER-2, and THR-9. Phosphorylation, which occurs by a random process, is most rapid at THR-9, is slower at SER-1 or -2, and occurs at the third site only on prolonged incubation. Phosphorylation by kinase C causes a progressive inhibition of the actin-activated Mg^{2+}-ATPase activity of heavy meromyosin previously phosphorylated by MLCK. This inhibition occurs through a decrease in affinity of heavy meromyosin for actin. Phosphorylation of the heavy meromyosin by kinase C alone has no effect on the actin-activated Mg^{2+}-ATPase, but it reduces the rate of subsequent phosphorylation by MLCK. However, to date, it is unclear whether the protein kinase C-catalyzed phosphorylation of myosin is of importance in the contractile regulation of smooth muscle.

5.7. Second-Site Phosphorylation of Myosin

Charge variants of myosin light chains have been detected by polyacrylamide gel electrophoresis of extracts of intact and skinned smooth muscle fibers, a finding that suggests variable extents of phosphorylation (e.g., Csabina *et al.*, 1986). Ikebe and Hartshorne (1985b) demonstrated that high concentrations of MLCK can catalyze phosphorylation of a second site, identified as THR-18 (Ikebe *et al.*, 1986), on the 20-kda light chain of turkey gizzard myosin. Second-site phosphorylation markedly enhanced the actin-activated Mg^{2+}-ATPase activity of myosin. The possibility that two-site phosphorylation of smooth muscle myosin may have physiological significance is suggested by Haeberle and Trockman (1986), who observed the formation of both mono- and diphosphorylated forms of LC_{20} on stimulation of glycerinated porcine carotid artery.

6. Mechanisms of Smooth Muscle Regulation Other Than MLCK

Whereas the central role of myosin light chain phosphorylation–dephosphorylation is well established in the regulation of smooth muscle contraction, biochemical and physiological evidence suggests the existence of additional control mechanisms. For example, in intact and skinned fibers, tension can be maintained during prolonged stimulation in spite of the fact that myosin becomes dephosphorylated (Dillon *et al.*, 1981; Aksoy *et al.*, 1982, 1983; Chatterjee and Murphy, 1983). This maintenance of tension without myosin phosphorylation, the "latch state," is achieved by noncycling or slowly cycling cross bridges. Latch bridges are Ca^{2+} dependent so that complete relaxation can be achieved on return of the cytosolic free Ca^{2+} to resting levels. More recently, more precise measurements indicated that low levels of myosin phosphorylation (significantly above the levels measured in fully relaxed muscle) occur during the latch state in muscle fibers (Hai and Murphy, 1988). It may be possible, therefore, to explain the formation and maintenance of latch bridges entirely on the basis of myosin phosphorylation, with the assumption that dephosphorylation of an attached cross bridge gives rise to a long-lasting, noncycling latch bridge that would conserve energy during prolonged tonic contractions.

The data are consistent with a dual calcium regulatory system. High calcium levels activate the MLCK and cause MLC phosphorylation and muscle contraction. At lower calcium levels the MLCs gradually dephosphorylate, but some remain in a "latch" position, cycle slowly, and maintain the contractile force. This distinction may explain the differences in the spontaneous contractility of the myometrium versus the extended tonic contractions of labor. The hormonal events of parturition may facilitate changes in cellular regulation to bring about this variation in myometrial contractile patterns.

6.1. Thin Filament Regulation: Caldesmon

Early studies of Ca^{2+}-mediated regulation of smooth muscle contraction provided indirect evidence for a thin-filament-linked regulatory mechanism similar to the vertebrate striated muscle troponin–tropomyosin system (smooth muscle contains tropomyosin but not troponin). The biochemical basis of such thin-filament-linked regulation is the subject of ongoing investigations (Hirata *et al.*, 1977; Marston *et al.*, 1980; Ngai *et al.*, 1987), and at present the caldesmon system is the best-understood example with a likely physiological role.

Caldesmon is a major smooth muscle protein that binds calmodulin in a Ca^{2+}-dependent manner and actin in a Ca^{2+}-independent manner and inhibits actin-activated myosin Mg^{2+}-ATPase activity (Sobue *et al.*, 1981a). Caldesmon is present in a variety of muscle and nonmuscle tissues associated with actin at a molar ratio of one caldesmon to 26 actin monomers (Marston and Lehman, 1985). Two classes of caldesmon have been distinguished by immunologic methods with subunits of 130–155 kda and 70–80 kda, respectively. The two isoforms are similar in their functional properties, which indeed are all retained in an 18-kda chymotryptic fragment of caldesmon (Szpacenko and Dabrowska, 1986).

The stoichiometry of Ca^{2+}-dependent binding of calmodulin is one calmodulin to one caldesmon (150-kda polypeptide) with $K_d = 10^{-6}$ M (Sobue *et al.*, 1981a,b; Smith *et al.*, 1987). Caldesmon binding to F-actin is Ca^{2+} independent and saturable, with maximal binding of one caldesmon per six to ten actin monomers (Bretscher, 1984; Clark *et al.*, 1986). Isolated caldesmon binds to high-affinity sites on actin with $K_d \sim 0.2-1$ μM and to actin/tropomyosin with $K_d \sim 50$ nM (Marston and Smith, 1985). In the presence of >1.0 μM Ca^{2+}, calmodulin and F-actin compete for binding to caldesmon; at lower Ca^{2+} concentrations, caldesmon binds exclusively to F-actin (Sobue *et al.*, 1981a; Bretscher, 1984; Clark *et al.*, 1986). However, at the physiological ratios of actin : caldesmon : calmodulin (26 : 1 : 3), most of the caldesmon is bound to the actin filaments even in the presence of Ca^{2+} (Clark *et al.*, 1986). In fact, gizzard thin filaments isolated in either the presence or absence of Ca^{2+} contain identical amounts of caldesmon (Lehman, 1986). Phosphorylation of caldesmon by a Ca^{2+}/calmodulin-dependent protein kinase blocks its inhibitory effect on the actin-activated myosin Mg^{2+}-ATPase (Ngai and Walsh, 1984, 1985, 1987). Caldesmon phosphorylation has been demonstrated in intact smooth muscle strips stimulated with carbachol or phorbol ester (Park and Rasmussen, 1986). Caldesmon appears to be associated with a "contractile unit" composed of actin, myosin, tropomyosin, myosin light chain kinase, and myosin light chain phosphatase, consistent with a functional role for caldesmon in the regulation of actin–myosin interaction (Small *et al.*, 1986).

6.2. Regulation of Smooth Muscle Contraction by Cyclic Nucleotides

Both cAMP and cGMP (cyclic 3′,5′-nucleotides) are recognized as important regulators of diverse cellular functions. They are formed from ATP and GTP, respectively, by the enzymes adenylate cyclase and guanylate cyclase, which are stimulated following ligand–receptor interaction on the cell membrane; e.g., β-adrenergic stimulation leads to activation of adenylate cyclase. This mechanism is the primary tocolytic pathway in the myometrium. The regulation of adenylate cyclase involves two distinct GTP-binding proteins, G_s and G_i, which respectively stimulate and inhibit the cyclase (Ross and Gilman, 1980). Both cAMP and cGMP are degraded by hydrolysis of the $3'$ bond by cyclic nucleotide phosphodiesterases to yield functionally inactive $5'$-AMP and $5'$-GMP, respectively. Most tissues contain at least two forms of cyclic nucleotide phosphodiesterase (Keravis *et al.*, 1980). One prefers cGMP to cAMP as substrate at low concentrations and is activated by Ca^{2+}/calmodulin; the other form prefers cAMP and is unaffected by Ca^{2+}/calmodulin. From the point of view of myometrial relaxation during pregnancy it is of interest that cAMP phosphodiesterases appear to be inhibited in the myometrium of pregnant women. Both forms of phosphodiesterase, whether from the uterus of nonpregnant, pregnant, or laboring women, showed identical K_m values, but in pregnancy, the V_{max} values of the enzymes were 75% inhibited (Kofinas *et al.*, 1987). This inhibition may be important in maintaining myometrial relaxation during gestation.

All known actions of cAMP in mammalian cells are mediated by the cAMP-dependent protein kinase (Krebs and Beavo, 1979). In the absence of cAMP, this enzyme exists as a tetramer of two regulatory and two catalytic subunits, R_2C_2, which is inactive. Two molecules of cAMP bind to each regulatory subunit causing dissociation of free active catalytic subunits ($4cAMP + R_2C_2 = R_2 \cdot cAMP_4 + 2C$). Elevations of cellular cAMP lead to activation of cAMP-dependent protein kinase, to protein phosphorylation(s), and, ultimately, to relaxation of the muscle.

One possible mechanism for relaxation involves the cAMP-dependent phosphorylation of smooth muscle MLCK (Adelstein *et al.*, 1978; Conti and Adelstein, 1981). Phosphorylation decreases the affinity of the kinase for calmodulin up to 20-fold. However, there are a number of inconsistencies with this mechanism (see Miller *et al.*, 1983), and it is possible that the primary action of cAMP is directed to a reduction in cytosolic free Ca^{2+} by increasing Ca^{2+} uptake by the SR or by increasing Ca^{2+} efflux from the cell. The prevalence of one or the other mechanism may vary with the physiological and endocrine condition of the myometrium. Using fura-2 to monitor intracellular free Ca^{2+} in guinea pig ileum strips, Parker *et al.* (1987) observed that the β-adrenergic agonist isoproterenol caused a reduction in the resting free Ca^{2+} from 180 nM to 130 nM and suppressed spontaneous Ca^{2+} transients. The effects of isoproterenol were mimicked by forskolin (which elevates intracellular cAMP concentration by direct activation of adenylate cyclase) and dibutyryl cAMP (a nonhydrolyzable analogue of cAMP). With respect to the potential role of cGMP, rises in intracellular cGMP levels generally correlate with inhibition of smooth muscle contraction (Rapoport and Murad, 1983), but no conclusive protein phosphorylation pattern or other evidence of direct correlation has been identified (Parks *et al.*, 1987).

6.3. Endocrine Regulation of Myometrial Contractility

Myosin light chain kinase has so far been shown to be influenced by two cellular regulators: calcium and cAMP. Intracellular free calcium must be present in concentrations of about 10^{-6} M to activate MLCK. MLCK interacts with calcium through calmodulin and cAMP may cause the phosphorylation of MLCK itself by a cAMP-dependent protein kinase as described above. This phosphorylation inhibits enzymatic activity by reducing the affinity of the kinase for the calmodulin–calcium complex.

Because cAMP is critically important in contractile regulation of the myometrium, the connection between estrogen and progesterone and between the enzymes of cAMP synthesis (adenylate cyclase) and cAMP degradation (phosphodiesterase) was investigated. In addition to the well-known adenylate cyclase stimulation by β-adrenergic agonists, α-adrenergic influence caused a decrease in cellular cAMP levels, most likely through activation of phosphodiesterase (Berg *et al.*, 1986). This finding may explain why the concentration of α-adrenergic receptors and myometrial contractility increase after estrogen treatment in rabbits. However, when progesterone was administered to estrogenized rabbits, there was an inhibition of the contractile activity mediated by a β-adrenergic response (Roberts *et al.*, 1981). This mechanism does not appear to be the dominant regulator because there was no decline in the myometrial β-adrenergic binding of β-adrenergic receptor concentrations during term and preterm labor (Dattel *et al.*, 1986).

The relative importance of various myometrial calcium sources in a given endocrine milieu or in labor remains to be elucidated. Contractile activity in the layers of rat myometrium has been observed during parturition (Anderson *et al.*, 1981). There are typical changes that consist of a transition from weak, irregular contractions to large, regular contractions and repetitive spike-type electrical discharges at term pregnancy. This transition is apparently necessary for normal parturition; if it does not occur, delivery is abnormal or delayed. Experiments directed to the contractile and electrical properties of myometrial strips of parturient rats demonstrated that the changes in electrical and contractile activity are related to the endocrine events that cause calcium modulation of the action potential (Bengtsson *et al.*, 1984a,b).

Oxytocin affects MLCK in mammary myoepithelial cells (Olins and Bremel, 1982). Nanomolar concentrations of oxytocin caused a threefold increase in the level of MLC phosphorylation if calcium was present in the culture medium. When the cells were incubated with oxytocin in a calcium-free medium, the increase in MLC phosphorylation was only transient. Thus, oxytocin facilitates entry of extracellular calcium.

Oxytocin has been shown to inhibit the (Ca^{2+}, Mg^{2+})-ATPase of sarcolemma with half-maximal inhibition at about 1 nM, which corresponds to the apparent K_d (equilibrium dissociation constant) of oxytocin binding to its myometrial receptors (Soloff and Sweet, 1982). At the time of the initiation of labor in rats (days 19 to 22), the suppressibility of the (Ca^{2+}, Mg^{2+})-ATPase by oxytocin has been increased about 10,000-fold compared to the inhibition on day 18, in parallel with the reported increase in the concentration of oxytocin receptors (Alexandrova and Soloff, 1980; Sakamoto and Huszar, 1984a). Whether this mechanism is predominant in maintaining the intracellular calcium milieu is not clear, because calcium channel blockers also delay the onset of labor and the rate of delivery in rats (Sakamoto and Huszar, 1984b). Indeed, simultaneous measurements of electrical and mechanical activities of myometrium from pregnant women indicated that oxytocin can increase spontaneous contractions supported by extracellular calcium, but oxytocin also releases calcium from intracellular sites to evoke longer contractions (Kawarabayashi *et al.*, 1986).

The effects of progesterone on the myometrium are characterized by a relative quiescence and uncoupling of the excitation–contraction process (Csapo, 1977). The action of progesterone may be due to a combination of (1) reduced activities of cell membrane function and cell-to-cell communication that diminish permeability to calcium, sodium, and potassium; (2) modulation of intracellular calcium binding that makes less calcium available for the calmodulin–MLCK system; or (3) regulatory influence on the phospholipids of the myometrial cells that attenuates phosphatidylinositol and prostaglandin biosynthesis. Indeed, progesterone caused diminished synthesis of prostaglandins and gap junctions (Jeremy and Dandona, 1986). Also, progesterone action clearly is related to the postreceptor events. For instance, in the rabbit myometrium progesterone increased the cellular response to β-adrenergic receptor stimulation, and the rate of cAMP synthesis was much higher under the influence of progesterone compared with that of estrogen (Riemer *et al.*, 1986).

Another line of evidence demonstrating the role of progesterone is based on RU 486 (mifepristone), a steroid with potent progesterone-antagonistic effects, which induces myometrial contractions at any stage of the pregnancy. Cabrol *et al.* (1985) have reported expulsion of human fetuses in cases of intrauterine death within 72 hr after administration of RU 486. Frydman *et al.* (1986) used RU 486 for medically indicated termination of early pregnancy; RU 486 also induced a "ripening" of the cervix, increased the Bishop score, and eased fetal–placental expulsion. These studies offered some evidence that the antiprogesterone may serve as a useful adjunct in the induction of labor.

Prostaglandins are components of the eicosenoid system, which is increasingly recognized to have an important role in the physiology of reproduction and gestation. Prostaglandins and the related acidic lipids all arise from the principal precursor arachidonic acid via three pathways, catalyzed by the enzymes cyclooxygenase (prostaglandins and prostacyclins), thromboxane synthetase (thromboxanes from prostaglandins), and lipooxygenase (leukotrienes) (Challis and Olson, 1988). Administration of aspirin and indomethacin (cyclooxygenase inhibitors) stops uterine contractions (Bygdeman, 1980). Amnion and chorion in women produce mostly PGE_2 while the decidua produces PGE_2 and $PGF_{2\alpha}$. The amnion, which has no blood supply, receives arachidonic acid from the fetus via amniotic fluid, whereas the chorion, which also lacks blood supply, receives arachidonic acid from the decidua.

On the basis of the association among the uterine contractile responses to prostaglandin administration to the mother, the increased prostaglandin production by the fetal membranes, and the elevated prostaglandin concentrations in the mother's serum and urine preceding the onset of labor or preterm labor, the conclusion has been drawn that prostaglandins are an important factor in labor. The association also can be extended to preterm labor caused by intrauterine infections: phospholipase A that originates in pathogenic bacteria causes the release of arachidonic acid that fuels prostaglandin biosynthesis (Lamont *et al.*, 1985; Romero *et al.*, 1986). Prostaglandins also cause increased myometrial contractility *in vitro*. In fact, it appears that there is even a regional sensitivity of the uterus in response to various prostaglandins that may be mediated by additional factors, e.g., the diversity of α- and β-adrenergic innervation. For instance, in the lower uterine segment PGE_2 caused relaxation rather than contraction. Also, contractility of cervical muscles was inhibited by $PGF_{2\alpha}$ (Bryman *et al.*, 1986).

Unlike most hormones and agonists, prostaglandins are synthesized at the site of action by the decidua, myometrium, and amnion of parturient women (Giannopoulis *et al.*, 1985). Prostaglandin biosynthesis is the penultimate step to increased uterine contractility of labor or preterm labor. Conversely, the administration of prostaglandin synthesis inhibitors delays the labor process (Bygdeman, 1980). Prostaglandin E_2 and $F_{2\alpha}$ are known to stimulate myometrial contractility, most likely by acting as calcium-ionophores, and they increase intracellular calcium. Neither the density nor the affinity of prostaglandin receptors appears to change during parturition (Okazaki *et al.*, 1981). Thus, during labor the increased contractile activity is directly related to the rise in prostaglandin E_2 and $F_{2\alpha}$ and to the production of other eicosanoids by the fetoplacental unit (Davidson *et al.*, 1987). The relations among the three major pathways of eicosanoid synthesis are dynamic, and the occurrence of various prostaglandins, thromboxanes, and leukotrienes may change according to the phases of the reproductive cycle (Skinner and Challis, 1985).

The regulation of prostaglandin metabolism in the uterus and cervix is clearly undefined. There are several proteins and protein factors that are implicated in the modulation of the various pathways. For instance, there is lipocortin, a protein of about 40 kDa, which inhibits phospholipase A activity. *In vivo* or *in vitro*, glucocorticoids increase lipocortin activity (Flower, 1986), whereas phosphorylation of the lipocortin mediated by various growth factors abolishes the inhibition of phospholipase A (Wilson *et al.*, 1985). Although the mechanism is still under investigation, for practical purposes one can conclude that lipocortins inhibit arachidonic acid release and prostaglandin synthesis. Lipocortins may promote the maintenance of pregnancy in that they are produced by the conceptus (Wallner *et al.*, 1986), are present in the amniotic fluid, and inhibit the release of arachidonic acid (thus prostaglandin biosynthesis) *in vitro*.

Overall, these findings suggest that prostaglandin $F_{2\alpha}$ and oxytocin enhance, whereas progesterone and cAMP diminish, intracellular calcium levels. The latter is followed by the declining rate of MLC phosphorylation and contractile state of the myometrium. *In vivo* findings support the experimental data: intracellular calcium concentration increases during contraction and decreases when the smooth muscle is relaxed after administration of β-adrenergic agents (Scheid *et al.*, 1979), phosphodiesterase inhibitors (Berg *et al.*, 1983), or forskolin (Muller and Baer, 1983), an activator of adenylate cyclase.

The inhibition of MLCK by cAMP-mediated phosphorylation offers an excellent model for direct hormonal regulation of actin–myosin interaction. This effect occurs in addition to the cAMP effect on cellular levels of free calcium because of the activation of the SR calcium pump (Nishikori and Maeno, 1979). The phosphorylation–dephosphorylation of MLC and MLCK suggests a dual relationship. When phosphorylation of the MLC occurs, actin–myosin interaction is enhanced and the contractile state of the muscle increases. If the MLCK is phosphorylated and kinase activity decreases, less MLC phosphorylation occurs, and the muscle relaxes. However, when the MLCK is dephosphorylated, light-chain kinase activity increases together with the contractility of the myometrium.

7. Integrated Model for Regulation of Smooth Muscle Contractility

We propose that the effects of several drugs and hormones on myometrial contractility can be explained on the basis of their relationship to the factors regulating MLCK activity. The main considerations are reviewed according to their relationship to the key process of MLC phosphorylation (Fig. 11):

1. In smooth muscles enzymatic phosphorylation of the 20-kda MLC is necessary in order for actin–myosin interaction to occur.
2. MLCK is the key enzyme for myosin phosphorylation and thus for regulation of myometrial contractility.
3. Calcium is essential for MLCK activation; calcium binds to the kinase as a calmodulin–calcium complex. A second, as yet undefined, calcium regulatory system causes a decline of cross-bridge turnover rate in contracting muscle. Thus, smooth muscles may retain tension at less than peak levels of cellular calcium and MLC phosphorylation.
4. Cytosolic free calcium concentrations are regulated at the level of the SR membrane and the sarcolemma. Both membranes contain several mechanisms that regulate transmembrane movements of Ca^{2+} in both directions (see Fig. 4).
5. The accumulation of calcium by the SR is an ATP-dependent enzymatic process that is modulated by various pharmacological agents and hormones.
6. MLCK is inhibited by cAMP-mediated phosphorylation of the enzyme itself. Phosphorylation of the MLCK diminishes its affinity for the calcium–calmodulin complex (Conti and Adelstein, 1981).
7. Cellular cAMP levels depend on the relative activities of two enzymes, adenylate cyclase (cAMP synthesis) and phosphodiesterase (cAMP breakdown). Activation and inhibition of these enzymes determine myometrial cAMP levels. For example, smooth muscle relaxation may be caused by activation of adenylate cyclase with β-adrenergic agonists or by inhibition of phosphodiesterase following the administration of theophylline or papaverine. The last two agents have recently been demonstrated to cause myometrial relaxation *in vitro* (Berg *et al.*, 1983). Myometrial contractility increases in response to α-adrenergic stimulation, which probably activates phosphodiesterase (Berg *et al.*, 1986).

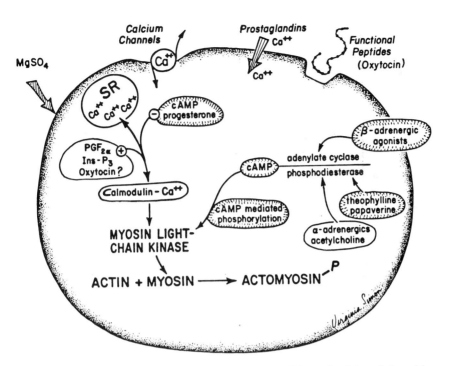

Figure 11. Cellular regulation of myometrial contractility. The MLCK is regulated through the calcium and cAMP pathways. Both calcium sequestration and cAMP levels in the cell are modulated by various drugs and hormones. Agonists circled with solid lines promote contractions; agonists in stippled areas promote relaxation. Specific sites that facilitate agonist interaction and have tocolytic potential include the β-adrenergic receptors, the calmodulin–MLCK interaction, the receptors for prostaglandins, the calcium channels, and the binding sites for functional peptides.

8. Prostaglandins affect myometrial contractility. At the present time, this can best be explained as the result of modulation of the calcium fluxes (Reiner and Marshall, 1976; Ohnishi and Devlin, 1979; Challis and Olson, 1988). Prostaglandins have been reported to change the calcium permeability of the membranes, thus influencing the levels of intracellular free calcium.

9. Various peptides and peptide hormones modulate myometrial function. For instance, as described in Section 6.3, oxytocin regulates intracellular calcium levels by affecting SR and the (Ca^{2+}, Mg^{2+})-ATPase of the myometrial cell membrane. Other data (Nishikori *et al.*, 1983) suggest that relaxin, an insulinlike peptide hormone, causes an increase in cellular cAMP levels with simultaneous inhibition of MLC phosphorylation and muscle relaxation. Also, there are peptides similar to the vasoactive intestinal peptide (VIP) that have a powerful relaxing effect on the myometrium (Ottesen *et al.*, 1980).

10. Finally, muscle cells in the myometrium are not isolated but are interconnected as a functional unit in simultaneous action during labor. The essential parts of this functional/metabolic coordination are the gap junctions. Modulation of functional unity among the myometrial smooth muscle cells through gap junctions, along with other associated cellular events, are regulated by estrogen and progesterone, as well as by other cellular agonists including prostaglandins, cAMP, and calcium (see Chapter 15).

From the point of view of tocolytic action, it is important that β-adrenergic drugs activate adenylate cyclase and increase the levels of cellular cAMP. The increased cAMP diminishes MLCK activity by two different inhibitory pathways: by reduction of cellular calcium levels and by modulation of phosphorylation of the MLCK. When myosin phosphorylation and actomyosin formation are reduced, the myometrium relaxes. The sequence and priority of the various myometrial regulatory processes are not known. The concept of cellular compartmentalization may explain the preferential activation of certain regulatory pathways. The β-adrenergic receptor–adenylate cyclase–cAMP–MLCK pathway constitutes the primary tocolytic (stopping myometrial contractility) pathway in the myometrium.

8. Preterm Birth and Tocolytic Therapy

Because preterm birth is the primary cause of perinatal morbidity and mortality, new approaches toward prevention and treatment of preterm labor, identification of maternal, fetal, and environmental factors, and development of new drugs and diagnostic procedures are primary goals of contemporary obstetrical research (Huszar, 1983).

On the basis of the mechanisms of cellular regulation of myometrial contractility described in this chapter, one can pinpoint five key pathways that present opportunities for tocolytic therapy (Fig. 11): (1) cAMP-mediated inhibition of contractility by β-adrenergic agonists; (2) inhibition of calmodulin–calcium function; (3) inhibition of prostaglandin biosynthesis; (4) inhibition of calcium influx by calcium channel-blocking agents; and (5) development and use of peptides that interfere with the myometrial contractile function.

Recently magnesium sulfate has also been introduced as a tocolytic agent (Petrie, 1981). The mechanism of this magnesium effect on myometrial contractility is not yet understood, but it is likely to be nonspecific and membrane related. The rate of calcium influx in smooth muscle is diminished by the administration of magnesium (Altura and Altura, 1981). The β-adrenergic pathway acting via cAMP has been described above; the action mechanisms of the other four drug groups are discussed briefly in the following sections.

8.1. Calcium Channel-Blocking Agents

Calcium channel-blocking agents, or calcium antagonists, selectively bind to cell membrane proteins that function as channels that allow Ca^{2+} entry into the cell and are likely to become the next generation of successful tocolytic agents. The binding of these drugs was quantified with radio tracers (Grover et al., 1984) and correlated well with the decrease in muscle tone in various studies (Bolger et al., 1982).

Several investigators have studied the role of calcium channel blockers in uterine physiology. With nicardipine, Csapo et al. (1982) showed a retardation of labor in rats ovariectomized during pregnancy. In recent experiments, a tocolytic effect on rats was demonstrated with another calcium channel blocker, nitrendipine (Sakamoto and Huszar, 1984b). Two groups of rats were treated with nitrendipine starting on days 20 and 21 of the pregnancy (term pregnancy in rats is 22 days). The mean delivery time (hours ± S.D., past 11 a.m. on day 22) in the untreated group was $9.7 ± 6.5$, whereas the groups that received nitrendipine from days 20 and 21 had mean delivery times of $18.9 ± 9.1$ ($P = 0.002$) and $12.8 ± 5.7$, respectively. Nitrendipine treatment did not appear to influence maternal or fetal outcomes. For example, the weights of the dams and pups or the number of offspring per dam were not different in the three groups. In order to investigate the effect of calcium channel blockers on the endocrine factors of labor, serum progesterone levels on days 20 and 22 (the period of progesterone withdrawal preceding labor in rats) were also measured in the control and experimental groups. Nitrendipine had no effect on the pattern of progesterone withdrawal, an observation that further indicates that the calcium channel blockers affect the contractile state of the myometrial muscle cells rather than the endocrine events underlying the initiation of labor (Carsten, 1974).

In nonpregnant human patients the calcium channel blocker nifedipine was beneficial in dysmenorrhea (Ulmsten et al., 1978; Sandahl et al., 1979). Stimulation of contractility in the postpartum uterus by methylergometrine, oxytocin, and prostaglandin $F_{2\alpha}$ has also been inhibited (Forman et al., 1982a). Clinical research with calcium channel-blocking agents is just beginning, and it is not clear whether these drugs will be used to stop premature labor or whether the major indication will be for prevention, either alone or in combination with β-adrenergic agonists (Ulmsten et al., 1980). In vitro studies suggest that combination therapies are likely to be successful because they utilize the tocolytic properties of more than one agent (Bird et al., 1987).

8.2. Prostaglandin Synthesis Inhibitors

Because prostanoids have a central role in the initiation of labor, drugs that inhibit prostaglandin synthesis are obvious choices for tocolytic therapy. The synthesis of prostaglandin does not occur in one step; instead, this process is catalyzed by a series of enzymes that are inhibited by various agents (meclofenamic acid, indomethacin, naproxen, phenylbutazone, and aspirin) with different efficiencies. The most extensive clinical experience thus far has been with indomethacin (Niebyl et al., 1980; Gammisans, 1984), which, along with aspirin, inhibits the enzyme cyclooxygenase. The effects of prolonged aspirin therapy have been demonstrated in rheumatic patients, who have an increased frequency of postmature deliveries (Lewis and Schulman, 1973).

Acceptance of the clinical administration of prostaglandin synthesis inhibitors has been slow, because the inhibitors cross the placenta and inhibit fetal prostaglandin synthesis, which may lead to fetal complications including pulmonary hypertension, premature closure of the ductus arteriosus, and blood coagulation disorders (Manchester et al., 1976; Bygdeman, 1980). At present, assessing the rate of complications is difficult because of the inconsistency in therapeutic regimens, differences in the duration of pregnancy among the women, and other associated factors (Niebyl and Witter, 1986). Prostaglandin synthesis inhibitors most likely will have a role in tocolytic management as a component of combination therapies. Side effects will be minimized when criteria for the use of these drugs are clarified, e.g., the week of gestation at which prostaglandin synthesis inhibitors are safe, the length of time they should be used, and how long before delivery the therapy should be terminated.

8.3. Calmodulin-Inhibiting Drugs

The interaction between calmodulin and MLCK may be inhibited by various phenothiazine drugs. When such drugs are added to actomyosin preparations of chicken gizzard or tracheal smooth muscles (Cassidy et al., 1980; Silver and Stull, 1983) or to sarcolemma-disrupted smooth muscle strips of rabbit ileum or rabbit pulmonary artery, contractility is inhibited by phenothiazines in proportion to the extent of inhibition of MLC phosphorylation. When an excess of calmodulin is supplied, the MLC phosphorylation and muscle tone are restored. The clinical potential of phenothiazines is increased by reports that nonionized forms of the phenothiazine drugs diffuse across plasma membranes (Chaturvedi *et al.*, 1978); thus, their reported muscle-relaxing effect is likely to occur through inhibition of the MLCK.

There are two major questions yet to be answered. First, because calmodulin is involved in several cell functions, can its action on myometrial contractility be selectively inhibited? Second, can drugs be developed that are specific for the calmodulin-mediated contractile process in the myometrium without causing effects on the central nervous system or elsewhere. With respect to the development of drugs that selectively inhibit myometrial function, this approach has definite potential by the development of organ-directed agents that are connected to a carrier molecule with affinity for a myometrial site. Examples of such tocolytics are prostaglandin synthesis inhibitors or phenothiazine-type calmodulin blockers attached to an oxytocin analogue that is recognized by the myometrial oxytocin receptors.

8.4. Functional Peptides

Various functional peptides, or peptide hormones, have been implicated in the modulation of uterine contractility. Best known and studied is oxytocin. In women (Fuchs *et al.*, 1982) and in experimental animals, increased oxytocin sensitivity at the time of the initiation of labor is related to an increase in the number of myometrial oxytocin receptors (Alexandrova and Soloff, 1980; Den *et al.*, 1981). In addition to inhibition of the (Ca^{2+}, Mg^{2+})-ATPase (the pump system that extrudes Ca^{2+} from the uterine smooth muscle cells) (Soloff and Sweet, 1982; Sakamoto and Huszar, 1984a), a second route of oxytocin action has been shown in rat and human myometrium and decidua, where an increased synthesis of prostaglandins E and $F_{2\alpha}$ was demonstrated in response to oxytocin (Husslein *et al.*, 1981).

A peptide hormone that is known to decrease myometrial contractility is relaxin. Recent data indicate that under conditions where relaxin inhibits uterine contractility, MLC phosphorylation also declines. *In vitro* experiments suggest that there is a relaxin-mediated inhibition of MLCK. At the present time, it is not clear whether relaxin acts directly on MLCK or perhaps via other cellular components involved in contractile regulation, e.g., cAMP (Nishikori *et al.*, 1983).

Peptide neurotransmitters such as the vasoactive intestinal peptide (VIP), a single chain of 28 amino acids, also modulate uterine contractility. It has been demonstrated by immunocytochemical methods that nerves supplying the vessels and smooth muscles in the uterus contain VIP (Larsson *et al.*, 1977; Ottesen *et al.*, 1981). Both the electrical and mechanical activities of myometrial explants were inhibited by systemically infused VIP even if the explants were stimulated by $PGF_{2\alpha}$ or oxytocin (Ottesen, 1983). This myometrial modulatory response is a part of gestational physiology since synthesis of VIP is modulated by steroid hormones. The inhibitory action of VIP on myometrial smooth muscle is not affected by phenoxybenzamine or propranolol (α- and β-adrenergic blockers), by atropine, or by blockers of nerve transmission (e.g., tetrodotoxin), a finding that suggests that VIP acts directly on the smooth muscle cells. The relaxing effect of VIP does not occur through competition with oxytocin or prostaglandin $F_{2\alpha}$ because in the presence of a large excess of these agents, the contractions are still inhibited. Thus, it is most likely that there are specific VIP receptors in uterine smooth muscle cells (Ottesen, 1983).

There is a strong possibility that synthesis of these functional peptides (e.g., VIP, relaxin) or their competitive nonfunctional analogues (e.g., oxytocin) will be a useful new approach in future tocolytic therapy. An example is the newly developed oxytocin analogue that has been shown to inhibit oxytocin action in strips of human myometrium and in parturient rats (Fuchs, 1986; Hahn *et al.*, 1987).

Since the etiology of preterm labor is as yet undetermined, it is not known whether the high failure rate (about 40%) of treatment is a consequence of a management problem or simply that there are patients with preterm labor in whom the condition is unrelated to the β-adrenergic receptor–cAMP pathway but who would respond to another therapeutic modality. It appears that better understanding of the cellular processes in the myometrium will help to select the most appropriate therapy for each patient.

For instance, it has become clear that continuous exposure of human myometrium to β-adrenergic agonists results in desensitization; the contractions eventually resume even in the presence of increasing concentrations of the drugs (Ke *et al.*, 1984). The reason for the loss of response appears to be a decrease in myometrial β-adrenergic receptors in women treated with tocolytic agents (Berg *et al.*, 1985). This phenomenon was studied further in the nonpregnant sheep, in which continuous infusion of long-acting (ritodrine) or short-acting (isoproterenol) β-adrenergic agonists could not sustain myometrial relaxation. However, intermittent treatment with isoproterenol prevented myometrial desensitization (Casper and Lye, 1986).

More recent, unexpected results on myometrial desensitization showed that simultaneously with β-adrenergic tocolytic therapy, there is an increase in prostaglandin biosynthesis, which may further diminish the action of tocolytic agents. When uterine segments of pregnant rats were treated with aminophylline *in vitro* (Laifer *et al.*, 1986), a significant decrease in frequency and force of contractions was observed initially. At the same time the synthesis of PGE_2 was increased by about 40%, whereas $PGF_{2\alpha}$ production was about 20% lower. In similar experiments on pregnant sheep, after isoproterenol infusion, plasma $PGF_{2\alpha}$ levels doubled without discernible changes in the PGE_2 concentrations (Casper and Lye, 1987).

Thus, there is an apparent relationship between increases in prostaglandin synthesis and uterine contractions during myometrial desensitization caused by β-adrenergic treatment. The modest but specific differences in the PGE_2 and $PGF_{2\alpha}$ responses detected between the rat and sheep models may be the result of species differences, the *in vivo–in vitro* condition differences (in the latter, membrane barriers would not prevent prostaglandin degradations), or perhaps the tissue origin of prostaglandins. The rat uterine segments did not contain membranes or decidua, which were shown to support varying patterns of prostaglandin biosynthesis (Skinner and Challis, 1985).

9. Cervix

The myometrium and cervix, two principal components of the uterus that have very different functions, respond in specific ways to the common endocrine regulation by estrogen, progesterone, prostaglandins, oxytocin, relaxin, and by other factors during pregnancy and labor. It has become increasingly evident that a close relationship between the cervix and myometrium is the basis for normal uterine function (Huszar, 1979, 1980, 1981, 1983, 1986; Huszar and Roberts, 1982; Huszar and Naftolin, 1984b). The lack of such coordination causes increased perinatal morbidity, whether in the form of inappropriate myometrial contractility (premature labor or postmaturity) or cervical dysfunction resulting from cervical incompetence or rigidity.

9.1. Biochemistry of Cervical Maturation

Cervical maturation, which converts the cervix from an unyielding to a distensible structure, is a key factor in the initiation of normal labor. During pregnancy, the cervix holds the uterine contents securely. The maturation process commences at about the 34th week of pregnancy (the time when the irregular Braxton–Hicks uterine contractions become more obvious). The cervix becomes soft, swollen, and flexible, while the cervical canal and cervical tissue become extensible. The obstetrician perceives the accompanying prelabor dilatation and effacement as the "ripening of the cervix." Among the three main structural components in the human cervix, changes in collagen and the connective tissue matrix ("ground substance") are the primary factors in ripening. The smooth muscle content is minor, only about 25, 16, and 6% in the upper, middle, and lower segments, respectively (Rorie and Newton, 1967). The recognition that changes in the connective tissue are key elements of cervical softening came from the work of Danforth et al. (1960), who demonstrated that during ripening collagen fibrils, which had previously been arranged in an orderly fashion, become disorganized. The main collagen types are I and III in the cervix of both nonpregnant and pregnant women (Minamoto et al., 1987). There are simultaneous changes in cervical compliance, and during ripening the flexibility of cervical tissue increases (Conrad and Ueland, 1979).

During cervical maturation, synthesis of collagenase occurs simultaneously with activation of the preformed zymogens (inactive preforms) and other proteolytic enzymes (Ito et al., 1977; Woessner, 1979; Martin et al., 1983). Once the collagenase and the other site-specific proteases break down the basic structure of collagen, the resulting collagen fragments can be cleaved further by various nonspecific enzymes such as cathepsins. A further control of cervical structure in the form of collagenase inhibitors exists in the cervical tissue and could play an important role in the coordination of cervical maturation (Woolley, 1979).

Experimental and clinical studies support the importance of glycosaminoglycans (molecules that bind collagen and the connective tissue matrix) in cervical ripening (Kleissl et al., 1978). The cervical concentrations of dermatan sulfate, chondroitin sulfate, and hyaluronic acid are unchanged during most of gestation in women. However, close to term, the concentration of hyaluronic acid increases from 6% in the nonpregnant state to 33% at the expense of dermatan sulfate. The increase in hyaluronic acid and its associated high water content further separates the structural elements and weakens the cervical structure; this change causes the soft, swollen appearance of the cervix (Cabrol et al., 1980; Uldbjerg et al., 1983). The study of glycosaminoglycans and collagen in the rat cervix before pregnancy, during parturition, and in involuting uteri provides a good example of such changes (Cabrol et al., 1981). At term (22nd day of gestation), cervical protein and collagen concentrations decrease about 40%. In the mature cervix the hyaluronic acid concentrations are about 2.5 times higher, and the dermatan sulfate concentrations two times lower than those of the 16-day pregnant rats. The decreases in collagen and dermatan sulfate concentrations were proportional during maturation.

The biochemical and mechanical events associated with cervical ripening are in good agreement. The extensibility modulus of the rat cervix shows no change until day 16 of pregnancy; then it increases rapidly in the final 5 days before delivery on day 22. Cervical extensibility multiplied by inner circumference, which closely describes cervical maturation, was 12, 91, 157, 208, and 320 on days 16, 18, 20, 21, and 22 of the pregnancy, respectively. The value then rapidly declined to 10 by the first postpartum day (Hollingsworth et al., 1979). In women there is a relative increase of cervical muscle concentration at term (Minamoto et al., 1987), and the contractile activity is modulated by PGE_2 and α-adrenergic agents. These findings indicate that cervical smooth muscle has an important role in cervical competence, dilatation, and effacement (Bryman et al., 1986).

These components of cervical ripening are interrelated in structure and function. During pregnancy, dermatan and chondroitin sulfates bind tightly to collagen fibers and secure them in the cervical structure (Obrink, 1973). The dense collagen framework and the associated glycosaminoglycans assure that the cervix remains firm and closed. At the end of pregnancy, the cervical matrix is disrupted as a result of two events: (1) collagen degradation increases as collagenase and other associated enzymes are activated, and (2) cervical dermatan sulfate proportionately diminishes along with collagen, and the cervix becomes swollen and soft because of increased hyaluronic acid and water content (Golichowski *et al.*, 1980). The latter accounts for the softness and fragility of the ripened cervix, whereas the loss of collagen and dermatan/chondroitin sulfates facilitates flexibility and distensibility. Simultaneously, there are cellular events associated with the initiation of labor in the myometrium, e.g., synthesis of estrogen and oxytocin receptors, formation of gap junctions, increased cellular calcium levels, and increased contractile activity, that in time lead to organized uterine contractility.

9.2. Hormonal Control of Cervical Maturation

The involuting uterus and explants of cervical and uterine tissues have served as experimental models for the study of steroid hormonal effects on collagenase activity and collagen breakdown. Estrogen increases collagenase formation and zymogen activation and promotes various myometrial events preceding labor. The inhibitory effect of progesterone on cervical maturation is well documented. In response to progesterone administration, collagen breakdown is diminished in the uteri of parturient rats (Tansey and Padykula, 1978), in guinea pig pubic symphysis ligament (Wahl *et al.*, 1977), and in cervical explants of the nonpregnant (Hillier and Wallis, 1981).

The action of prostanoids has been demonstrated by intraaortic infusion of PGE_2 and intracervical administration of $PGF_{2\alpha}$ and PGE_2, which produced maturational changes in the sheep cervix in the absence of uterine contractions (Fitzpatrick, 1977; Stys *et al.*, 1981). Effects of prostaglandins also have been demonstrated in women (Ekman *et al.*, 1983; Prins *et al.*, 1983; Hulka and Chepko, 1987). Intracervical administration of PGE_2 caused cervical softening and ultrastructural changes identical to those preceding labor (Theobald *et al.*, 1982). The stretch modulus of cervical tissue strips was reduced as well in patients who received PGE_2 or who were in spontaneous labor in comparison with tissues from the nonpregnant cervix (Conrad and Ueland, 1979). The contractility of cervical smooth muscle is influenced by prostaglandin action. Incubation of cervical strips with PGE_2 caused an increase in the stretch response and distensibility (Bryman *et al.*, 1984).

The importance of local cervical prostaglandin action in the absence of myometrial contractions has been demonstrated in clinical studies. In one study, two groups of patients (four women each) were investigated; the patients who received treatment with PGE_2 vaginal suppositories for 6 hr prior to interruption of pregnancy had about two times more advanced cervical dilatation than did patients given oxytocin induction (Forman *et al.*, 1982b).

The possible role of relaxin in cervical changes was based on the original observation that connective tissue changes in pregnant rats occurred after treatment with estrogen and relaxin (Kroc *et al.*, 1959). Whereas prostaglandin administered to pigs caused a relaxin surge from the ovaries (Sherwood *et al.*, 1976), no such effect was observed in women (Hochman *et al.*, 1978). Attempts to demonstrate relaxin receptors in the human uterus have only recently been successful (Mercado-Simmen *et al.*, 1980). Relaxin and progesterone cause a decrease in the contractility of myometrial and cervical smooth muscle *in vitro*. Therefore, it appears possible that relaxin acts in parallel with progesterone to support early pregnancy (Szlachter *et al.*, 1980; Norstrom *et al.*, 1984). In recent studies, local administration of purified relaxin to women has been shown to increase cervical dilatation (Maclennan *et al.*, 1980).

In efforts to facilitate the dilation of the cervix and improve cervical ripening, various clinical approaches have been developed. Intracervical laminaria (Gold *et al.*, 1980), urea (Droegemueller *et al.*, 1978), and Foley catheters (Ezimokham and Nwabinelli, 1980) were advantageous prior to instrumental cervical dilatation. The connection between some of these maneuvers and the factors underlying physiological changes of the cervix seems straightforward, because balloon-induced dilatation of the lower uterine segment of term patients is accompanied by cervical softening and an increase in levels of prostaglandin $F_{2\alpha}$ in the amniotic fluid (Manabe *et al.*, 1982). Ultrastructural studies also have demonstrated break-down of collagen and loss of glycosaminoglycans in the cervices of women following injection of urea (Kischer *et al.*, 1980).

The use of hormones to facilitate cervical ripening is important in clinical practice. Labor induction was conducted after administration of PGE_2 cervical suppositories (Calder, 1980; Bernstein *et al.*, 1987). There were multiple benefits such as shortened delivery time, lower frequency of cesarean section, and decreased incidence of maternal fever and fetal asphyxia (Calder, 1980). Systemic injection of dehydroepiandrosterone sulfate (DHEA) was advantageous with respect to cervical dilatation, cervical effacement, and promotion of uterine contractility, thus shortening the duration of labor (Mochizuki and Tojo, 1980; Sasaki *et al.*, 1982; Zuidema *et al.*, 1986). The DHEA is converted to estradiol by the placenta; thus, this treatment raises the levels of local estrogen, which is known to promote cervical maturation and myometrial contractility. However, administration of estradiol alone (Zuidema *et al.*, 1986) or in addition to PGE_2 gels provided no benefit (Williams *et al.*, 1988).

9.3. Relationship between Myometrial Contractility and Cervical Maturation

It is increasingly evident that under normal conditions myometrial contractility and cervical maturation are subject to concordant endocrine regulation (i.e., myometrial quiescence and cervical firmness versus increased myometrial activity and cervical extensibility). The information thus far reviewed designates estrogen, estrogen/progesterone ratios, prostanoids, and relaxin as important factors in cervical ripening. At the cellular level, changes have been shown to occur in cervical collagen and proteoglycans. During initiation of labor, changes in the myometrium include increased interaction among the muscle cells and among the actin, myosin, and MLCK that is regulated by calcium and cAMP.

The relationship between myometrial contractility and cervical maturation in pregnancy and labor is further demonstrated by consideration of patients with prolonged pregnancies. In most instances these women have unfavorable, unripe cervices. In an analysis of 197 patients with a gestational duration of 42 weeks, the Bishop cervical response score (on a scale of 10) was only 3.9 ± 2.4 (S.D.) (Harris *et al.*, 1983). Only 8% of the group had Bishop scores >7.

In a logical progression from the clinical point of view, it is also evident that assessment of the cervix can be used to predict the status of the myometrium. In a retrospective study by Lange *et al.* (1982), about 1200 women were analyzed for a correlation between cervical status and inducibility of labor. Among all cervical criteria, dilatation and effacement have been the best predictors of the onset of labor. Whether the assessment and grading of the cervix could be important in the prevention and management of preterm labor has been investigated in a group of 132 patients with twin pregnancies who had a 32% incidence of preterm labor (Houlton *et al.*, 1982). The length and dilatation of the cervical canal were not different during the 7 days prior to labor whether the patients had preterm or term labor. Thus, cervical maturation occurs preceding term or preterm labor, and changes in cervical compliance may be used in the prediction of preterm labor before the onset of uterine contractions. A new instrument, a "cervicoflexometer," for the detection of such cervical changes has recently been developed (Huszar, 1984).

The main factors governing the relationship between uterine contractility and cervical ripening are summarized in Fig. 12. Many regulatory features are common:

1. Progesterone dominance during pregnancy is associated with a firm closed cervix, few myometrial gap junctions, lower calcium levels in the muscle cells, and a quiescent myometrium.
2. At term, estrogen or a rising estrogen/progesterone ratio has been shown to be important in increased uterine contractility and in cervical ripening. The myometrium exhibits a marked rise in the concentration of estrogen and oxytocin receptors, which coincides with gap junction formation and cervical ripening.

3. In rats, ovariectomy or luteolysis induced by administration of $PGF_{2\alpha}$ leads to a decline in progesterone concentrations, increased myometrial estrogen and oxytocin receptors, increased formation of gap junctions, and premature labor (Mochizuki and Tojo, 1980; Alexandrova and Soloff, 1980). Although estrogen receptors are present in the human cervix (Sanborn et al., 1975), fluctuations in their concentrations in connection with pregnancy and labor have not yet been reported.

4. The various effects of eicosanoids on the myometrium and cervix are well established. Prostaglandins appear to increase myometrial contractility and cervical maturation. Prostaglandins E_2 and $F_{2\alpha}$ stimulate myometrial contractility, but PGE_2 is much more effective than $PGF_{2\alpha}$. Also, there is a regional responsiveness of the uterus to prostaglandins. The upper uterine segment responds to PGE_2 and the lower segment to $PGF_{2\alpha}$. During labor it appears that PGE_2 is the main initiator of contractility and $PGF_{2\alpha}$ does not seem to elicit much response. Although prostaglandins at low levels cause cervical maturation, the administration of PGE_2 and PGF_α in larger amounts will induce myometrial contractions in pregnant women at any stage of the gestation. Related to this issue is the recent finding that factors affecting eicosanoid biosynthesis originate in the fetal urine not only in the form of ACTH but also as protein factors such as growth factors or proteins of the lipocortin system (Casey et al., 1983). This finding highlights the role of the fetus in the initiation of labor, cervical maturation, and increased myometrial contractility.

5. The role and mechanism of action of oxytocin in promoting myometrial contractility are well known. Oxytocin-mediated decidual prostaglandin synthesis (Fuchs et al., 1982) could be an additional example of common regulation of myometrial and cervical functions.

6. Effects of cAMP are studied more easily in the myometrium than in the cervix. There is, however, the possibility of further, still unknown, roles of cAMP in cervical physiology and tocolytic management based on reports that relaxin increases cellular cAMP levels and that administration of β-adrenergic agonists, such as ritodrine (Hanssens et al., 1983) and isoxsuprine (Csapo and Herczeg, 1977), caused a significant rise in circulating progesterone and a significant decrease in mean serum estradiol.

Most of the hormones and agonists reviewed affect the myometrium and cervix by acting at multiple levels within the cell and between cells. For instance, estrogen plays a role in the following processes: increased myometrial contractility, biosynthesis of various hormones and

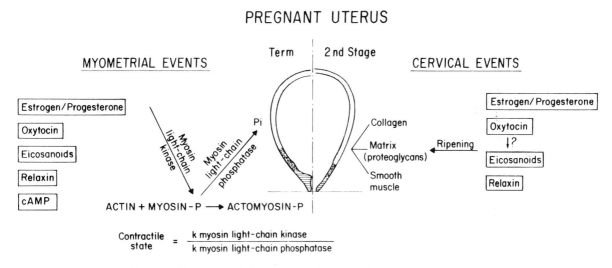

Figure 12. Common regulation of myometrial contractility and cervical ripening.

hormone receptors in the myometrium and cervix, biosynthesis of prostaglandins, regulation of myometrial levels of calcium and protein phosphorylation, collagenase synthesis and activation, collagen breakdown, and other events of cervical ripening.

10. References

Adelstein, R. S., Conti, M. A., Hathaway, D. R., and Klee, C. B., 1978, Phosphorylation of smooth muscle myosin light chain kinase by the catalytic subunit of adenosine $3':5'$-monophosphate-dependent protein kinase, *J. Biol. Chem.* **253**:8347.

Aksoy, M. O., Murphy, R. A., and Kamm, K. E., 1982, Role of Ca^{2+} and myosin light chain phosphorylation in regulation of smooth muscle, *Am. J. Physiol.* **242**:C109.

Aksoy, M. O., Mras, S., Kamm, K. E., and Murphy, R. A., 1983, Ca^{2+}, cAMP, and changes in myosin phosphorylation during contraction of smooth muscle, *Am. J. Physiol.* **245**:C255.

Alexandrova, M., and Soloff, M. S., 1980, Oxytocin receptors and parturition. I. Control of oxytocin receptor concentration in the rat myometrium at term, *Endocrinology* **106**:730.

Altura, J. M., and Altura, B. T., 1981, Magnesium modulates calcium entry and contractility in vascular smooth muscle, in: *The Mechanism of Gated Calcium Transport Across Biological Membrane* (F. Ohnishi and M. Endo, eds.), Academic Press, New York, p. 137.

Anderson, G., Kawarabayashi, T., and Marshall, J. M., 1981, Effect of indomethacin and aspirin on uterine activity in pregnant rats: Comparison of circular and longitudinal muscle, *Biol. Reprod.* **24**:359.

Armstrong, D., and Eckert, R., 1987, Voltage-activated calcium channels that must be phosphorylated to respond to membrane depolarization, *Proc. Natl. Acad. Sci. U.S.A.* **84**:2518.

Bagby, R. M., 1983, Organization of contractility/cytoskeletal elements, in: *Biochemistry of Smooth Muscle,* Vol. I (N. L. Stephens, ed.), CRC Press, Boca Raton, FL, pp. 1–85.

Baker, P. F., 1975, *Calcium Movement in Excitable Cells,* Pergamon Press, Oxford, pp. 9–53.

Batra, S., 1982, Uptake and energy-dependent extrusion of calcium in the rat uterus, *Acta Physiol. Scand.* **114**:447.

Bengtsson, B., Chow, E. M., and Marshall, J. M., 1984a, Activity of circular muscle of rat uterus at different times in pregnancy, *Am. J. Physiol.* **246**:C216.

Bengtsson, B., Chow, E. M., and Marshall, J. M., 1984b, Calcium dependency of pregnant rat myometrium: Comparison of circular and longitudinal muscle, *Biol. Reprod.* **30**:869.

Berg, G., Andersson, R. G., and Ryden, G., 1983, *In vitro* study of phosphodiesterase-inhibiting drugs: A complement to β-sympathomimetic drug therapy in premature labor, *Am. J. Obstet. Gynecol.* **145**:802.

Berg, G., Andersson, R. G. G., and Ryden, G., 1985, β-Adrenergic receptors in human myometrium during pregnancy: Changes in the number of receptors after β-mimetic treatment, *Am. J. Obstet. Gynecol.* **151**:392.

Berg, G., Andersson, R. G. G., and Ryden, G., 1986, α-Adrenergic receptors in human myometrium during pregnancy, *Am. J. Obstet. Gynecol.* **154**:601.

Bernstein, P., Leyland, N., Gurland, P., and Gare, D., 1987, Cervical ripening and labor induction with prostaglandin E_2 gel: A placebo-controlled study, *Am. J. Obstet. Gynecol.* **156**:336.

Berridge, M. J., and Irvine, R. F., 1984, Inositol trisphosphate, a novel second messenger in cellular signal transduction, *Nature* **312**:315.

Bird, L. M., Anderson, N. C., Chandler, M. L., and Young, R. C., 1987, The effects of aminophylline and nifedipine on contractility of isolated pregnant human myometrium, *Am. J. Obstet. Gynecol.* **157**:171.

Bitar, K. N., Bradford, P., Putney, J. W., Jr., and Makhlouf, G. M., 1986a, Cytosolic calcium during contraction of isolated mammalian gastric muscle cells, *Science* **232**:1143.

Bitar, K. N., Bradford, P. G., Putney, J. W., Jr., and Makhlouf, G. M., 1986b, Stoichiometry of contraction and Ca^{2+} mobilization by inositol 1,4,5-trisphosphate in isolated gastric smooth muscle cells, *J. Biol. Chem.* **261**:16591.

Blumentalh, D. K., Takio, K., Edelman, A. M., Charbonneau, H., Titani, K., Walsh, K. A., and Krebs, E. G., 1985, Identification of the calmodulin-binding domain of skeletal muscle myosin light chain kinase, *Proc. Natl. Acad. Sci. U.S.A.* **82**:3187.

Bolger, G. T., Gengo, P. J., Luchowski, E. M., Siegel, H., Triggle, D. J., and Janis, R. A., 1982, High affinity binding of a calcium channel antagonist to smooth and cardiac muscle, *Biochem. Biophys. Res. Commun.* **104**:1604.

Bond, M., and Somlyo, A. V., 1982, Dense bodies and actin polarity in vertebrate smooth muscle, *J. Cell Biol.* **95**:403.

Bretscher, A., 1984, Smooth muscle caldesmon. Rapid purification and F-actin cross-linking properties, *J. Biol. Chem.* **259**:12873.

Brum, G., Osterreider, W., and Trautwein, W., 1984, β-Adrenergic increase in the calcium conductance of cardiac myocytes studied with the patch clamp, *Pflugers Arch.* **401**:111.

Bryman, I., Sahni, S., Norstrom, A., and Lindblom, B., 1984, Influence of prostaglandins on contractility of isolated human cervical muscle, *J. Obstet. Gynecol.* **63**:280.

Bryman, I., Norström, A., and Lindblom, B., 1986, Influence of prostaglandins and adrenoceptor agonists on contractile activity in the human cervix at term, *Obstet. Gynecol.* **67**:574.

Bygdeman, M., 1980, Clinical applications, in: *Advances in Prostaglandin and Thromboxane Research,* Vol. 6 (B. Samuelsson, P. W. Ramwell, and R. Paoletti, eds.), Raven Press, New York, p. 87.

Cabrol, D., Breton, M., Berrou, E., Vissier, A., Sureau, C., and Picard, J., 1980, Variation in the distribution of glycosaminoglycans in the uterine cervix of pregnant women, *Eur. J. Obstet. Gynecol. Reprod. Biol.* **10**:281.

Cabrol, D., Huszar, G., Romero, R., and Naftolin, F., 1981, Gestational changes in the rat uterine cervix: Protein, collagen and glycosaminoglycan content, in: *The Cervix in Pregnancy and Labour: Clinical and Biochemical Investigations* (D. A. Ellwood and A. B. M. Anderson, eds.), Churchill Livingstone, Edinburgh, p. 34.

Cabrol, D., Bouvier, and D'Yvoire, M., 1985, Induction of labor with mifepristone after intrauterine fetal death [letter], *Lancet* **2**:1019.

Calder, A. A., 1980, Pharmacological management of the unripe cervix in the human, in: *Dilatation of the Uterine Cervix: Connective Tissue Biology and Clinical Management* (F. Naftolin and P. G. Stubblefield, eds.), Raven Press, New York, p. 317.

Carsten, M. E., 1974, Hormonal regulation of myometrial calcium transport, *Gynecol. Invest.* **5**:269.

Casey, M. L., Cutrer, S., and Mitchell, M. D., 1983, Origin of prostanoids in human amnionic fluid: Prostanoids, *Am. J. Obstet. Gynecol.* **147**:547.

Casper, R. F., and Lye, S. J., 1986, Myometrial desensitization to continuous but not to intermittent β-adrenergic agonist infusion in the sheep, *Am. J. Obstet. Gynecol.* **154**:301.

Casper, R. F., and Lye, S. J., 1987, β-Adrenergic receptor agonist infusion increases plasma prostaglandin F levels in pregnant sheep, *Am. J. Obstet. Gynecol.* **157**:998.

Cassidy, P. S., Hoar, P. E., and Kerrick, W. G. L., 1979, Irreversible thiophosphorylation and activation of tension in functionally skinned rabbit ileum strips by [^{35}S]ATPγS, *J. Biol. Chem.* **254**:11148.

Cassidy, P., Hoar, P. E., and Kerrick, W. G., 1980, Inhibition of calcium-activated tension and myosin light chain phosphorylation in skinned smooth muscle strips by the phenothiazines, *Pflugers Arch.* **387**:115.

Casteels, R., Wuytack, F., Himpens, B., and Raeymaekers, L., 1986, Regulatory systems for the cytoplasmic calcium concentration in smooth muscle, *Biomed. Biochim. Acta* **45**:S147.

Chacko, S., 1981, Effects of phosphorylation, calcium ion, and tropomyosin on actin-activated adenosine 5′triphosphatase activity of mammalian smooth muscle myosin, *Biochemistry* **20**:702.

Chacko, S., Conti, M. A., and Adelstein, R. S., 1977, Effect of phosphorylation of smooth muscle myosin on actin activation and Ca^{2+} regulation, *Proc. Natl. Acad. Sci. U.S.A.* **74**:129.

Challis, J. R. G., and Olson D. M., 1988, Parturition, in: *The Physiology of Reproduction* (E. Knobil, J. Neill, *et al.,* eds.), Raven Press, New York, p. 2177.

Chatterjee, M., and Murphy, R. A., 1983, Calcium-dependent stress maintenance without myosin phosphorylation in skinned smooth muscle, *Science* **221**:464.

Chaturvedi, A. K., Landon, E. J., and Sastry, B. V., 1978, Influence of chlorpromazine on calcium movements and contractile responses of guinea pig ileum longitudinal smooth muscle to agonists, *Arch. Int. Pharmacodyn.* **236**:109.

Clark, T., Ngai, P. K., Sutherland, C., Gröschel-Stewart, U., and Walsh, M. P., 1986, Vascular smooth muscle caldesmon, *J. Biol. Chem.* **261**:8028.

Conrad, J., and Ueland, K., 1979, The stretch modulus of human cervical tissue in spontaneous, oxytocin-induced, and prostaglandin E_2-induced labor, *Am. J. Obstet. Gynecol.* **133**:11.

Conti, M. A., and Adelstein, R. S., 1981, The relationship between calmodulin binding and phosphorylation of smooth muscle myosin kinase by the catalytic subunit of 3′:5′ cAMP-dependent protein kinase, *J. Biol. Chem.* **256**:3178.

Craig, R., Smith, R., and Kendrick-Jones, J., 1983, Light-chain phosphorylation controls the conformation of vertebrate non-muscle and smooth muscle myosin molecules, *Nature* **302**:436.

Csabina, S., Mougios, V., Bárány, M., and Bárány, K., 1986, Characterization of the phosphorylatable myosin light chain in rat uterus, *Biochim. Biophys. Acta* **871**:311.

Csapo, A. I., 1977, The "see-saw" theory of parturition, in: *The Fetus and Birth,* Ciba Foundation Symposium (J. Knight and M. O'Connor, eds.), Elsevier, Amsterdam, p. 159.

Csapo, A. I., and Herczeg, J., 1977, Arrest of premature labor by isoxsuprine, *Am. J. Obstet. Gynecol.* **129:**482.

Csapo, A. I., Puri, C. P., Tarro, S., and Henzl, M. R., 1982, Deactivation of the uterus during normal and premature labor by the calcium antagonist nicardipine, *Am. J. Obstet. Gynecol.* **142:**483.

Cummins, P., and Perry, S. V., 1974, Chemical and immunochemical characteristics of tropomyosins from striated and smooth muscle, *Biochem. J.* **141:**43.

Curtis, B. M., and Catterall, W. A., 1986, Reconstitution of the voltage-sensitive calcium channel purified from skeletal muscle transverse tubules, *Biochemistry* **25:**3077.

Dabrowska, R., Hinkins, S., Walsh, M. P., and Hartshorne, D. J., 1982, The binding of smooth muscle myosin light chain kinase to actin, *Biochem. Biophys. Res. Commun.* **107:**1524.

Danforth, D. N., Buckingham, J. C., and Roddick, J. W., 1960, Connective tissue changes incident to cervical effacement, *Am. J. Obstet. Gynecol.* **80:**939.

Dattel, B. J., Lam, F., and Roberts, J. M., 1986, Failure to demonstrate decreased β-adrenergic receptor concentration or decreased agonist efficacy in term or preterm human parturition, *Am. J. Obstet. Gynecol.* **154:**450.

Davidson, B. J., Murray, R. D., Challis, J. R. G., and Valenzuela, G. J., 1987, Estrogen, progesterone, prolactin, prostaglandin E_2, prostaglandin $F_{2\alpha}$, 13,14-dihydro-15-keto-prostaglandin $F_{2\alpha}$, and 6-keto-prostaglandin $F_{1\alpha}$ gradients across the uterus in women in labor and not in labor, *Am. J. Obstet. Gynecol.* **157:**54.

DeFeo, T. T., and Morgan, K. G., 1985, Calcium–force relationships as detected with aequorin in two different vascular smooth muscles of the ferret, *J. Physiol. (Lond.)* **369:**269.

Den, K., Sakamoto, H., Kimura, S., and Takaji, S., 1981, Study of oxytocin receptor. II. Gestational changes in oxytocin activity in the human myometrium, *Endocrinol. Jpn.* **28:**375.

Dillon, P. F., Aksoy, M. O., Driska, S. P., and Murphy, R. A., 1981, Myosin phosphorylation and the cross-bridge cycle in arterial smooth muscle, *Science* **211:**495.

Droegemueller, W., Chvapil, M., Vining, J., Whitaker, L., and Christian, C. D., 1978, Urea and dilatation of the cervix, *Am. J. Obstet. Gynecol.* **132:**775.

Ekman, G., Forman, A., Marsal, K., and Ulmsten, U., 1983, Intravaginal versus intracervical application of prostaglandin E_2 in viscous gel for cervical priming and induction of labor at term in patients with an unfavorable cervical state, *Am. J. Obstet. Gynecol.* **147:**657.

Endo, M., 1977, Calcium release from the sarcoplasmic reticulum, *Physiol. Rev.* **57:**71.

Ezimokham, M., and Nwabinelli, J. N., 1980, The use of Foley's catheter in ripening the unfavourable cervix prior to induction of labour, *Br. J. Obstet. Gynaecol.* **87:**281.

Fatigati, V., and Murphy, R. A., 1984, Actin and tropomyosin variants in smooth muscles. Dependence on tissue type, *J. Biol. Chem.* **259:**14383.

Filo, R. S., Bohr, D. F., and Rüegg, J. C., 1965, Glycerinated skeletal and smooth muscle: Calcium and magnesium dependence, *Science* **147:**1581.

Fitzpatrick, R. J., 1977, Changes in cervical function at parturition, *Ann. Rech. Vet.* **8:**438.

Fliegel, L., Ohnishi, M., Carpenter, M. R., Khanna, V. K., Reithmeier, R. A. F., and MacLennan, D. H., 1987, Amino acid sequence of rabbit fast-twitch skeletal muscle calsequestrin deduced from cDNA and peptide sequencing, *Proc. Natl. Acad. Sci. U.S.A.* **84:**1167.

Flower, R. J., 1986, The mediators of steroid action, *Nature* **320:**20.

Forman, A., Gandrup, P., Andersson, K.-E., and Ulmsten, U., 1982a, Effects of nifedipine on spontaneous and methylergometrine-induced activity postpartum, *Am. J. Obstet. Gynecol.* **144:**442.

Forman, A., Ulmsten, U., Banyai, J., Wingerup, L., and Uldbjerg, N., 1982b, Evidence for a local effect of intracervical prostaglandin E_2-gel, *Am. J. Obstet. Gynecol.* **143:**756.

Foster, C., Van Fleet, M., and Marshak, A., 1986, Tryptic digestion of myosin light chain kinase produces an inactive fragment that is activated on continued digestion, *Arch. Biochem. Biophys.* **251:**616.

Foyt, H. L., Guerriero, V., Jr., and Means, A. R., 1985, Functional domains of chicken gizzard myosin light chain kinase, *J. Biol. Chem.* **260:**7765.

Frydman R., Taylor, S., Fernandez, H., Pons, J. C., Forman, R. G., and Ulmann, A., 1986, Obstetrical indication of mifepristone (RU 486) [Abstract]. Presented at the sixth annual meeting of the Society for Advances in Contraception, Chicago, Society for the Advances in Contraception.

Fuchs, A. R., 1986, The role of oxytocin in parturition, in: *The Physiology and Biochemistry of the Uterus* (G. Huszar, ed.), CRC Press, Boca Raton, FL, pp. 163–184.

Fuchs, A. R., Fuchs, F., and Husslein, P., 1982, Oxytocin receptors and human parturition: A dual role for oxytocin in the initiation of labor, *Science* **215:**1396.

Fukunaga, K., Yamamoto, H., Matsui, K., Higashi, K., and Miyamoto, E., 1982, Purification and characterization of a Ca^{2+} and calmodulin-dependent protein kinase from rat brain, *J. Neurochem.* **39:**1607.

Furukawa, K.-I., and Nakamura, H., 1984, Characterization of the $(Ca^{2+} + Mg^{2+})$-ATPase purified by calmodulin-affinity chromatography from bovine aortic smooth muscle, *J. Biochem. (Tokyo)* **96**:1343.

Galizzi, J.-P., Qar, J., Fosset, M., Van Renterghem, C., and Lazdunski, M., 1987, Regulation of calcium channels in aortic muscle cells by protein kinase C activators (diacylglycerol and phorbol esters) and by peptides (vasopressin and bombesin) that stimulate phosphoinositide breakdown, *J. Biol. Chem.* **262**:6947.

Gallis, B., Edelman, A. M., Casnellie, J. E., and Krebs, E. G., 1983, Epidermal growth factor stimulates tyrosine phosphorylation of the myosin regulatory light chain from smooth muscle, *J. Biol. Chem.* **258**:13089.

Gammisans, O., 1984, The effects of prostaglandin synthesis inhibitors on preterm labor, in: *Preterm Birth: Cases, Prevention, Management* (F. Fuchs and P. Stubblefield, eds.), Macmillan, New York, p. 223.

Garfield, R. E., Kannan, M. S., and Daniel, E. E., 1980, Gap junction formation in myometrium: Control by estrogens, progesterone and prostaglandins, *Am. J. Physiol.* **238**:C81.

Garfield, R. E., Puri, C. P., and Csapo, A. I., 1982, Endocrine, structural, and functional changes in the uterus during premature labor, *Am. J. Obstet. Gynecol.* **142**:21.

Garfield, R. E., Gasc, J. M., and Baulieu, E. E., 1987, Effects of antiprogesterone RU 486 on preterm birth in the rat, *Am. J. Obstet. Gynecol.* **157**:1281.

Giannopoulis, G., Jackson, K., Kredentser, J., and Tulchinsky, D., 1985, Prostaglandin E_2 and $F_{2\alpha}$ receptors in human myometrium during the menstrual cycle and in pregnancy and labor, *Am. J. Obstet. Gynecol.* **153**:904.

Gold, J., Schulz, K. F., and Cates, W., Jr., 1980, The safety of laminaria and rigid dilator for cervical dilation prior to suction curettage for first trimester abortion: A comparative analysis, in: *Dilatation of the Uterine Cervix, Connective Tissue Biology and Clinical Management* (F. Naftolin and P. G. Stubblefield, eds.), Raven Press, New York, p. 363.

Golichowski, A. M., King, S. R., and Mascaro, K., 1980, Pregnancy-related changes in rat cervical glycosaminoglycans, *Biochem. J.* **192**:1.

Grover, A. K., Kwan, C. Y., Luchowski, E., Daniel, E. E., and Triggle, D. J., 1984, Subcellular distribution of [^{3}H]nitrendipine binding in smooth muscle, *J. Biol. Chem.* **4**:2223.

Grynkiewicz, G., Poenie, M., and Tsien, R. Y., 1985, A new generation of Ca^{2+} indicators with greatly improved fluorescence properties, *J. Biol. Chem.* **260**:3440.

Guerriero, V., Jr., Russo, M. A., Olson, N. J., Putkey, J. A., and Means, A. R., 1986, Domain organization of chicken gizzard myosin light chain kinase deduced from a cloned cDNA, *Biochemistry* **25**:8372.

Haeberle, J. R., and Trockman, B. A., 1986, Two-site phosphorylation of the 20,000 dalton myosin light chain of glycerinated porcine carotid artery smooth muscle, *Biophys. J.* **49**:389a.

Haeberle, J. R., Hathaway, D. R., and DePaoli-Roach, A. A., 1985, Dephosphorylation of myosin by the catalytic subunit of a type-2 phosphatase produces relaxation of chemically skinned uterine smooth muscle, *J. Biol. Chem.* **260**:9965.

Hahn, D. W., Demarest, K. T., Ericson, E., Homm, R. E., Capetola, R. J., and McGuire, J. L., 1987, Evaluation of 1-deamino-[D-Tyr(O ethyl)^2,Thr^4,Orn^8]vasotocin, an oxytocin antagonist, in animal models of uterine contractility and preterm labor: A new tocolytic agent, *Am. J. Obstet. Gynecol.* **157**:977.

Hai, C.-M., and Murphy, R. A., 1988, Cross-bridge phosphorylation and regulation of latch state in smooth muscle, *Am. J. Physiol.* **254**:C99.

Haluska, G. J., Stanczyk, F. Z., Cook, M. J., and Novy, M. J., 1987, Temporal changes in uterine activity and prostaglandin response to RU 486 in rhesus macaques in late gestation, *Am. J. Obstet. Gynecol.* **157**:1487.

Hammer, J. A. III, Sellers, J. R., and Korn, E. D., 1984, Phosphorylation and activation of smooth muscle myosin by *Acanthamoeba* myosin I heavy chain kinase, *J. Biol. Chem.* **259**:3224.

Hanssens, M. C., Selby, C., Filshie, G. M., Gilbert, B. J., and Symonds, E. M., 1983, Changes in plasma steroid hormones during treatment of preterm labour with ritodrine-HC1, *Br. J. Obstet. Gynaecol.* **90**:847.

Harris, B., Jr., Huddleston, J. F., Sutliff, G., and Perlis, H. W., 1983, The unfavorable cervix in prolonged pregnancy, *J. Obstet. Gynecol.* **62**:171.

Hartshorne, D. J., 1987, Biochemistry of the contractile process in smooth muscle, in: *Physiology of the Gastrointestinal Tract,* second edition (L. R. Johnson, ed.), Raven Press, New York, pp. 423–482.

Hashimoto, T., Hirata, M., Itoh, T., Kanmura, Y., and Kuriyama, H., 1986, Inositol 1,4,5-trisphosphate activates pharmacomechanical coupling in smooth muscle of the rabbit mesenteric artery, *J. Physiol. (Lond.)* **370**:605.

Hidaka, H., Asano, M., Iwadare, S., Matsumoto, I., Totsuka, T., and Aoki, M., 1978, A novel vascular relaxing agent, N-(aminohexyl)5-chloro-1-naphthalene-sulfonamide, which affects vascular smooth muscle actomyosin, *J. Pharmacol. Exp. Ther.* **207**:8.

Hidaka, H., Yamaki, T., Naka, M., Tanaka, T., Hayashi, H., and Kobayashi, R., 1980, Calcium-regulated modulator protein interacting agents inhibit smooth muscle calcium-stimulated protein kinase and ATPase, *Mol. Pharmacol.* **17**:66.

Hidaka, H., Asano, M., and Tanaka, T., 1981, Activity–structure relationship of calmodulin antagonists. Naphthalenesulfonamide derivatives, *Mol. Pharmacol.* **20**:571.

Higashi, K., Fukunaga, K., Matsui, K., Maeyama, M., and Miyamoto, E., 1983, Purification and characterization of myosin light-chain kinase from porcine myometrium and its phosphorylation and modulation by cyclic AMP-dependent protein kinase, *Biochim. Biophys. Acta* **747**:232.

Hillier, K., and Wallis, R., 1981, Prostaglandins, steroids and the human cervix, in: *The Cervix in Pregnancy and Labour: Clinical and Biochemical Investigations* (D. A. Ellwood, and A. M. Anderson, eds.), Churchill Livingstone, Edinburgh, p. 34.

Hirata, M., Mikawa, T., Nonomura, Y., and Ebashi, S., 1977, Ca^{2+} regulation in vascular smooth muscle, *J. Biochem. (Tokyo)* **82**:1793.

Hoar, P. E., Kerrick, W. G. L., and Cassidy, P. S., 1979, Chicken gizzard: Relation between calcium-activated phosphorylation and contraction, *Science* **204**:503.

Hoar, P. E., Pato, M. D., and Kerrick, W. G. L., 1985, Myosin light chain phosphatase. Effect on the activation and relaxation of gizzard smooth muscle skinned fibers, *J. Biol. Chem.* **260**:8760.

Hochman, J., Weiss, G., Steinetz, B. G., and O'Byrne, E. M., 1978, Serum relaxin concentrations in prostaglandin- and oxytocin-induced labor in women, *Am. J. Obstet. Gynecol.* **130**:473.

Hokin, M. R., and Hokin, L. E., 1953, Enzyme secretion and the incorporation of P^{32} into phospholipides of pancreas slices, *J. Biol. Chem.* **203**:967.

Holbrook, R. H., Jr., Lirette, M., and Katz, M., 1987, Cardiovascular and tocolytic effects of nicardipine HC1 in the pregnant rabbit: Comparison with ritodrine HC1, *Obstet. Gynecol.* **69**:83.

Hollingsworth, M., Isherwood, C. N. M., and Roster, R. W., 1979, The effects of oestradiol benzoate, progesterone, relaxin and ovariectomy on cervical extensibility in the late pregnant rat, *J. Reprod. Fertil.* **56**:471.

Holz, G. G., Rane, S. G., and Dunlap, K., 1986, GTP-binding proteins mediate transmitter inhibition of voltage-dependent calcium channels, *Nature* **319**:670.

Houlton, M. C. C., Marivate, M., and Philpott, R. H., 1982, Factors associated with preterm labour and changes in the cervix before labour in twin pregnancy, *Br. J. Obstet. Gynaecol.* **89**:190.

Hulka, J. F., and Chepko, M., 1987, Vaginal prostaglandin E_1 analogue (ONO-802) to soften the cervix in first trimester abortion, *Obstet. Gynecol.* **69**:57.

Hurwitz, L., 1986, Pharmacology of clacium channels and smooth muscle, *Annu. Rev. Pharmacol. Toxicol.* **26**:225.

Husslein, P., Fuchs, A. R., and Fuchs, F., 1981, Oxytocin and the initiation of human parturition, I. Prostaglandin release during induction of labor by oxytocin, *Am. J. Obstet. Gynecol.* **141**:688.

Huszar, G., 1979, Cellular aspects of labor, in: *Proceedings 15th Mead Johnson Symposium on Premature Labor* (J. C. Sinclair, J. B. Warshaw, and R. S. Bloom, eds.), Mead Johnson and Company, Evansville, IN, p. 16.

Huszar, G., 1980, The relationship between myometrial contractility and cervical ripening in parturition, in: *Dilatation of the Uterine Cervix: Connective Tissue Biology and Clinical Management* (P. Stubblefield and F. Naftolin, eds.), Raven Press, New York, p. 371.

Huszar, G., 1981, Biology and biochemistry of myometrial contractility and cervical maturation, *Preterm Parturition, Semin. Perinatol.* **5**:216.

Huszar, G., 1983, Physiology of myometrial contractility and of cervical dilatation, in: *Preterm Birth: Causes, Prevention and Management* (F. Fuchs and P. Stubblefield, eds.), Macmillan, New York, p. 21.

Huszar, G., 1984, Method for Determining the Extensibility of Selected Non-Excised Tissue of the Uterine Cervix, Ear or Skin, *U.S. Patent 4,432,376.*

Huszar, G., 1986, Cellular regulation of myometrial contractility and essentials of tocolytic therapy, in: *The Physiology and Biochemistry of the Uterus* (G. Huszar, ed.), CRC Press, Boca Raton, FL, pp. 107–126.

Huszar, G., and Bailey, P., 1979a, Relationship between actin–myosin interactions and myosin light-chain phosphorylation in human placental smooth muscle, *Am. J. Obstet. Gynecol.* **135**:718.

Huszar, G., and Bailey, P., 1979b, Isolation and characterization of myosin in the human term placenta, *Am. J. Obstet. Gynecol.* **135**:707.

Huszar, G., and Naftolin, F., 1984, Myometrium and cervix: The physiologic basis of labor and tocolytic management, *N. Engl. J. Med.* **311**:571.

Huszar, G., and Roberts, J. R., 1982, Biochemistry and pharmacology of the myometrium and labor: Regulation at the cellular and molecular levels, *Am. J. Obstet. Gynecol.* **142**:225.

Huszar, G., and Vigue, L., 1986, The structure of myosin heavy chain in various smooth muscles, *Biophys. J.* **49**:184a.

Huszar, G., Cabrol, D., and Naftolin, F., 1986, The relationship between myometrial contractility and cervical maturation in pregnancy and labor, in: *The Physiology and Biochemistry of the Uterus* (G. Huszar, ed.), CRC Press, Boca Raton, FL, pp. 201–223.

Huxley, H. E., 1971, The structural basis of muscular contraction, *Proc. R. Soc. Lond. [Biol.]* **178**:131.

Ikebe, M., and Hartshorne, D. J., 1984, Conformation-dependent proteolysis of smooth-muscle myosin, *J. Biol. Chem.* **259**:11639.

Ikebe, M., and Hartshorne, D. J., 1985a, Proteolysis of smooth muscle myosin by *Staphylococcus aureus* protease: Preparation of heavy meromyosin and subfragment 1 with intact 20,000-dalton light chains, *Biochemistry* **24**:2380.

Ikebe, M., and Hartshorne, D. J., 1985b, Phosphorylation of smooth muscle myosin at two distinct sites by myosin light chain kinase, *J. Biol. Chem.* **260**:10027.

Ikebe, M., Ogihara, S., and Tonomura, Y., 1982, Nonlinear dependence of actin-activated Mg^{2+}-ATPase activity on the extent of phosphorylation of gizzard myosin and H-meromyosin, *J. Biochem. (Tokyo)* **91**:1809.

Ikebe, M., Hinkins, S., and Hartshorne, D. J., 1983, Correlation of enzymatic properties and conformation of smooth muscle myosin, *Biochemistry* **22**:4580.

Ikebe, M., Hartshorne, D. J., and Elzinga, M., 1986, Identification, phosphorylation, and dephosphorylation of a second site for myosin light chain kinase on the 20,000-dalton light chain of smooth muscle myosin, *J. Biol. Chem.* **261**:36.

Ikebe, M., Hartshorne, D. J., and Elzinga, M., 1987a, Phosphorylation of the 20,000-dalton light chain of smooth muscle myosin by the calcium-activated, phospholipid-dependent protein kinase. Phosphorylation sites and effects of phosphorylation, *J. Biol. Chem.* **262**:9569.

Ikebe, M., Stepinska, M., Kemp, B. E., Means, A. R., and Hartshorne, D. J., 1987b, Proteolysis of smooth muscle myosin light chain kinase. Formation of inactive and calmodulin-independent fragments, *J. Biol. Chem.* **262**:13828.

Irvine, R. F., and Moor, R. M., 1986, Micro-injection of inositol 1,3,4,5-tetrakiphosphate activates sea urchin eggs by a mechanism dependent on external Ca^{2+}, *Biochem. J.* **240**:917.

Ito, A., Naganeo, K., Mori, Y., Mirakawa, S., and Hayashi, M., 1977, PZ-peptidase activity in human uterine cervix in pregnancy at term, *Clin. Chim. Acta* **78**:267.

Itoh, T., Ueno, H., and Kuriyama, H., 1985, Calcium-induced calcium release mechanism in vascular smooth muscles—assessments based on contractions evoked in intact and saponin-treated skinned muscles, *Experientia* **41**:989.

Janis, R. A., Bárány, K., Bárány, M., and Sarmiento, J. G., 1981, Association between myosin light chain phosphorylation and contraction of rat uterine smooth muscle, *Mol. Physiol.* **1**:3.

Janis, R., and Triggle, D., 1986, Effects of calcium channel antagonists on the myometrium, in: *The Physiology and Biochemistry of the Uterus* (G. Huszar, ed.), CRC Press, Boca Raton, FL, pp. 201–223.

Jeremy, J. Y., and Dandona, P., 1986, RU 486 antagonizes the inhibitory action of progesterone on prostacyclin and thromboxane A_2 synthesis in cultured rat explants, *Endocrinology,* **119**:665.

Jorgensen, A. O., and Jones, L. R., 1986, Localization of phospholamban in slow but not fast canine skeletal muscle fibers. An immunocytochemical and biochemical study, *J. Biol. Chem.* **261**:3775.

Kaczmarek, L. K., 1986, Phorbol esters, protein phosphorylation and the regulation of neuronal ion channels, *J. Exp. Biol.* **124**:375.

Kamm, K. E., and Stull, J. T., 1985, The function of myosin and myosin light chain kinase phosphorylation in smooth muscle, *Annu. Rev. Pharmacol. Toxicol.* **25**:593.

Kamps, M. P., Taylor, S. S., and Sefton, B. M., 1984, Direct evidence that oncogenic tyrosine kinases and cyclic AMP-dependent protein kinase have homologous ATP-binding sites, *Nature* **310**:389.

Kanamori, M., Naka, M., Asano, M., and Hidaka, H., 1981, Effects of N-(6-aminohexyl)-5-chloro-1-naphthalene-sulfonamide and other calmodulin antagonists (calmodulin interacting agents) on calcium-induced contraction of rabbit aortic strips, *J. Pharmacol. Exp. Ther.* **217**:494.

Kawamoto, S., and Adelstein, R. S., 1987, Characterization of myosin heavy chains in cultured aorta smooth muscle cells. A comparative study, *J. Biol. Chem.* **262**:7282.

Kawarabayashi, T., Kishikawa, T., and Sugimori, H., 1986, Effect of oxytocin on spontaneous electrical and mechanical activities in pregnant human myometrium, *Am. J. Obstet. Gynecol.* **155**:671.

Ke, R., Vohra, M., and Casper, R., 1984, Prolonged inhibition of human myometrial contractility by intermittent isoproterenol, *Am. J. Obstet. Gynecol.* **149**:841.

Kemp, B. E., and Pearson, R. B., 1985, Spatial requirements for location of basic residues in peptide substrates for smooth muscle myosin light chain kinase, *J. Biol. Chem.* **260**:3355.

Kemp, B. E., Pearson, R. B., and House, C., 1982, Phosphorylation of a synthetic heptadecapeptide by smooth muscle myosin light chain kinase, *J. Biol. Chem.* **257**:13349.

Kemp, B. E., Pearson, R. B., and House, C., 1983, Role of basic residues in the phosphorylation of synthetic peptides of myosin light chain kinase, *Proc. Natl. Acad. Sci. U.S.A.* **80**:7471.

Kemp, B. E., Pearson, R. B., Guerriero, V., Jr., Bagchi, I. C., and Means, A. R., 1987, The calmodulin binding domain of chicken smooth muscle myosin light chain kinase contains a pseudosubstrate sequence, *J. Biol. Chem.* **262**:2542.

Keravis, T. M., Wells, J. N., and Hardman, J. G., 1980, Cyclic nucleotide phosphodiesterase activities from pig coronary arteries. Lack of interconvertibility of major forms, *Biochim. Biophys. Acta* **613**:116.

Kerrick, W. G., and Hoar, P. E., 1981, Inhibition of smooth muscle tension by cyclic AMP-dependent protein kinase, *Nature* **292**:253.

Kirchberger, M. A., Tada, M., and Katz, A. M., 1974, Adenosine 3':5'-monophosphate-dependent protein kinase-catalyzed phosphorylation reaction and its relationship to calcium transport in cardiac sarcoplasmic reticulum, *J. Biol. Chem.* **249**:6166.

Kischer, C. W., Droegemueller, W., Shetlar, M., Chvapil, M., and Vining, J., 1980, Ultrastructural changes in the architecture of collagen in the human cervix treated with urea, *Am. J. Pathol.* **99**:525.

Klee, C. B., 1980, Calmodulin: Structure–function relationships, in: *Calcium and Cell Function,* Vol. 1 (W. Y. Cheung, ed.), Academic Press, New York, pp. 59–78.

Kleissl, H. P., Van der Rest, M., Naftolin, F., Glorieux, F. H., and DeLeon, A., 1978, Collagen changes in the human uterine cervix at parturition, *Am. J. Obstet. Gynecol.* **130**:748.

Kofinas, A. D., Rose, J. C., and Meis, P. J., 1987, Changes in cyclic adenosine monophosphate-phosphodiesterase activity in nonpregnant and pregnant human myometrium, *Am. J. Obstet. Gynecol.* **157**:733.

Krebs, E. G., and Beavo, J. A., 1979, Phosphorylation–dephosphorylation of enzymes, *Annu. Rev. Biochem.* **48**:923.

Kroc, R. L., Steinetz, B. G., and Beach, V. L., 1959, The effects of estrogens, progestagens and relaxin in pregnant and nonpregnant laboratory rodents, *Ann. N.Y. Acad. Sci.* **75**:942.

Laifer, S. A., Ghodgoankar, R. B., Zacur, H. A., and Dubin, N. H., 1986, The effect of aminophylline on uterine smooth muscle contractility and prostaglandin production in the pregnant rat uterus *in vitro, Am. J. Obstet. Gynecol.* **155**:212.

Lamont, R. F., Rose, M., and Elder, M., 1985, Effect of bacterial products on prostaglandin E production by amnion cells, *Lancet* **2**:1331.

Lange, A. P., Secher, N. J., Westergaard, J. G., and Skovgard, I., 1982, Prelabor evaluation of inductibility, *Obstet. Gynecol.* **60**:137.

Larsson, L. I., Fahrenkrug, J., and Schaffalitzky de Muckadel, O. B., 1977, Vasoactive intestinal polypeptide occurs in nerve of the female genitourinary tract, *Science* **197**:1374.

Lebowitz, E. A., and Cooke, R., 1979, Phosphorylation of uterine smooth muscle myosin permits actin-activation, *J. Biochem. (Tokyo)* **85**:1489.

Lehman, W., 1986, Caldesmon association with smooth muscle thin filaments isolated in the presence and absence of calcium, *Biochim. Biophys. Acta* **885**:88.

Lema, M. J., Pagani, E. D., Shemin, R., and Julian, F. J., 1986, Myosin isozymes in rabbit and human smooth muscles, *Circ. Res.* **59**:115.

LePeuch, C. J., Haiech, J., and Demaille, J. G., 1979, Concerted regulation of cardiac sarcoplasmic reticulum calcium transport by cyclic adenosine monophosphate dependent and calcium-calmodulin-dependent phosphorylations, *Biochemistry* **18**:5150.

Leung, A. T., Imagawa, T., and Campbell, K. P., 1987, Structural characterization of the 1,4-dihydropyridine receptor of the voltage-dependent Ca^{2+} channel from rabbit skeletal muscle, *J. Biol. Chem.* **262**:7943.

Levin, R. M., and Weiss, B., 1979, Selective binding of antipsychotics and other psychoactive agents to the calcium-dependent activator of cyclic nucleotide phosphodiesterase, *J. Pharmacol. Exp. Ther.* **208**:454.

Lewis, R. B., and Schulman, J. D., 1973, Influence of acetylsalicylic acid, an inhibitor of prostaglandin synthesis, on the duration of human gestation and labour, *Lancet* **2**:1159.

Lukas, T. J., Burgess, W. H., Prendergast, F. G., Lau, W., and Watterson, D. M., 1986, Calmodulin-binding domains: Characterization of a phosphorylation and calmodulin binding site from myosin light chain kinase, *Biochemistry* **25**:1458.

Maclennan, A. H., Green, R. C., Bryant-Greenwood, G. D., Greenwood, F. C., and Seamark, R. F., 1980, Ripening of the human cervix and induction of labor with purified porcine relaxin, *Lancet* **1**:220.

MacLennan, D. H., Campbell, K. P., and Reithmeier, R. A. F., 1983, Calsequestrin, in: *Calcium and Cell Function,* Vol. 4 (W. Y. Cheung, ed.), Academic Press, New York, pp. 151–173.

Manabe, Y., Manabe, A., and Takahashi, A., 1982, F prostaglandin levels in amniotic fluid during balloon-induced cervical softening and labor at term, *Prostaglandins* **23**:247.

Manchester, D., Margolis, H. S., and Sheldon, R. E., 1976, Possible association between maternal indomethacin therapy and primary pulmonary hypertension of the newborn, *Am. J. Obstet. Gynecol.* **126**:467.

Marston, S. B., and Lehman, W., 1985, Caldesmon is a Ca^{2+} regulatory component of native smooth-muscle thin filaments, *Biochem. J.* **231**:517.

Marston, S. B., and Smith, C. W. J., 1985, The thin filaments of smooth muscles, *J. Muscle Res. Cell Motil.* **6**:669.

Marston, S. B., Trevett, R. M., and Walters, M., 1980, Calcium ion-regulated thin filaments from vascular smooth muscle, *Biochem. J.* **185**:355.

Martin, A., Fara, J. F., Alallon, W., Thoulon, J. M., Dumont, M., and Louisot, P., 1983, Enzymatic screening of human uterine cervical biopsies in nonpregnant and pregnant women at parturition, *Am. J. Obstet. Gynecol.* **145**:44.

Mercado-Simmen, R. C., Bryant-Greenwood, G. D., and Greenwood, F. C., 1980, Relaxin receptor in the rat myometrium: Regulation by estrogen and relaxin, *Endocrinology* **110**:220.

Michell, R. H., 1975, Inositol phospholipids and cell surface receptor function, *Biochim. Biophys. Acta* **415**:81.

Miller, J. R., Silver, P. J., and Stull, J. T., 1983, The role of myosin light chain kinase phosphorylation in beta-adrenergic relaxation of tracheal smooth muscle, *Mol. Pharmacol.* **24**:235.

Minamoto, T., Arai, K., Hirakawa, S., and Nagai, Y., 1987, Immunohistochemical studies on collagen types in the uterine cervix in pregnant and nonpregnant states, *Am. J. Obstet. Gynecol.* **156**:138.

Miyata, H., and Chacko, S., 1986, Role of tropomyosin in smooth muscle contraction: Effect of tropomyosin binding to actin on actin activation of myosin ATPase, *Biochemistry* **25**:2725.

Mochizuki, M., and Tojo, S., 1980, Effect of dehydroepiandrosterone sulfate on softening and dilatation of the uterine cervix in pregnant women, in: *Dilatation of the Uterine Cervix: Connective Tissue Biology and Clinical Management* (F. Naftolin and P. G. Stubblefield, eds.), Raven Press, New York, p. 267.

Morgan, J. P., and Morgan, K. G., 1982, Vascular smooth muscle: The first recorded Ca^{2+} transients, *Pflugers Arch.* **395**:75.

Movsesian, M. A., Nishikawa, M., and Adelstein, R. S., 1984, Phosphorylation of phospholamban by calcium-activated, phospholipid-dependent protein kinase. Stimulation of cardiac sarcoplasmic reticulum calcium uptake, *J. Biol. Chem.* **259**:8029.

Mrwa, U., Güth, K., Rüegg, J. C., Paul, R. J., Boström, S., Barsotti, R., and Hartshorne, D., 1985, Mechanical and biochemical characterization of the contraction elicited by a calcium-independent myosin light chain kinase in chemically skinned smooth muscle, *Experientia* **41**:1002.

Muller, M. J., and Baer, H. P., 1983, Relaxant effects of forskolin in smooth muscle: Role of cyclic AMP, *Arch. Pharmacol.* **322**:78.

Ngai, P. K., and Walsh, M. P., 1984, Inhibition of smooth muscle actin-activated myosin Mg^{2+}-ATPase activity by caldesmon, *J. Biol. Chem.* **259**:13656.

Ngai, P. K., and Walsh, M. P., 1985, Properties of caldesmon isolated from chicken gizzard, *Biochem. J.* **230**:695.

Ngai, P. K., and Walsh, M. P., 1987, The effects of phosphorylation of smooth-muscle caldesmon, *Biochem J.* **244**:417.

Ngai, P. K., Scott-Woo, G. C., Lim, M. S., Sutherland, C., and Walsh, M. P. 1987, Activation of smooth muscle myosin Mg^{2+}-ATPase by native thin filaments and actin/tropomyosin, *J. Biol. Chem.* **262**:5352.

Niebyl, J. R., and Witter, F. R., 1986, Neonatal outcome after indomethacin treatment for preterm labor, *Am. J. Obstet. Gynecol.* **155**:747.

Niebyl, J. R., Blake, D. A., White, R. D., Kumor, K. M., Dubin, N. H., Robinson, J. C., and Egner, P. G., 1980, The inhibition of premature labor with indomethacin, *Am. J. Obstet. Gynecol.* **136**:1014.

Nishikawa, M., Hidaka, H., and Adelstein, R. S., 1983, Phosphorylation of smooth muscle heavy meromyosin by calcium-activated phosopholipid-dependent protein kinase. The effect on actin-activated Mg^{2+}-ATPase activity, *J. Biol. Chem.* **258**:14069.

Nishikori, K., and Maeno, H., 1979, Close relationship between adenosine $3':5'$-monophosphate-dependent endogenous phosphorylation of a specific protein and stimulation of calcium uptake in rat uterine microsomes, *J. Biol. Chem.* **254**:6009.

Nishikori, K., Weisbrodt, N. W., Sherwood, O. D., and Sanborn, B. M., 1983, Effects of relaxin on rat uterine myosin light chain kinase activity and myosin light chain phosphorylation, *J. Biol. Chem.* **258**:2468.

Nishizuka, Y., 1984, The role of protein kinase C in cell surface signal transduction and tumour promotion, *Nature* **308**:693.

Noiman, E. S., 1980, Phosphorylation of smooth muscle myosin light chains by cAMP-dependent protein kinase, *J. Biol. Chem.* **255**:11067.

Norstrom, A., Bryman, I., Wiqvist, N., Swadesh, S., and Lindblom, B., 1984, Inhibitory action of relaxin on human cervical smooth muscle, *J. Clin. Endocrinol. Metab.* **59**:379.

Obrink, B., 1973, A study of the interactions between monomeric tropocollagen and glycosaminoglycans, *Eur. J. Biochem.* **33**:387.

Ohnishi, S. T., and Devlin, T. M., 1979, Calcium ionophore activity of a prostaglandin B_1 derivative (PGB), *Biochem. Biophys. Res. Commun.* **89**:240.

Okazaki, T., Casey, M. L., Okita, J. R., MacDonald, P. C., and Johnston, J. M., 1981, Initiation of human parturition. XII. Biosynthesis and metabolism of prostaglandins in human fetal membranes and uterine decidua, *Am. J. Obstet. Gynecol.* **139**:373.

Olins, G. M., and Bremel, R. D., 1982, Phosphorylation of myosin in mammary myoepithelial cells in response to oxytocin, *Endocrinology* **110**:1933.

Onishi, H., and Wakabayashi, T., 1982, Electron microscopic studies of myosin molecules from chicken gizzard muscle. 1: The formation of the intramolecular loop in the myosin tail, *J. Biochem. (Tokyo)* **92**:871.

Ottesen, B., 1983, Vasoactive intestinal polypeptide as a neurotransmitter in the female genital tract, *Am. J. Obstet. Gynecol.* **147**:208.

Ottesen, B., Wagner, G., and Fahrenkrug, J., 1980, Vasoactive intestinal polypeptide (VIP) inhibits prostaglandin $F_{2\alpha}$-induced activity of the rabbit myometrium, *Prostaglandins* **19**:427.

Ottesen, B., Larsen, J. J., Fahrenkrug, J., Stjernquist, M., and Sundler, F., 1981, Distribution and motor effect of VIP in female genital tract, *Endocrinol. Metab.* **3**:E32.

Park, S., and Rasmussen, H., 1986, Carbachol-induced protein phosphorylation changes in bovine tracheal smooth muscle, *J. Biol. Chem.* **261**:15734.

Parker, I., Ito, Y., Kuriyama, H., and Miledi, R., 1987, β-Adrenergic agonists and cyclic AMP decrease intracellular resting free-calcium concentration in ileum smooth muscle, *Proc. R. Soc. Lond. [Biol.]* **30**:207.

Parks, T. P., Nairn, A. C., Greengard, P., and Jamieson, J. D., 1987, The cyclic nucleotide-dependent phosphorylation of aortic smooth muscle membrane proteins, *Arch. Biochem. Biophys.* **255**:361.

Pato, M. D., and Adelstein, R. S., 1980, Dephosphorylation of the 20,000-dalton light chain of myosin by two different phosphatases from smooth muscle, *J. Biol. Chem.* **255**:6535.

Pato, M. D., and Kerc, E., 1985, Purification and characterization of a smooth muscle myosin phosphatase from turkey gizzards, *J. Biol. Chem.* **260**:12359.

Pato, M. D., and Kerc, E., 1986, Limited proteolytic digestion and dissociation of smooth muscle phosphatase-1 modifies its substrate specificity, *J. Biol. Chem.* **261**:3770.

Payne, M. E., Elzinga, M., and Adelstein, R. S., 1986, Smooth muscle myosin light chain kinase. Amino acid sequence at the site phosphorylated by adenosine cyclic 3',5'-phosphate-dependent protein kinase whether or not calmodulin is bound, *J. Biol. Chem.* **261**:16346.

Pearson, R. B., Jakes, R., John, M., Kendrick-Jones, J., and Kemp, B. E., 1984, Phosphorylation site sequence of smooth muscle myosin light chain (M_r = 20,000), *FEBS Lett.* **168**:108.

Pearson, R. B., Misconi, L. Y., and Kemp, B. E., 1986, Smooth muscle myosin kinase requires residues on the COOH-terminal side of the phosphorylation site. Peptide inhibitors, *J. Biol. Chem.* **261**:25.

Persechini, A., and Hartshorne, D. J., 1981, Phosphorylation of smooth muscle myosin: Evidence for cooperativity between the myosin heads, *Science* **213**:1383.

Persechini, A., Kamm, K. E., and Stull, J. T., 1986, Different phosphorylated forms of myosin in contracting tracheal smooth muscle, *J. Biol. Chem.* **261**:6293.

Petrie, R. H., 1981, Tocolysis using magnesium sulfate, *Semin. Perinatol.* **5**:226.

Pope, B., Hoh, J. F. Y., and Weeds, A., 1980, The ATPase activities of rat cardiac myosin isoenzymes, *FEBS Lett.* **118**:205.

Popescu, L. M., and Ignat, P., 1983, Calmodulin-dependent Ca^{2+}-pump ATPase of human smooth muscle sarcolemma, *Cell Calcium* **4**:219.

Potter, J. D., Strang-Brown, P., Walker, P. L., and Iida, S., 1983, Ca^{2+} binding to calmodulin, *Methods Enzymol.* **102**:135.

Prins, R. P., Bolton, R. N., Mark, C., Neilson, D. R., and Watson, P., 1983, Cervical ripening with intravaginal prostaglandin E_2 gel, *Obstet. Gynecol.* **61**:459.

Raeymaekers, L., and Jones, L. R., 1986, Evidence for the presence of phospholamban in the endoplasmic reticulum of smooth muscle, *Biochim. Biophys. Acta* **882**:258.

Rapoport, R. M., and Murad, F., 1983, Endothelium-dependent and nitrovasodilator-induced relaxation of vascular smooth muscle: Role of cyclic GMP, *J. Cyclic Nucleotide Protein Phosphor. Res.* **9**:281.

Reiner, O., and Marshall, J. M., 1976, Action of prostaglandin, $PGF_{2\alpha}$, on the uterus of the pregnant rat, *Arch. Pharmacol.* **292**:243.

Riemer, R. K., Jacobs, M. M., Wu, Y. Y., and Roberts, J. M., 1986, Progesterone-induced rabbit myometrial beta-adrenergic response is accompanied by increased concentration and expression of stimulatory adenylate cyclase coupling protein (Gs). Program of the 33rd Annual Meeting of the Society for Gynecologic Investigation, Toronto, Canada, p. 171 (abstract 274P).

Roberts, J. M., Insel, P. A., and Goldfein, A., 1981, Regulation of myometrial adrenoceptors and adrenergic response by sex steroids, *Mol. Pharmacol.* **20**:52.

Romero, R., Emamian, M., Quintero, R., Wan, M., Hobbins, J. C., and Mitchell, M, 1986, Amniotic fluid prostaglandin levels and intra-amniotic infections, *Lancet* **1**:1380.

Rorie, D. K., and Newton, M., 1967, Histologic and chemical studies of the smooth muscle in the human cervix and uterus, *Am. J. Obstet. Gynecol.* **99**:466.

Ross, E. M., and Gilman, A. G., 1980, Biochemical properties of hormone-sensitive adenylate cyclase, *Annu. Rev. Biochem.* **49**:533.

Rossier, M. F., Capponi, A. M., and Vallotton, M. B., 1987, Metabolism of inositol 1,4,5-trisophosphate in permeabilized rat aortic smooth muscle cells. Dependence on calcium concentration, *Biochem. J.* **245**:305.

Rovner, A. S., Thompson, M. M., and Murphy, R. A., 1986, Two different heavy chains are found in smooth muscle myosin, *Am. J. Physiol.* **250**:C861.

Rüegg, J. C., DiSalvo, J., and Paul, R. J., 1982, Soluble relaxation factor from vascular smooth muscle: A myosin light chain phosphatase? *Biochem. Biophys. Res. Commun.* **106**:1126.

Saito, Y., Sakamoto, H., MacLusky, N. J., and Naftolin, F., 1985, Correlation between gap junctions and steroid hormone receptors in myometrial tissue of pregnant and postpartum rats, *Am. J. Obstet. Gynecol.* **151**:805.

Sakamoto, H., and Huszar, G., 1984a, A mechanism for action of oxytocin in parturition, *Proc. Soc. Gynecol. Invest.* 176a.

Sakamoto, H., and Huszar, G., 1984b, Nitrendipine prolongs rat parturition: No changes occur in progesterone withdrawal, *Endocrinology* **115**:959.

Sanborn, B. M., Held, B., and Kuo, H. S., 1975, Specific estrogen binding proteins in human cervix, *J. Steroid Biochem.* **6**:1107.

Sandahl, B., Ulmsten, U., and Andersson, K.-E., 1979, Trial of the calcium antagonist nifedipine in the treatment of primary dysmenorrhoea, *Arch. Gynecol.* **227**:247.

Sanders, C., Burtnick, L. D., and Smillie, L. B., 1986, Native chicken gizzard tropomyosin is predominantly a βγ-heterodimer, *J. Biol. Chem.* **261**:12774.

Sasaki, K., Nakano, R., Kadoya, M., Iwao, K., and Sowa, S. M., 1982, Cervical ripening with dehydroepiandrosterone sulphate, *Br. J. Obstet. Gynaecol.* **89**:195.

Scheid, C. R., Honeyman, T. W., and Fay, F. S., 1979, Mechanism of β-adrenergic relaxation of smooth muscle, *Nature* **277**:32.

Seidel, J. C., 1980, Fragmentation of gizzard myosin by α-chymotrypsin and papain, the effects on ATPase activity, and the interaction with actin, *J. Biol. Chem.* **255**:4355.

Sellers, J. R., Pato, M. D., and Adelstein, R. S., 1981, Reversible phosphorylation of smooth muscle myosin, heavy meromyosin and platelet myosin, *J. Biol. Chem.* **256**:13137.

Sellers, J. R., Chock, P. B., and Adelstein, R. S., 1983, The apparently negatively cooperative phosphorylation of smooth muscle myosin at low ionic strength is related to its filamentous state, *J. Biol. Chem.* **258**:14181.

Sherry, J. M. F., Gorecka, A., Aksoy, M. O., Dabrowska, R., and Hartshorne, D. J., 1978, Roles of calcium and phosphorylation in the regulation of the activity of gizzard myosin, *Biochemistry* **17**:4411.

Sherwood, O. D., Change, C. C., BeVier, G. W., Diehl, J. R., and Dziuk, P. J., 1976, Relaxin concentrations in pig plasma following the administration of prostaglandin $F_{2\alpha}$ during late pregnancy, *Endocrinology* **98**:875.

Shigekawa, M., Finegan, J.-A., and Katz, A. M., 1976, Calcium transport ATPase of canine cardiac sarcoplasmic reticulum. A comparison with that of rabbit fast skeletal muscle sarcoplasmic reticulum, *J. Biol. Chem.* **251**:6894.

Silver, P. J., and Stull, J. T., 1983, Effects of the calmodulin antagonist, fluphenazine, on phosphorylation of myosin and phosphorylase in intact smooth muscle, *Mol. Pharmacol.* **23**:665.

Singh, T. J., Akatsuka, A., and Huang, K.-P., 1983, Phosphorylation of smooth muscle myosin light chain by five different kinases, *FEBS Lett.* **159**:217.

Skinner, K. A., and Challis, J. R. G., 1985, Changes in the synthesis and metabolism of prostaglandins by human fetal membranes and decidua at labor, *Am. J. Obstet. Gynecol.* **151**:519.

Small, J. V., 1977, The contractile apparatus of the smooth muscle cell, in: *The Biochemistry of Smooth Muscle* (N. L. Stephens, ed.), University Park Press, Baltimore, MD, p. 379.

Small, J. V., Fürst, D. O., and DeMey, J., 1986, Localization of filamin in smooth muscle, *J. Cell Biol.* **102**:210.

Smith, C. W. J., Pritchard, K., and Marston, S. B., 1987, The mechanism of Ca^{2+} regulation of vascular smooth muscle thin filaments by caldesmon and calmodulin, *J. Biol. Chem.* **262**:116.

Sobieszek, A., and Small, J. V., 1977, Regulation of the actin–myosin interaction in vertebrate smooth muscle: Activation via a myosin light-chain kinase and the effect of tropomyosin, *J. Mol. Biol.* **112**:559.

Sobue, K., Muramoto, Y., Fujita, M., and Kakiuchi, S., 1981a, Purification of a calmodulin-binding protein from chicken gizzard that interacts with F-actin, *Proc. Natl. Acad. Sci. U.S.A.* **78:**5652.

Sobue, K., Muramoto, Y., Fujita, M., and Kakiuchi, S., 1981b, Calmodulin-binding protein from chicken gizzard that interacts with F-actin, *Biochem. Int.* **2:**469.

Soloff, M. S., and Sweet, P., 1982, Oxytocin inhibition of (calcium–magnesium)-ATPase activity in rat myometrial plasma membranes, *J. Biol. Chem.* **275:**10687.

Somlyo, A. P., 1985, Excitation contraction coupling and the ultrastructure of smooth muscle, *Circ. Res.* **57:**497.

Somlyo, A. P., and Somlyo, A. V., 1974, Ultrastructure of smooth muscle, in: *Methods in Pharmacology,* Vol. 3 (E. E. Daniels and D. M. Paton, eds.), Plenum Press, New York, p. 3.

Somlyo, A. P., Somlyo, A. V., Shuman, H., and Endo, M., 1982, Calcium and monovalent ions in smooth muscle, *Fed. Proc.* **41:**2883.

Somlyo, A. V., 1980, Ultrastructure of vascular smooth muscle, in: *The Handbook of Physiology. The Cardiovascular System,* Vol. II, *Vascular Smooth Muscle* (D. F. Bohr, A. P. Somlyo, and H. V. Sparks, eds.) American Physiological Society, Washington, pp. 33–67.

Somlyo, A. V., Butler, T. M., Bond, M., and Somlyo, A. P., 1981, Myosin filaments have non-phosphorylated light chains in relaxed smooth muscle, *Nature* **294:**567.

Somyalo, A. V., Bond, M., Somlyo, A. P., and Scarpa, A., 1985, Inositol trisphosphate induced calcium release and contraction in vascular smooth muscle, *Proc. Natl. Acad. Sci. U.S.A.* **82:**5231.

Spät, A., Fabiato, A., and Rubin, R. P., 1986, Binding of inositol triphosphate by a liver microsomal fraction, *Biochem. J.* **233:**929.

Stull, J. T., Nunnally, M. H., and Michnoff, C. H., 1986, in: *The Enzymes,* Vol. XVII, Academic Press, New York, pp. 113–166.

Stys, S. J., Dresser, B. L., Otte, T. E., and Clark, K. E., 1981, Effect of prostaglandin E_2 on cervical compliance in pregnant ewes, *Am. J. Obstet. Gynecol.* **140:**415.

Sumimoto, K., and Kuriyama, H., 1986, Mobilization of free Ca^{2+} measured during contraction–relaxation cycles in smooth muscle cells of the porcine coronary artery using quin-2, *Pflugers Arch.* **406:**173.

Suzuki, H., Kamata, T., Onishi, H., and Watanabe, S., 1982, Adenosine triphosphate-induced reversible change in the conformation of chicken gizzard myosin and heavy meromyosin, *J. Biochem. (Tokyo)* **91:**1699.

Szlachter, N. B., O'Byrne, E. M., Goldsmith, L., Steinetz, B. G., and Weiss, G., 1980, Myometrial-inhibiting activity of relaxin-containing extracts of human corpora lutea of pregnancy, *Am. J. Obstet. Gynecol.* **136:**584.

Szpacenko, A., and Dabrowska, R., 1986, Functional domain of caldesmon, *FEBS Lett.* **202:**182.

Tada, M., and Katz, A. M., 1982, Phosphorylation of the sarcoplasmic reticulum and sarcolemma, *Annu. Rev. Physiol.* **44:**401.

Takahashi, M., Seagar, M. J., Jones, J. F., Reber, B. F. X., and Catterall, W. A., 1987, Subunit structure of dihydropyridine-sensitive calcium channels from skeletal muscle, *Proc. Natl. Acad. Sci. U.S.A.* **84:**5478.

Takio, K., Blumenthal, D. K., Edelman, A. M., Walsh, K. A., Krebs, E. G., and Titani, K., 1985, Amino acid sequence of an active fragment of rabbit skeletal muscle myosin light chain kinase, *Biochemistry* **24:**6028.

Takio, K., Blumenthal, D. K., Walsh, K. A., Titani, K., and Krebs, E. G., 1986, Amino acid sequence of rabbit skeletal muscle myosin light chain kinase, *Biochemistry* **25:**8049.

Tanabe, T., Takeshima, H., Mikami, A., Flockerzi, V., Takahashi, H., Kangawa, K., Kojima, M., Matsuo, H., Hirose, T., and Numa, S., 1987, Primary structure of the receptor for calcium channel blockers from skeletal muscle, *Nature* **328:**313.

Tansey, R. R., and Padykula, H. A., 1978, Cellular responses to experimental inhibition of collagen degradation in the postpartum rat uterus, *Anat. Rec.* **191:**287.

Theobald, P. W., Rath, W., Kuhnle, H., and Kuhn, W., 1982, Histologic and electron-microscopic examinations of collagenous connective tissue of the non-pregnant cervix, the pregnant cervix, and the pregnant prostaglandin-treated cervix, *Arch. Gynecol.* **231:**241.

Triggle, D. J., and Janis, R. A., 1987, Calcium channel ligands, *Annu. Rev. Pharmacol. Toxicol.* **27:**347.

Trybus, K. M., and Lowey, S., 1985, Mechanism of smooth muscle myosin phosphorylation, *J. Biol. Chem.* **260:**15988.

Trybus, K. M., Huiatt, T. W., and Lowey, S., 1982, A bent monomeric conformation of myosin from smooth muscle, *Proc. Natl. Acad. Sci. U.S.A.* **79:**6151.

Tsien, R. W., 1983, Calcium channels in excitable cell membranes, *Annu. Rev. Physiol.* **45:**341.

Tuazon, P. T., and Traugh, J. A., 1984, Activation of actin-activated ATPase in smooth muscle by phosphorylation of myosin light chain with protease-activated kinase I, *J. Biol. Chem.* **259:**541.

Uldbjerg, N., Ekman, G., Malmstrom, A., Olsson, K., and Ulmsten, U., 1983, Ripening of the human uterine cervix related to changes in collagen, glycosaminoglycans, and collagenolytic activity, *Am. J. Obstet. Gynecol.* **147**:662.

Ulmsten, U., Andersson, K.-E., and Forman, A., 1978, Relaxing effects of nifedipine on the nonpregnant human uterus *in vitro* and *in vivo*, *Obstet. Gynecol.* **52**:436.

Ulmsten, U., Andersson, K.-E., and Wingerup, L., 1980, Treatment of premature labor with the calcium antagonist nifedipine, *Arch. Gynecol.* **229**:1.

Van Breemen, C., Aaronson, P., Loutzenhiser, R., and Meisheri, K., 1982, Calcium fluxes in isolated rabbit aorta and guinea pig tenia coli, *Fed. Proc.* **41**:2891.

Van Breemen, C., Leijten, P., Yamamoto, H., Aaronson, P., and Cauvin, C., 1986, Calcium activation of vascular smooth muscle, *Hypertension* **8**[Suppl. II]:II–89.

Vandekerckhove, J., and Weber, K., 1979, The complete amino acid sequence of actins from bovine aorta, bovine heart, bovine fast skeletal muscle, and rabbit slow skeletal muscle. A protein-chemical analysis of muscle actin differentiation, *Differentiation* **14**:123–133.

Verhoeff, A., and Garfield, R., 1986, Ultrastructure of the myometrium and the role of gap junctions in myometrial function, in: *The Physiology and Biochemistry of the Uterus in Pregnancy and Labor* (G. Huszar, ed.), CRC Press, Boca Raton, FL, p. 73.

Wahl, L. M., Blandau, R. J., and Page, R. C., 1977, Effect of hormones on collagen metabolism and collagenase activity in the pubic symphysis ligament of the guinea pig, *Endocrinology* **10**:571.

Walker, J. W., Somlyo, A. V., Goldman, Y. E., Somlyo, A. P., and Trentham, D. R., 1987, Kinetics of smooth and skeletal muscle activation by laser pulse photolysis of caged inositol 1,4,5-trisphosphate, *Nature* **327**:249.

Wallner, B. P., Mattaliano, R. J., Hession, C., et al., 1986, Cloning and expression of human lipocortin, a phospholipase A_2 inhibitor with potential anti-inflammatory activity, *Nature* **320**:77.

Walsh, M. P., 1985, Limited proteolysis of smooth muscle myosin light chain kinase, *Biochemistry* **24**:3724.

Walsh, M. P., Hinkins, S., Flink, I. L., and Hartshorne, D. J., 1982a, Bovine stomach myosin light chain kinase: Purification, characterization and comparison with the turkey gizzard enzyme, *Biochemistry* **21**:6890.

Walsh, M. P., Dabrowska, R., Hinkins, S., and Hartshorne, D. J., 1982b, Calcium-independent myosin light chain kinase of smooth muscle: Preparation by limited chymotryptic digestion of the Ca^{2+}-dependent enzyme, purification and characterization, *Biochemistry* **21**:1919.

Walsh, M. P., Bridenbaugh, R., Hartshorne, D. J., and Kerrick, W. G. L., 1982c, Phosphorylation-dependent activated tension in skinned gizzard muscle fibers in the absence of Ca^{2+}, *J. Biol. Chem.* **257**:5987.

Walsh, M. P., Bridenbaugh, R., Kerrick, W. G. L., and Hartshorne, D. J., 1983, Ca^{2+}-independent myosin light chain kinase: Evidence in favor of the phosphorylation theory of regulation in smooth muscle, *Fed. Proc.* **42**:45.

Wathes, D. C., and Porter, D. G., 1982, Effect of uterine distension and oestrogen treatment on gap junction formation in the myometrium of the rat, *J. Reprod. Fertil.* **65**:497.

Werth, D. K., Haeberle, J. R., and Hathaway, D. R., 1982, Purification of a myosin phosphatase from bovine aortic smooth muscle, *J. Biol. Chem.* **257**:7306.

Williams, D. A., and Fay, F. S., 1986, Calcium transients and resting levels in isolated smooth muscle cells as monitored with quin-2, *Am. J. Physiol.* **250**:C779.

Williams, D. A., Fogarty, K. E., Tsien, R. Y., and Fay, F. S., 1985, Calcium gradients in single smooth muscle cells revealed by the digital imaging microscope using fura-2, *Nature* **318**:558.

Williams, D. A., Becker, P. L., and Fay, F. S., 1987, Regional changes in calcium underlying contraction of single smooth muscle cells, *Science* **235**:1644.

Williams, J. K., Lewis, M. L., Cohen, G. R., and O'Brien, W. F., 1988, The sequential use of estradiol and prostaglandin E_2 topical gels for cervical ripening in high-risk term pregnancies requiring induction of labor, *Am. J. Obstet. Gynecol.* **158**:55.

Wilson, T., Liggins, G. C., Aimer, G. P., and Skinner, S. J. M., 1985, Partial purification and characterization of two compounds from amniotic fluid which inhibit phospholipase activity in human endometrial cells, *Biochem. Biophys. Res. Commun.* **131**:22.

Woessner, J. F., Jr., 1979, Total, latent and active collagenase during the course of postpartum involution of the rat uterus, *Biochem. J.* **180**:95.

Woolley, D. E., 1979, Human collagenases: Comparative and immunolocalization studies, *Ciba Found. Symp.* **75**:69.

Wuytack, F., Raeymaekers, L., Verbist, J., De Smedt, H., and Casteels, R., 1984, Evidence for the presence in smooth muscle of two types of Ca^{2+}-transport ATPase, *Biochem. J.* **224**:445.

Wuytack, F., Raeymaekers, L., and Casteels, R., 1985, The Ca^{2+}-transport ATPases in smooth muscle, *Experientia* **41**:900.

Wuytack, F., Raeymaekers, L., Verbist, J., Jones, L. R., and Casteels, R., 1987, Smooth-muscle endoplasmic reticulum contains a cardiac-like form of calsequestrin, *Biochem. Biophys. Acta* **899:**151.

Yamaguchi, K., Hirata, M., and Kuriyama, H., 1987, Calmodulin activates inositol 1,4,5-trisphosphate 3-kinase activity in pig aortic smooth muscle, *Biochem. J.* **244:**787.

Zuidema, L. J., Khan-Dawood, F., Dawood, M. Y., and Work, B. A., 1986, Hormones and cervical ripening: Dehydroepiandrosterone sulfate, estradiol, estriol, and progesterone, *Am. J. Obstet. Gynecol.* **155:**1252.

Electrophysiological Properties of Uterine Smooth Muscle

C. Y. KAO

14

Until recently almost all knowledge of the electrophysiological properties of the myometrium and other mammalian smooth muscles was based on descriptive observations of some natural phenomena or on modifications of such phenomena by changes in the ionic environment or produced by hormonal and pharmacological agents. Although much of value has been learned about the resting and action potentials and their relationship to contractions, the information derived from such approaches was limited because of the nature of the methods. In the previous edition of this book, substantial revisions were incorporated into this chapter to include advances then being made with the introduction of certain analytical methods for studying the electrophysiological properties of mammalian smooth muscles. For instance, basic electrical properties of some smooth muscle preparations were being unmasked by the polarization method of Abe and Tomita (1968), and the nature of the ionic currents, their equilibrium potentials, and some aspects of the ionic conductances were being identified by use of the double-sucrose-gap voltage-clamp method (Anderson, 1969; Kao and McCullough, 1975; Inomata and Kao, 1976). All that information, fulfilling a need then existing, was also flawed, because it had to be obtained on multicellular preparations, which presented formidable technical obstacles to an unambiguous understanding of the underlying cellular processes.

It is gratifying that not long before the preparation of this chapter, powerful new methods have become available that allow the study of electrophysiological properties of single mammalian smooth muscle cells and of single ionic channels in the living cellular membrane. Although the amount of new information for the myometrium is still limited, sufficient general knowledge about single smooth muscle cells has now been gathered to permit an attempt to bridge observations of tissue phenomena with cellular phenomena, and of both with single-channel phenomena occurring in the protein molecules of ionic channels.

C. Y. KAO • Department of Pharmacology, State University of New York Downstate Medical Center, Brooklyn, New York 11203.

As with prior editions of this chapter, the current version is not an encyclopedic coverage of the vast topic of the electrophysiological properties of the myometrium and other smooth muscles. Instead, it is a sketchy tale biased towards a few threads of continuity that can extend from tissue-level observations all the way through cellular phenomena to single-channel events. It is too early for the tale to have an ending, but there should be a sufficient beginning to help direct the reader's interest to an important emerging phase of smooth muscle research.

1. Review of Methodology

1.1. Comparison of Uterine, Cardiac, and Skeletal Muscles

It is generally acknowledged that much more is known about the electrophysiological properties of skeletal and cardiac muscles than about those of uterine or other mammalian smooth muscles. A serious difficulty of working with smooth muscles, which contributes to this paucity of knowledge, is that the individual smooth muscle cells are much smaller than cells in the other two types of muscles. Figure 1 illustrates this point. Assume a sheetlike preparation of each of the three types of muscles, measuring $10 \times 1 \times 0.1$ mm, with a volume of 1 mm³. From well-known information about the extracellular spaces and the sizes of individual cells in each type of muscle, it is readily evident that occupying the same 1-mm³ volume would be about 17 skeletal muscle fibers and about 1700 cardiac myocytes. For the myometrium or another mammalian visceral smooth muscle, there would be about 100,000 times as many cells. To impale with a capillary microelectrode a tapering cell that is 6 μm in its largest diameter is quite a different problem from impaling one that is 80 μm in diameter for most of its length.

The small size of smooth muscle cells also produces a volume/surface ratio that is about one-tenth that of skeletal or cardiac muscles. Stated differently, for each unit cell volume, there is about ten times more surface in a smooth muscle cell than in a cell of the other two muscles. For this reason, much more extensive passive electrolyte shifts can be expected in isolated preparation of the myometrium (e.g., Kao and Siegman, 1963). Finally, it would be hard to expect the very large cell population in a myometrial preparation to be homogeneous in chemical composition or uniform in physiological state. Where knowledge of cellular function is desired, such inhomogeneity can lead to considerable variations in observations.

Another important difference is the interconnections among individual cells in the three

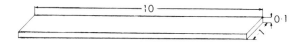

Muscle	Diameter of each cell (mm)	Length of each cell (mm)	Relative cell volume (%)	Cells /mm³	V/A (μ)
Skeletal	0·08	10	88	17	10·3
Cardiac	0·02	0·2	75	1200	7·1
Uterine	0·006	0·03	65	2·3x10⁶	0·9

Figure 1. Some comparisons of skeletal, cardiac, and uterine smooth muscles based on a hypothetical preparation of each type of muscle measuring 10 by 1 by 0.1 mm with a volume of 1 mm³.

different preparations (see Eisenberg and Johnson, 1970). In skeletal muscle, each individual fiber is a distinct cell not connected to fibers surrounding it. An electric current applied at a point in a skeletal muscle fiber will become dissipated along that fiber according to classical cable properties (see, e.g., Katz, 1966; Jack *et al.*, 1974). In cardiac and smooth muscles, however, individual cells are electrically interconnected with one another not only on one plane but also in three dimensions. Whereas cable analysis can be made successfully in some cardiac tissue preparations, in most smooth muscles, the interconnections are so numerous and so complex that reliable analysis based on cable properties became possible only with the introduction of a technique that forced massive amounts of current through the entire cross section of a preparation (Abe and Tomita, 1968).

Related to this problem is the generally more complex geometry of the smooth muscle preparations. It is still not entirely clear how current is spread within a smooth muscle preparation, and such uncertainty has a limiting effect on our understanding of how impulses are generated and propagated in the myometrium and the uterus as an organ or in other similar smooth muscle organs. The interstitial space among the individual smooth muscle cells is also arranged in a complex pattern (if, indeed, any pattern can be discerned). From an electrophysiological point of view, in a multicellular preparation the electrical resistance of the interstitial fluid surrounding individual cells is a major source of error in any voltage-clamp study. No doubt, these are all serious disadvantages of a multicellar smooth muscle preparation, but so long as they are kept in mind they should not be insurmountable obstacles to reasonable investigations of smooth muscle functions. The danger lies in a lack of awareness of these problems, which leads to unreasonable expectations of imperfect techniques.

Recently, however, appropriate procedures have been developed to dissociate myometrial or other smooth muscle cells into free individual cells. Such individual cells can be studied with newer electrophysiological techniques to yield direct information on cellular functions without the problems encountered in studying multicellular preparations. Surprisingly, many fundamental properties of smooth muscles first observed on multicellular preparations have been confirmed by recent observations on single individual cells (e.g., Yamamoto *et al.*, 1988b,c).

1.2. A Brief Statement of the Ionic Theory of Excitation

The ionic theory of excitation (Hodgkin, 1951; Hodgkin and Huxley, 1952) is a successful integration of the ionic distribution patterns, ionic movements, and various electrical phenomena in excitable cells. Many accounts are available summarizing the theory in its classical form (e.g., Hodgkin 1951, 1964; Katz, 1966; Brinley, 1980) or with important elaborations of recent advances in single-channel studies (e.g., Hille, 1984). A very brief account is given here to facilitate the presentation of some material in subsequent sections.

1.2.1. Resting Potential

Under resting conditions, a potential difference exists across the surface membrane of an excitable cell, the interior of the cell being some 50–100 mV negative with respect to the exterior. This potential difference is referred to as the *resting potential*. Within certain limitations, the magnitude of this resting potential is reasonably well related to the ratio of the concentrations of the two most abundant cations in the tissues, potassium and sodium. In all animal cells, the interior of the cell has a high potassium and a low sodium content, and the extracellular fluid has a high sodium and a low potassium content. In mammalian tissues, the approximate values are: (1) intracellular potassium concentration, $[K^+]_i = 150$ mEq/liter cell water; (2) intracellular sodium concentration, $[Na^+]_i = 25$ mEq/liter cell water; (3) extracellular potassium concentration, $[K^+]_0 = 5$ mEq/liter water; and (4) extracellular sodium concentration, $[Na^+]_0 = 145$ mEq/liter water.

The first formulation relating ionic distribution to resting potential was made by Bernstein in 1902 (see Hodgkin, 1951; Hille, 1984) when he considered the cell membrane to be permeable only to potassium ions and the relationship between ion concentration and membrane potential to be

$$E = \frac{RT}{F} \ln \frac{[K^+]_o}{[K^+]_i} \tag{1}$$

where R, T, and F are physical constants with their usual meanings, and the entire term has a value of 58 mV at 25°C if the ratio of the concentrations is expressed on a log scale to the base 10. From the foregoing values of ionic concentrations, a value of -86 mV for E would result, the inside of the cell being negative. The relationship also predicts that the resting potential should vary as a log function of the ratio of potassium concentrations outside and inside of the cell and that the function should have a slope of 58 mV for every tenfold change in the concentration ratio. When carefully tested on various cells, the observable relationship does not agree completely with this simple prediction. The slope of the function is somewhat less, and the deviation from the theoretical value is particularly manifest at low values of $[K^+]_0$.

These discrepancies were explained by Hodgkin (1951) on the basis that the membrane is permeable not only to potassium ions but also slightly to sodium ions, so that the relationship between resting potential and ion concentrations is

$$E = \frac{RT}{F} \ln \frac{[K^+]_o + b[Na^+]_o}{[K^+]_i + b[Na^+]_i} \tag{2}$$

where $b = P_{Na}/P_K$, the ratio of the permeabilities of sodium and potassium through the membrane.

Consider the value of E in a case in which only the ratio of sodium concentrations is important. From the foregoing concentration values, a value of 44 mV, inside positive, would result. Thus, there are two extreme values of membrane potentials, with opposite signs, that depend on the permeability of the membrane to the particular cation. By measuring the resting potential under special conditions in which internal and external ionic concentrations are known, Hodgkin and Horowicz (1959) concluded that in frog sartorius muscle fiber, b, the ratio of permeabilities of sodium and potassium, has a value of 0.01. In other words, P_{Na} is only 1/100 of P_K. In rabbit myometrium, from experimentally observed values of E and various ionic concentrations under conditions of equilibrium, b was estimated to be about 0.1 (Kao and Nishiyama, 1964). A similar value was found for the rat myometrium (Casteels and Kuriyama, 1965). The effect of this slight degree of permeability to sodium is to reduce the resting potential from that expected from equation 1 toward a new level somewhat less negative. If b were 0.01, the foregoing ionic concentrations would lead to a resting potential of -79 mV. If b were 0.1, the resting potential would be -52 mV.

1.2.2. Action Potential

The essence of the ionic theory of excitation is that changes in membrane potential result from changes in the permeability of the excitable membrane to sodium and potassium. Before proceeding to a more detailed description of these changes, it would be wise to consider the conditions existing in the resting cell as dynamic equilibria. Potassium is distributed in such a way that the chemical (concentration) forces tend to drive it from the interior of the cell toward the exterior, whereas the internal electrical negativity tends to prevent the outward movement of the positively charged potassium ion. If the chemical forces and electrical forces are equal and opposite, then the distribution of the potassium ions is strictly passive and in accord with the requirements of the Gibbs–Donnan distribution. Such a potential difference, at which the potassium ions are in electrochemical equilibrium, is referred to as the *potassium equilibrium potential* (E_K). If for any reason the resting potential becomes less negative, then to achieve equilibrium, intracellular potassium moves outward through the cell membrane. This movement is *passive* or *downhill* in the sense that it follows electrochemical gradients and does not require the expenditure of metabolic energy.

For sodium the conditions are somewhat different. Under resting conditions the chemical forces tend to drive sodium ions inward, and the internal electrical negativity tends to act in the same direction. Thus, under resting conditions, the distribution of sodium ions cannot be in electrochemical equilibrium. With the usual values of $[Na^+]_i$ and $[Na^+]_0$, electrochemical equilibrium can be attained only when the interior of the cell is positive with respect to the exterior. The potential difference at which the chemical and electrical driving forces for sodium are equal and opposite is referred to as the *sodium equilibrium potential* (E_{Na}). To maintain the usual concentration pattern of sodium in the resting cell against electrochemical gradients, metabolic energy must be expended. The process is often referred to as the *sodium pump* or, better, the *sodium–potassium pump*, that is, the *active extrusion* of sodium from the interior of the cell, which is coupled with some *active uptake* of potassium. This process is not immediately involved in excitation, but it is indirectly involved in the sense that it keeps the concentration patterns in a condition that allows excitation to occur.

Without discussing the evidence in detail (see Hodgkin *et al.*, 1952), it can be stated that when the resting potential is increased (*hyperpolarized*) there is an inward current flow. The interpretation is that when the internal negativity is increased, there is an inward movement of positive charges that tends to restore the membrane potential to the original state. When the resting potential is decreased (*depolarized*) by a few millivolts, there is an outward current flow. This is explained by the fact that when the internal negativity is slightly reduced, there is an outward flow of positive charges, tending again to restore the membrane to the original state. Such responses to perturbations are expected of stable physical systems.

When the resting potential is depolarized by about 10–15 mV, however, there is a large inward current. This change is opposite to that expected of a stable system, because the inward current causes further depolarization, which leads to more inward current. In this sense the change is regenerative, and the level of membrane potential at which the change is triggered is known as the *spike threshold*. The inward current during the regenerative change has been considered a result of inward movement of sodium ions under the existing electrochemical gradients; i.e., the movement is passive and downhill. Theoretically, inward sodium movement stops only when the interior of the cell is sufficiently positive to balance the chemical driving forces, that is, at the sodium equilibrium potential.

According to the ionic theory of excitation, these current flows result from changes in membrane permeability to sodium. In the resting state, when b (equation 2) is relatively small, the membrane potential approaches the potassium equilibrium potential. On threshold depolarization, some unknown molecular alterations take place in the excitable membrane, resulting in an increase of b by several hundredfold. As a result, the potential difference approaches the sodium equilibrium potential.

This change is not sustained, nor is it the only change that takes place. Almost as soon as the increase in sodium permeability begins, another process, known as sodium *inactivation*, begins to oppose the increase. Also, shortly after the beginning of the increase in sodium permeability, the potassium permeability increases, and this change is more sustained than that for sodium permeability. The process of sodium inactivation has the effect of limiting the extent of the increase in sodium permeability; consequently, the membrane potential approaches but does not reach the sodium equilibrium potential. The increase in potassium permeability allows an outward flow of positive charges, which brings the membrane potential back to the resting value, a process known as *repolarization*. The entire observable electrical change is a transient positive-going signal termed the *spike* or the *action potential*.

These basic concepts have since been found to apply to the movement of a variety of other ions through the excitable membrane, notably calcium, which replaces sodium as the charge carrier of inward current in many smooth muscles. Thus, such terms as sodium action potentials or calcium action potentials are used. There are important differences in the properties of sodium currents and calcium currents, and these are discussed in subsequent sections.

1.2.3. Current Status

The idea of rapid changes in membrane permeability to different ions was initially a convenient conceptual way of handling the known biophysical information. There had been no evidence of any chemical or structural features of the excitable membrane that could support such functions. In the mid-1960s two natural toxins, tetrodotoxin and saxitoxin, became available, which selectively affected the sodium channel (see Kao, 1966). Because of their specificity of action, they ushered in a new phase of biochemical studies of excitable membranes. With the use of these toxins, it soon became possible to isolate the channel macromolecule for detailed chemical studies. From such studies, the amino acid composition and sequence of the sodium channel has been established through molecular biological methods. Thus, studies of excitation phenomena are no longer based narrowly on electrophysiological approaches alone but must include considerations of protein structures as well. Such an approach can be found in a recent conference monograph on the sodium channel (Kao and Levinson, 1986). On the basis of similar approaches using specific ''handles,'' other ionic channels also are being studied actively.

It is now generally accepted that the ionic channels occur in integral protein molecules that project through the cell membrane, extending from the cytoplasmic side to the extracellular side. Although the details are still unknown, it is believed that under appropriate changes in electric fields, some parts of the protein molecule, perhaps in the lining of the channel, undergo conformational changes. After all, a 20-mV change across a 50-Å-thick cell membrane (such as that occurring in depolarizing from the resting potential to the spike threshold) is equivalent to a change of 40,000 V across a 1-cm distance, the usual measure of electric fields. Such conformational changes are considered to be at the root of the *gating* process, which controls the opening and closing of the channel to ion passage. Ion channels that respond in this way are known collectively as *voltage-gated ionic channel,* in contradistinction to the *ligand-gated ionic channels,* which respond to interaction with specific chemical modulators such as acetylcholine. Opening gating is called *activation*; closing of the same opened gate is called *deactivation. Inactivation* is believed to be a separate process occurring in sites different from those of activation.

In addition to advances in studying the chemical structure of channel proteins, new developments in electrophysiological techniques have made it possible to observe a single ionic channel in a living membrane opening or closing under appropriate stimuli (see Hamill *et al.,* 1981). By and large, the opening of a resting (and closed) channel is always to the same level; only rarely are there sublevels of opening. The probability of a channel opening is variable, as is the duration of its remaining open. Taken on a population basis of many channels in the cell membrane of an entire cell, the *macroscopic* current carried by any particular ion, such as potassium, sodium, or calcium, is then the sum total of the statistical behavior of individual channels. As is made clear in Section 3.2.4b, single-channel events of one type of potassium channel appropriately summed and averaged show remarkable similarities to the potassium current observed on an intact single smooth muscle cell, which in turn closely resembles the potassium current elicited from multicellular preparations under classical voltage-clamp conditions (Hu *et al.,* 1988a). A similar correlation between single-channel events and a calcium inward current has also been demonstrated (Yoshino and Yabu, 1985).

Because of the small sizes of individual cells and their complex interconnections with one another, electrophysiological investigations of the myometrium and other smooth muscles were confined, until recently, almost entirely to recordings of the resting potential or spontaneous action potentials. Attempts to investigate basic electrical properties of smooth muscles by means of techniques that had become commonplace in studies of other tissues (such as constant-current analysis of cable properties) have been much less successful.

In 1968, Abe and Tomita introduced a method whereby current applied to a strip of smooth muscle can be distributed fairly uniformly throughout the cross section of the preparation. With this technique, electrophysiological studies of smooth muscles advanced from a status of observing natural phenomena only to one in which consequences of planned perturbations also can be studied. As important an advance as it was for smooth muscle work, there were inherent limitations to any constant-current methods. When applied outward currents depolarized the smooth muscle membrane to spike threshold, action potentials ensued. Furthermore, transmembrane movements of charge-carrying ions are influenced by both the driving force and the conductance of the membrane. In constant-current analysis, both factors can change, making it difficult to arrive at direct answers to some basic questions.

Another important advance was made by Anderson (1969) when he successfully adapted a voltage-clamp technique to a small strip of myometrium. Even though there are serious limitations to this technique when applied to such multicellular smooth muscle preparations, for the first time it became possible to approach some fundamental electrophysiological problems in these preparations by a rather direct route. For instance, by separating the influences of driving force from those of conductance, it was possible to clarify the nature of the ionic currents responsible for the action potential (Anderson *et al.,* 1971; Kao and McCullough, 1975; Inomata and Kao, 1976) and to study certain pharmacological responses (Kao *et al.,* 1976).

The difficulty in voltage-clamp studies of multicellular smooth muscle preparations lies chiefly in the problem of series resistance, which can be viewed as the collection of electrical resistances in the small extracellular clefts immediately surrounding the cell membrane (Section 1.1). Electric current applied through an electrode in the bath solution can reach the cell membrane only by passing through the extracellular cleft; the cleft resistance therefore is in series with the resistance of the cell membrane. If the series resistance component is a substantial part of the total, then significant errors are involved. Since there is no easy way around this obstacle, the information obtained from such studies is also limited (see Johnson and Lieberman, 1971).

In the last few years, it has become possible to dissociate individual smooth muscle cells from multicellular preparations by various regimens of enzymatic digestion. Such individual cells have been voltage clamped with capillary microelectrodes and most recently with a new technique based on the formation of an extremely high-resistance seal between the cell surface and the electrode tip.

Since appropriate recording is common to all electrophysiological studies of mammalian smooth muscles, some discussion of the common methods is made in the following sections of this chapter. The different types of recording methods available provide different types of information, which, when taken together, form a rounded picture of the electrical activities of the tissue. No single recording method is all-embracing and totally superior to all others in all requirements. For example, as powerful as single-channel recordings are for understanding the molecular events in channel proteins, to use them alone without any associated knowledge of whole-cell currents would be like examining a microscopic slide with the highest magnification without first gleaning some idea of the general topography of the section. Even voltage-clamp data are not entirely satisfying unless they help to explain familiar physiological observations based on action potentials.

1.3.1. Surface Recording

As the name "surface recording" implies, all of these methods record activity from the surface of myometrial cells, which, like all other excitable cells, show a relative surface negativity when they are active. Such surface negativity can be recorded as potential changes of the region under study with respect to another region that does not undergo such a change. The electrode at the second region may or may not be grounded; it may be placed on another part of the myometrial preparation or on some different tissue. If the second electrode is not grounded and is placed at another site on a myometrial preparation, activity of cells under this electrode also can be recorded, although the polarity of the signals should be the opposite of those under the first electrode.

1.3.1a. Wire and Wick Electrodes. These electrodes can be fashioned from appropriate material of various sizes. Wick electrodes are usually saturated with an electrolyte, through which they are connected to a recording amplifier. Wire electrodes may be connected directly to an amplifier, but not all metallic wires can be used for recording purposes. The primary requirement of a wire electrode is that it be nonpolarizable, a requirement that limits bare metallic wires generally to the noble metals. A simple and convenient way of making a nonpolarizable electrode is to use an appropriate silver wire that is coated electrolytically with chloride; bare silver is undesirable because of its toxicity to cells. Wick electrodes are nonpolarizable, since the conducting element is an electrolyte solution. Unlike a wire electrode, a wick electrode cannot be of exact external diameter. Usually it is difficult to make wick electrodes smaller than 100 μm in diameter, but wire electrodes appropriately held in some rigid material can be made from fine wires 20–40 μm in diameter that can be purchased commercially. Glass capillaries, with tips several micrometers in diameter, filled with electrolytes also can be used.

Depending on the size of the electrode, the recordings obtained vary because the number of cells from which activity originates is different. With a large electrode (0.5–1 mm), the activity of a few cells may be buried in a mass of "noise." With a small electrode, it may take considerable exploration to locate a few active cells. In any event, the activity recorded would be the combined activity of more than one cell, and the amplitude of the compound spike would be a rough indication of the number of cells active at any time. The rate of rise and the duration of a spike would be determined largely by the temporal dispersion of the individual spikes. If the spikes of individual active cells are synchronous, a fast rising velocity, a high amplitude, and a short duration result. If the individual spikes are asynchronous, the rising velocity is slow, the amplitude is low, multiple peaks are apparent, and the total duration of activity is long.

The underlying principle of surface recording is that when an action potential is generated at one point, there is a current flowing on the inside of the cell longitudinally toward the resting region of the cell. Since the membrane is not a perfect insulator, some current will leak outward across the membrane and flow along the extracellular fluid back towards the current source. Surface recordings are not recordings of the voltage changes in the cell membrane itself but are recordings of the voltage drop, i.e., the *IR* change, produced by the flow of current in the interstitial fluid. Hence, their amplitude is proportional to the external (or interstitial) resistance. The voltage drop is proportional to the sum of the external resistance (r_o) and the longitudinal resistance of the inside of the cell (r_i). Therefore, as in the case of a voltage divider, the amplitude of the surface-recordable voltage change is dependent on the ratio of the external resistance to the sum of the external and internal resistances [$r_o/(r_i + r_o)$].

Since the extracellular resistance is usually much lower than the intracellular resistance, the recordable signals are usually quite small, at best a few millivolts. There are two ways of increasing the amplitude of the voltage signal, both of which depend on increasing the ratio. The first is to increase the membrane voltage change by causing the synchronous discharge of many individual cells, simultaneously reducing the number of inactive cells that serve only as external shunting paths. This method may not always be possible in smooth muscles, and the variability of the externally recorded voltage signal is an indication of the number of cells active during any one action potential. A second way of increasing the ratio of the resistances is to increase the external shunting resistance. When the external resistance is high but still finite, it will be possible to increase the amplitude of the surface-recordable voltage signal. Such an effect is the basis of the sucrose-gap method of recording.

Surface recording with wire and wick electrodes is a very useful method for studying electrical activities of the myometrium as long as one is aware of its limitations and does not draw conclusions that are obviously beyond the capabilities of the method. Because the signal is usually small, noise must be controlled by careful shielding. Some reasonable applications of the method are to the study of patterns of excitability in the myometrium during pregnancy or under various hormonal influences. It has been employed successfully to study the patterns of excitation in the pregnant human uterus (Wolfs and van Leeuwen, 1979).

1.3.1b.   Sucrose-Gap Method.   One of the most convenient techniques of recording from myometrial or other smooth muscle preparations is the sucrose-gap method (Stämpfli, 1954), the principle of which is simply to increase extracellular resistance. Although several other methods to accomplish the same objective have been used by a number of investigators on various tissues, none of them has been so useful for smooth muscle work as Stämpfli's method.

In this method, the preparation is bathed in a saline solution at each end and in a high-resistance isotonic sucrose solution in the middle (Fig. 2). Thus, the preparation is separated into two electrically interconnected segments. The electrodes, placed at the junctions of the sucrose and the saline solutions, record the potential difference between the two end segments, i.e., across the sucrose gap. Since the external resistance of the sucrose is considerably higher

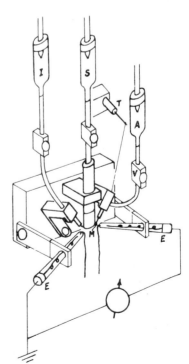

Figure 2. Schematic representation of single sucrose-gap chamber and associated parts used in author's laboratory (approximately to scale; see Kleinhaus and Kao, 1969). Solutions in reservoirs (not shown) enter three channels of apparatus via drop counters and flow-regulating valves (at top of figure). A, Active channel through which flows Krebs solution or a test solution; S, sucrose channel, closed at bottom with polyethylene cap (6 mm diameter), which is pierced with two small holes horizontally just above bottom closure; I, inactive channel through which flows Krebs solution or K_2SO_4; T, mechanotransducer for recording tension; M, small bundle of smooth muscle preparation, which passes through two small holes in the polyethylene cap of sucrose channel; ends of muscle preparation are in both A and I channels; E, electrodes with Ag–AgCl wire in KCl-agar and wicks at ends for drawing emerging solutions from channels to dampen flow artifacts.

than that of the natural interstitial fluid that it replaced, the potential difference, or the *IR* change, would be larger.

For constant-current and voltage-clamp studies, the sucrose-gap method has been modified to what is generally known as the *double sucrose-gap method*. As the name implies, the preparation is now separated by two sucrose gaps into three electrically interconnected segments, which are bathed in saline solutions, two at the ends and one in the center. By means of appropriate connections, it is possible to pass current between one end and the center segment and to record the consequent voltage changes between the center segment and the remaining end. A schematic representation is shown in Fig. 3. There are some variants of the sucrose-gap method in which rubber diaphragms with small holes are used to partition the segments, to keep the sucrose and saline solutions around the preparation from direct contact. In my experience, there is no particular advantage to having such extraneous material, which serves only to impede thorough washout by sucrose of the interstitial space under the diaphragm (of about 100 μm thickness).

Although the principles of the sucrose-gap methods are relatively simple, there are many associated details that are important for successful recording from a smooth muscle preparation. First, it is of utmost importance that the flow rates of various solutions be constant, particularly in the double sucrose-gap method. Otherwise, there will be considerable fluctuations in the recording, which in their mildest form would be misleading and in more severe forms would render the recording meaningless. For single-gap work (e.g., Kleinhaus and Kao, 1969), we have been successful in using gravity feed and screw-type pinchcocks to regulate flow rates. However, it should be recognized that any pinchcock regulates in part because of the elasticity of the tube that it pinches and that the elasticity of the tube is a highly variable and uncertain property on which to depend for regulation of high precision. In double-gap work (e.g., Kao and McCullough, 1975), particularly that type in which the sucrose–saline interface is dependent entirely on continuously flowing solutions of different densities, pinchcocks are totally unsatisfactory. Needle valves with fine controls are essential for maintaining constant flow rates.

The sucrose solution used must be of very high resistance if it is to serve its purpose. In earlier work, we have used water of very high resistivity (2 MΩ-cm) to make sucrose solutions and assumed the final solution to be of adequate quality. It is now evident that even chemically pure sucrose contains enough contaminants to degrade the high resistance appreciably (to approximately 0.5 MΩ-cm). In recent work, we have continued to prepare sucrose in high-resistance water and have additionally passed the sucrose solution through an ion-exchange resin column immediately before the sucrose enters the experimental chamber. Moreover, until just before the experiment, the sucrose solution is pump-recirculated through the ion-exchange column to increase further the resistance. With such high-resistivity solutions, absorption of atmospheric carbon dioxide is sufficient to degrade their qualities. Therefore, the sucrose solution must be appropriately protected from atmospheric carbon dioxide through a breather tube containing a mixture of calcium hydroxide and lithium hydroxide, to maintain a resistivity around 2 MΩ-cm. With such a sucrose solution, it is not uncommon to record spikes as high as 60 mV.

In double sucrose-gap work the quality of the sucrose is especially important, because shunting through low-resistance sucrose solutions can vitiate any attempt at recording from or controlling the center region. This problem is illustrated vividly in the records shown by Bolton (1975), who added a small amount of calcium chloride to the sucrose under the misconception that it could improve the viability of his preparations. His experience undoubtedly biased his personal attitude towards a useful technique (Bolton *et al.*, 1981). To be sure, isotonic sucrose is unphysiological, and long, drawn-out experiments allow the diffusion of sucrose into the cell, which, by increasing core resistance, degrades the experimental control of the preparation. The approach we have adopted is to avoid long experiments, and in our experience (see records in Kao and McCullough, 1975; Inomata and Kao, 1976, 1979, 1985) reasonable work can be done in spite of the problem.

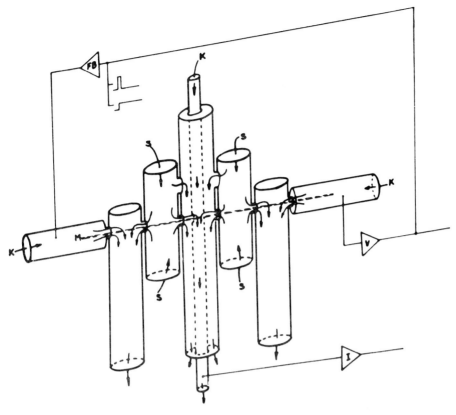

Figure 3. Schematic representation (not to scale) of double sucrose-gap chamber used in author's laboratory (see Kao and McCullough, 1975). Associated accessories such as reservoirs and flow-regulating needle valves are not shown. Small bundle of smooth muscle (M) traverses five vertical channels, with its ends resting in two horizontal channels at outer edges. Horizontal channel for muscle is 0.6 mm. Three central vertical channels are each 1 mm except at ends, where they are enlarged to receive connecting polyethylene tubing. Flanking vertical channels are two drainage channels that are closed at top. Operation of chamber is best appreciated by following flow of solutions, as indicated by arrows: K, Krebs solution or other test solutions; S, sucrose. In use, muscle bundle is separated into three interconnected segments in Krebs or test solution by two cuffs of high-resistance sucrose, and interfaces are produced by these flowing solutions. At flow rate of about 2 drops/min, differences in density of sucrose and Krebs produce stable interfaces in the central channel, resulting in a "node" of muscle bundle readily adjustable to 60 μm width. All solutions drain out from side drainage channels as well as central vertical channel. Sucrose–Krebs interfaces are also present in side drainage channels. For stability of flow pattern, total cross-sectional area of inlet channels should be roughly equal to that of outlet channels. Electrical connections are shown. Center vertical channel is at virtual ground, with an operational amplifier connected as a current-to-voltage converter (*I*). Voltage monitoring (*V*) at one end. Clamp amplifier is in negative feedback configuration (FB), taking commands on input and feeding output to preparation at other end. Electrodes (not shown) are connected at sucrose–Krebs interfaces, in side drainage channels, and upstream to muscle preparation in central channel. To reduce the series resistance of the narrow column of Krebs solution in the central channel between muscle bundle and electrode, an electrically floating segment of hypodermic needle is inserted in the channel just upstream to the muscle. Additional details in text.

A third important detail in the practical use of the sucrose-gap method is that the various solutions should be passed through drop counters placed upstream but close to the experimental chamber. Although these drop chambers (see Fig. 2) serve as a convenient way of checking flow rates, they are also important for breaking the electrical continuity between the experimental chamber and the reservoir bottles containing the solutions. Unless the electrical continuity is broken, the reservoir bottles will serve as effective antennas for picking up extraneous noise signals. An alternative to drop counters would be the more inconvenient and less effective method of shielding all the bottles of solutions.

1.3.1c.   Problems Peculiar to the Double Sucrose-Gap Method.   In this method, there are some special problems that require attention. As mentioned, the preparation is separated into three electrically interconnected segments by two streams of isotonic sucrose. The important region under study is the center segment, which, by analogy with the myelinated nerve axon, is often called the "node," meaning an artificial node of Ranvier. Electrically, the node is set at virtual ground; current can be passed between this point and one end, and the resultant changes can be measured between it and the other end. Ideally, the cells in the node should be relatively uniform, and the only way to achieve that quality is by limiting the amount of tissue in the node. To be anywhere close to being manageable, the width of the node (or the length of the segment along the preparation) should not exceed 80 μm (see also Anderson, 1976). The size of the node can be measured with an ocular micrometer, but a more reliable measure is the total capacitance of the node, assuming that all of the capacitance is in the lipid material in the cell membrane. We have found that nodes with capacitance of 0.1 to 0.15 μF are relatively easy to prepare and work with. Nodes with capacitance of about 0.07 μF or less do not survive well, whereas nodes larger than 0.2 μF tend to contain too much tissue. Large nodes pose another problem. Suprathreshold depolarizations or depolarizing drugs tend to cause visible contractions in the nodal tissue and cause substantial changes in the total capacitance, which must indicate that the cell membrane under study is not constant. Nodes of about 0.1 μF rarely cause such problems.

To produce nodes of 80 μm or less in width, the central pool of saline must be narrow, with the result that the series resistance is higher than in the case of a wider central pool. The series resistance consists of two components, one in the narrow column of saline solution between the center electrode and the preparation and the other in the cleft resistance in the interstitial spaces. Although there are methods to compensate for the series resistance, they are based on introducing a certain amount of positive feedback into the circuit. For this reason, the series resistance cannot be fully compensated for, because oscillations then tend to occur. Such compensation would work well for the first type of series resistance in the solution but would not be of much value for the cleft resistance, which must be accepted as the unavoidable cost of using this method. In our work, we have used an electronic compensation method for the series resistance in the solution but have preferred to work without it because the positive feedback circuit tended to introduce an extra level of noisiness into the recording.

The undesirability of series resistance is not confined to voltage-clamp studies, where it could cause substantial errors, but also applies to constant-current work, where it appears as an instantaneous jump in the voltage record at the make and break of the current step. To arrive at some acceptable compromise between controllable node size and acceptable series resistance, we shunt the high resistance of the narrow column of saline solution (ca. 100 kΩ) with a short segment of 20-gauge hypodermic needle tubing through which the saline flows. By this simple maneuver, nodes of 50 to 60 μm width can be produced easily with a series resistance of less than 10 kΩ, which resides almost entirely in the cleft resistance.

In making a recording with the sucrose-gap appartus, both end channels can be filled with a physiological saline solution. It is more convenient, however, to depolarize one end of the preparation completely and then record the surface negativity of an active region against the depolarized region. This measurement is similar to a demarcation potential, and some idea of the magnitude of the resting potential can be gained in this way. The depolarization is best produced with an isotonic solution of potassium sulfate (2.1%). It should be kept in mind that, because the composition of this solution is very different from that of a saline solution such as Krebs bicarbonate, there will be a significant difference in the liquid junction potentials at the two ends of the sucrose solution. Absolute measurements of resting potential by this method are difficult unless one can be certain of the magnitude of the liquid junction potentials. This uncertainty does not reduce the usefulness of the method in recording changes in membrane potential produced during activity or by drugs. Spike activity thus recorded from a smooth muscle preparation, however, should not be interpreted as having originated in a single cell. The recorded spike sometimes can resemble that obtained with an intracellular microelectrode, but just as often it can have multiple peaks indicating a plural origin. What appears to be activity of a single cell may reflect only a temporal synchrony of several cells. In double-gap work, the objective is to keep studying the same group of cells under control and experimental conditions. If the size of the node is appropriately small, that group of cells should respond virtually in unison.

For studying the actions of drugs on myometrium or other smooth muscles, this is probably one of the most convenient methods. Since most drugs are employed in relatively low concentrations, compared with those of the electrolytes in a saline solution, there will be no significant effect on liquid junction potentials. Certain subtle mechanisms of action, such as the modulation of excitability properties, would be discernible only by use of some constant-current or voltage-clamp methods. In spite of some real and serious limitations, very useful exploratory work can be done through the judicious use of this method.

1.3.2. Intracellular Recording

1.3.2a. Microelectrodes for Impalement. Intracellular recordings are usually made with an electrolyte-filled glass capillary drawn out to a tip of less than 0.5 µm in diameter. Generally such electrodes are now made from capillary glass of about 1 mm diameter by use of an electrode puller, which has an electrical heating coil to soften the glass and some mechanical contrivance to stretch and thin the softened segment into the required microtip. Consequently, there are three distinct parts to a microelectrode: the *shank* is the unreduced capillary tube, which usually serves to make connection to some electrode holder; the *shaftlet* is the thinned segment, which tapers at the free end into the *tip*, which usually further tapers more abruptly to the desired 0.5 µm or less.

For most recording purposes, the conducting fluid is 3 M KCl, to improve conductivity and to reduce junction potentials. As shown by the originators of this technique, tips of 0.5 µm, when inserted through the cell membrane, do not cause substantial injury (Ling and Gerard, 1949). For smooth muscle work, the general experience is that the tip should be 0.25 µm or less. With such small tips, the resistance is generally over 30 MΩ, and a significant DC potential can be found on the tip. A tip potential of more than 5 mV can usually be reduced if the 3 M KCl is acidified to pH 2 with HCl (Riemar *et al.*, 1974).

Traditionally, such capillary microelectrodes are filled by boiling in the filling solution under reduced pressure for about 5 min. On reintroduction of atmospheric pressure, a fair proportion of the electrode is well filled. There are often some that contain small air bubbles. If the electrodes are stored with the tip down (such as by strapping them to a microscopic slide and storing the slide in an ordinary histology staining jar) in a chilled solution, most of these air bubbles will make their way up to the end of the shank of the electrode, where they can be readily removed. Problems in filling microelectrodes have been greatly simplified with the wide commercial availability of capillaries containing a thin filament of glass fiber. Electrodes are fashioned in a puller in the usual manner. Filling is accomplished by first leaving the tips in the filling solution for some 20 min, when the tips and the shaftlet are filled by capillary action. Then the shank of the electrode is back-filled by use of a long, thin hypodermic needle (30 gauge, 2 or 3 inches length), beginning from the fluid level already in the shaftlet. Sometimes, a small air bubble is trapped between the fluid levels. This bubble usually can be dislodged by manipulating with a length of fine wire (250 µm diameter tungsten wire will have the stiffness for the purpose).

In our work, 30 or 40 electrodes are pulled at one sitting and then stored unfilled in covered staining jars, strapped by dental rubber bands about ten to a slide, always tips pointing down. Filling is done just before the day's run of experiments. In use, each electrode is checked for absence of air bubbles, and then selected from those with resistance of 30–60 MΩ.

Capillary microelectrodes are used not only for recording but also for passing current. For the latter purpose, very little current can be passed through electrodes with resistances of over 10 MΩ. To remedy this limitation, the filling solution is often changed to 4 M potassium citrate or some other polyionic solute. Further, the tip is often larger than that of the recording electrode, or it could be beveled, either on a special apparatus or in a stirred slurry of a fine carborundum particles. For many excitable tissues, these are rather standardized techniques, but for smooth muscles, because of the small size of individual cells, impalement with more than one electrode in the same cell has only rarely been successful (see notable exception in Walsh and Singer, 1980, 1987).

Because of such difficulties, which are also encountered in cells in complex tissues, several techniques are now available by which stimulation and recording can be done through a single microelectrode. One of these relies on using a Wheatstone bridge to balance out the stimulating current and recording the ensuing cell response. Another depends on a chopped electronic circuit, which alternates between recording and current passing, and could be used for some voltage-clamp work. Additional information on the latter method can be found in a recent monograph (Smith *et al.*, 1985).

A rarely used variant that is of value in some special circumstances is the phase-plane analysis. In this method, the action potential is recorded with a capillary microelectrode, and the voltage signal is differentiated by external circuitry and then displayed as dV/dt versus V. The method can provide some information on total membrane current and on some membrane conductances and equilibrium potentials, and it has been used to check on some of the conclusions about smooth muscle properties based on double sucrose-gap studies (Specht, 1976).

Although very little injury is evident when impalement is done properly, the quality of the recording is still dependent on the quality of the membrane seal around the penetrating tip of the microelectrode. The reason is that the seal resistance and the membrane resistance form a parallel circuit, and what can be recorded across the membrane resistance is influenced by what is shunted by the seal resistance.

1.3.2b.   Tight-Seal Suction Microelectrodes.   Within the last decade, an important new technique has been introduced that allows faithful recording from single cells chiefly because of the very tight seal the electrode forms on the cell surface. The technique is frequently referred to as the *patch-clamp* method, because the electrode–membrane seal is so tight and mechanically strong that the electrode can be retracted from the cell surface and break off a patch of the cell membrane with it for studying single ionic channels within the detached patch. Details of this new technique can be found in a review article by Hamill *et al.* (1981). Briefly, microelectrodes are made with tips of 2 to 5 μm diameter and are then heat-polished under microscopic observation to 1–2 μm (or larger, depending on the nature of the study). The cell on which such a technique is to be applied must have its surface "cleaned" through some enzymatic digestion process that also frees the cell from the multicellular matrix. Such individual cells could either be freshly isolated from multicellular preparations or be grown in culture. The principal enzyme used is collagenase, which probably serves to help disperse individual cells. However, quite probably, the "cleansing" of the surface is accomplished by some nonspecific protease activity. Unless the cell surface is clean, it is impossible to form tight seals with resistances in the gigaohm range (10^9 Ω).

The tight-seal is formed by gentle suction on the shank end of the electrode after its tip is brought to rest on the cleaned cell surface. The method can be used either in the whole-cell mode or in the patch mode with the patch attached to the cell or detached from it. In the whole-cell mode, the cell surface must be broken by some pulsatile suction, which differs from the seal-forming suction in its abruptness and greater magnitude. Once the cell surface is broken, the electrode has literally gained access to the interior of the cell, as in the case of penetration with a finer tip, except that now the access is through a much lower resistance, which allows better recording and current application for both current-clamp and voltage-clamp studies. Also, because of the larger diameter of the electrode tip, the diffusible cellular components readily reach an equilibrium with the solutes in the electrode. Thus, a form of controllable perfusion of the intracellular phase is possible.

In smooth muscle work, recording from patches is easier than recording from whole cells, especially in freshly dispersed cells. From our experience, we believe that the membrane in freshly dispersed smooth muscle cells has a tendency to reseal after initial rupture, and unless some means is devised to prevent resealing, stable whole-cell recordings are difficult to make. Yamamoto *et al.* (1988b) describe a method in which a strong vacuum is applied through solenoid valves in controlled bursts of short pulses (of about 25 msec duration each) until the rupture is apparently wide enough that resealing becomes rare and improbable.

The tight-seal technique has made it possible to study the properties of single channel proteins in a patch of living membrane, whether and how they open and close, the influence of membrane voltage, ionic composition, drugs, and neurotransmitters, and other features. Ionic currents in whole cells, which underlie action potentials, are really the summed manifestations of the currents in many individual ionic channels. By themselves, however, single-channel events are frequently so far removed from familiar physiological properties that a clear connection between the two levels of observations cannot be made easily. In smooth muscle studies especially, where the reservoir of knowledge of cellular ionic-channel events is quite limited, the emergence of many ''new'' types of single channels has created a situation in which many physiological phenomena cannot yet be explained by the fruits of the new technique, and many observations of single-channel functions appear to be dangling with no physiological relevance. What is needed now, as more and more patch-clamp studies on smooth muscles are being conducted, is a thoughtful and deliberate approach to problems that will incorporate examinations of cellular as well as single-channel functions, so that physiological phenomena could find their appropriate molecular explanations.

1.3.3. Selection of a Method

The selection of a method for recording or stimulation depends on the nature of the problem to be studied. In clinical studies, there is little alternative to using a surface recording method. In laboratory investigation, a wide range of possible techniques is available. Some years ago, when observations of natural phenomena consumed much attention, it was important to know the magnitude of the resting potential, because many aspects of excitation phenomena were influenced by the membrane potential. Now, however, with voltage-clamp methods available, knowledge of the resting potential is no longer a pressing issue, because the membrane potential can be set by the voltage clamp. In fact, the ionic composition is often distorted deliberately for specific experimental objectives, and the membrane potential is controlled entirely by the clamp.

For descriptive work on the tissue level, the sucrose-gap techniques deserve more use for their relative ease of utilization, lack of trauma to the cells, and a measure of statistical validity for including multiple cells. For cellular and single-channel work, clearly only the enzymatically dissociated cells and the tight-seal suction electrode would provide the necessary technical base.

2. *Ionic Distribution as the Basis of Electrophysiological Phenomena*

2.1. *Studies in Ionic Contents and Distribution*

2.1.1. *Changed Nature of Problems in Ionic Distribution Studies*

Since the driving forces for ionic movements underlying all electrical phenomena in smooth muscle cells are closely dependent on ionic concentrations inside and outside of the cells, it is essential to have reliable data on the contents and distribution of some of the quantitatively abundant or functionally important ions. Such knowledge generally is derived from data on contents of whole tissues, appropriately partitioned into intracellular and extracellular components. There is a voluminous literature on the ionic contents and distributions in the myometrium and other smooth muscles (see, for instance, Casteels, 1970). Lengthy accounts on this topic were incorporated in the previous editions of this chapter, in large part because descriptive electrophysiological properties of the smooth muscles were intimately dependent on the existing driving forces that could be estimated from the chemical concentrations. Thus, the estimated resting potential, the calculated potassium equilibrium potential, and even the estimated sodium and calcium reversal potentials were appropriate topics of attention at a time when most electrophysiological studies consisted of recording natural phenomena. At present, when voltage-clamp techniques can be successfully applied to smooth muscle tissues or cells, the need for an accurate knowledge of the intracellular or extracellular concentrations of ions is no longer so compelling. The reason is that within some wide boundaries of concentrations, the driving force for transmembrane movements of ions can now be controlled by the experimentally selected membrane potential. Two examples illustrate this point.

The first example illustrates how the voltage-clamp technique can bypass an unresolvably controversial issue that depended on chemical analyses and partitioning of ionic contents. For some years, an accurate estimate of the potassium equilibrium potential consumed considerable effort in smooth muscle studies. The reason is that the information was needed to assess the resting potentials measured by impalement microelectrodes. The problems, however, involved accurate analyses of the total potassium content of the tissues and estimations of the extracellular fluid volume, because these two factors determined the final concentration of potassium assigned to the intracellular compartment. Because there was no way to establish objectively one chemical method as being superior to another on estimations of the extracellular fluid volume, controversies were unending. With the voltage-clamp technique, however, the potassium equilibrium potential in smooth muscle preparations can be determined unequivocally as the zero-current potential for potassium current (Kao and McCullough, 1975; Inomata and Kao, 1976). Moreover, the procedure was easily accomplished by connecting several points in a current–voltage plot at which I_K was inwards with several points at which it was outwards (almost always with a straight line) and then reading off the intersection with the voltage axis as the potassium equilibrium potential. To the disappointment of some vociferous critics of the double sucrose-gap method, because there is no current at this potential, there is not even error that could be attributed to the unavoidable series resistance.

Another example illustrates how highly unphysiological ionic compositions can be used in voltage-clamp studies to provide pivotal evidence on the properties of important ionic channels. Thus, to identify the charge carrier for the late outward current in the myometrium (Kao and McCullough, 1975) and the guinea pig taenia coli (Inomata and Kao, 1976), an extracellular medium was used in which all the extracellular Na^+ of the usual Krebs bicarbonate solution was replaced by K^+ (over 140 mM). In such a medium, the smooth muscle cells were totally depolarized. If one were to record only natural phenomena, one would have recorded no more than a few millivolts of internal negativity in the steady state and perhaps a transient burst of action potentials, lasting no more than a few seconds, before the steady state was reached. With the voltage-clamp technique, however, an artifical membrane potential close to the natural resting potential of -50 mV could be imposed. When the channel responsible for the late current was gated open by appropriate depolarization, what had previously been an outward current was now reversed to an inward current. The only ion that could account for the current was readily identified as K^+.

2.1.2. Pitfalls in Ionic Distribution Studies

As mentioned in previous editions of this chapter, two important pitfalls in analyses for ionic contents and distribution in smooth muscles should be carefully avoided. Analytical technology for the major ionic species has advanced so much that there is no problem with their sensitivity or reliability. The pitfalls are in the biological preparations. Smooth muscle cells have large surface-to-volume ratios, and passive loss of cellular potassium from isolated preparations occurs readily. Such a loss can be both variable and extensive. To maintain osmotic balance, the lost potassium is replaced by sodium whenever the tissue is in contact with artificial saline solution. Unless close attention is paid to this point, one is likely to collect highly variable data on the ionic contents. Needless to say, if the focus of interest is on the muscle cells, there is not much point in analyzing samples of muscle tissues mixed with large amounts of endometrial connective or epithelial tissues.

The second pitfall concerns the choice of an appropriate substance as a marker of the extracellular fluid volume. For readers unfamiliar with this type of study, it might be useful to recall that the smooth muscle cells are too small to permit direct analyses of the intracellular ionic concentrations. The elegant technique of x-ray spectroscopy is inappropriate for general use. Total ionic contents in tissue specimens are determined chemically on ashed or appropriately extracted samples. The total water content of the samples is also determined, which is then partitioned into intracellular and extracellular components in which the ionic solutes are dissolved. Therefore, a marker for the extracellular phase is necessary. If the solute concentrations in the extracellular fluid are in equilibrium with those in the bathing fluid (or serum), the fraction of the total contents assignable to the extracellular phase can be readily determined. By calculating the difference between the total and extracellular fractions and the intracellular water volume, the intracellular ionic concentrations can be deduced.

The thorny problem, however, is that there is no universally acceptable marker for the extracellular fluid volume. A marker either might be found in substantial amounts in the intracellular phase (such as chloride and probably ethanesulfonate) or is not distributed completely throughout all extracellular fluid compartment (such as [131I]-labeled albumin and probably [60Co]-EDTA) (Brading and Jones, 1969). In my own experience both with such analytical studies and with voltage-clamp studies, the commonly used inulin is still the best estimate of extracellular fluid volume in the myometrium and possibly also in some other mammalian smooth muscles. The reason for this conclusion is that certain ionic equilibrium potentials can be determined in the voltage clamp without any need to know the extracellular fluid volume. From the known extracellular ionic concentrations, the intracellular concentrations (at least the functionally significant portions) can be estimated directly from the zero-current equilibrium potential. When the intracellular concentrations derived by this approach are compared with those determined analytically, only those estimated on the basis of inulin space turn out to provide generally reasonable and good agreement.

2.2. Ionic Contents and Intracellular Concentrations

The focus of this chapter is the electrophysiological properties of the myometrium and some other mammalian smooth muscles. For this interest, some knowledge of the ionic concentrations is necessary. However, because the successful application of the voltage-clamp technique to smooth muscles has fundamentally altered the nature of the problems in this field, the present version is much shorter than previous versions (e.g., Kao, 1977), including only material that bears directly on our understanding of the electrophysiological properties.

Table 1 lists some information on the total contents of the three most abundant monovalent ions, and Table 2 their respective intracellular concentrations. Most of the information is self-evident and needs no further comment. One exception is that the intracellular content of potassium is so high that a straightforward computation of its intracellular concentration leads to values that would result in significant hyperosmolarity of the intracellular phase. Actually, for intracellular concentrations of sodium and potassium, a correction is necessary to exclude a fraction of each ion species that appears to be tightly bound and is liberated only on ashing or extraction in acid. Such bound amounts are probably not osmotically or electrochemically active. In the rabbit myometrium, the quantities of bound ions per kilogram of wet tissue are 29 mEq Na^+ and 14 mEq K^+ for the estrogen-dominated state and 9 mEq Na^+ and 4 mEqK$^+$ for the progestrone-dominated state (Kao, 1961). In mixed endometrial and myometrial samples of rabbit and cat uteri, Daniel and Daniel (1957) also found 13–16 mEq of the total tissue sodium to be unextractable in sucrose or choline chloride and thus presumably bound. The problem of bound ions is difficult and complex, but it certainly needs to be studied further. In one instance, a hyperpolarization induced by catecholamines has been found to be accom-

Table 1. Contents of Water, Sodium, Potassium, and Chloride in Myometrium

Species and preparation	Water (g/kg)	Total ions (mEq/kg)			References
		Na^+	K^+	Cl^-	
Rabbit					
Estrogen-dominated					
In situ[a]	812	77	102	59	Kao and Siegman, 1963
Isolated; 20 min[b]	831	112	61	78	Kao and Siegman, 1963
Isolated; 2 hr[b]	850	111	59	79	Kao and Siegman, 1963
Isolated; 4 hr[b]	846	110	72	83	Kao and Siegman, 1963
Isolated[c]	843	79	74	57	Daniel, 1958
Isolated[c]	—	71	76	—	Horvath, 1954
Progesterone-dominated					
In situ[a]	814	86	104	62	Kao and Siegman, 1963
Isolated; 20 min[b]	831	115	64	82	Kao and Siegman, 1963
Isolated; 2 hr[b]	839	108	74	84	Kao and Siegman, 1963
Isolated; 4 hr[b]	835	101	85	79	Kao and Siegman, 1963
Isolated[c]	830	74	79	49	Daniel, 1958
Isolated[c]	—	71	73	—	Horvath, 1954
Rat[d]					
Anestrus	—	86–90	63–66	89–93	Casteels and Kuriyama, 1965
Estrus	—	87	61	91	Casteels and Kuriyama, 1965
Pregnant; 15 days	—	84	59	91	Casteels and Kuriyama, 1965
Pregnant; 12–20 days	—	85–90	62–67	91–95	Casteels and Kuriyama, 1965
Postpartum; ½ day	—	89	54	92	Casteels and Kuriyama, 1965
Postpartum; 1 day	—	93	51	94	Casteels and Kuriyama, 1965
Cat					
Anestrus; isolated[c]	766	110	59	71	Daniel, 1958
Estrogen; isolated[c]	806	94	64	76	Daniel, 1958
Progesterone; isolated[c]	804	84	72	72	Daniel, 1958
Pregnant[c]	810	89	56	83	Daniel, 1958

[a]Preparation kept from saline solution during dissection.
[b]Incubation in Krebs bicarbonate solution at 25°C.
[c]Handling conditions not clear. For pregnant cat myometrium, stage of pregnancy unknown.
[d]All rat tissues were isolated and incubated for at least 90 min at room temperature in Kregs bicarbonate solution.

Table 2. Intracellular Ionic Concentrations of Sodium, Potassium, and Chloride in Myometrium

Species and preparation	Extracellular space (ml/kg)	Concentration (mEq/liter cell water)			References
		Na⁺	K⁺	Cl⁻	
Rabbit					
Estrogen-dominated					
In situ	322[a]	7	194	71	Kao, 1961
Isolated; 20 min	390[a]	59	102	59	Kao and Siegman, 1963; Kao and Nishiyama, 1964
Isolated; 2 hr	390[a]	54	93	59	Kao and Siegman, 1963; Kao and Nishiyama, 1964
Isolated; 4 hr	390[a]	53	120	68	Kao and Siegman, 1963; Kao and Nishiyama, 1964
Progesterone-dominated					
In situ	312[a]	60	221	83	Kao, 1961
Isolated; 20 min	380[a]	111	129	73	Kao and Siegman, 1963; Kao and Nishiyama, 1964
Isolated; 2 hr	380[a]	94	148	76	Kao and Siegman, 1963; Kao and Nishiyama, 1964
Isolated; 4 hr	380[a]	79	174	59	Kao and Siegman, 1963; Kao and Nishiyama, 1964
Rat					
Anestrus	387–398[a]	56–70	110–114	65–73	Casteels and Kuriyama, 1965
	564–569[b]	22–33	154–163	35–43	Casteels and Kuriyama, 1965
Estrus	402[a]	58	106	68	Casteels and Kuriyama, 1965
Pregnant, 15 days	399[a]	52	103	67	Casteels and Kuriyama, 1965
Pregnant, 10–20 days	365–376[a]	59–66	104–113	66–78	Casteels and Kuriyama, 1965
	557–570[b]	22–29	149–162	41–48	Casteels and Kuriyama, 1965
Postpartum, ½ day	473[a]	50	107	60	Casteels and Kuriyama, 1965
Postpartum, 1 day	484[a]	57	102	62	Casteels and Kuriyama, 1965
	616[b]	27	140	33	Casteels and Kuriyama, 1965

[a]Inulin space.
[b]Ethanesulfonate space.

panied by an increase in the intracellular potassium concentration, a change that could have resulted from a change in binding to liberate more electrochemically active potassium ions (Kao *et al.*, 1976).

Readers who work or wish to work with the rat myometrium are likely to rely on the data of Casteels and Kuriyama (1965) for information on ionic distributions. In the previous edition of this chapter (Kao, 1977), I discussed in some detail a fundamental flaw in the values of the total water content assumed by those investigators in that work (900–910 ml/kg wet tissue). Such water contents have never been reported for any muscular tissues and are some 100 ml/kg higher than those reported for the myometrium by other investigators. Although it is possible to recalculate the intracellular concentrations from their data on the basis of the usual water content of about 800 ml/kg wet tissue, such information will necessarily be somewhat vague for lack of knowledge of the bound fractions.

The usefulness of information on the intracellular concentrations is that limiting values of ionic equilibrium potentials can be calculated to guide electrophysiological investigations. Some of these values are shown in Table 3. When the calculated equilibrium potentials are compared with those determined in voltage-clamp experiments, the E_{Na} of about 25 mV is consistent with that observed, as is the E_K of about −75 to −80 mV. The low E_{Cl} values

Table 3. Resting and Action Potentials of Myometrium[a]

Species and preparation	Resting potential	Action potential	References
Rabbit			
Nonpregnant			
Estrogen-dominated	−49.8 ± 0.3	—	Kao and Kishiyama, 1964
Estrogen-dominated	*ca.* −43	—	Goto and Csapo, 1959
Estrogen-dominated	−38 to −46	9–25	Kuriyama and Csapo, 1961
Progesterone-dominated	−48.9 ± 0.4	—	Kao and Nishiyama, 1964
Progesterone-dominated	*ca.* −55	—	Goto and Csapo, 1959
Pregnant			
20–26 days, placental	−53.4 ± 0.9	—	Goto and Csapo, 1959
20–26 days, nonplacental	−42.3 ± 0.9	—	Goto and Csapo, 1959
30–31 days	−54	33–66	Kuriyama and Csapo, 1961
Postpartum			
6–12 hr	−50	35–65	Kuriyama and Csapo, 1961
Rat			
Castrated			
Untreated	−35.2 ± 1.2	—	Marshall, 1959
Estrogen-dominated	−57.6 ± 0.5	65.3 ± 0.7	Marshall, 1959
Progesterone-dominated	−63.8 ± 0.5	—	Marshall, 1959
Nonpregnant			
Anestrus and estrus	−42 ± 0.7[b] −38 ± 0.5[b]	*ca.* 35[c]	Casteels and Kuriyama, 1965 (Fig. 1; Table 4a)
Pregnant			
6–9 days	−63	—	Marshall and Miller, 1964
15–16 days	−60.5 ± 0.5	*ca.* 63[c]	Casteels and Kuriyama, 1965
18–20 days	−52 ± 0.6	36–68	Kuriyama and Csapo, 1961
18–20 days	*ca.* −57[c]	*ca.* 64[c]	Casteels and Kuriyama, 1965
20–21 days	−54.5 ± 0.5[b] −58.0 ± 0.8 −56.5 ± 0.2	*ca.* 57[c] — —	Casteels and Kuriyama, 1965 (Table 3) (Table 4b)
20–22 days	−62.8 ± 0.8	71.8 ± 1.3	Marshall, 1962
20–22 days	−58	70	Marshall and Miller, 1964
Parturient	−48 ± 0.5	44 ± 0.5	Kuriyama and Csapo, 1961
Postpartum			
6 hr	−48 ± 0.5	—	Kuriyama and Csapo, 1961
12 hr	*ca.* −50[c]	*ca.* 58[c]	Casteels and Kuriyama, 1965
24 hr	−40 ± 0.7	—	Csapo and Kuriyama, 1963
2–3 days	*ca.* −42[c]	*ca.* 40[c]	Casteels and Kuriyama, 1965
Mouse			
Pregnant			
18–20 days	−53 ± 0.8	42 ± 0.8	Kuriyama, 1961
Postpartum			
6 hr	−46 ± 0.7	41 ± 0.7	Kuriyama, 1961

[a]All values are in millivolts, expressed as mean. Standard error of the mean is given wherever the distribution is indicated.
[b]In these instances, several values were given in the same paper.
[c]These values are estimated from a graph in the original paper.

follow directly from the relatively high intracellular concentration of chloride (Kao, 1961). The function of the high chloride concentration is still unknown, but it could well be involved in some ionic channel activity. For one thing, any substantial permeability of the resting membrane to chloride would easily move the resting potential towards less negative voltages than the potassium equilibrium potential.

2.3.1. On Ionic Contents and Distribution

Because of the ready response of uterine tissues to ovarian hormones, there is much interest in the influences of these hormones on the ionic contents and distribution in these tissues. As shown in Table 1, unlike the influence of estrogen on whole uterus, this hormone did not significantly change the total contents of sodium, potassium, and chloride per unit wet weight from those in the immature rabbit uterus (Kao, 1961). There was also no marked difference when the myometrium was additionally subjected to the influence of progesterone.

There is a claim that under progesterone domination, the intracellular potassium concentration of rabbit myometrium becomes significantly lower than it is in the estrogen-dominated state (Horvath, 1954). For a number of years, this claim served as the basis for a hypothesis that the progesterone-dominated myometrium had a smaller resting potential than did the estrogen-dominated myometrium and for a corollary hypothesis that a progesterone block existed because the myometrium membrane was depolarized in the progesterone-dominated state (Csapo, 1956). There were some serious flaws in Horvath's analyses (see Kao, 1977), and later work on the rabbit myometrium under estrogen or progesterone domination (Kao, 1961; Kao and Siegman, 1963) and on the rat myometrium during estrus and anestrus (Casteels and Kuriyama, 1965) showed no difference between the total contents and distributions of potassium, sodium, and chloride in these hormonal states.

2.3.2. On Electrical Properties

It has generally been observed that whereas the resting potential of immature myometrium is low in rabbits and rats, it is readily increased by estrogen treatment. Although there is no available information on the ionic contents in the immature myometrial cells, the increase in resting potential is probably caused by a real increase in the $[K^+]_i$ in the estrogen-primed state. The resting potential of the estrogen-dominated myometrium is around -45 to -50 mV in rabbits (Goto and Csapo, 1959; Kao and Nishiyama, 1964), and -42 to -58 mV in rats (Marshall, 1959, 1963; Kuriyama, 1961; Csapo and Kuriyama, 1963; Casteels and Kuriyama, 1965). Some very negative values reported by Jung (1961, 1964) for the rat myometrium were probably tainted by some technical flaws (see Kao, 1977).

There was at one time some controversy whether progesterone altered the resting potential of estrogen-dominated myometrial cells. The controversy was related to the "progesterone-block" hypothesis (Csapo, 1961), which sought to explain the apparent lower excitability of the myometrial cells under the influence of progesterone and during midpregnancy. Evidence was provided to show that the resting potential of the progesterone-dominated myometrium was both less (Csapo, 1956) and more (Marshall and Csapo, 1961) negative than that of the estrogen-dominated myometrium. Other investigators have found no significant differences between the resting potentials of myometrial cells in the two hormonal states (Kao and Nishiyama, 1964). A detailed critique of the "progesterone-block" hypothesis was given in the previous edition of this chapter (Kao, 1977). The main defect of that hypothesis is that it relied on a simplistic view of the excitability properties of the myometrium that could not stand the test of objective evidence.

There is no doubt that the excitability properties of the myometrium during midpregnancy, when progesterone influence is profound, are rather different from those at term. Available information excludes differences in ionic distributions and resting potentials as the basis for such different properties. The question has not been resolved, and the answers probably lie in the subtler properties of the various ionic channels in the myometrial cell membrane as they are influenced by the ovarian hormones. Another line of current thinking on the question relates to the effects of progesterone on intercellular gap junctions and the spread of electric currents in the myometrium (see Section 3.3).

3. Electrical Activity of the Myometrium and Other Mammalian Smooth Muscles

Mammalian smooth muscles are varied in nature, and there are many differences in the electrophysiological behavior of individual types of smooth muscle. A common error among those not familiar with smooth muscles is to assume that all smooth muscles are alike. This view is quite misleading because the variations range from smooth muscles that normally discharge bursts of action potentials to those that cannot produce action potentials under physiological conditions and from smooth muscle cells that depend exclusively on Ca^{2+} for carrying the early inward current to those that have both Na^+ and Ca^{2+} components to this current. With further developments and extensions of studies into other types of smooth muscles, additional differences will surely be uncovered.

The myometrium is a visceral smooth muscle, sharing many similarities with some intestinal smooth muscles and possibly some urinary tract smooth muscles but also possessing unique and complex properties of its own. All these smooth muscles differ from the vascular smooth muscles. In this section, I discuss some electrical activities in the myometrium as well as those in an intestinal muscle (the guinea pig taenia coli). Areas of similarities and differences are illustrated.

3.1. Descriptive Phenomena

The characteristic electrical activity of the myometrium and the taenia coli are spontaneous bursts of spike discharges at irregular intervals (Fig. 4a). In the myometrium, the frequency of the burst discharges and the number of spikes in each burst vary considerably and are readily influenced by hormonal and gestational factors as well as by ionic environment and pharmacological agents. There are also some species differences: the isolated rabbit myometrium is usually only infrequently active, whereas that of the rat or mouse is active at much higher rates. In the guinea pig taenia coli, repetitive spikes are frequent and markedly influenced by the degree of stretch applied to the isolated preparation.

3.1.1. Simple Spontaneous Spikes

The basic individual spike is a transient positive-going signal lasting about 50 msec at around 37°C. The amplitude of the spike is somewhat variable, in part affected by the resting potential. In the nonpregnant rat myometrium, the spikes are 30–40 mV (Casteels and Kuriyama, 1965). Similar simple-peaked spikes can be seen in the immediately postpartum myometrium (Fig. 4e,f). In the guinea pig taenia coli, such simple-peaked individual spikes are readily seen in the single dispersed cell, where total amplitudes of just over 60 mV are quite common (Yamamoto et al., 1988b; Fig. 5). Similar properties have been seen in the single dispersed cells of the guinea pig urinary bladder (Klöckner and Isenberg, 1985). The depolarizing phase of such spikes usually rises at a velocity of 4–5 V/sec but can be faster under a variety of conditions. The repolarizing phase begins right after the peak, without any intervening plateau such as those seen in some cardiac tissues (see the following exception) and usually proceeds at a rate rather close to that of the rising phase. The total duration of the

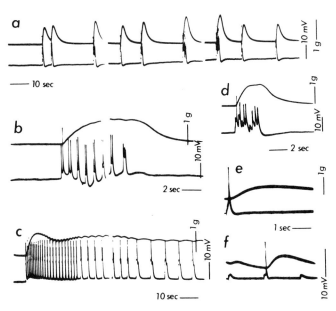

Figure 4. Different forms of spontaneous electrical activity in myometrium. All frames are from pregnant rabbit myometrium. Bottom trace in each frame represents electrical activity, and top trace represents associated contractile activity. Frames a–d were obtained with single sucrose-gap recording. Frames e and f were obtained with intracellular microelectrodes. (a) A 29-day pregnant myometrium, placental site preparation. Bursts of spikes are seen at irregular intervals. Each burst contains many individual spikes, the number of individual spikes directly influencing the force of contraction. From Kleinhaus and Kao (1969). (b) A 30-day pregnant myometrium, interplacental site. Most spikes are double-peaked. (c) A 30-day pregnant myometrium, interplacental site. Note that tension declined when the rate of spike discharge was highest, and tension was higher when spike discharge rate was slightly lower. (d) A 27-day pregnant myometrium. The complex appearance with many peaks suggests asynchronous activity of many cells. (e,f) A 29-day pregnant myometrium, intracellular microelectrode recordings, resting potential −46 mV, spike height 57 mV. Except where noted, these results are from unpublished records obtained with A. L. Kleinhaus.

spike at body temperature is about 50 msec. In sucrose-gap recordings from multicellular preparations, the duration of the spike is slightly longer because of some temporal dispersion of the spikes of individual cells in the recording.

An interesting exception to the simple spike just described is that observed in the circular myometrium of the rat (Osa, 1974; Chamley and Parkington, 1984). Microelectrode recordings from single cells enmeshed in this tissue show that the action potential resembles that in the cardiac Purkinje fiber: following a rapid spike phase with partial repolarization, there is a plateau lasting several seconds when the membrane potential remains close to −10 mV. Then repolarization ensues. There is some species difference: in the uterus of the pregnant ewe, the action potential in the circular myometrium has the simple spike form, without any plateau.

Usually there is no appreciable negative afterpotential (afterdepolarization), but it may become evident when spikes follow one another in rapid succession. In such a case, cumulation of incomplete repolarizations becomes manifested as a sustained depolarization (see Figs. 4 and 7). Not infrequently, the repolarization phase continues beyond the original resting potential to give a brief phase of undershoot (afterhyperpolarization). In spontaneously spiking preparations, this feature is highly variable; some spikes in a burst may show it and others not, or a group of spikes may show it at one moment but not a few minutes later.

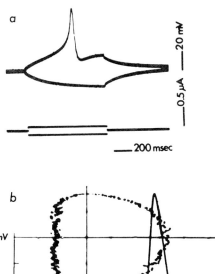

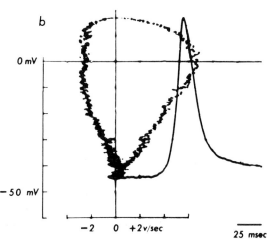

Figure 5. Two electrically elicited spikes from pregnant rat myometrium. (a) An 18-day pregnant myometrium recorded in double sucrose-gap arrangement in current-clamp mode. The bottom two traces are applied currents: upward step is outward current, and downward step is inward current. The top two traces are voltage responses of myometrium to applied current. Inward current produced hyperpolarization (downward) with its characteristic *RC* waveform. Outward current produced depolarization (upward), which triggered discharge of a single spike. Note that the spike is about 100 msec in duration because of some temporal dispersion of spikes from individual cells. The repolarizing phase of the spike produced a transient dip in the voltage trace, indicating the presence of lowered membrane resistance caused by activation of potassium channels (unpublished record). (b) Propagated spike recorded in a single myometrial cell with an intracellular microelectrode. Propagation is indicated by the flat baseline and exponential nature of the foot of the spike. Resting potential −44 mV; spike height 62 mV. Elliptical trace to left is a phase-plane display of spike (dV/dt versus V) from which some membrane currents and membrane properties can be deduced (see also Specht, 1976).

3.1.2. Complex Spikes

In a broad consideration of the electrical activities of the myometrium, single spikes are the exception rather than the rule. They occur in appreciable numbers only at parturition, and they are rarely seen at other times in either the pregnant or nonpregnant uterus. Outside of parturition, the spikes are usually more complex. They may vary from relatively simple coupled discharges of two or three peaks to forms of great complexity. These complex action potentials may be the only form of electrical activity in a preparation, or they may be interspersed with simple spikes. Such complex spikes and variabilities in form have been recorded with intracellular microelectrodes as well as with the sucrose-gap method. Some of them are the result of asynchronous activity of a number of cells that have some electrical interconnections.

3.1.3. Elicited Spikes

Until the double sucrose-gap technique was successfully used on the myometrium (Anderson, 1969; Kao and McCullough, 1975) and the taenia coli (Inomata and Kao, 1976), it had been difficult to elicit spikes in a reproducible manner. As has been discussed (Section 1.1), the difficulty arises from the complex interconnections within the smooth muscles. Under appropriate conditions in the double sucrose-gap method, it is possible repeatedly to cause a group of smooth muscle cells to respond synchronously. The spikes so elicited are always simple, and the phenomenon of afterhyperpolarization as a result of persistent potassium conductance is readily seen (Fig. 5a). Using the Abe–Tomita method of extrapolar stimulation, Chamley and Parkington (1984) were able to elicit the interesting spike-with-plateau type of response in the circular myometrium of the rat. It is often observed that the amplitude of the spike varies with the strength or the duration of the applied current. These phenomena are explainable on the basis of series resistance in such multicellular preparations that causes the spike threshold for individual cells to be reached at slightly different levels of applied current and at different times because of some differences in the membrane time constant.

In dispersed single myocytes of either the myometrium or the taenia coli, spikes elicited by applied current are always of the simple type (Fig. 5).

3.1.4. Pacemakers and Pacefollowers

In many records made with intracellular microelectrodes or the sucrose-gap method, it is possible to see slow depolarizations that lead into spike discharges (Fig. 6). These spikes are probably similar to the pacemakers in the heart and in some other smooth muscles. As in all autorhythmic tissues, the frequency of firing of the pacemaker spikes sets the frequency of activity of the tissue. In the myometrium, two types of frequencies can be discerned. One type has a long period, which is on the order of several seconds to tens of seconds, ending in each case with a burst of spike discharges (Figs. 6 and 14). Another type has a shorter period of 0.1–1 sec and is associated with the repetitive firing of spikes in a single burst. The mechanical consequences of these spike discharges and the influences of hormones, ions, and drugs on these two types of periodicity are discussed in later sections. For the moment, it might be appropriate to point out that the long periodicity that is associated with the appearance of bursts of spike discharges determines the frequency of "contractions" as encountered in clinical

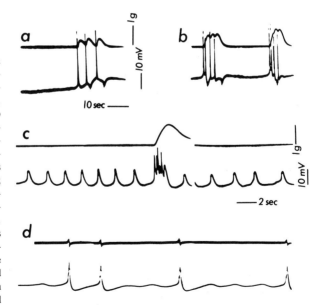

Figure 6. Pacemaker activity in pregnant rabbit myometrium. (a) Interplacental myometrium from 30-day pregnant uterus. Note the slow, gradual depolarization leading into three spikes, each followed by a contraction. (b) Same preparation. Absence of any distinct pacemaker potentials suggests that these spikes may be conducted from another site; i.e., these cells may be pacefollowers. (c) A 29-day pregnant myometrium, placental-site preparation. Consecutive sweeps of spontaneous activity. Note pacemaker depolarization leading to each discharge. The first four discharges have rounded peaks; the fifth, sixth, and seventh have slightly larger amplitudes and faster rates of rise. The eighth consists of complex spikes capable of producing contraction. Remaining discharges are similar to the first four. (d) A 29-day pregnant myometrium. Pacemaker spikes are mixed with abortive pacemakers.

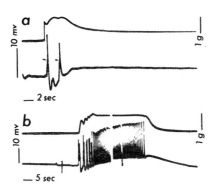

Figure 7. Stretch-induced and KCl-induced spike discharges. (a) Stretch response; estrogen-dominated nonpregnant rabbit myometrium. Stretch is indicated by quick tension rise (top trace). The spike initiated by stretch has its foot on a rising phase (arrow), which probably represents the depolarization that subsequently triggered the spike. Following the spike, there is a contraction, as there is also following the second spike. Note the large undershoot following the first spike and the small spike during this phase that is still in the relative refractory period left by the first spike. (b) A KCl-induced burst in rabbit myometrium. Interplacental myometrium from a 29-day pregnant uterus. The burst was initiated by 12 mM KCl in the bathing medium; the time of introduction is shown by the vertical artifact on the lower trace. Note the change of spike forms from complex to simple. Removal of high $[K^+]_o$ is indicated by the second artifact. Undershoots are present with the first five complex spikes but are not obvious after the preparation became depolarized. Compare the duration and amplitude of simple spikes with those of complex spikes. Note the slight decline in tension in the early part of the sustained contraction when the spike discharge rate was high.

experience. The short periodicity, which determines the rate of firing of individual spikes in each burst, profoundly affects the intensity of each contraction.

Not all myometrial cells are pacemakers because not all spikes are preceded by pacemaker depolarizations. Many spikes arise abruptly out of the resting potential (Fig. 6b) and generally are considered to be spikes conducted from a pacemaker somewhere else (see also Kuriyama, 1961). The conduction probably results from spread of local circuit current, which gates open the voltage-dependent ionic channel for the inward current in the cell under observation. Such cells may be termed ''pacefollowers'' to distinguish them from the pacemakers. Unlike the situation in the heart, however, pacemakers and pacefollowers in the myometrium are not anatomically discrete. Each myometrial cell is capable of being a pacefollower or, for unknown reasons, becoming a pacemaker. This potentiality is responsible for the observation that pacemaker sites in a myometrial preparation frequently shift from one area to another (Kao, 1959; Marshall, 1959).

Pacemaker activities may be initiated by stretch (Fig. 7), and the frequency of spike discharges in any one preparation is dependent to some extent on the degree of stretch applied. These properties have been known since Bozler's (1947) classical study and are similar to those described for some other smooth muscles (see Burnstock *et al.*, 1963). Although not proven yet by direct observations at the whole-cell or tissue levels, they may well have their origin in certain single membrane ionic channels that are opened by stretch (Kirber *et al.*, 1987). In the myometrium, the most effective form of stretch to initiate spikes seems to be a relatively small but quick stretch, which apparently causes some depolarization before initiating spikes (Fig. 7a). Under extreme stretch in some preparations, especially those from a parturient uterus, spike discharges may become continuous.

3.2. Ionic Basis of Electrical Activity

3.2.1. The Voltage-Clamp Technique and Its Application to Smooth Muscles

A major advance in understanding the electrophysiological properties of the myometrium and of other smooth muscles was made when Anderson (1969) successfully adapted a double sucrose-gap voltage-clamp technique to the rat myometrium. In spite of some serious limitations, the importance of that advance cannot be overstated. In his original paper, Anderson (1969) warned of the fundamental difficulties of applying the technique to multicellular prepa-

rations. However, in the absence of any alternative methods, it was a most valuable tool for **429**
providing interim information to advance smooth muscle studies from mere description to an

ELECTRO-
PHYSIOLOGY

analytical level. The criticisms leveled against the method (Bolton *et al.*, 1981) were entirely
of a general nature, based on expected impossibilities rather than on specific deficiencies in the
collected data, as the critics themselves were never able to use the technique properly (e.g.,
Bolton, 1975). Not surprisingly, as shall become clear later, the broad outlines of the ionic
currents and conductances discovered in the myometrium and the taenia coli using the double
sucrose-gap method have since been confirmed in studies on single cells from these tissues.
From that point of view, as imperfect as the double sucrose-gap technique might be in some
respects, it still forms a most important link that bridges observations on molecular events at
the single-channel level with familiar physiological phemonena at the tissue level.

The two most important advantages of the voltage-clamp technique over other techniques
are that (1) it completely controls the excitable membrane so that the variable factor, the
membrane current, is a graded response, changing according to changes in the controlled
membrane voltage, and (2) it minimizes the complex interference of the capacitive current and
reduces membrane current to ionic currents. By the first advantage, it is possible to separate
changes in membrane properties from changes in driving forces and to study each independently of the other. Such an important condition cannot be achieved when action potentials are
allowed to develop. By the second advantage, it is easier to identify the nature of the ionic
current and to understand some of the principles that govern their movements.

Fundamentally, the voltage-clamp technique is an electronic technique by which a negative feedback system controls and maintains (hence the term "clamp") the membrane voltage.
Even on suprathreshold stimulation that otherwise would have produced some all-or-none
action potential, the membrane voltage is controlled and clamped at some desired level, and
the underlying current is measured. The time resolution of the voltage-clamp technique is very
fast. In studying the nature of the ionic currents in smooth muscle, it is not difficult to resolve
characteristics of sodium and potassium currents down to milliseconds. If these ionic currents
were to be resolved by measuring the actual ionic fluxes, many minutes would be needed.
From some general principles of the ionic theory (see Section 1.2), it is possible to manipulate
experimentally the membrane to reveal some ideal properties and to make relatively accurate
estimates of some fundamental properties such as the equilibrium potentials.

Voltage clamp is not simply a powerful technique capable of resolving otherwise un-
answerable questions. It entails an entire methodology that leads to a level of understanding of
the excitable membrane far beyond that afforded by simple phenomenological descriptions.
The same underlying principles prevail whether the technique is applied to multicellular tissue
preparations or to single channels in the patch-clamp technique. Unfortunately, in smooth
muscle studies, there is a degree of misconception about voltage-clamp studies that leads on
one hand to frustrations and overreactions and on the other hand to unreal expectations and
overreaching conclusions. The objective of this section is to attempt to find an even keel on
which our understanding of the electrophysiological properties of some mammalian smooth
muscles can be based without building up unrealistic expectations.

3.2.2. Holding Potential and Holding Current

Voltage commands can be in the form of long-lasting steady-state voltage levels. Under
physiological conditions, smooth muscle cells in a multicellular preparation or in an isolated
dispersed form have resting potentials at which potassium ions are closest to being in electrochemical equilibrium. The net membrane current at that potential would be lowest. If the
membrane were held at the resting potential by voltage command, the holding current would
be very small or practically nil. If the membrane potential were to be held at a more negative
level, then an inward holding current would be needed; the more negative from resting
potential, the more current would be required. On the other hand, if the membrane were to be

held at a less negative potential than the resting potential, then an outward current would be needed.

Similarly, if the cell were to be depolarized by say 150 mM K^+ externally to a membrane potential of only a few millivolts inside negative, then the holding current at that voltage would be minimal. However, if the cell were to be held at -50 mV, the original physiological resting potential, then a sizable inward holding current would be needed. One of the basic tenets in the ionic theory is that the properties of the ionic channels are dependent only on the membrane voltage and not on the chemical composition of the environment. So, holding such a depolarized cell back to its original physiological membrane potential presumably restores all the essential properties of the ionic channels. In studies of single-channel activities in the patch-clamp technique, frequently voltage changes are made as changes in holding potential. Then the frequency of channel opening or closing can be observed at a steady voltage for prolonged periods.

3.2.3. Step Voltage Changes and Associated Currents

A widely used form of voltage command is a step function that alters the membrane voltage from the holding potential abruptly to another predetermined steady level of any desired duration and then again abruptly either to the original holding potential or to some different voltage level. Although other forms of transient voltage commands, such as ramp or sinusoidal functions, are also used sometimes, the present discussion focuses on the currents associated with the step commands.

When membrane voltage is stepped from one level (e.g., holding potential) to another, whether the new level is more or less negative, the first current is a surge of capacitive current that is proportional to the product of membrane capacity and the rate of change of the voltage ($C_m dV/dt$). The current corresponds to displacement of charges on the membrane dielectric and not to any ionic movements. It normally lasts only a very short time, and the rate of decay of the capacitive current provides a good means of determining the size of the membrane capacity, which is one way of estimating the amount of membrane surface involved under the voltage-clamp. In a properly run double sucrose-gap experiment, a multicellular preparation would have a total capacitance of about 1×10^{-7} F. In a single smooth muscle cell, the total capacitance would be about 5×10^{-11} F. Following the capacitive current, a more persistent current lasts for as long as the new membrane voltage is maintained. Since dV/dt at the new steady voltage level is zero, so is capacitive current. All the persistent current, then, is ionic current. It is the amount, polarity, and kinetics of such ionic currents that are most revealing of the ionic channels in the whole cell and tissues.

Figure 8 illustrates some typical currents of this type. The preparation was held at resting potential and required very little holding current. Step voltage commands were then applied, at 5-mV increments, alternately to hyperpolarize (increased intracellular negativity) and depolarize (decreased intracellular negativity). The currents occurring at the beginning and end of the voltage steps are the short surges of capacitive current. Ideally, the peak of the capacitive current should be very large. In practice, it is always limited because of series resistance, which actually can be estimated from the peak current. During the voltage step, there is a steady ionic current. With increasing hyperpolarizing pulses, the currents increase accordingly, but not necessarily in a linear proportion. These currents are inward, with a negative sign. With depolarizing pulses, the currents are complex. With small depolarizations, the currents, which are outward with a positive sign, are almost mirror images of the corresponding inward currents caused by hyperpolarization. However, when larger depolarizations are imposed, the membrane current is no longer simple, nor does it remain outward. At some voltage level (corresponding to the spike threshold), abruptly an inward current develops immediately following the capacitive current. This early inward current is transient and is

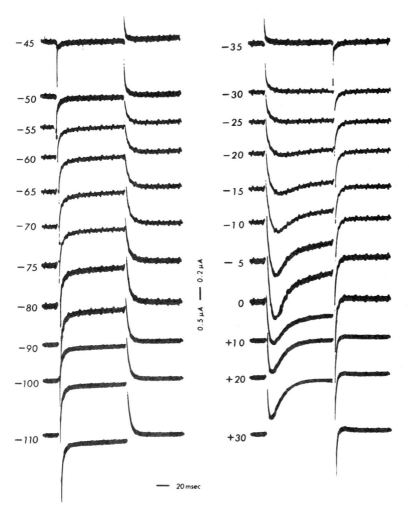

Figure 8. Membrane currents in a voltage-clamped preparation of rat myometrium; 19-day pregnant uterus. Left column shows currents caused by hyperpolarizing steps. Right column shows currents caused by depolarizing steps. The preparation was held at −40 mV, which was its natural resting potential, and the number attached to each current trace indicates the membrane voltage attained during the command step. Voltage steps have been omitted, and current traces are mounted close together to save space. In each case, a step voltage change is accompanied by a surge of capacitive current, which was not completely recorded, followed by ionic current. Hyperpolarization produced inward currents (negative current). Depolarization produced transient inward current followed by late outward current (positive current). At steps −20 mV to 0 mV, the initial current is clearly inward. At a step of +10 mV, it is inward and very small. At steps of +20 and +30 mV, it is outward. These are net total currents, so there must be some overlap of inward and outward currents. For further details, see text.

followed by a late outward current. The relationship between membrane voltage and the early current is complex: with increasing depolarization, it is inward and increases up to a point; with further depolarization, the early current declines and eventually reverses direction to become outward. The relationship between the late outward current and membrane voltage is simpler: with increasing depolarization, the outward current progressively increases. These features are best seen in a graph of the current–voltage relationship (Fig. 9).

It now can be said on the basis of considerable evidence that the observed currents result

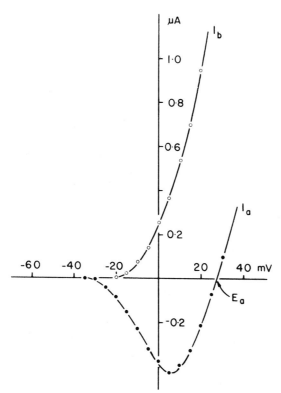

Figure 9. Current–voltage relationship of a voltage-clamped multicellular rat myometrial preparation. Actual currents are shown in Fig. 8. Currents in this graph have been corrected for leakage and residual capacitive current. Filled circles denote early current (I_a), which is inward (negative) from -35 mV to 28 mV and outward (positive) from 28 mV on. Zero-current voltage (28 mV) represents the apparent reversal potential of the early current. Because of overlap with the outward current, this reversal potential (E_a) probably is an underestimate of the actual reversal potential. An accurate estimate of the reversal potential requires blocking of the outward current to eliminate such error (see Fig. 11). Unfilled circles denote late current (I_b), which is outward.

from voltage-activated openings of specific ionic channels and consequent downhill movements of ions (see Section 1.2). The early current corresponds to openings of a sodium or a calcium channel and inward movements of extracellular Na^+ or Ca^{2+} ions down their electrochemical gradients. The late current corresponds to openings of a potassium channel, allowing outward movements of intracellular K^+ ions. The total current is the result of highly patterned sequences of changes in different ionic channels. Such changes are probably conformational changes in the channel proteins.

Many important and interesting details of the properties of excitable membranes are known as a result of voltage-clamp studies. At this time, it would be relevant just to mention a few basic points. With the assumption that the total area of cell membrane under study is constant, the magnitude of an ionic current would be a reflection of the amount of the ion crossing the membrane. Also, the voltage at which no net current flows across the membrane represents the point of balance between the electrical and chemical driving forces, in other words, the equilibrium potential for that particular ion. This point is also referred to as the reversal potential, because the current changes from being inward to being outward, or vice versa, at this voltage. This term is often preferred to equilibrium potential for a specific ion because it does not presume that the selectivity of the channel is exclusively for that particular ion.

3.2.2. Problems Encountered in Voltage-Clamp Studies of Smooth Muscles

As has been pointed out earlier (Section 1.3), voltage-clamp studies on multicellular preparations of smooth muscles are fraught with difficulties arising from uncertainties in the membrane area under study and the appreciable series resistance. These problems are virtually insoluble, but they can be bypassed adequately by using the method for comparing membrane properties under one condition with those under another. Thus, although the total membrane area cannot be known exactly in multicellular preparations, it can be maintained the same under different conditions, so that properties of the same amount of membrane can be compared. A sensitive and reliable means of estimating membrane area indirectly is a measure of the total membrane capacity (see Kao and McCullough, 1975; Inomata and Kao, 1976, 1979, 1985).

The series resistance in multicellular preparations resides primarily in the narrow intercellular clefts. It can be reduced to a rather low level but not eliminated or fully compensated for. Although it causes errors, these errors can be minimized by working with small preparations that give limited amounts of currents. Again, if it can be maintained relatively constant, observations under two different conditions can still be compared. In part because of the series resistance, the voltage imposed on individual cells might be different, and the currents elicited might show a considerable degree of overlap.

In an attempt to check on the usefulness of the multicellular studies, Specht (1976), working in my laboratory, used the phase-plane analysis (Section 1.3.2a) to derive the magnitude of the inward current and compared it with what was found in the multicellular studies. An example of those records is shown in Fig. 5b. He found that the inward current in a single myometrial cell was about 12 $\mu A/\mu F$ of membrane capacitance. From very recent information on the specific membrane capacitance (1.15 $\mu F/cm^2$ membrane area, Yamamoto et al., 1988b; see also general comments in Section 3.2.4), this value would correspond to about 14 $\mu A/cm^2$. In multicellular studies, the maximum inward current was around 6 $\mu A/\mu F$. Two reasons could account for the shortfall: (1) in the multicellular preparation, some of the capacitance resides in nonexcitable membranes, such as injured cells on the periphery of the preparation, and (2) temporal overlap of outward current would have significantly reduced the inward current. Such imperfections are expected of multicellular work, but the basic information generated by those studies was valid. It is interesting that Specht's work was based on the spontaneous or electrically elicited action potential, which contained some overlap of the underlying inward and outward currents. In recent studies on dispersed single cells in which the inward current was isolated, current densities of 20 $\mu A/cm^2$ (urinary bladder myocyte, Klöckner and Isenberg, 1985) and 19 $\mu A/cm^2$ (taenia coli myocyte, Yamamoto et al., 1988b) have been found.

3.2.3. Identification of the Ionic Currents in the Myometrium

3.2.3a. The Early Current. Under physiological conditions, when membrane potential can change as a result of current flow across the membrane, the early inward current is responsible for the rising (depolarizing) phase of the action potential, whereas the late outward current is responsible for the falling (repolarizing) phase. There was considerable controversy as to the ion responsible for the rising phase of the action potential in smooth muscles, which can now be rephrased as ''the ion responsible as the charge carrier for the early current.'' In spite of some early evidence that in an intestinal smooth muscle spontaneous or drug-induced spike discharges were abolished by drastically lowering $[Na^+]_o$ (e.g., Holman, 1957; Bülbring and Kuriyama, 1963), some later observations showed that the effects on spike discharges of such changes in $[Na^+]_o$ were considerably less than those of changing $[Ca^{2+}]_o$ (Brading et al., 1969). The conclusion from the later observations was that the ion responsible for the rising phase of the spike was Ca^{2+} and not Na^+. This conclusion has been extended to the myometrium on the basis of similar experimental observations (Osa, 1971).

The conclusion of Osa was in agreement with some earlier observations of Daniel and Singh (1958) and Csapo and Kuriyama (1963), whose main reason was that spontaneous spike discharges in cat or rat myometrium persisted for several hours in sodium-free media. As pointed out in the first edition of this chapter (Kao, 1967), one of the problems of the latter experiments was that relatively thick preparations containing both endometrium and myometrium were used, and insufficient time was allowed for adequate washout of extracellular sodium ions. Additional problems, which have become evident as a result of voltage-clamp studies, are that on removal of extracellular sodium some hyperpolarization developed, and the membrane resistance tended to increase (Inomata and Kao, 1976), probably because of a reduction in the leakage conductance normally present. Since a fraction of the normal sodium channels is inactivated at the usual resting potential of around -50 mV (also see Anderson and Ramon, 1972, 1976), the hyperpolarization tended to reduce that fraction. Moreover, by Ohm's law, in a membrane with increased resistance, even a reduced flux of sodium ions would still be capable of producing an action potential, possibly one even larger than that in normal solutions. This feature would hold true for myometrium as well as for the taenia coli. Therefore, the question of whether Na^+ or Ca^{2+} is the main charge carrier simply cannot be answered on the basis of descriptive recordings of the action potentials alone.

By using the voltage-clamp technique, many of the difficulties associated with earlier investigations can be avoided, and answers to some basic questions can be obtained relatively directly with reasonably independent control over complex, interdependent factors. The identification of the species of ion responsible for any current is still most readily accomplished by replacing that ion with a substituent that is unable to cross the membrane through that specific channel. For the early current, when the $[Na^+]_o$ is lowered in the medium, there is a reduction in the magnitude of the early current as well as a shift of the equilibrium potential towards a less positive level. These changes have been observed in myometrium obtained from nonpregnant rats that had been oophorectomized and primed with estradiol (Anderson, 1969; Anderson et al., 1971) and in myometrium obtained from pregnant rats close to term (Kao and McCullough, 1975). The substituent ions replacing Na^+ were dimethyldiethanolammonium ion (Kao and McCullough, 1975), choline, and Tris (Anderson et al., 1971), and these had no apparent effect on the outcome. The interpretation of the observations is as follows: when $[Na^+]_o$ was reduced, the electrochemical driving force for inward movement of Na^+ was lowered. As a result, the inward current was less, and the equilibrium potential was less positive.

In comparing these observations with those observations on the effects of sodium removal on spike discharges, the advantages of the voltage-clamp studies are readily apparent. Even though sodium removal produced some hyperpolarization that could have reduced the fraction of inactivated channels, the voltage-clamp technique can readily reset the membrane potential to the original resting potential to obviate this possible complication. Also, what was observed was the current, a direct manifestion of charges moving across the membrane, and not a consequence of such movement across the membrane resistance.

To go further, other experimental manipulations can be made to clinch the conclusion. One type of experiment is based on the quantitative relationship between changes in the inward current and in the early current equilibrium potential and changes in $[Na^+]_o$. Thus, from a straightforward physical–chemical relationship for a sodium-sensitive membrane, a 50% reduction of $[Na^+]_o$ at 37°C should cause a shift of 18.4 mV of the equilibrium potential towards the negative. In the broadest view, a 50% reduction of $[Na^+]_o$ should halve the inward current. The actual experimental observations of the effect of a 50% reduction of $[Na^+]_o$ were that the shift of the equilibrium potential was 17.2 mV towards the negative and the magnitude of inward current was reduced to 0.5 of the original (Kao and McCullough, 1975). Since these changes took place without any significant alterations in the early-current conductance of the membrane, it can be concluded that the changes are to be attributed to changes in the driving force.

A second type of experiment provides somewhat different proof for this conclusion. It should be recalled that the intracellular sodium concentration $[Na^+]_i$ in the myometrium is around 25–50 mmole/liter cell water (Section 2). Under physiological conditions, when $[Na^+]_o$ is about 150 mM, the existing electrochemical driving forces would produce an inward movement of sodium and hence the early inward current. After the small strip of myometrium was washed in a sodium-free solution for 10 min, when $[Na^+]_o$ was expected to be less than $[Na^+]_i$, the early current, which had been inward, reversed direction and became outward, indicating that the movement of Na^+ was now from intracellular phase to the extracellular phase (Kao and McCullough, 1975). Since all of these various observations were made in media containing the usual concentration of Ca^{2+}, the only conclusion they all lead to is that the charge carrier for the early current in the pregnant rat myometrium at term must be primarily Na^+.

What are the roles of Ca^{2+} in the early current of the myometrium? How could the above conclusion be reconciled with other observations pointing to the role of Ca^{2+} as the main charge carrier? Some answers to these questions have been obtained through experiments similar to those just described except that attempts to reverse the direction of the early current could not be done because $[Ca^{2+}]_i$ is so low that the membrane is damaged when $[Ca^{2+}]_o$ is lowered to 1 μM using a Ca^{2+}-buffering system. The remaining experiment is to test the effect of lowering $[Ca^{2+}]_o$. Since this is a divalent ion, comparable effects on the equilibrium potential and inward current would be expected when $[Ca^{2+}]_o$ is reduced to 25% of the original. In 25% $[Ca^{2+}]_o$, the magnitude of the early current was reduced to 0.5 of the original, not the expected 0.25, and the equilibrium potential was shifted by 20.2 mV, exceeding the theoretical maximum of 18.4 mV (Kao and McCullough, 1975). Moreover, the early current conductance was lowered significantly by reduction in $[Ca^{2+}]_o$. These observations suggest that the effects were produced not through effects on driving force alone but at least partly through significant effects on the conductance properties of the early current.

Another place where reduction of $[Ca^{2+}]_o$ has a greater influence than reduction in $[Na^+]_o$ is in the kinetics of the opening of the early-current channel. Such a change is deduced from the appreciably later peaking of the early current when $[Ca^{2+}]_o$ is reduced than when $[Na^+]_o$ is reduced. From all the observations, it seems appropriate to conclude that as important as its roles are, Ca^{2+} is probably not the main charge carrier of the early current in the pregnant rat myometrium at term.

Anderson et al. (1971) attempted to resolve the nature of the early current in a different manner. They depended heavily on agents and polyvalent cations that for some other tissues seemed to have selective blocking actions on the early channel. One of these is tetrodotoxin, which has been clearly established as a highly potent and specific blocking agent for the early channel (see Kao, 1966). In the nonpregnant rat myometrium, tetrodotoxin in concentrations 1000–10,000 times higher than the effective concentration for nerve membrane had no effect at all on the early current. This finding is consistent with historical observations on the effects of tetrodotoxin on mammalian smooth muscles (see Kao, 1966). As recognized by Anderson et al., this observation did not necessarily indicate that the early current was not carried by Na^+, because the tetrodotoxin blockade depended on the molecular configuration of the early channel and not on the species of ions passing through the channel (for other details, see Kao, 1966).

Polyvalent ions, La^{3+}, Co^{2+}, and Mn^{2+}, have been shown to block the early channels in some tissues through which a calcium current flows. These polyvalent ions did reduce the early current of the rat myometrium, an observation that led Anderson et al. (1971) to the conclusion that some calcium influx was involved in the early current, which was carried by both Na^+ and Ca^{2+}. Confusingly, these polyvalent ions also caused a significant reduction of the late outward potassium current. We now know that a good part of the potassium current is activated or enhanced by an increase in the intracellular calcium activity and that the reduction in the potassium current is associated with the blockage of the calcium influx.

Mironneau (1974) worked with the myometrium from pregnant rat uterus. Using choline to replace Na^+ and polyvalent cations Mn^{2+} and La^{3+} as well as lowering and raising $[Ca^{2+}]_o$, he concluded that the early current can be attributed to both Na^+ and Ca^{2+}. In attempting to establish the possible presence of a calcium current more clearly, Kao (1978) worked with the pregnant rat myometrium in a medium containing the usual $[Na^+]_o$ of 138 mM, 5 mM of tetraethylammonium to reduce outward potassium current, and chloride replaced by ethanesulfonate to reduce the chloride shunt. In the same group of myometrial cells, when $[Ca^{2+}]_o$ was increased from 1.8 mM to 9.5 mM, there was a significant increase in the early inward current and a highly significant shift of the reversal potential to a level 12 mV more positive.

Nakai and Kao (1983) used a slightly different approach to show the presence of a calcium current in the pregnant rat myometrium. They first found the early inward current in a medium containing 138 mM of Na^+ and 1.8 mM of Ca^{2+}. They then depolarized the preparation in a solution containing 138 mM of K^+ and 1.8 mM of Ca^{2+} and held the membrane back to the original resting potential. Under these conditions, a slowly developing inward current, the magnitude of which was directly affected by $[Ca^{2+}]_o$, was found. Assuming the fast early current to be I_{Na} and the slow inward current to be I_{Ca}, they found that in midpregnancy, the ratio of I_{Ca}/I_{Na} was 0.57, whereas at term that ratio was 0.31. They interpreted the results to indicate that both sodium and calcium channels were present in the myometrium and that the relative contribution of each to the total inward current varied at different times of pregnancy. Thus, at midterm, contributions of calcium current appear to be more important than those from sodium current, but at term, there is an increase in the role of the sodium current. This finding is consistent with the observation that the action potential of the myometrium at term always rose significantly faster than that during midpregnancy.

Vassort (1975), working with the nonpregnant, estrogen-primed guinea pig myometrium, found that the early current was not responsive to changes in $[Na^+]_o$ but was responsive to changes in $[Ca^{2+}]_o$. He concluded that the early current in the guinea pig myometrium was carried by Ca^{2+}. Although this work has not been confirmed, the conclusion is plausible. In another smooth muscle of this species, the taenia coli, the inward current is entirely Ca^{2+} (Inomata and Kao, 1976), an observation that has now been confirmed in the isolated single myocyte (Yamamoto et al., 1988b).

3.2.3b.   The Early Current in the Taenia Coli.   As an instructive contrast to the myometrium, the intestinal smooth muscle from the taenia coli provides a very different picture. Reducing $[Na^+]_o$ did not reduce the size of the early current or shift its reversal potential, but reducing $[Ca^{2+}]_o$ produced both expected effects (Inomata and Kao, 1976). Recently, it has been shown that in dispersed single myocytes of the taenia coli, no inward Na^+ current could be found even in a Ca^{2+}-free environment containing 140 mM of Na^+ (Yamamoto et al., 1988b). Usually under such conditions, some Na^+ could be made to move inwards through the calcium channel.

3.2.3c.   The Late Current.   In marked contrast to the controversy involving the nature of the early current, there is almost no difference of opinion among investigators on smooth muscles about the nature of the late current. There is universal acceptance that K^+ is the charge carrier. Ironically for this extraordinary unanimity, there was no direct supportive evidence until the problem was studied in the voltage-clamped preparation.

An identification of K^+ as the charge carrier for any smooth muscle was first made by Kao and McCullough (1975) in the pregnant rat myometrium. A myometrial strip was studied first in a normal solution. As $[K^+]_i$ was about 150 mM and $[K^+]_o$ 6 mM, the late current was always outward when its channel was opened. The same group of myometrial cells was then treated with an isotonic K_2SO_4 solution (149 mM), which reduced the membrane potential to nearly zero. The depolarized preparation can be held back to the original resting potential thereby imposing a new set of electrochemical driving forces (see Section 1.2). By opening the late current channel with appropriate depolarizing steps, the late current now flowed inward up to the depolarized membrane potential and then became outward. Since the concentration of

Ca^{2+} was the same as before, the only charge carrier that could account for this pattern had to be K^+.

Another way of identifying K^+ as the charge carrier is to make use of tail-current analysis for the equilibrium potential. In this method, while the late current channel was opened with an appropriate depolarization arising out of the holding potential, the membrane potential was returned abruptly to a level close to but different from the holding potential. The opened channel would close, but the rate of closure lagged behind the voltage change. Consequently, a transient current flowed either in the inward direction or in the outward direction: inward when the potential was more negative and outward when it was less negative than the equilibrium potential. In multicellular preparations of the pregnant rat myometrium (Kao and McCullough, 1975) and the guinea pig taenia coli (Inomata and Kao, 1976), the equilibrium potential so found was usually 15–20 mV more negative than the usual resting potential, i.e., about −70 mV. This value is lower than the expected equilibrium potential for a highly selective K^+ channel, about −85 mV, and the shortfall has been attributed to some imperfect selectivity. Still, K^+ is the only major ion species that could account for the observation. In recent studies on freshly dissociated single smooth myocytes of the guinea pig taenia coli, where the Nernst potential for K^+ is −86 mV, the observed equilbrium potential was −85 mV, indicating a very high degree of selectivity for K^+ (Yamamoto et al., 1988c).

In the guinea pig myometrium, Vassort (1975) found that the outward current showed a very prominent hump and then declined. A similar but less striking observation was made by Mironneau (1974). On the basis of such recordings, these investigators concluded separately that there were at least two different potassium currents, one fast and one slow, and that these currents also could be distinguished by susceptibility to different blocking agents such as tetraethylammonium ion and 4-aminopyridine. Although different potassium channels have since then been identified in many other tissues, I believe the observations made in those studies basically were artifactual, caused by the inclusion of too much tissue in the "node" under study. Using their methods, but very small multicellular tissues, M. Wakui and I never saw any significant humps in the outward current and never found different susceptibility of the early part of the outward current from the late part (unpublished observations). The large hump on the K^+ current clearly was caused by temporal overlap with the large Na^+ and/or Ca^{2+} current when a rather large amount of tissue was included in the clamped region. Although critics of the double sucrose-gap method have made much of this problem (Bolton et al., 1981), appreciable current overlaps have now been shown to occur even in the single smooth myocyte (Yamamoto et al., 1988b). In other words, the problem was always less in the multicellular nature of the preparation than in some intrinsic properties of ionic currents of individual cells. Current overlap is not unique to mammalian smooth muscles; it occurs in such single cells as the squid giant axon, the node of Ranvier, and single skeletal muscle fibers. Resolution of individual ionic currents requires blocking one of the overlapping currents by specific and appropriate methods, such as uniquely acting toxins or other pharmacological agents (see Hille, 1984).

3.2.4. Recent Findings on Single Cells and Single Channels

Dispersed single smooth muscle cells are providing a new realm for studies of ionic channel functions on a truly cellular basis. These cells generally are prepared by incubating small pieces of tissues in collagenase along with some form of mechanical agitation. With appropriate care, single cells can be prepared that have the various electrophysiological properties known to exist in single cells enmeshed in tissue matrices. The dispersed cells are free of restricted extracellular clefts and embedded nerve endings; they are also readily accessible to surface-applied agents.

These cells can be impaled with conventional glass microelectrodes, which must have very fine tips and hence very high resistances. The high-resistance electrodes introduce difficult technical problems (see Walsh and Singer, 1980). The dispersed cells often are studied better by using the new tight-seal patch-clamp technique (see Section 1.3.2b). With one notable exception, most smooth muscle tissues yield myocytes that have their surfaces rather well "cleaned" by the enzymic treatment. Consequently, the cell surface can form a seal with a glass micropipette having mechanical strength and high electrical resistance. This is the essence of the new tight-seal patch-clamp technique (see Hamill *et al.*, 1981). The exception is the myometrial cell from the pregnant uterus. These cells frequently are coated with a thin layer of some optically transparent gelatinous material that prevents a proper tight seal from being formed. There is no published information on freshly dissociated myometrial cells at present, but some on myometrial cells in tissue culture (Mollard *et al.*, 1986; Stefani *et al.*, 1988). The myometrial cell can be rather labile, undergoing profound functional changes within a matter of a few hours. Some examples of such functional changes are the appearance and disappearance of gap junctions just at the time of parturition, changes of the electrical length constant, and changes in the conduction of impulses (see Section 3.3). Although studies on the cultured cells possess intrinsic significance, the functional observations on them may not reflect the properties of fresh myometrial cells without a more thorough comparison of cells under the two conditions. Therefore, the following account is based chiefly on intestinal smooth muscle, supported in appropriate places by information available on other mammalian smooth muscle cells.

3.2.4a. The Calcium Current.   In the whole-cell mode (Yamamoto *et al.*, 1988b; Fig. 10), the net ionic currents of the individual taenia myocyte, on depolarization, are an inward Ca^{2+} current initially and transiently and an outward K^+ current more slowly and more sustained. At about 33°C, the inward Ca^{2+} current in single taenia myocytes reaches a maximum at around 2 msec, but its duration cannot be determined properly because the outward K^+ current develops rapidly enough to cause appreciable overlap. Such an overlap is reminiscent of the happenings in the multicellular preparation, but with the patch-clamp method it is possible to introduce high concentrations of Cs^+ into the cell interior by simply incorporating Cs^+ in the pipette solution. Because of the fairly large rupture in the cell membrane when a whole-cell recording is made, there is a rapid equilibration of the solutes in the cell interior with those of the pipette solution. The predominant effect of intracellular Cs^+ is to block the K^+ channels. Then the Ca^{2+} current can be isolated for detailed analysis (Fig. 11).

The key findings are: (1) the Ca^{2+} current is first activated at around -30 mV and reaches a maximal value between $+10$ to $+20$ mV; (2) it activates and deactivates with unexpectedly fast kinetics, the time constants being around 1 msec; (3) it has a reversal potential of around $+75$ mV, but this value is believed to result in part from Cs^+ moving outwards through the Ca^{2+} channel under the drive of the strongly positive imposed voltage (in other words, the $+75$ mV value is most probably not the equibrium potential of Ca^{2+}); (4) the steady-state inactivation properties are such that at the usual resting potential of -50 mV, over 90% of the Ca^{2+} channels are available for opening on threshold depolarization; (5) half of the Ca^{2+} channels are inactivated when the membrane potential is at -30 mV; (6) the kinetics of inactivation is complex, suggesting the presence of more than a single type of Ca^{2+} channel; (7) half-recovery from inactivation occurs in about 75 msec, corresponding roughly to the refractory period following an action potential; and (8) the influx of Ca^{2+} during an action potential is so large that it would be capable of raising the intracellular [Ca^{2+}] into micromolar ranges if no calcium-buffering system were present inside the myocyte.

Single-channel studies (Yoshino *et al.*, 1988; Yamamoto *et al.*, 1988a) show that there are at least two types of calcium channels: (1) a large type with a unit conductance of about 6 pS, using Ca^{2+} as the charge carrier, and (2) a small type with a unit conductance that is probably around one-fifth of the large type. Multiple types of calcium channels with distinctive activation and inactivation properties have been described for neurons and cardiac myocytes (e.g., McClesky *et al.*, 1986). The two types we see in the taenia myocyte have some resemblance to those in other tissues, but they have significant differences also. Thus, the two types in the taenia myocyte cannot be distinguished from each other by any appreciable differences in activation properties. The large Ca^{2+} channels in the taenia inactivate, whereas the small type do not or do so only very slowly. At present, we believe that the large channel is most involved in physiologically functional roles such as generating action protentials and providing the Ca^{2+} for such intracellular events as contraction and activation of K^+ channels.

3.2.4b. The Potassium Current. Because of the overlap of Ca^{2+} current and K^+ current in the whole cell, to study the latter, it is necessary to block the former by applying Co^{2+} to the outside of the myocyte. The K^+ current in the whole cell has two components: one that is dependent on $[Ca^{2+}]_i$ and another dependent on membrane potential. The K^+ current activates more slowly than the Ca^{2+} current, with a voltage-dependent time constant

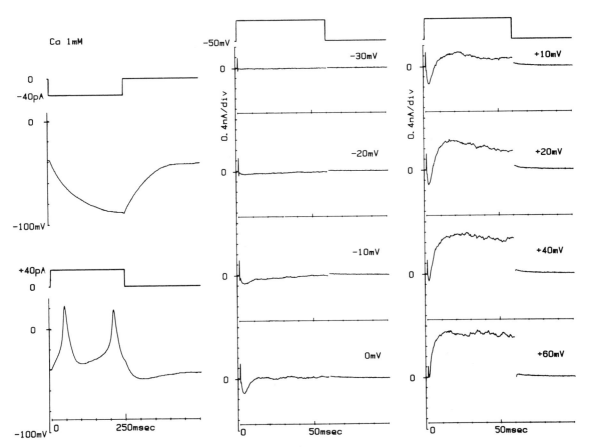

Figure 10. Response of a dispersed single myocyte of guinea pig taenia coli to current clamp and voltage clamp. Left column: current-clamp responses. Top panel: resting potential −40 mV; inward current (downward step in top trace) produced hyperpolarization with characteristic *RC* waveform, with a time constant of 77 msec. Bottom panel: outward current (upward step in top trace) produced depolarizing waveform, which triggered action potentials. Height of first spike, 62 mV. Note the large afterhyperpolarization following the second spike because of residual increased potassium conductance. Middle and right columns: voltage-clamp responses. Cell was held at −50 mV and stepped to voltage levels indicated in each panel (top trace of columns). Inward and outward currents are similar to those seen in multicellular preparations (Fig. 8). Note that the duration of inward current is shortened when outward current appeared because of overlap.

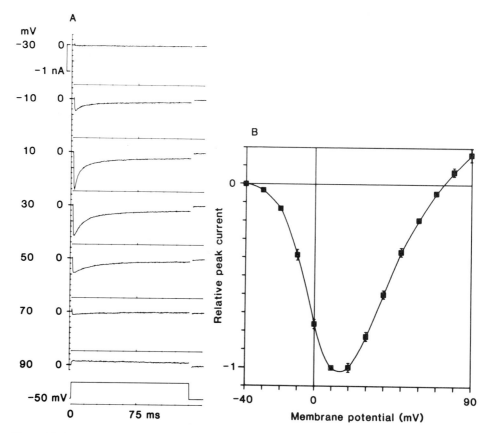

Figure 11. Current–voltage relationship of initial inward current of single myocyte of taenia coli. (A) Actual currents. Holding potential −50 mV; voltage step indicated by number to left of each panel; voltage protocol at bottom of panel. This cell was recorded with an electrode containing Cs⁺, which blocked the outward K⁺ current. Note that the duration of the inward current is much longer than that in a preparation or cell in which outward current was present (e.g., Figs. 8 and 10). (B) Current–voltage relationship of inward current. In the taenia myocyte, inward current is carried entirely by Ca^{2+}.

of about 10 msec at a membrane potential of 0 mV, shortening to about 2 msec at +70 mV. The Ca^{2+}-activated K⁺ current has a voltage dependence that is very similar to that of the Ca^{2+} current itself, with a peak current occurring at a voltage where I_{Ca} tends to be maximum. By tail-current analysis (see Section 3.2.3b), the E_K is determined to be −85 mV, compared with an expected Nernst potential of −86 mV. Thus, the selectivity of the channel for K⁺ is very high. The form of the I_K, its activation kinetics, and its selectivity for K⁺ all suggest that it is comparable with, if not identical to, the delayed rectifier previously demonstrated in multicellular preparations (Kao and McCullough, 1975; Inomata and Kao, 1976).

In single-channel recordings (Hu *et al.,* 1988a,b), three types of K⁺ channels can be recognized, having unit conductances of *ca.* 150, 95, and 65 pS, respectively. The 150-pS channel is the most abundant and most active. Its current–voltage relationships, activation kinetics, sensitivity to $[Ca^{2+}]_i$, permeation properties to other monovalent cations, and blockade by Cs⁺ and tetraethylammonium ion all suggest strongly that it is the molecular basis of the delayed rectifier channel. The experimental basis for this conclusion comes from an analysis of the probability of the channel being in the open state as a function of membrane voltage, using cell-detached membrane patches. The open probability is lowest at −30 mV but rapidly increases (according to the Boltzmann distribution) when the membrane is made more positive. The channel activity is then characterized by more frequent openings and longer open times.

Significantly, these channel openings can be observed not only with changes in holding potentials but also in response to step depolarizations of the type that has been used in voltage-clamp studies on multicellular preparations and on single myocytes. By summing many traces of single-channel currents and averaging them for different step depolarizations, we have reproduced current traces that are very similar to the I_K recorded in whole-cell mode from isolated taenia myocytes (Fig. 12). All these currents at the different levels of organization share the common properties of a gradual onset, a maintained amplitude during the depolarizing voltage step, and an acceleration of the rate of activation with increasing depolarization. Therefore, we believe at this time that the 150-pS K^+ channel that is Ca^{2+} activated is the delayed rectifier channel.

Another physiological role subserved by the 150-pS channel is in the regulation of the resting potential. As mentioned, the probability of the channel being in the open state is lowest at -30 mV. When the membrane patch is made more negative, the open probability increases again, reaching a maximal value at around -50 mV, the natural resting potential. The pattern

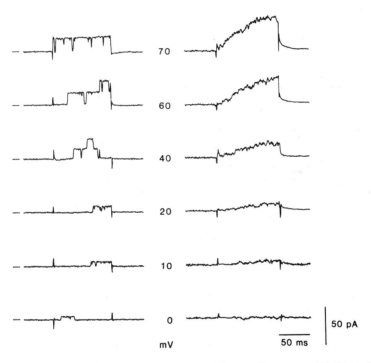

Figure 12. Activities of a single Ca^{2+}-activated K^+ channel in a taenia myocyte. Cell-detached inside-out patch in solution with $[K^+]_o = 6$ mM and $[K^+]_i = 135$ mM. Holding potential -50 mV, stepped to voltages indicated by number attached to each trace. Traces in the left column are single sweeps. Timing of the voltage step can be recognized from the capacitive artifacts at the beginning and end of each step. In the left column, at 0, 10, and 20 mV, one single channel opens during the depolarizing step. Some outward rectification is already exhibited, with current increasing in size. In steps 40 and 60 mV, two single channels open simultaneously, one on top of the other. Also, open time is longer than before. At 70 mV, the channel stays open almost continuously during the step. Traces in the right column are averaged currents of 60 to 100 single sweeps at each voltage step of the type shown in the left column. Compared with the outwardly rectifying K^+ current in whole cell (Fig. 11) and multicellular tissue preparation (Fig. 8), these averaged currents share similar gradual onset, a maintained magnitude, and an accelerated rate of activation with increasing depolarization. For these and other reasons, this Ca^{2+}-activated K^+ channel is believed to be the single-channel basis of the physiologically familiar phenomenon of delayed rectification (see Hu *et al.*, 1988a).

of the channel activity, however, is now different from that at voltages more positive than -30 mV. In place of the long open times, the channel now opens frequently (with short closed time) and with short open times. Because the channel activity deviates from the Boltzmann distribution, we termed this part of the probability–voltage relationship the anomalous activity region. At present, we believe that this type of activity could well be involved in the regulation of the resting potential.

We have estimated that in each taenia myocyte, there are probably 3300 such Ca^{2+}-activated K^+ channels.

From this short account of some of the recent studies of single-channel functions, it should be readily apparent that there is a continuous spectrum of worthy information extending from familiar physiological phenomena in multicellular preparations to the opening and closing of single molecules of channel proteins. By itself, the information on single channels is novel and important, but its significance is enhanced manyfold when it can be read and appreciated within a context of physiological relevance.

3.3. Tissue Phenomena

Most cells in the body do not function independently of one another, particularly in a tissue such as the myometrium that must rely on some intercellular coordination to accomplish its biological functions. In recent years much new information on cellular functions has been gained through the use of new techniques and concepts. In the area of integrated intercellular coordination, however, much remains to be explored.

3.3.1. Pattern of Excitation in the Whole Uterus

One reason for the relative paucity of information in this area is that when experiments were carried out on whole uteri, or on pieces of myometrium large enough to provide information on integrated cellular activities, the number of recording sites was limited to one or two small spots (Jung, 1955; Kao, 1959). Jung's work was based on acute experiments on the rat uterus. My own experiments (Kao, 1959) and those of several other investigators (e.g., Csapo et al., 1963; Demianczuk et al., 1984) were based on chronic experiments on live and conscious rabbits, using implanted small surface-recording electrodes in the uterine wall. In these chronic experiments, if the electrodes were properly affixed, they could record the activity of the same group of myometrical cells through various functional states over relatively long periods of observation. For instance, although no action potentials were seen in the myometrium of oophorectomized rabbits, a single injection of 50 μg of estradiol brought forth spontaneous bursts of spike discharges in 24 hr (Kao, 1959). During pregnancy, the frequency of spike discharges was relatively low until about 12 hr before parturition, when the spike frequency rapidly increased to a maximum (Kao, 1959; Csapo et al., 1963; Csapo and Takeda, 1965; Demianczuk et al., 1984). Another interesting observation was made when one uterine horn was made sterile before mating, and pregnancy occurred in only one horn. Throughout the course of pregnancy and during parturition, the sterile horn, in spite of the absence of a placenta and placental progesterone, was consistently three to five times less active in spike discharges than the pregnant horn (Kao, 1959).

Wolfs and van Leeuwen (1979) have conducted a detailed study of the electrical activities of the human uterus in conjunction with recordings of intrauterine pressure. Because their electrodes were built into a fine catheter that was introduced into the uterine cavity through the cervix, the records were taken from the endometrial surface of the myometrium. Whether these recorded electrical activities are entirely comparable with those of the longitudinal myometrial layer of the rabbit is not known, especially now that some differences between the logitudinal and circular layers have been recognized in the uteri of several species (see below). However, the organization of the layers of the myometrium in the human uterus is not so distinct as that in the rat or rabbit uterus. Also, the differences in the two layers of the myometrium reside chiefly in certain details such that they are not likely to affect the overall character of Wolfs and van Leeuwen's observations.

Since there is no other work on the human uterus of the same comprehensiveness and quality, we shall consider the observations of Wolfs and van Leeuwen in some detail. They showed that the electrical activity of the human myometrium, *in situ,* occurred in cyclic bursts that usually preceded contractions. Confirming an earlier observation (Wolfs and Rottinghuis, 1970), Wolfs and van Leeuwen (1979) again showed that although some electrical potential changes can be recorded via cutaneous electrodes placed on the abdominal wall, the recorded signals only rarely correlated with myometrial spike activities recorded via intrauterine electrodes. Moreover, such cutaneous recordings had a large component of artifacts. Thus, the "electrohysterograms" of the 1950s and 1960s are basically uninterpretable tracings of no physiological relevance.

Of some interest in this clinical study is the observation that in prelabor frequent and short bursts of small spikes were recorded, some of them occurring without accompanying contractions. As labor progressed, the actual bursts became less frequent, but each burst lengthened, and there developed a closer correlation between the electrical activity and the following contraction (see also Sakaguchi and Nakajima, 1973). These observations have been interpreted to mean that the intercontraction bursts of spikes represented local and relatively uncoordinated activity and that the coordination throughout the entire uterus improved as labor progressed. The amplitude of the spikes in each burst also increased markedly as labor progressed toward full cervical dilation. The only means of measurement available to Wolfs and van Leeuwen was what they termed "cumulative-peak-to-peak EMG amplitude," which increased from 3 mV in early stage 1 of labor to 14 mV at full cervical dilation. Since the spike activities were recorded with surface electrodes, the amplitude change actually reflected an increasing number of myometrial cells firing relatively synchronously (see Section 1.3.1a). The number of spikes in each burst also increased appreciably, so there was actually a marked increase in electrical activity that could not be fully described by a simple numerical designation.

The records clearly showed that the frequency of contractions was dependent on the frequency of bursts of spikes, whereas the force of the contraction is related to the number of spikes in each burst. By simultaneously recording intrauterine pressure, Wolfs and van Leeuwen (1979) were able to show that pressure changes of 10 mm Hg or less were usually not felt subjectively, even though they could be preceded, accompanied, or followed by electrical spike activities of low amplitude. With progression of labor and increasing force of contraction, the pressure waveform changed from a relatively symmetrical type with about equal rates of rise and fall to an asymmetric type with the rise significantly faster than the fall. Contractions with a force of 20 mm Hg could easily be felt subjectively, and at full dilation forces exceeding 70 mm Hg were encountered. Correlated with such increases in force of contractions and rates of rise of the pressure, the bursts of spike activity became more and more confined to the initial phase of the contraction. The electrical spike activity usually preceded the contraction, often coinciding with the rising phase of the pressure increase, and was almost always absent on the falling phase as well as between contractions.

In a few women in whom oxytocin was administered to induce labor, continuous spike activities were sometimes elicited between what had been distinct bursts of spikes. Mechanically, the interauterine pressure remained elevated between distinct peaks of contraction, resulting in the clinical state of hypertonia. The continuous spike activity and hypertonia can be reversed by reducing the rate of infusion of oxytoxin.

Another point of some interest concerns the possible existence of pacemaker regions in the whole uterus. On finding the tubal end of the rat uterus electrically more active than the vaginal end, Jung (1955) suggested that the former might be the pacemaker region. I found the tubal and vaginal ends equally active and concluded that no special anatomic area was exclusively pacemaker (Kao, 1959). A similar conclusion was reached by Wolfs and Rottighuis (1970) and Wolfs and van Leeuwen (1979) in the human uterus.

3.3.2. Problems of Impulse Conduction in the Myometrium

The myometrium is one of the smooth muscles that form a physiological syncytium of individual cells. To attain intercellular coordination, there must be some means of "crosstalk" between individual cells. Some idea of this coordination was obtained by Melton and Saldivar (1964), who studied impulse conduction by surface recording at five different sites of the isolated uterus from estrogen-primed rats. Instead of relying on spontaneous action potentials, they studied electrically elicited impulses and avoided the complication of shifting pacemaker areas during spontaneous activity. Electrical stimuli were applied to the tubal end of the uterus or its longitudinal muscle, and action potentials were recorded at varying distances from the stimulated site. Unlike the situation in skeletal and cardiac muscles, impulses in the myometrium were not always conducted in a nondecremental manner. Although nondecremental impulses were seen on occasion, more often impulses originating in one area were extinguished after being conducted for 1–2 cm. The longitudinal layer of the myometrium also was organized into functionally distinct bundles, because impulses could travel in separate bundles quite independently of one another. Some interconnections existed between bundles, for impulses in one bundle could spread to another bundle, although the latency between the impulses was rather long compared with that between impulses traveling longitudinally in the same bundle.

In the mouse (Osa, 1974) and the rat (Osa and Katase, 1975), there is evidence for myogenic interactions between the longitudinal and circular layers of the myometrium. In both species, the circularly arranged myometrial fibers showed comparatively more slow waves and fewer spike discharges than did the longitudinal fibers. The length constant was also shorter in the circular myometrium, and the conduction velocity was slower. Electrical signals applied to the longitudinal myometrial fibers could be recorded in the circular fibers and vice versa. Such interactions were not blocked by the potent axonal blocking agent tetrodotoxin and therefore could not be attributed to neural elements. Coincident spike discharges often occurred in the two layers, and such synchronous activity was enhanced by longitudinal stretch or increase in intraluminal pressure. In the ewe, Parkington (1985) observed that at about midpregnancy, the circular muscle had a short length constant and scattered pacemakers. At term, the length constant increased about fivefold, and impulse conduction improved.

By analogy with some other tissues, the gap junction between individual myometrial cells has long been suspected as being the site where intercellular interactions occur. The gap junction (nexus of Dewey and Barr, 1964) is a specialized area of intimate contact between two adjacent cells at which some structural modifications have taken place. In the myometrium, however, its presence and possible role in overall uterine function were controversial until a correlation was found between the number of gap junctions and labor (Garfield et al., 1977). Since then, it has been shown repeatedly in experimental animals and in women that the number of gap junctions increases rapidly as labor approaches, remains abundant throughout labor, and declines post-partum (e.g., Sims et al., 1982; Demianczuk et al., 1984). Significantly, Sims et al., by measuring the longitudinal impedance of myometrial strips taken from animals before or during labor, found that whereas the myoplasmic resistance remained constant before and during labor, the gap-junction resistance during labor was about a third of that before labor. They proposed that together with the much larger number of gap junctions present, the lowered gap resistance facilitated the spread of electrical impulse throughout the whole uterus.

3.4.1. Oxytocin and Other Oxytocic Drugs

It is well known that oxytocin increases the frequency as well as the force of contractions of the uterus. There are numerous studies of the electrophysiological actions of oxytocin on isolated rat and rabbit myometrium (Jung, 1957; Soto, 1960; Marshall and Csapo, 1961; Kuriyama, 1961; Kuriyama and Csapo, 1961; Marshall, 1963). The general conclusion from those studies was that, in most situations, when the membrane potential was more negative to the spike threshold, oxytocin caused depolarization of the myometrial membrane and thereby increased the frequency of spike discharges and increased contractile activities.

One difficulty with most of those studies was that the doses of oxytocin used to produce observable effects were in the milliunit per milliliter range, whereas threshold contractile effects might be induced by doses in the nanounit range (see Berde, 1968, for references). At concentrations of 50–500 μU/ml, oxytocin never produced any depolarization (Kleinhaus and Kao, 1969). Its actions are fourfold: (1) it can initiate spike discharges in quiescent preparations; (2) it can increase the frequency of burst discharges; (3) it can increase the number of spikes in any one burst; and (4) it can increase the amplitude of individual spikes when these are low.

Figures 13a and 14 illustrate the first three actions. The preparation was quiescent and did not respond to 50 μU of oxytocin/ml, but shortly after application of 500 μU of oxytocin/ml, spike dicharges began. As described earlier (Section 3.1.4 on pacemakers), there was a long periodicity of fluctuation in the membrane potential, each upswing leading to a burst of spike discharges. Initially there were only a few spikes in a burst, but with time more and more spikes appeared per burst. The contractile activities were closely related to the electrical discharges. Each burst of spikes produced a contraction, and the intensity of each contraction was directly dependent on the number of spikes in each burst, there having been summation of the contractions produced by each spike. As oxytocin was removed, the interval between the bursts lengthened, and all discharges eventually ceased. Interestingly, very similar observations have been observed in the human uterus *in situ* (Wolfs and van Leeuwen, 1979). Both bursts and the number of spikes in each burst increased on infusion of oxytocin, with resultant increases in contractions. When the electrical activity became continuous, with spike discharges between the usual bursts, a clinical condition of hypertonia resulted, with a long-maintained increased intrauterine pressure.

An additional feature of the actions of oxytocin as shown in Fig. 13b. This preparation was active, with relatively small spikes. When 50 μU of oxytocin/ml was applied, the frequency of such low spikes was readily increased. Additionally, fast-rising, large spikes appeared. Since the recording was made on a multicellular preparation, these larger spikes can only be interpreted to indicate that more individual myometrial cells have been induced into synchronous discharges. A similar conclusion has been reached with the pregnant mouse myometrium, because the spread of excitation was improved by oxytocin (Osa and Taga, 1973).

When recordings were made with intracellular microelectrodes from individual myometrial cells, oxytocin often increased the amplitude as well as the maximum rate of rise of electrically elicited spikes (Kleinhaus and Kao, 1969). Because the doses of oxytocin did not alter the resting potential, it was possible to ask whether oxytocin altered the relationship between the maximum rate of rise of the spike and the resting potential of the myometrial cells. It should be recalled that these experiments were done before a voltage-clamp method was adapted to mammalian smooth muscles. The question aimed at resolving a problem of possible membrane currents that could not be approached by other techniques available at the time. The basis of the question is as follows. From considerations of the classical cable equation, membrane current is proportional to the second derivative of membrane voltage with respect to

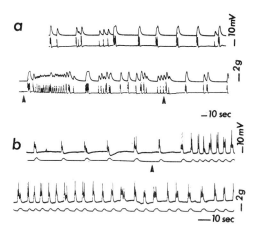

Figure 13. Increase of spike activity by oxytocin. Continuous sucrose-gap recordings. (a) A 29-day pregnant myometrium, spontaneously active preparation from placental region. At the first arrowhead, oxytocin, 50 μU/ml, was introduced, leading to increased burst and spike activities. At the second arrowhead, oxytocin was removed, followed by a gradual return to the original pattern of activity. (b) A 19-day pregnant myometrium, placental site preparation. At the arrowhead, oxytocin, 50 μU/ml, was introduced. Oxytocin increased not only the frequency of bursts and spikes but also the amplitude of spikes. High-amplitude spikes were of very short duration, suggesting the possibility of a single-cell origin. From Kleinhaus and Kao (1960).

time ($I_m \propto d^2V/dt$). Since membrane current is made up of the ionic current and the capacitive current ($I_m = I_i + C_m dV/dt$), when $I_m = 0$, $I_i = -C_m dV/dt$. This condition is satisfied at the peak of dV/dt. Because this condition is reached rather early in the spike, maximum dV/dt is often taken as reflecting the current through the early channel (whether sodium or calcium), even though strictly it is only a measure of total ionic current.

The relationship between the maximum dV/dt and the resting potential of the rabbit myometrial cell is rather flat (Fig. 15). At membrane potentials of -50 mV (the natural resting potential) and more negative levels, the maximum dV/dt reached a plateau value of *ca.* 5 V/sec. Similar rates have been observed in a number of other smooth muscles. For excitable membranes, these are very low rates, an observation that suggests that sodium (or calcium) channels are rather sparse in the cell membrane of the myometrial and other smooth myocytes. On action of oxytocin, the curve was steepened and shifted toward more positive voltages. Thus, at the natural resting potential, the maximum dV/dt was nearly doubled. On the basis of this evidence, Kleinhaus and I (Kleinhaus and Kao, 1969) proposed that the action of oxytocin on the pregnant rabbit myometrium was to increase the number of openable sodium channels. By such a mechanism, all the observed electrophysiological actions of oxytocin could be explained. The increased spike amplitude would be a direct result. The initiation of spike activity and the increase in the number of bursts and spike discharges can be explained by an

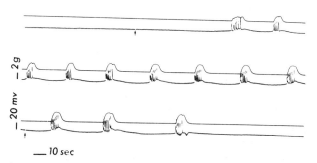

Figure 14. Initiation of electrical and mechanical activities by oxytocin. Continuous sucrose-gap record; 30-day pregnant myometrium, interplacental preparation; quiescent preparation. At the arrow in the top row, 500 μU oxytocin/ml was introduced. One minute later, spikes were initiated in a characteristic burst pattern. Individual spikes increased from six in the first burst to 12 in the ninth burst (end of second row). The membrane potential gave characteristic swinging long-period fluctuations but no lasting depolarization. At the arrow in the third row, oxytocin was removed. Note the progressive decrease in the number of individual spikes in each burst and the lengthening of the interval between bursts. The membrane potential after oxytocin and at maximal negativity between bursts was the same as before oxytocin. Top traces in each row are contractile activity. The force of contraction is directly related to the number of spikes in each burst. From Kleinhaus and Kao (1969).

Figure 15. Relationship between maximum rate of rise of spikes and resting potential. Recordings were made on single rabbit myometrial cells in a strip of longitudinal myometrium with intracellular microelectrodes. The maximum rate of rise is an indication of total membrane current. In an untreated preparation, the maximum rate of rise is about 5 V/sec. Treatment with oxytocin, while not altering the resting potential, significantly increased the maximum rate of rise and steepened the relationship, suggesting that oxytocin increased the number of openable channels for early current. Other details in text. From Kleinhaus and Kao (1969).

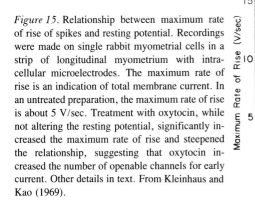

increased probability of successful spikes arising out of pacemaker potentials that, in the absence of oxytocin, would have been abortive.

The oxytocin effect of increasing spike amplitude has been confirmed for the rat myometrium (Chamley and Parkington, 1984). This working hypothesis has been tested on a voltage-clamped multicellular myometrial preparation (Mironneau, 1976). An increased initial inward current was observed, which would be consistent with opening of more channels under the influence of oxytocin. However, with the recent advances in studies of the ionic channels of mammalian smooth muscles, the working hypothesis should be tested more thoroughly.

An interesting detail of oxytocin action requires some comment because of its controversial nature and uncritical citation in a standard reference (Marshall, 1974). In conjunction with his progesterone block hypothesis, Csapo (1961) proposed that the action of oxytocin was voltage dependent. If the membrane potential was more negative to the spike threshold, oxytocin would have a depolarizing action, taking the membrane potential to the spike threshold and producing activity. Such a condition would exist in the myometrium of the term uterus. If the membrane potential were highly negative, as in midpregnancy, then oxytocin would be ineffective, because it could not depolarize the membrane enough to reach spike threshold. If the membrane potential were slightly less negative to the spike threshold, as might be produced experimentally by lowering $[Ca^{2+}]_o$, oxytocin would be effective because it could reverse its depolarizing action by repolarizing the membrane potential to the spike threshold (Kuriyama and Csapo, 1961). However, if the membrane potential were considerably less negative than the spike threshold, as might exist in immature and spayed animals, then oxytocin would be ineffective because it could not repolarize enough to reach spike threshold. Out of these observations came the conclusion that a prerequisite for oxytocin to be effective is that the membrane potential must be close to the spike threshold (Marshall, 1974).

The idea that oxytocin can be depolarizing as well as repolarizing, both towards some assumed spike threshold, is simplistic and apparently based on a misapplication of the concept of reversal potential in some ligand-gated ionic channel (see Katz, 1966). It is unclear what combination of ionic selectivities and equilibrium potentials in the myometrial cell would lead to a reversal potential of around -40 mV, the presumed spike threshold, for serious supporting evidence for that hypothesis simply does not exist. As stated before, the depolarizing actions of oxytocin were observed only with unphysiologically high doses of oxytocin and not when microunit ranges of oxytocin were used (Kleinhaus and Kao, 1969; Osa and Taga, 1973; Mironneau, 1976; Chamley and Parkington, 1984). The alleged repolarizing action of oxytocin, produced in media containing lowered $[Ca^{2+}]_o$, could not be reproduced by Kleinhaus and Kao (1969). Moreover, rabbit myometrium slightly depolarized either by slight elevation of $[K^+]_o$ or by K^+-free media responded readily to oxytocin with increased spike discharges without any observable changes in existing resting potential (Kleinhaus and Kao, 1969). Similarly, in the rat myometrium depolarized with excess $[K^+]_o$, oxytocin did not have any repolarizing action (Marshall, 1968).

Considerably less information is available on the actions of other oxytocic drugs, but ergonovine, ergotamine, and sparteine all increased the frequency of spike discharges in a manner similar to that of oxytocin (Kleinhaus, 1968).

3.5.2. Autonomic Drugs

Most uteri respond with some depolarization or increased spike discharges to acetylcholine and more stable choline esters such as methacholine (Kleinhaus, 1968) and carbachol (Osa and Taga, 1973).

The responses to adrenergic agents are variable and depend on both the species and the hormonal state. In some species such as the rabbit, epinephrine or norepinephrine caused spike discharges and contractions (Kleinhaus, 1968). In other species such as the rat, these agents caused a hyperpolarization, cessation of spike discharges, and relaxation (Marshall, 1974). In still others, such as the cat, epinephrine caused a contraction in the nongravid state and relaxation in the gravid state.

Some comments will be made on the hyperpolarizing action of catecholamines on the rat myometrium. A similar phenomenon occurs in an intestinal muscle, the guinea pig taenia coli. From some current-clamp experiments, Bülbring and Tomita (1969) suggested that epinephrine specifically increased K^+ conductance, thereby moving the membrane potential towards E_K, which is more negative. In voltage-clamp studies of multicellular preparations of both the rat myometrium and the guinea pig taenia coli, however, no conductance changes could be detected (Kao et al., 1976). In fact, Magaribuchi and Osa (1971), using the Abe–Tomita constant-current method on the mouse myometrium, had already found that catecholamines shifted the current–voltage relationship of the myometrium in a parallel way (i.e., same conductance) towards more negative membrane potentials. In our voltage-clamp studies, in place of a conductance change, there was a change in the electromotive force of K^+, with the potassium equilibrium potential (E_K) becoming about 15 mV more negative. Chemical analysis of myometrial strips showed an increase in $[K^+]_i$ of about 20 mmole/liter of cell water, an amount that is consonant with the increase in the E_K. The hyperpolarizing effect of catecholamine is mediated through the β-adrenergic receptor because it can be blocked by β-adrenergic blockers (Kao et al., 1976; Magaribuchi and Osa, 1971) and because phenylephrine, an α-adrenergic agent, has no such effect (Kao et al., 1976).

The implication of our observations is that for smooth muscles with small individual cells, electrical changes can be produced by alternative routes to biophysical actions on the membrane, such as by biochemical and metabolic changes resulting in changes in ionic concentrations. Suggested in 1976, the proposal was considered radical, and the work was not even cited in a recent review (Bülbring and Tomita, 1987). However, in view of recent studies on the relationship between protein phosphorylation and ionic channel functions in many other excitable membranes (Levitan, 1985), the entire question of the catecholamine hyperpolarization of mammalian smooth muscles deserves a reexamination with newer techniques.

3.5.3. Prostaglandins

Descriptive accounts of the actions of the prostaglandins E and F on the isolated myometrium abound, no doubt because of their clinical usefulness. However, because these accounts were based mostly on effects on the resting potential and spontaneous action potentials, they are not directly informative about the underlying mechanism(s) of action. In low doses, PGE_2 and $PGF_{2\alpha}$ increased the frequency of burst and spike discharges without any depolarization, but in higher doses depolarization was prominent (Osa et al., 1974; Reiner and

Marshall, 1976). By eliciting action potentials in the circular myometrial layer of the rat, Chamley and Parkington (1984) found that $PGF_{2\alpha}$ increased the amplitude and the duration of the plateau of the action potential without much significant effect on the spike portion. If the calcium influx during an action potential in a myometrial cell is similar to that in the taenia myocyte (see Section 3.2.4a and Yamamoto et al., 1988b), then the prolonged plateau would indeed provide more calcium for contraction. What remain to be clarified are the ionic channel activities underlying the plateau.

The prostaglandin PGE_1 is often described as reducing myometrial tension. In the pregnant rat myometrium, it did not affect the resting and action potentials (Osa and Kuriyama, 1975), but in a double sucrose-gap study, Grosset and Mironneau (1977) found that it reduced the duration of the action potential. In the voltage-clamped rat myometrial bundle, it did not affect the magnitude of the calcium current or its inactivation properties. All of these changes in electrical properties of the membrane were accompanied by a marked increase in contractile force. In view of the seemingly incongruous observations of the electrical and mechanical consequences, Grosset and Mironneau (1977) proposed that PGE_1 increased the intracellular calcium concentration by translocation from membrane-bound microvesicles. Clearly, this is a default conclusion propelled by negative results that require more work.

4. Summary and Concluding Remarks

As in all mammalian tissues, the myometrial cell has a high concentration of potassium and a low concentration of sodium intracellulary. Compared with those of skeletal and cardiac muscles, the intracellular concentrations of sodium and chloride in the myometrium are higher. The distribution of chloride between the intracellular and extracellular phases does not appear to be passive but may involve some active accumulation mechanism.

The resting potential of the myometrial cell is about 50 mV inside negative. It is influenced by some permeability of the membrane to sodium and most probably also to chloride. The resting potential of myometrium deprived of estrogenic stimulation is low, and administration of estrogens causes an increase of the resting potential to -50 mV. There is some question whether additional treatment with progesterone further increases the resting potential.

The characteristic action potentials of the myometrium appear as irregular bursts of spikes. Two types of pacemaker activities set the pattern of excitation: one, of a periodicity on the order of tens of seconds, initiates the burst discharges; the other, of a periodicity in the range of 0.5–1 sec, controls the number of individual spikes in each burst. Direct in situ recordings from women in labor confirm many of the observations made on experimental animals. The bursts determine the frequency of ''contractions'' in clinical practice, and the number of individual spikes in each burst, by causing partially summated contractions, influence the force of the contractions. The forms of the spikes are usually complex because of asynchronous discharges of neighboring cells; at parturition they become synchronous and simple. The improved synchronization is now attributed in part to the apparance of gap junctions between myometrial cells.

Voltage-clamp studies on mammalian smooth muscles have now progressed to the stage of studies on single myocytes and single ionic channels. However, there is as yet no published work on the freshly isolated myometrial cell. By analogy with observations made on an intestinal myocyte, the newer information on single cells has confirmed much of that obtained on small multicellular preparations. In the myometrium, the initial inward current apparently is carried by both Na^+ and Ca^{2+}, with a possibility that their relative contributions vary at different stages of pregnancy. The outward current is mediated by efflux of K^+. In the model cell used for analogy, the myocyte of the guinea pig taenia coli, the inward current is carried entirely by Ca^{2+}, and single-channel recordings show that there are two types of Ca^{2+} channels. In the taenia myocyte, three types of K^+ channels have been observed, but only one, a Ca^{2+}-activated K^+ channel with a unit conductance of 150 pS, has been shown to be involved closely in known physiological functions. It is believed to be responsible for the macroscopic current for repolarization of the action potential and important in the regulation of the resting potential.

Oxytocin is capable of initiating spike discharges in quiescent myometrial preparations and of increasing the frequency of burst discharges as well as prolonging the duration of each burst. It also can increase the amplitude of spikes. The maximum rate of rise of the action potential of the myometrium cell is rather low but can be increased by the action of oxytoxin. The relationship between the maximum rate of rise and the resting potential is steepened by oxytocin and shifted toward more positive levels. This mechanism is believed to be capable of explaining the electrophysiological actions of oxytocin.

Although some progress was made in the last decade in studies of the ionic channels of the myometrial and other mammalian smooth muscle cells, hopes of advances were largely unrealized because of exaggerated criticisms of voltage-clamp studies of multicellular preparations. Now that voltage-clamp studies on single cells and single channels have confirmed observations on multicellular preparations and made other studies possible, it is to be hoped that real strides can henceforth be made toward better understanding of the properties of ionic channels in smooth muscles.

ACKNOWLEDGMENTS. All work from my laboratory, published or unpublished, was supported by a grant from the National Institute of Child Health and Human Development (HD00378).

5. References

Abe, Y., and Tomita, T., 1968, Cable properties of smooth muscles, *J. Physiol. (Lond.)* **196**:87–100.

Anderson, N. C., 1969, Voltage clamp studies on uterine smooth muscle, *J. Gen. Physiol.* **54**:145–165.

Anderson, N. C., 1976, Membrane potential oscillations in smooth muscle, in: *Smooth Muscle Pharmacology and Physiology* (M. Worcel and G. Vassort, eds.), Institute Nationale de la Santé et de la Recherche Medicale, Paris, pp. 113–124.

Anderson, N. C., and Ramon, F. C., 1972, Transient current inactivation in uterine smooth muscle, *Fed. Proc.* **31**:829.

Anderson, N. C., and Ramon, F. C., 1976, Interaction between pacemaker electrical behavior and action potential mechanism in uterine smooth muscle, in: *Physiology of Smooth Muscle* (E. Bülbring and M. F. Shuba, eds.), Raven Press, New York, pp. 53–63.

Anderson, N. C., Ramon, F. C., and Snyder, A., 1971, Studies in calcium and sodium in uterine smooth muscle excitation under current-clamp and voltage-clamp conditions, *J. Gen. Physiol.* **58**:322–339.

Berde, B. (ed.), 1968, *Handbook of Experimental Pharmacology,* Vol. 23, *Neurohypophyseal Hormones and Similar Polypeptides,* Springer-Verlag, Berlin.

Bolton, T. B., 1975, Effects of stimulating the acetylcholine receptor on the current–voltage relationship of the smooth muscle membrane studied by voltage clamp of potential recorded by microelectrode, *J. Physiol. (Lond.)* **250**:175–202.

Bolton, T. B., Tomita, T., and Vassort, G., 1981, Voltage clamp and the measurement of ionic conductances in smooth muscle, in: *Smooth Muscles: An Assessment of Current Knowledge* (E. Bülbring, A. F. Brading, A. W. Jones, and T. Tomita, eds.), Edward Arnold, London, pp. 47–63.

Bozler, E., 1947, The response of smooth muscle to stretch, *Am. J. Physiol.* **149**:299–301.

Brading, A. F., and Jones, A. W., 1969, Distribution and kinetics of CoEDTA in smooth muscle, and its use as an extracellular marker, *J. Physiol. (Lond.)* **200**:387–401.

Brading, A. F., Bülbring, E., and Tomita, T., 1969, The effect of sodium and calcium on the action potential of the smooth muscle of the guinea-pig taenia coli, *J. Physiol. (Lond.)* **200**:637–654.

Brinley, F. J., 1980, Excitation and conduction in nerve fibers, in: *Medical Physiology* (V. B. Mountcastle, ed.), C. V. Mosby, St. Louis, pp. 46–81.

Bülbring, E., and Kuriyama, H., 1963, Effects of changes in external sodium and calcium concentration on spontaneous electrical activity in guinea-pig taenia coli, *J. Physiol. (Lond.)* **166:**29–58.

Bülbring, E., and Tomita, T., 1969, Increase of membrane conductance by adrenaline in the smooth muscle of the guinea-pig taenia coli, *Proc. R. Soc. Lond. [Biol.]* **172:**89–102.

Bülbring, E., and Tomita, T., 1987, Catecholamine action on smooth muscle, *Pharmacol. Rev.* **39:**49–96.

Burnstock, G., Holman, M. E., and Prosser, C. L., 1963, Electrophysiology of smooth muscle, *Physiol. Rev.* **43:**482–527.

Casteels, R., 1970, The relation between the membrane potential and the ion distribution in smooth muscle cells, in: *Smooth Muscle* (E. Bülbring, A. F. Brading, A. W. Jones, and T. Tomita, eds.), Williams & Wilkins, Baltimore, pp. 70–99.

Casteels, R., and Kuriyama, H., 1965, Membrane potential and ionic content in pregnant and non-pregnant rat myometrium, *J. Physiol. (Lond.)* **177:**263–287.

Chamley, W. A., and Parkington, H. C., 1984, Relaxin inhibits the plateau component of the action potential in the circular myometrium of the rat, *J. Physiol. (Lond.)* **353:**51–65.

Csapo, A. I., 1956, The relation of threshold to the K gradient in the myometrium, *J. Physiol. (Lond.)* **133:**145–158.

Csapo, A. I., 1961, Defence mechanism of pregnancy, in: *Progesterone and the Defence Mechanism of Pregnancy* (G. E. W. Wolstenholme and M. A. Cameron, eds.), Little, Brown, Boston, pp. 3–31.

Csapo, A. I., and Kuriyama, H., 1963, Effects of ions and drugs on cell membrane activity and tension in the postpartum rat myometrium, *J. Physiol. (Lond.)* **165:**575–592.

Csapo, A. I., and Takeda, H., 1965, Effect of progesterone on the electrical activity and intrauterine pressure of pregnant and parturient rabbits, *Am. J. Obstet. Gynecol.* **91:**221–321.

Csapo, A. I., Takeda, H., and Wood, C., 1963, Volume and activity of the parturient rabbit uterus, *Am. J. Obstet. Gynecol.* **85:**813–818.

Daniel, E. E., 1958, Smooth muscle electrolytes, *Can. J. Biochem. Physiol.* **36:**805–818.

Daniel, E. E., and Daniel, B. N., 1957, Effects of ovarian hormones on the content and distribution of cation in intact and extracted rabbit and cat uterus, *Can. J. Biochem. Physiol.* **35:**1205–1223.

Daniel, E. E., and Singh, H., 1958, The electrical properties of the smooth muscle cell membrane, *Can. J. Biochem. Physiol.* **36:**959–975.

Demianczuk, N., Towell, M. E., and Garfield, R. E., 1984, Myometrial electrophysiologic activity and gap junctions in the pregnant rabbit, *Am. J. Obstet. Gynecol.* **149:**485–491.

Dewey, M. M., and Barr, L., 1964, A study of the structure and distribution of the nexus, *J. Cell Biol.* **23:**553–585.

Eisenberg, R. S., and Johnson, E. A., 1970, Three-dimensional electric field problems in physiology, *Prog. Biophys. Mol. Biol.* **20:**1–65.

Garfield, R. E., Sims, S., and Daniel, E. E., 1977, Gap junctions: Their presence and necessity in myometrium during parturition, *Science* **198:**958–960.

Goto, M., 1960, The effects of oxytocin on the transmembrane potential of the rat myometrium, *Jpn. J. Physiol.* **10:**427–435.

Goto, M., and Csapo, A. I., 1959, The effect of the ovarian steroids on the membrane potential of the uterine muscle, *J. Gen. Physiol.* **43:**455–466.

Grosset, A., and Mironneau, J., 1977, An analysis of the actions of prostaglandin E_1 on membrane currents and contraction in uterine smooth muscle, *J. Physiol. (Lond.)* **270:**765–784.

Hamill, O. P., Marty, A., Neher, E., Sakmann, B., and Sigworth, F. J., 1981, Improved patch-clamp techniques for high-resolution current recording from cells and cell-free membrane patches, *Pflugers Arch.* **391:**85–100.

Hille, B., 1984, *Ionic Channels of Excitable Membranes,* Sinauer Associates, Sunderland, MA.

Hodgkin, A. L., 1951, The ionic basis of electrical activity in nerve and muscle, *Biol. Rev.* **26:**339–409.

Hodgkin, A. L., 1964, *The Conduction of the Nerve Impulse,* Charles C. Thomas, Springfield, IL.

Hodgkin, A. L., and Horowicz, P., 1959, The influence of potassium and chloride on the membrane potential of a single muscle fiber, *J. Physiol. (Lond.)* **148:**127–160.

Hodgkin, A. L., and Huxley, A. F., 1952, A quantitative description of membrane current and its application to conduction and excitation in nerve, *J. Physiol. (Lond.)* **116:**424–448.

Hodgkin, A. L., Huxley, A. F., and Katz, B., 1952, Measurement of current voltage relations in the membranes of the giant axon of *Loligo*, *J. Physiol. (Lond.)* **136:**569–584.

Holman, M. E., 1957, The effect of changes in sodium chloride concentration on the smooth muscle of the guinea pig's taenia coli, *J. Physiol. (Lond.)* **136:**569–584.

Horvath, B., 1954, Ovarian hormones and the ionic balance of uterine muscle, *Proc. Natl. Acad. Sci. U.S.A.* **40:**515–521.

Hu, S. L., Yamamoto, Y., and Kao, C. Y., 1988a, The Ca^{2+}-activated K^+ channel and its functional roles in smooth muscle cells of guinea-pig taenia coli, *J. Gen. Physiol.* (in press).

Hu, S. L., Yamamoto, Y., and Kao, C. Y., 1988b, Permeation, selectivity, and blockade of the Ca^{2+}-activated K^+ channel of the guinea-pig taenia coli myocyte, *J. Gen. Physiol.* (in press).

Inomata, H., and Kao, C. Y., 1976, Ionic currents in the guinea pig taenia coli, *J. Physiol. (Lond.)* **255**:347–378.

Inomata, H., and Kao, C. Y., 1979, Ionic mechanisms of repolarization in guinea-pig taenia coli as revealed by the actions of Sr^{2+}, *J. Physiol. (Lond.)* **297**:443–462.

Inomata, H., and Kao, C. Y., 1985, Actions of Ba^{2+} on ionic currents of the guinea-pig taenia coli, *J. Pharmacol. Exp. Ther.* **233**:112–124.

Jack, J. J. B., Noble, D., and Tsien, R. W., 1974, *Electric Current Flow in Excitable Cells,* Clarendon, Oxford.

Johnson, E. A., and Lieberman, M., 1971, Heart: Excitation and contraction, *Annu. Rev. Physiol.* **33**:479–532.

Jung, H., 1955, Aktionspotentiale am schwangeren und nicht schwangeren Uterus, *Pfluegers Arch. Ges. Physiol.* **262**:13–22.

Jung, H., 1957, Über den Wirkungsmechanismus des Oxytocins, *Arch. Gynaekol.* **190**:194–206.

Jung, H., 1961, Zur Erregungsphysiologishen Steuerung des Uterusmuskels durch Oestradiol, Oestrone, und Oestriol, *Klin. Wochenschr.* **39**:1169–1174.

Jung, H., 1964, Die Wirkung der Ovarial- und der Placentar-Hormone, in: *Pharmacology of Smooth Muscle* (E. Bülbring, ed.), Macmillan, New York, pp. 113–126.

Kao, C. Y., 1959, Long-term observations of spontaneous electrical activity of the uterine smooth muscle, *Am. J. Physiol.* **196**:343–350.

Kao, C. Y., 1961, Contents and distribution of potassium, sodium and chloride in uterine smooth muscle, *Am. J. Physiol.* **201**:717–722.

Kao, C. Y., 1966, Tetrodotoxin, saxitoxin, and their significance in the study of excitation phenomena, *Pharmacol. Rev.* **18**:997–1049.

Kao, C. Y., 1967, Ionic basis of electrical activity in uterine smooth muscle, in: *Cellular Biology of the Uterus* (R. M. Wynn, ed.), Appleton–Century–Crofts, New York, pp. 386–448.

Kao, C. Y., 1977, Electrophysiological properties of the uterine smooth muscle, in: *Biology of the Uterus* (R. M. Wynn, ed.), Plenum Press, New York, pp. 423–496.

Kao, C. Y., 1978, A calcium current in the rat myometrium, *Jpn. J. Smooth Muscle Res.* (Suppl.) **14**:9–10.

Kao, C. Y., and Levinson, S. R. (eds.), 1986, Tetrodotoxin, saxitoxin, and the molecular biology of the sodium channel, *Ann. N.Y. Acad. Sci.* **479**:1–448.

Kao, C. Y., and McCullough, J. R., 1975, Ionic currents in the uterine smooth muscle, *J. Physiol. (Lond.)* **246**:1–36.

Kao, C. Y., and Nishiyama, A., 1964, Ovarian hormones and resting potentials of uterine smooth muscle, *Am. J. Physiol.* **207**:793–799.

Kao, C. Y., and Siegman, M. J., 1963, Nature of electrolyte exchange in isolated uterine smooth muscle, *Am. J. Physiol.* **205**:674–680.

Kao, C. Y., Inomata, H., McCullough, J. R., and Yuan, J. C., 1976, Voltage clamp studies of the actions of catecholamines and adrenergic blocking agents on mammalian smooth muscles, in: *Smooth Muscle Pharmacology and Physiology* (M. Worcel and G. Vassort, eds.), Institute National de la Santé et de la Recherche Medicale, Paris, pp. 165–176.

Katz, B., 1966, *Nerve, Muscle, and Synapse,* McGraw-Hill, New York.

Kirber, M. T., Singer, J. J., and Walsh, J. V., 1987, Stretch-activated channels in freshly dissociated smooth muscle cells, *Biophys. J.* **51**:252a.

Kleinhaus, A. L., 1968, *Electrophysiological actions of oxytocic drugs,* Ph.D. thesis, State University of New York Downstate Medical Center, Brooklyn, NY.

Kleinhaus, A. L., and Kao, C. Y., 1969, Electrophysiological actions of oxytocin on the rabbit myometrium, *J. Gen. Physiol.* **53**:758–780.

Klöckner, U., and Isenberg, G., 1985, Action potentials and net membrane currents of isolated smooth muscle cells (urinary bladder of the guinea pig), *Pfluegers Arch.* **405**:329–339.

Kuriyama, H., 1961, The effect of progesterone and oxytocin on the mouse myometrium, *J. Physiol. (Lond.)* **159**:26–39.

Kuriyama, H., and Csapo, A. I., 1961, A study of the parturient uterus with the microelectrode technique, *Endocrinology* **68**:1010–1025.

Levitan, I. B., 1985, Phosphorylation of ion channels, *J. Membr. Biol.* **87**:177–190.

Ling, G. N., and Gerard, R. W., 1949, The normal membrane potential of frog sartorius muscle, *J. Cell. Comp. Physiol.* **34**:383–396.

Magaribuchi, T., and Osa, T., 1971, Effect of catecholamines on electrical and mechanical activities of the pregnant mouse myometrium, *Jpn. J. Physiol.* **21**:627–643.

Marshall, J. M., 1959, Effects of estrogen and progesterone on single uterine muscle fiber in the rat, *Am. J. Physiol.* **194**:935–942.

Marshall, J. M., 1962, Regulation of activity in uterine smooth muscle, *Physiol. Rev.* **42**(Suppl. 5):213–227.

Marshall, J. M., 1963, Behavior of uterine muscle in Na^+-deficient solutions: Effect of oxytocin, *Am. J. Physiol.* **204**:732–738.

Marshall, J. M., 1968, Relation between the ionic environment and the action of drugs on the myometrium, *Fed. Proc.* **27**:115–119.

Marshall, J. M., 1974, Effect of neurohypophyseal hormones on the myometrium, in: *Handbook of Physiology,* Sect. 7 *Endocrinology,* Vol. IV, Part I, American Physiological Society, Bethesda, MD. pp. 469–492.

Marshall, J. M., and Csapo, A. I., 1961, Hormonal and ionic influences on the membrane activity of uterine smooth muscle cells, *Endocrinology* **68**:1026–1035.

Marshall, J. M., and Miller, M. D., 1964, Effects of metabolic inhibitors on the rat uterus and on its response to oxytocin, *Am. J. Physiol.* **206**:437–443.

McClesky, E. W., Fox, A. P., Feldman, D., and Tsien, R. W., 1986, Different types of calcium channels, *J. Exp. Biol.* **124**:177–190.

Melton, C. E., and Saldivar, J. T., 1964, Impulse velocity and conduction pathways in rat myometrium, *Am. J. Physiol.* **207**:279–285.

Mironneau, J., 1974, Voltage clamp analysis of the ionic currents in uterine smooth muscle using the double sucrose gap method, *Pfluegers Arch.* **352**:197–210.

Mironneau, J., 1976, Effects of oxytocin on ionic currents underlying rhythmic activity and contraction in uterine smooth muscle, *Pfluegers Arch.* **363**:113–118.

Mollard, P., Mironneau, J., Amedee, T., and Mironneau, C., 1986, Electrophysiological characterization of single pregnant myometrial cells in short-term primary culture, *Am. J. Physiol.* **250**:C47–C54.

Nakai, Y., and Kao, C. Y., 1983, Changing properties of Na^+ and Ca^{2+} components of the early inward current in the rat myometrium during pregnancy, *Fed. Proc.* **42**:313.

Osa, T., 1971, Effect of removing the external sodium on the electrical and mechanical activities of the pregnant mouse myometrium, *Jpn. J. Physiol.* **21**:607–625.

Osa, T., 1974, An interaction between the electrical activities of longitudinal and circular smooth muscles of pregnant mouse uterus, *Jpn. J. Physiol.* **24**:189–203.

Osa, T., and Katase, T., 1975, Physiological comparison of the longitudinal and circular muscles of the pregnant rat uterus, *Jpn. J. Physiol.* **25**:153–164.

Osa, T., and Kuriyama, H., 1975, Electrophysiological and mechanical investigations on the dual action of prostaglandin E, in the pregnant rat myometrium *in vitro, Jpn. J. Physiol.* **25**:357–369.

Osa, T., and Taga, F., 1973, Effects of external Na and Ca on the mouse myometrium in relation to the effects of oxytocin and carbachol, *Jpn. J. Physiol.* **23**:97–112.

Osa, T., Suzuki, H., Katase, T., and Kuriyama, H., 1974, Excitatory action of synthetic prostaglandin E_2 on the electrical activity of pregnant mouse myometrium in relation to temperature changes and external sodium and calcium concentrations, *Jpn. J. Physiol.* **24**:233–248.

Parkington, H. C., 1985, Some properties of the circular myometrium of the sheep throughout pregnancy and during labor, *J. Physiol. (Lond.)* **359**:1–15.

Reiner, O., and Marshall, J. M., 1976, Action of progstaglandin $PGF_{2\alpha}$ on the uterus of the pregnant rat, *Pfluegers Arch.* **292**:243–250.

Reimar, J., Mayer, C. J., and Ulbrecht, G., 1974, Determination of membrane potential in smooth muscle cells using microelectrodes with reduced tip potentials, *Eur. J. Physiol.* **349**:267–275.

Sakaguchi, M., and Nakajima, A., 1973, Electromyogram of the human uterus in labor, *J. Appl. Physiol.* **35**:423–426.

Sims, S. M., Daniel, E. E., and Garfield, R. E., 1982, Improved electrical coupling in uterine smooth muscle is associated with increased numbers of gap junctions at parturition, *J. Gen. Physiol.* **80**:353–375.

Smith, T. G., Lecar, H., Redman, S. J., and Gage, P. W. (eds.), 1985, *Voltage and Patch Clamping with Microelectrodes,* American Physiology Society, Washington.

Specht, P. C., 1976, Phase-plane analysis of action potentials in uterine smooth muscle, *Eur. J. Physiol.* **367**:89–95.

Stämpfli, R., 1954, A new method for measuring membrane potentials with external electrodes, *Experientia* **10**:508–509.

Stefani, E., Toro, L., and Erulkar, S. D., 1988, Calcium currents in single uterine smooth muscle cells, *Biophys. J.* **53**:553a.

Vassort, G., 1975, Voltage-clamp analysis of transmembrane ionic currents in guinea-pig myometrium: Evidence for an initial potassium activation triggered by calcium influx, *J. Physiol. (Lond.)* **252**:713–734.

Walsh, J. V., and Singer, J. J., 1980, Calcium action potentials in single freshly isolated smooth muscle cells, *Am. J. Physiol.* **239**:C162–174.

Walsh, J. V., and Singer, J. J., 1987, Identification and characterization of major ionic currents in isolated smooth muscle cells using the voltage-clamp technique, *Pfluegers Arch.* **408**:83–97.

Wolfs, G., and Rottinghuis, H., 1970, Electrical and mechanical activity of the human uterus during labor, *Arch. Gynaekol.* **208**:375–385.

Wolfs, G. M. J. A., and van Leeuwen, M., 1979, Electromyographic observations on the human uterus during labor, *Acta Obstet. Gynecol. Scand. [Suppl.]* **90**:1–62.

Yamamoto, Y., Hu, S. L., and Kao, C. Y., 1988a, Demonstration of multiple types of calcium channels in smooth muscle cells of the guinea-pig taenia coli, *Biophys. J.* **53**:594a.

Yamamoto, Y., Hu, S. L., and Kao, C. Y., 1988b, The inward current in single smooth muscle cells of the guinea-pig taenia coli, *J. Gen. Physiol.* (in press).

Yamamoto, Y., Hu, S. L., and Kao, C. Y., 1988c, The outward current in single smooth muscle cells of the guinea-pig taenia coli, *J. Gen. Physiol.* (in press).

Yoshino, M., and Yabu, H., 1985, Single Ca channel currents in mammalian visceral smooth muscle cells, *Pfluegers Arch.* **404**:285–286.

Yoshino, M., Someya, T., Nishio, A., and Yabu, H., 1988, Whole-cell and unitary Ca channel currents in mammalian intestinal smooth muscle cells: Evidence for the existence of two types of Ca channels, *Pfluegers Arch.* **411**:229–231.

15

Ultrastructure of the Myometrium

W. C. COLE and R. E. GARFIELD

The concept that a well-developed appreciation of structure is an essential prerequisite to an understanding of function permeates research into all physical processes but is especially true for the biological sciences. The electron microscopic and x-ray diffraction studies conducted on the myometrium during the past 25 years have provided important insights into the physiology of this organ. This chapter reviews our understanding of the ultrastructure of the myometrium. Particular emphasis is placed on the development and functional significance of gap junctions between myometrial cells, a topic not covered in previous editions of this book because of its relatively recent development. We believe that the observation that gap junctions appear in large numbers between myometrial cells during the onset and progression of labor (Garfield *et al.*, 1977) was a major step forward in our understanding of the circumstances that control parturition. We also provide a detailed description of the structure of the contractile apparatus and its relationship to the plasma membrane and cytoskeleton. Several important observations have been made in this area since the last edition of this book.

1. Cellular Organization of the Myometrium

The myometrium is composed of smooth muscle cells, fibroblasts, nerves, and blood vessels that lie in an extracellular matrix containing large numbers of collagen fibers and lesser numbers of elastic fibers. An outer layer of longitudinally oriented smooth muscle cells is

W. C. COLE ● Division of Cardiovascular Sciences, St. Boniface Research Institute, Department of Physiology, University of Manitoba, Winnipeg, Manitoba R2H 2A6, Canada.   R. E. GARFIELD ● Departments of Neurosciences and Obstetrics and Gynecology, McMaster University, Health Sciences, Hamilton, Ontario L8N 3Z5, Canada.

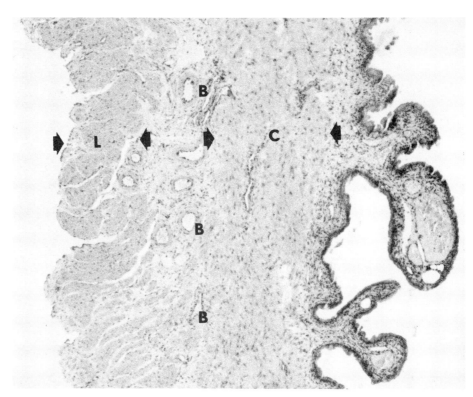

Figure 1. Light micrograph of a cross section through the uterine wall from a pregnant rat. Note the thickness of the smooth muscle layers indicated by arrows (longitudinal, L, and circular, C) as well as the vascular plexus containing blood vessels (B) between the layers (×75). From Garfield *et al.* (1988), with permission.

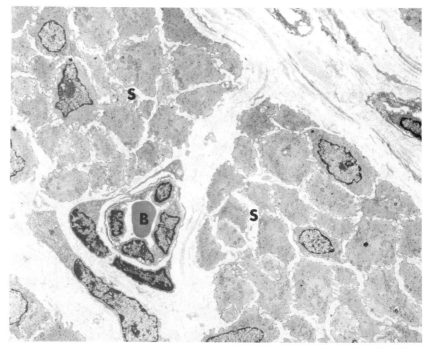

Figure 2. Electron micrograph of a cross section through the longitudinal myometrium of a rabbit, illustrating two bundles of smooth muscle cell (S) and a blood vessel (B) (×3000) From Garfield (1984), with permission.

separated from an inner, circular layer of more transversely oriented muscle cells by an extensive vascular and nerve plexus (Figs. 1 and 2). Small arterioles exit on either side of this plexus to form networks of capillaries, which penetrate into and feed the muscle layers. Axons containing varicosities follow the arterioles and capillaries into the interior of the muscle layers. Most of the fibers remain associated with the blood vessels and are likely to be involved in control of blood flow to the myometrium (Figs. 3 and 4). Some fibers also possess varicosities that are closer to bundles of myometrial cells (Fig. 5). Whether this innervation is important to control of uterine contractility has been debated considerably and dismissed by most authors. However, an indirect influence through control of vascular flow should not be ignored (Garfield, 1986).

The nerve fibers found within the myometrium include adrenergic axons containing small vesicles with small electron-dense cores, cholinergic axons with agranular vesicles, and some fibers containing large dense-cored vesicles with an unknown content (Buchanan and Garfield, 1984; Garfield, 1986). Several recent studies have provided strong evidence for the loss of this innervation to the myometrium during pregnancy (Sporrong et al., 1978; Thorbert, 1979; Wikland et al., 1984; Buchanan and Garfield, 1984; Garfield, 1986). The cause of the

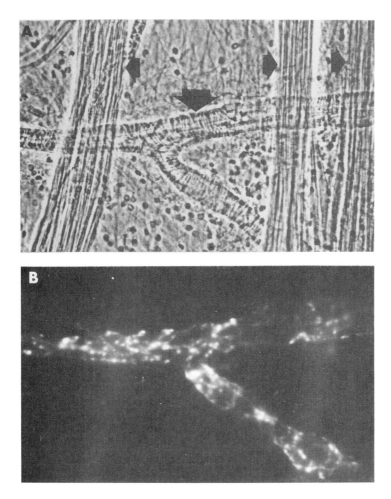

Figure 3. Light micrographs of a whole-mount preparation of the uterine wall. Three bundles of smooth muscle (small arrows) and a branching blood vessel (large arrow) are shown in phase contrast in the upper micrograph (A) (×80). The lower micrograph (B) shows the corresponding fluorescence in the tissues after glyoxylic acid staining for noradrenergic nerves. The fluorescence is most dense surrounding the blood vessel (×80).

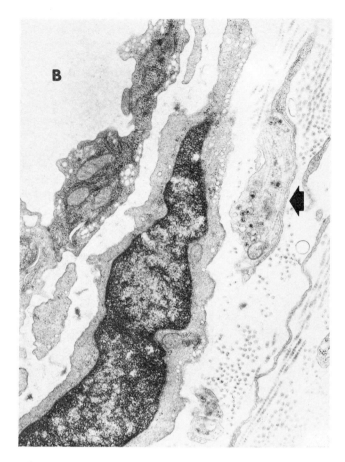

Figure 4. Electron micrograph of a nerve varicosity containing dense-cored vesicles (arrow) next to a blood vessel (B) in rat myometrium (×18,700).

degeneration is unknown, but increased distention caused by fetal growth may be involved (Garfield, 1986).

2. Ultrastructure of Myometrial Smooth Muscle Cells

2.1. Size and Shape

Uterine smooth muscle cells are spindle-shaped, occasionally branching cells ranging in size from 2 to 10 µm in diameter and 200–600 µm in length, depending on the species and hormonal state of the individual (Figs. 6 and 7). The muscle cells are largest during the later stages of pregnancy, primarily because of the stimulatory influence of the steroid hormones and distention caused by fetal growth (Bergman, 1968; Bo *et al.*, 1968; Ross and Klebanoff, 1967). The average volume of a myometrial cell has been estimated at 21,000 µm³ (Csapo, 1962), but this value obviously varies considerably, depending on the age and hormonal state of the individual. A value for the surface area of about 23,000 µm has been calculated on the basis of a surface-to-volume ratio of 0.9 (Garfield and Somlyo, 1985).

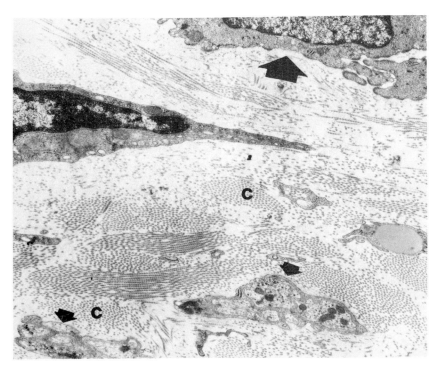

Figure 5. Electron micrograph of nerve varicosities containing dense-cored vesicles (small arrows) near a bundle of smooth muscle (large arrow). Note also the bundles of collagen fibers (C) (×11,500). From Garfield and Somlyo (1985), with permission.

2.2. Organelles

2.2.1. Sarcoplasmic Reticulum

Myometrial smooth muscle cells, like cells in other smooth muscles, have an intracellular system of tubules and flattened cisternae or sacs referred to as sarcoplasmic reticulum (SR) (see Fig. 8 and 9; for a review see A. V. Somlyo, 1980). This system occupies a variable percentage of the volume of the cytoplasm in different types of smooth muscles, ranging from about 2% to over 7% (A. V. Somlyo and Somlyo, 1975; A. P. Somlyo, 1985). The SR in myometrial smooth muscle of pregnant or estrogen-treated animals is among the most extensive (Garfield and Somlyo, 1985). That the SR is a closed system and not continuous with the extracellular space is evident from the fact that extracellular markers such as ferritin, horseradish peroxidase, and lanthanum are excluded from its tubules (A. P. Somlyo, 1985). Moreover, electron microprobe analysis has shown that the content of Na and Cl within SR tubules is the same as that in the cytoplasm and different from that in the extracellular space (Kowarski *et al.*, 1985). As in other cell types, the SR may be divided into smooth and rough varieties based on the absence and presence, respectively, of ribosomes attached to the cytoplasmic surface of the SR membrane. The two varieties of SR differ in function and in their general distribution within myometrial cells, but it is important to note that their tubules are continuous.

The majority of agranular SR tubules may be found just under the plasma membrane (Fig. 8), although they are also present within the interior of the cytoplasm, and a continuity between SR tubules and the nuclear envelope has been described (Gabella, 1981). Devine *et al.* (1972) originally suggested that the SR of smooth muscle has a relationship to the plasma

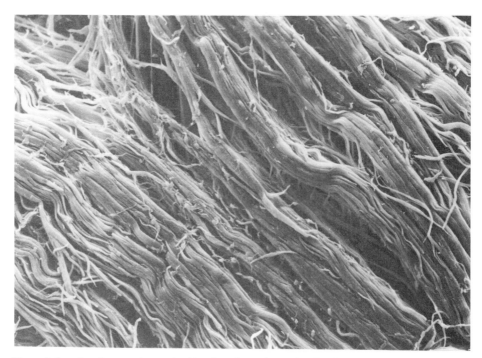

Figure 6. Scanning electron micrograph of bundles of smooth muscle cells. Note the spindle-shaped individual smooth muscle cells (×550). Courtesy of Drs. S. Ward and K. Sanders (unpublished).

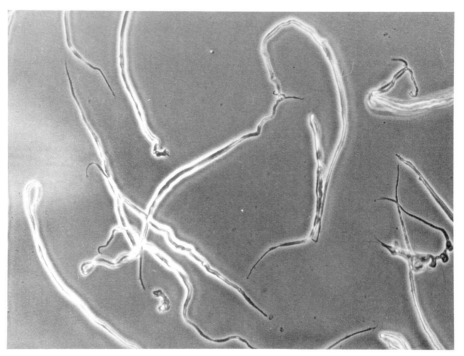

Figure 7. Light micrograph of freshly dispersed, isolated smooth muscle cells (×500). Courtesy of Drs. P. Langton and K. Sanders (unpublished).

membrane similar to that seen in cardiac muscle and in triadic junctions between terminal SR cisternae and T-tubules of skeletal muscle. That is, the SR tubules frequently establish structurally similar close couplings with the plasma membrane (e.g., Somner and Johnson, 1980; Franzini-Armstrong, 1970; A. V. Somlyo, 1979). The SR of smooth muscle also makes close contacts with the caveolae (Fig. 8) and gap junctions of the plasma membrane (Garfield and Somlyo, 1985).

At the sites of contact with the plasma membrane, the 12- to 20-nm space separating the two membranes contains periodically spaced electron-opaque "bridging" structures (A. P. Somlyo et al., 1971; A. V. Somlyo, 1979; A. P. Somlyo, 1985). These structures have been studied in detail in quick-frozen, deep-etched samples of smooth muscle, where they appear as single strands linking the two membranes (see Fig. 4b of A. V. Somlyo and Franzini-Armstrong, 1985). Their function remains unknown, although A. V. Somlyo and Franzini-Armstrong (1985) speculate that they may serve a mechanical function, maintaining the SR and its calcium stores close to the excitable plasma membrane. These authors also describe the presence of a globular material within the lumen of the SR, which they suggest may represent a Ca^{2+}-binding protein.

In a series of studies using a variety of different techniques, Somlyo and Somlyo and their co-workers (A.V. Somlyo and Somlyo, 1971; A.P. Somlyo et al., 1979, 1982; A.V. Somlyo et al., 1981; Bond et al., 1984a,b; Kowarski et al., 1985) have clearly established that the agranular SR of smooth muscle functions as an intracellular storage site for regulating cytoplasmic levels of Ca^{2+} (see A. P. Somlyo, 1984). These studies, and those employing electron probe and electron energy loss analysis in particular, have been reviewed in detail by

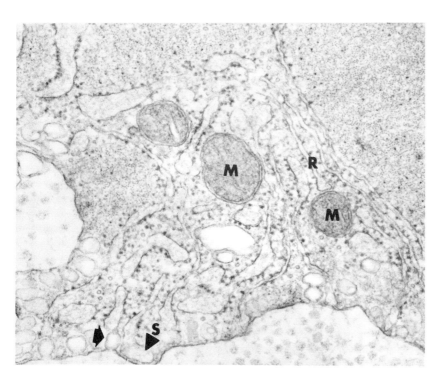

Figure 8. Electron micrograph of a portion of a longitudinal myometrial smooth muscle cell in the uterus of a pregnant guinea pig. Note the continuity between the granular (R) and agranular (S) sarcoplasmic reticulum as well as the close association of these tubules with mitochondria (M) and surface caveolae (arrows) ($\times 37,500$). From Garfield (1984), with permission.

Garfield and Somlyo (1985). Vascular muscle cells analyzed by electron probe methods show high concentrations of Ca^{2+} within the agranular SR (A. P. Somlyo *et al.*, 1977, 1978, 1979) and release of Ca^{2+} from these stores following stimulation by norepinephrine or caffeine (A. P. Somlyo *et al.*, 1982). Moreover, it seems likely that the areas of the SR that show close contact with the plasma membrane may be "hot spots" for uptake and release of Ca^{2+} (Bond *et al.*, 1984a).

The granular SR of smooth muscle is somewhat less abundant than the agranular tubules under most conditions, but it has a markedly increased prominence in estrogen-treated or pregnant myometrial tissues (Garfield and Somlyo, 1985). Presumably, this abundance is related to the synthesis of new extracellular components, most notably collagen, required during pregnancy (Shoenberg, 1978). Granular SR is typically associated with mitochondria and Golgi saccules in the perinuclear poles (Figs. 8–10).

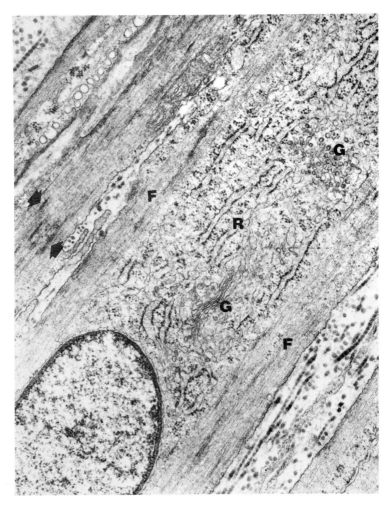

Figure 9. Longitudinal section through the perinuclear region of a myometrial smooth muscle cell. Note the Golgi saccules (G) associated with granular sarcoplasmic reticulum (R) in the polar cap. Myofilaments (F) also can be seen to run longitudinally in the peripheral cytoplasm. Cytoplasmic dense bodies (arrows) are evident in an adjacent cell (×22,000). From Garfield (1984), with permission.

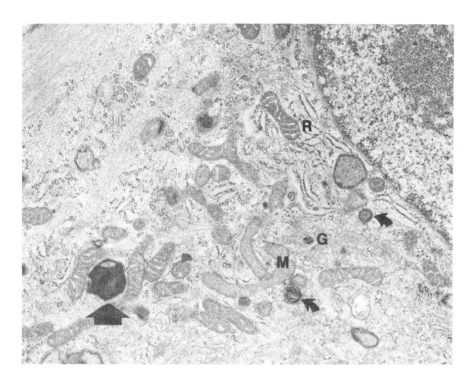

Figure 10. Longitudinal section through the perinuclear region of a smooth muscle cell in the longitudinal myometrium of a rat. Mitochondria (M), granular sarcoplasmic reticulum (R), Golgi saccules (G), lysosomes (large arrow), and residual bodies (small arrows) are distributed in the perinuclear region (×11,000).

2.2.2. *Mitochondria*

Mitochondria have been found to occupy a volume of about 3–9% in different varieties of smooth muscle (A. V. Somlyo, 1980; Gabella, 1981). In general, they are found either in small clusters at the perinuclear poles along with granular SR and the Golgi apparatus or oriented longitudinally between myofilaments, frequently in close association with tubules of agranular SR or caveolae (Figs. 8 and 10; A. P. Somlyo *et al.,* 1971, 1974; Devine and Rayns, 1975). The gap between the mitochondrial membrane and SR or caveolar membranes can be quite small (4–5 nm according to Shoenberg, 1978); however, bridging structures such as those between the SR and plasma membrane are never observed (Gabella, 1981).

Mitochondria in myometrial muscle cells, like those in other muscles and cells, are sites of oxidative phosphorylation (Chance, 1963; Lehninger, 1965). Despite early indications that smooth muscle mitochondria can accumulate strontium and barium (A. P. Somlyo and Somlyo, 1971) or calcium by an active transport mechanism (Vallieres *et al.,* 1975; Wikstrom *et al.,* 1975) and that they are capable of storing calcium (Batra, 1973), they do not appear to function in the physiological regulation of intracellular Ca^{2+} levels in smooth muscle cells (A. P. Somlyo, 1985).

Wikstrom *et al.* (1975) demonstrated that in the presence of physiological concentrations of Mg^{2+}, the apparent affinity constant of myometrial mitochondria for Ca^{2+} is 10–17 μM. This value is too low to permit Ca^{2+} accumulation under normal levels of cytoplasmic Ca^{2+} and probably even during a maximal contraction when the levels approach 1–5 μM. Consistent with this idea is the observation of A. P. Somlyo *et al.* (1979) that vascular smooth muscle tissues maintained under maximal tension for extended periods of time do not show evidence of mitochondrial Ca^{2+} accumulation. Nor do they accumulate Ca^{2+} when the cytoplasmic levels of this ion are maintained at or below 1 μM (A. P. Somlyo *et al.*, 1982). Calcium loading of mitochondria can occur, however, under pathological conditions either when the cells are damaged (A. P. Somlyo *et al.*, 1979) or when cytoplasmic levels of the ion are abnormally elevated (A. P. Somlyo *et al.*, 1982). In the rat myometrium it seems likely that mitochondria may function to regulate Ca^{2+} when the cytoplasmic levels are very high but that the SR is more important when the levels are lower.

2.2.3. Golgi Apparatus

Myometrial smooth muscle cells have an extensive Golgi apparatus consisting of numerous stacks of lamellae and vacuoles (Figs. 9 and 10). Although the function of the Golgi apparatus has never been studied in smooth muscle, it is likely that it participates in secretory, synthetic, and degradation processes as well as in the glycosylation of membrane proteins (Beams and Kessel, 1968; Hand and Oliver, 1977; Leblond and Bennett, 1977; Novikoff and Novikoff, 1977). The association among the Golgi membranes, granular SR, and lysosomes at the perinuclear poles of myometrial cells (Fig. 10) is consistent with such an interpretation. Moreover, it has been suggested that the ability of the Ca^{2+} ionophore, X537A, to dilate Golgi saccules in vascular smooth muscle cells results from an inhibition of glycoprotein synthesis (A. P. Somlyo *et al.*, 1975; Garfield and Somlyo, 1977).

2.2.4. Lysosomes and Residual and Multivesicular Bodies

Although lysosomes and other structures associated with degradation processes, such as multivesicular and residual bodies, occur in the myometrium (Fig. 10) and are subject to hormonal influences (Sloane, 1980), they have not been studied in great detail. They are particularly noticeable in tissues that are in a predominantly anabolic state or are undergoing extensive degeneration, such as in pregnant and postpartum myometria, respectively (Brandes and Anton, 1969; Chamley-Campbell *et al.*, 1979; Sloane, 1980).

2.2.5. Ribosomes and Glycogen Granules

Ribosomes are generally found at the perinuclear poles along with the Golgi complexes, granular SR, and mitochondria. Glycogen particles are found throughout the cytoplasm, and, given the importance of anaerobic metabolism to energy production in smooth muscle, it is not surprising that these structures are particularly abundant (Fig. 11).

2.3. The Plasma Membrane

The plasma membrane of myometrial smooth muscle cells is similar to that of other smooth muscles and cell types. It is separated from the basal lamina that surrounds each myometrial cell by an electron-lucent area traversed by filamentous material. The plasma membrane is a trilaminar structure of about 8–9 nm thickness, and when viewed *en face* in replicas of freeze–fractured tissues, it displays numerous integral membrane particles (Fig. 12). When plasma membranes, as well as other double-layered membrane systems of cells, are cleaved during freeze–fracture, the fracture plane generally passes along the midregion of the membrane bilayer. Such cleavage divides the membrane into halves and exposes the inner surfaces, or faces, of both the inner or protoplasmic (P) half and the outer or external (E) half of the membrane.

Integral membrane proteins seem to remain preferentially within the protoplasmic half of

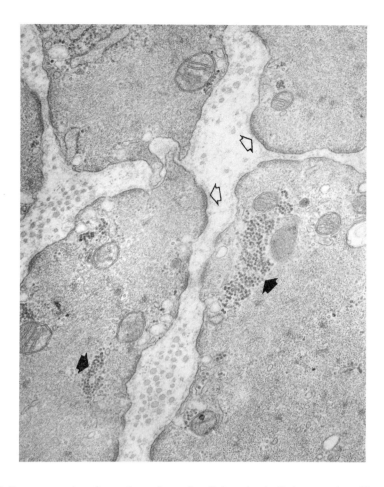

Figure 11. Transverse section of several smooth muscle cells in rat longitudinal myometrium. Glycogen particles (arrows) are grouped together in the periphery of the cytoplasm, and several membrane dense bands are
evident (open arrows) (×30,800).

the membrane, as the number of these particles is generally greater on the P than on the E face
(Devine and Rayns, 1975). The majority of particles are 8–9 nm in diameter. In some cases
the E face may show pits indicating the sites where the proteins fit into the outer leaflet prior to
membrane fracture. There is also a suggestion that the particles are more numerous in regions
around the caveolae than under the membrane-associated dense bands (Devine and Rayns,
1975; Gabella, 1984). The particles probably represent receptors, ion pumps, or other enzymes
within the membrane.

   The most striking aspect of the plasma membrane of freeze–fractured smooth muscle
cells is the abundance of regular, longitudinally oriented arrays of caveolae (Figs. 12 and 13),
which may occupy more than a third of the surface of smooth muscle cells (Verity and Bevan,
1966; Goodford, 1970; Gabella, 1981). The necks of the caveolae usually are cross-fractured
by the cleavage plane and are about 35 nm across (Figs. 12 and 13). When perfectly transected
in thin-sectioned samples of tissue, caveolae appear as flask-shaped infoldings of the membrane that are uniform in size (about 70 nm across and 120 nm long) and spacing (Fig. 8).
When sectioned away from the plane of the neck, they look like small vesicles, not unlike
pinocytotic vesicles seen in a variety of other cell types.

   The function of such caveolae is uncertain. Several authors have suggested that they are

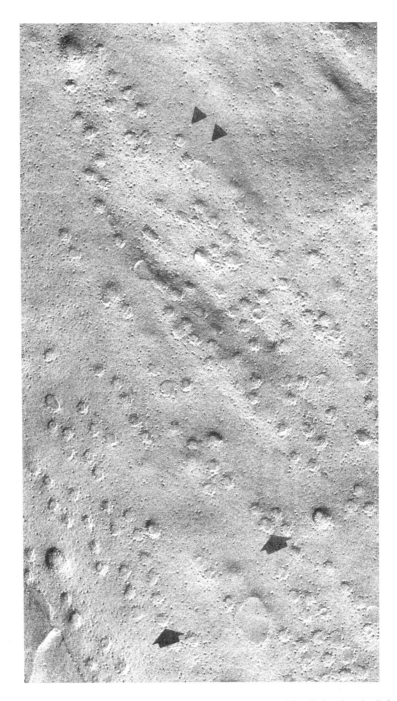

Figure 12. Freeze–fracture replica of parturient rat longitudinal myometrial cell showing the P face of the plasma membrane *en face* and exposing integral membrane protein particles (arrowheads) and rows of caveolae (arrows). Note the relative absence of caveolae in the membrane in the upper right corner.

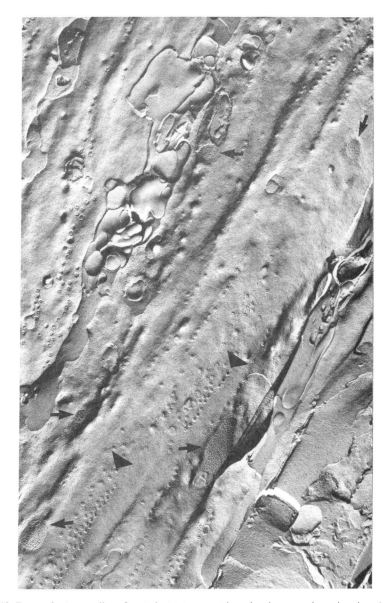

Figure 13. Freeze–fracture replica of parturient rat myometrium showing several gap junctions (arrows) and longitudinally oriented rows of caveolae on the membrane (arrowheads) (×23,000).

involved in ion transport (e.g., A. V. Somlyo *et al.*, 1969; Goodford and Wolowyk, 1972; Garfield and Daniel, 1977a,b; Popescu and Diculescu, 1975), but this idea remains to be proved experimentally. It is interesting that their numbers and size do not change with the degrees of contraction or relaxation (Gabella and Blundell, 1978), and this finding probably reflects their importance to normal cell function.

The areas of the plasma membrane between the longitudinal rows of caveolae are occupied by sites for the attachment of the cytoskeletal and contractile apparatus on the inner plasma membrane surface and cell-to-cell adhesion on its outer surface. The internal aspect of the membrane shows the accumulation of a granular and filamentous electron-opaque material, referred to as membrane-associated dense bands (or attachment plaques), into which insert thin

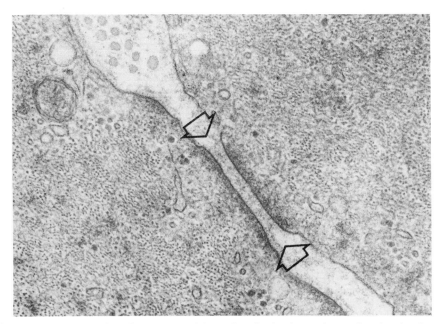

Figure 14. Transverse section of two myometrial muscle cells showing an intermediate junction (between arrows) connecting their plasma membranes. Note the densification of the cytoplasmic surface of the membrane along the junction and the row of material within the narrow extracellular space separating the membranes (×30,800). From Garfield (1985), with permission.

filaments of the contractile apparatus and intermediate filaments of the cytoskeleton (Fig. 11). The dense bands are discussed in detail in Section 4.3. The outer surface and intervening space between the two membranes at sites where there are symmetrically opposed dense bands are also associated with filamentous material. The entire structure is referred to as an intermediate junction (Fig. 14).

Myometrial muscle cells, like cells in other smooth muscle tissues, form extensive cell-to-cell junctions that function to permit the many individual cells that comprise the tissue to perform a variety of functions in unison. Structural adhesion and cell-to-cell force transmission are achieved in smooth muscle, at least in part, through the presence of such intermediate junctions. The direct flow of electrical and metabolic signals between cells is achieved by another class of cell-to-cell junctions, the so-called gap junctions, which are discussed in detail in Section 3.

Intermediate junctions are characterized by thickening of the plasma membrane as a result of the dense-band material on the inner aspect of the membrane and the presence of a layer of electron-dense material with a faint filamentous appearance within the 50-nm gap separating the cells (Fig. 14). This material appears to be a continuation of the basal laminar substance, but it is more electron dense, appears to have some periodic substructure, and is of unknown chemical composition.

2.4. Effects of Hormones and Pregnancy

The hormonal state and distention of the myometrium by the uterine contents during pregnancy have a profound effect on the smooth muscle cells. Estrogen in particular has been shown to play an important role in the regulation of growth and differentiation of myometrial muscle cells (Bergman, 1968; Ross and Klebanoff, 1967; Frederici and DeCloux, 1968).

Unfortunately, almost all structural studies performed to document these alterations in the myometrium have been qualitative instead of quantitative. The exceptions are the morphometric studies of myometrial gap junctions that show a dramatic rise in the number and size of the structures at the end of gestation and during labor (see Section 3). Precise morphometric measurements of changes in other cell components by electron microscopic stereological techniques are required.

In general, steroid hormones stimulate the myometrium to expand the cellular machinery for synthesis of intracellular and extracellular components and secretion of the latter. Large increases in numbers of mitochondria, Golgi saccules, ribosomes, and granular SR are noted in the perinuclear poles following estrogen treatment (Ross and Klebanoff, 1967; Frederici and DeCloux, 1968). In general, similar changes in ultrastructure accompany sexual maturation and the onset of pregnancy (Dessouky, 1968, 1976; Althoff and Albert, 1970).

Immediately postpartum myometrial smooth muscle cells contain large numbers of lysosomes and residual bodies, although the granular SR and Golgi apparatuses of the cells still appear highly active at this stage (Dessouky, 1971). There can be no doubt that these cells are actively involved in the degradation of intracellular and extracellular components.

3. Gap Junctions and Cell-to-Cell Communication in the Myometrium

At the end of pregnancy the myometrium becomes increasingly active and sensitive to stimulatory agents to reach a state of contractile activity that will forcefully expel the fetus and other contents of the uterus. Labor is thought to be achieved when the weak contractions of different regions of the myometrium become stronger, more frequent, and synchronous.

As is described in considerable detail in Chapter 14, the contractile activity of the uterus is largely dependent on the underlying electrical activity in the smooth muscle cells. The frequency, magnitude, and strength of myometrial contractions are dependent on the frequency of action potential discharge, the duration of the periods when action potentials are fired repetitively (i.e., trains of discharges), and the total number of cells that are simultaneously active (Marshall, 1962). Therefore, cell-to-cell propagation of action potentials throughout the myometrium from pacemaker regions or areas influenced by stimulatory agonists is of fundamental importance to the regulation of uterine excitability and contractility. This section summarizes what is known concerning the structure, presence, function, and control of gap junctions in myometrial smooth muscle. For a detailed review of the distribution and structure of gap junctions the interested reader is referred to the excellent papers by Larsen (1977a, 1983). Techniques for the study of the structure and function of gap junctions in the myometrium are discussed in detail elsewhere (Cole and Garfield, 1986a).

3.1. Gap Junction Structure

Gap junctions were first differentiated from other cell-to-cell junctional specializations by Revel and Karnovsky (1967). These authors applied a lanthanum infiltration technique to delineate the substructure of gap junctions by transmission electron microscopy. The regions of close cell–cell contact stood out in negative image and were revealed to possess hexagonally organized connections 8–9 nm in diameter that bridged the narrow 2- to 3-nm extracellular space between the opposing membranes (Fig. 14). The characteristic five- or seven-lined morphology of the gap junction (Fig. 15), demonstrated in Figs. 16 and 17, has subsequently been observed in a wide variety of different tissues stained *en bloc* with uranyl acetate.

The hexagonal pattern of the gap-junctional subunits has also been observed in replicas of tissues prepared for freeze–fracture electron microscopy (Kreutziger, 1968; Figs. 18 and 19)

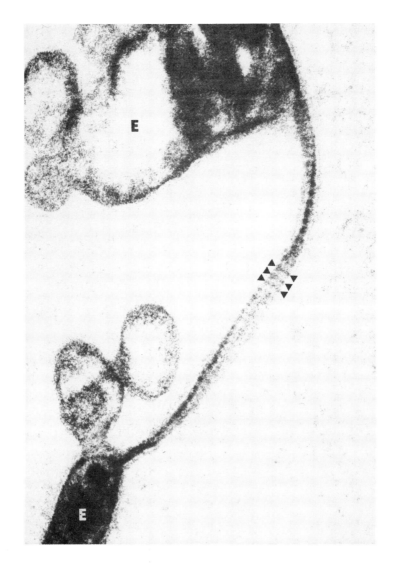

Figure 15. Transverse section of a gap junction after fixation in glutaraldehyde and 8% tannic acid. Note that the electron-dense tannic acid in the extracellular space (E) penetrates between the junctional membranes to outline the connexons bridging this space in negative image (arrowheads) (×328,000). From Garfield (1984), with permission.

and in studies that attempted to describe the structure of isolated gap junctions by negative staining (Benedetti and Emmelot, 1968), optical diffraction (Unwin and Zampighi, 1980), and x-ray diffraction (Caspar *et al.*, 1977). That integral membrane protein particles within the respective opposing halves of the gap junction membrane are paired precisely across the extracellular space was originally observed in mirror-image replicas of freeze–fractured tissues (Chalcroft and Bullivant, 1970) and later confirmed in the abovementioned optical and x-ray diffraction studies. A diagrammatic representation of a gap junction is shown in Fig. 20.

The bridging units that span between cells at the gap junction are generally referred to as "connexons" (Goodenough and Stoeckinius, 1972). Each such bridge is believed to harbor an aqueous cell-to-cell channel or pore about 1.5 nm in diameter that permits a direct exchange of small molecules and ions between the connected cells. Unequivocal evidence for the presence

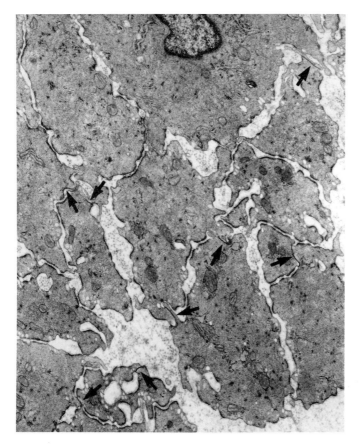

Figure 16. Low-magnification transverse section of smooth muscle cells illustrating several gap junctions (arrows) (×12,800). From Garfield (1984), with permission.

of this channel has not yet been obtained, although there is substantial indirect functional evidence. Each connexon appears to have a sixfold symmetry (i.e., is composed of six identical subunits), and there is some evidence for flaplike appendages at the cytoplasmic surfaces of the pore (Makowski, 1985) (Fig. 20). These latter structures are thought to represent gating structures, which might regulate access to the pore interior and, as a result, control the cell-to-cell movements of molecules through the channel (Fig. 20).

3.2. Gap Junctions in the Myometrium

Gap junctions were first observed in myometrium only 10 years ago, when they were found to be present in large numbers and sizes for the brief period of time associated with labor and delivery of the fetuses at parturition (Garfield *et al.,* 1977). Since that time they have been observed in the myometria of several species, including mice (Dahl and Berger, 1978), sheep (Garfield *et al.,* 1979), guinea pigs (Garfield *et al.,* 1982), rabbits (Demianczuk *et al.,* 1984), bats (Buchanan and Garfield, 1984), and humans (Garfield and Hayashi, 1981). In all instances, they were found to possess a structure comparable to that described for gap junctions in other smooth muscles (Gabella 1979b, 1981) and tissues (Larsen, 1977a, 1983). Figures 13 and 15–19 show gap junctions in thin-sectioned, freeze–fractured and negatively stained (i.e., with tannic acid) preparations of myometrial tissues.

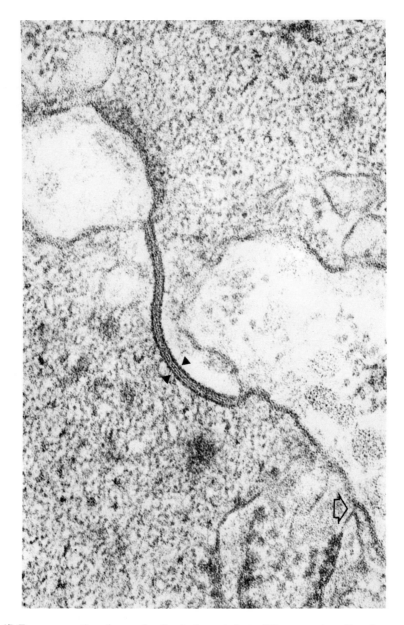

Figure 17. Transverse section of a gap junction in the parturient rabbit myometrium. Note the seven-lined appearance (four dark and three pale lines) of the junction between the arrowheads and the close approach of an agranular sarcoplasmic tubule to the plasma membrane (open arrow) ($\times 146,000$). From Garfield (1984), with permission.

Gap junctions increase in frequency and size at the end of gestation, immediately prior to the onset of the coordinated contractility associated with labor (Garfield *et al.*, 1977, 1978) (Fig. 21). They are infrequent and small in the nonpregnant and pregnant, nonparturient myometrium of the rat, rarely occupying more than 0.001% of the plasma membrane surface area. In contrast, tissues removed from animals delivering fetuses contain large, numerous gap junctions; each cell has at least 1000 junctions with an average diameter of 0.2 μm (range 0.08–0.5 μm) that occupy a total of 0.2–0.4% of the cell surface (Fig. 21). The development

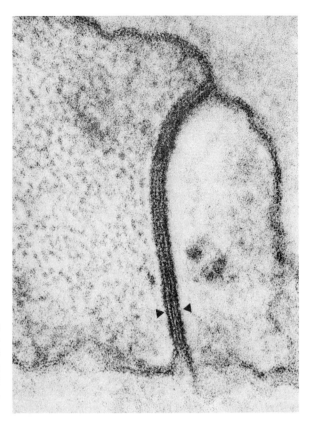

Figure 18. Transverse section of a gap junction in the parturient rat myometrium. The seven-lined appearance of the junction is especially evident in this micrograph (between arrowheads) (×246,000). From Garfield (1985), with permission.

of gap junctions in the myometrium at term was first described in the rat but has since been documented for several different mammalian species (Fig. 22).

Initial attempts to identify gap junctions in myometrium failed, largely because only tissues from nonpregnant or pregnant, nonparturient animals were used for study (Garfield and Daniel, 1974; Daniel *et al.*, 1976). It is extremely difficult to identify the junctions in these tissues because of the extremely small size of the regions of cell-to-cell contact. In most cases, they are only point contacts that fail to demonstrate the characteristic multilayered structure in thin section and consist of only a few particles arranged as small maculae or linear rows in replicas of freeze-cleaved tissues (Fig. 23).

These types of junctions are generally observed only by exhaustive and patient study, and in most instances, such studies have not been done. Indeed, failure to identify junctions adequately in myometrium and other smooth muscles (as discussed by Gabella, 1981), in which cell-to-cell electrotonic coupling and action potential propagation are observed, has led to the controversial claim that other structures must subserve these electrical interactions.

3.3. Function of Gap Junctions

Given the multicellular nature of the myometrium, a mechanism must be present to synchronize the activities of individual cells and facilitate the coordinated movements observed during labor. In 1870, Engelmann (described by Bozler, 1938, 1940) first postulated that electrical excitation propagates from cell to cell in smooth muscle. The subsequent studies by Bozler (1938, 1940) on propagation in uterine muscle confirmed the observations of

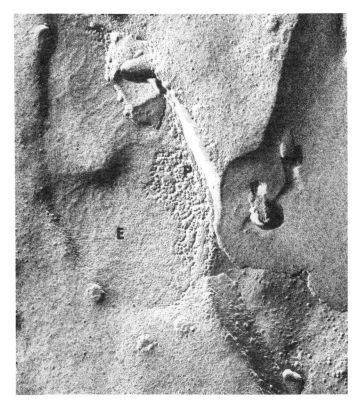

Figure 19. Freeze–fracture replica of an oval-shaped gap junction in the myometrium of a parturient rat. The exoplasmic or E face (E) and the protoplasmic or P face (P) of the junction are indicated. Note the hexagonal arrangement of the pits on the E face (×83,000). From Garfield (1985), with permission.

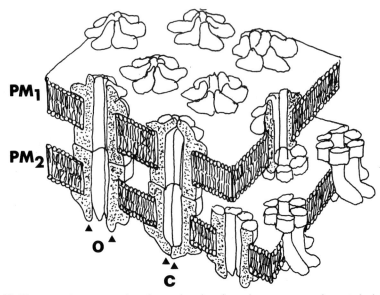

Figure 20. Diagrammatic representation of a gap junction. Several connexons are shown to be integrated into the phospholipid bilayers (PM_1 and PM_2). The cell-to-cell channels of two adjacent connexons are shown in the open (O) and closed (C) conformations. Hypothetical gates at the ends of the channels (arrowheads) move to prevent access to the channel in the closed state. Each connexon comprises two hemichannels, and each hemichannel is made up of six connexin proteins. Modified from Makowski *et al.* (1984).

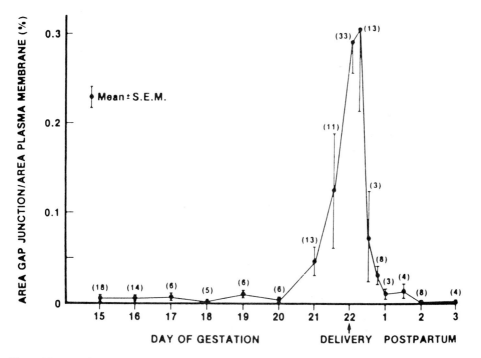

Figure 21. Area of gap junctions in the myometrium as a percentage of the plasma membrane area before, during, and after parturition in the rat. The number of tissues studied for each day is indicated in parentheses.

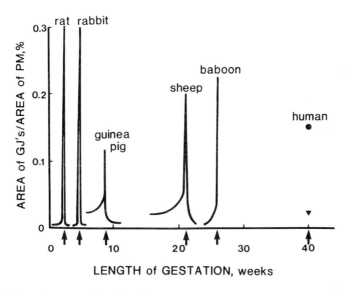

Figure 22. The change in myometrial gap junctions at term in several mammalian species. Area of gap junctions as a percentage of the plasma membrane is compared with the length of gestation for the rat, guinea pig, sheep, and baboon. Human data: ●, at term and in labor; ▼, at term but not in labor. From Garfield (1984), with permission.

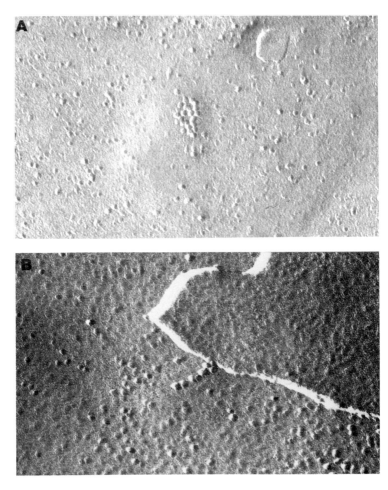

Figure 23. Freeze–fracture replicas of very small gap junctions with a macular (A) or linear (B) array of intramembrane protein particles (A, ×105,000; B, ×150,000).

Engelmann and showed coordinated movements in the absence of any neuronal input. He proposed that excitation was conducted from cell to cell in a manner exactly similar to that observed in cardiac muscle, that is, as though there were "a protoplasmic continuity between the muscle fibers" and the tissue acted as if it were a functional syncytium.

It is now generally accepted that electrical excitation propagates in smooth muscle by cell-to-cell flow of electrotonic currents via low-resistance pathways between cells. Gap junctions (then called nexuses) were originally thought by Dewey and Barr (1962) to be the morphological correlate of this pathway. Since 1962 a variety of evidence has been obtained, largely from study of the myometrium, to support the concept that gap junctions facilitate direct intercellular communication in smooth muscle; i.e., they mediate electrical coupling through the transfer of small ions, primarily potassium ions, as well as metabolic coupling, involving cell-to-cell diffusion of low-molecular-weight metabolites, second messengers, regulatory molecules, and high-energy phosphates between myometrial cells. The functional significance of electrical coupling is evident, but the role of metabolic coupling remains speculative.

3.3.1. Electrical Coupling

Electrical coupling between individual fibers is believed to exist in all smooth muscles, but the evidence for this claim is largely indirect. Electrical coupling generally is assessed with two intracellular microelectrodes. One microelectrode is used to pass current and record the amplitude of the voltage response or electrotonic potential within the injected cell (V_a), and a second serves to measure the amplitude of the propagating voltage response in cells at various distances from the site of injection (V_b). The ratio (V_b/V_a) of the amplitudes of the electrotonic potentials at the source (V_a) and in a distant cell (V_b) is referred to as the coupling coefficient. If the cells are well coupled, then the intercellular (i.e., gap junctional) resistance is negligible, and this ratio approaches unity. In contrast, if the cells are poorly coupled and therefore electrically isolated, the ratio nears zero.

Unfortunately, however, most intact preparations of smooth muscle, including myometrium, possess a complex three-dimensional arrangement of cells. Because of this geometry, it is generally difficult to record propagating electrotonic potentials more than a few tens of millimeters from the site of intracellular current injection with a microelectrode. For this reason a direct measure of the extent of current flow and electrical coupling between smooth muscle cells cannot be obtained by such an approach. It has been necessary to study the propagation of electrotonic potentials in myometrium by a technique referred to as the Abe–Tomita method (Abe and Tomita, 1968). This method employs large extracellular plate electrodes to stimulate one portion of a length of tissue and reduce the complex geometry to that of a one-dimensional cable. The amplitude of propagating electrotonic potentials can be measured with microelectrodes and be shown to fall exponentially with distance from the plate electrodes, as predicted by the cable equations. An indirect measure of the extent of cell-to-cell coupling can be achieved by calculating the value of the length constant for the tissue. It represents the distance required for the electrotonic potential amplitude to decay to $1/e$ of its value at the stimulus site. The length constant for different smooth muscles ranges from 0.5 to 3.8 mm (Tomita, 1975; Creed, 1979; Sims et al., 1982). Because the average cell length is 0.2–0.3 mm, it is evident that electronic potentials may propagate over several cells; hence, the cells must be coupled by low-resistance pathways.

The change in electrical coupling associated with the elaboration of gap junctions in the parturient myometrium has been demonstrated by this technique (Sims et al., 1982). The length constant was assessed in longitudinal myometrial tissues from rats at different times during pregnancy and parturition and postpartum. Careful attention was paid to appropriate categorization of the tissues according to the day of pregnancy and to the maintenance of *in vivo* length (i.e., stretch). It was shown that the length constant was significantly greater in tissues from parturient animals (3.7 ± 1.0 mm) compared with animals not in labor (2.6 ± 1.0 mm). Separate experiments that analyzed the impedance of similar tissues to alternating current flow yielded results consistent with the idea that the intercellular resistance is lower during delivery (Sims et al., 1982). Gap junctions were measured in some of the tissues used for the electrophysiological experiments and were found to increase about 50-fold.

The relationship between changes in the length constant and structural coupling in the myometrium is consistent with the view that gap junctions facilitate cell-to-cell coupling in smooth muscle. However, there remain many observations of relatively good electrical coupling, as indicated by a long length constant, in smooth muscles that have been described to possess few or no gap junctions. For example, gap junctions occupy only 0.01% or less of the cell membrane of myometrial cells in pregnant, nonparturient rats, but the length constant is 2.6 mm. Gap junctions are described as absent or as rare point contacts 10 nm in length in thin sections and 50–600 nm in diameter in freeze–fracture replicas of taenia coli smooth muscle (Gabella, 1979b), yet the length constant is 1.5 mm (Abe and Tomita, 1968). Observations such as these have led to the controversial claim that other structures must subserve the function of low-resistance contacts in smooth muscle (Daniel *et al.*, 1976; Gabella, 1981). However, it should be understood that most small gap junctions such as those just considered are very difficult to identify unequivocally in thin sections or freeze–fracture replicas. To complicate matters further, it is also possible that single, completely dispersed connexons may permit functional coupling. Under these conditions one can easily see that it is not possible to ascertain accurately the number of gap-junctional channels between coupled cells in smooth muscle by routine electron microscopic techniques. Future experiments utilizing antibodies or other probes to label gap junction proteins in the plasma membrane definitely will aid in the resolution of this controversy. It should be kept in mind that the gap junction is the only cell-to-cell coupling structure that has been shown to subserve low-resistance electrical communication in other tissues.

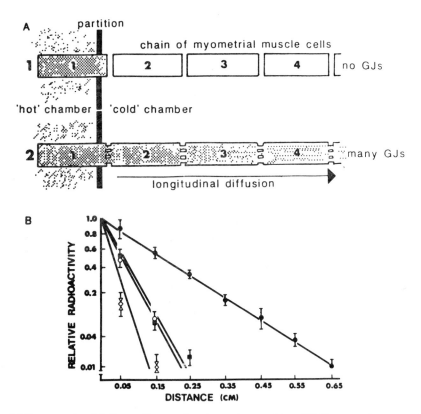

Figure 24. Summary of metabolic coupling experiments on rat myometrium. (A) Diagrammatic representation of the two-compartment bathing chamber used to study longitudinal diffusion of 2-deoxyglucose (stippling) in myometrial tissues with and without gap junctions between the smooth muscle cells. (B) The distribution of radioactive 2-deoxyglucose in the cold chamber (relative to tissue in the hot chamber) after 5 hr for longitudinal diffusion is shown as a function of distance along muscle strips from delivering (solid circles), preterm (open circles), and postpartum (solid squares) rats. The distribution of tracer is clearly greater in the parturient tissues that had large numbers of gap junctions. The distribution of an extracellular tracer was not different in the three tissues (parturient, diamond; preterm, triangle; postpartum, inverted triangle). (C) The apparent diffusion coefficient for 2-deoxyglucose (bar graph) and relative area of gap junctions (open circles) in rat myometrium as a function of the day of gestation. Note that there is an association between the alterations in structural coupling and cell-to-cell communication. From Cole *et al.* (1986), with permission.

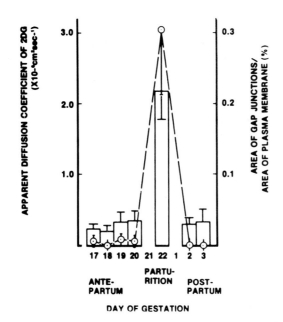

Figure 24. (Continued)

3.3.2. Metabolic Coupling

Gap junctions in other tissues also mediate the direct cell-to-cell transfer of low-molecular-weight small molecules up to about 1000 daltons or 1.5 nm in diameter. Recent studies using radiolabeled metabolites (Cole *et al.*, 1985; Cole and Garfield, 1986b, 1988), or membrane-impermeant fluorescent dyes (Blennerhassett *et al.*, 1987) provide evidence that myometrial gap junctions facilitate this type of communication as well.

A two-compartment bathing chamber was used to show enhanced cell-to-cell exchange of radioactive phosphorylated [^{3}H]-2-deoxy-D-glucose in longitudinal myometrium of parturient animals (Cole *et al.*, 1985) (Fig. 24). One portion of small strips of myometrium from pregnant rats, days 17–20 (few gap junctions), and rats in the midst of delivering fetuses (many gap junctions) were exposed to the tracer, and its distribution within the tissues was assessed after time for longitudinal diffusion (Fig. 24A). The tracer enters the myometrial cells by substituting for glucose and, once inside, is phosphorylated. In this form it is neither metabolized further nor can recross the plasma membrane but provides a diffusible pool of tracer in the cells within the labeled compartment. If appropriate cell-to-cell pathways are present in the tissue, the tracer will diffuse longitudinally from the labeled into unlabeled tissue (Fig. 24A).

The distribution of radiolabeled 2-deoxyglucose was found to be considerably greater in tissues removed from delivering animals (Fig. 24B). This finding implies that the rate of tracer movement is greater in tissues containing large numbers of gap junctions, as reflected in quantitative terms by an almost tenfold increase in the apparent diffusion coefficient for 2-deoxyglucose (Fig. 24C). Similar experiments employing tracers that did not enter the intracellular compartment demonstrated that extracellular diffusion can not account for the redistribution of 2-deoxyglucose (Fig. 24B).

Direct study of molecular exchange between myometrial cells has been performed using *ex situ* preparations of longitudinal muscle from rat myometrium (Blennerhassett *et al.*, 1987). The fluorescent dye Lucifer yellow (457 mol. wt.) was injected into the intracellular compart-

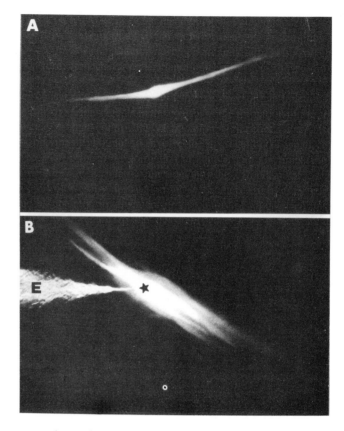

Figure 25. Fluorescence micrographs of Lucifer yellow dye injection experiments. The dye that spread into adjacent myometrial cells after intracellular injection via a microelectrode is shown to be limited in preterm tissues (A) but extensive in parturient tissues (B). The positions of the microelectrode (E) and injected myometrial cell (star) are shown in B. Note the bipolar shape of the muscle cells (×220).

ment of myometrial cells with a microelectrode, and its cell-to-cell movement was visualized by fluorescent light microscopy. If tissues from parturient and nonparturient animals are compared, only those from the former group show rapid cell-to-cell dye transfer (Fig. 25).

It is evident from radioactive and fluorescent tracer studies that there is a marked upswing in the capability of myometrial cells for metabolic coupling as a consequence of increased numbers of gap junctions. The significance of this exchange in myometrial physiology is ill defined at present. In other tissues metabolic exchange is thought to permit ionic and osmotic homeostasis and synchronization of metabolic activities in cell populations as a result of the absence of variations of important metabolites, regulatory molecules, or both within the tissue (Peracchia, 1980; Loewenstein, 1981). It is also possible that coordinated responses in cell populations arise from the exchange of regulatory or intercellular signal molecules such as small peptides, cyclic nucleotides, and vitamins. In the myometrium, this exchange could contribute to the coordination of metabolic activities during labor by ensuring that high-energy phosphates and other molecules are in adequate supply throughout the muscle syncytium.

3.4. Control of Myometrial Junctional Communication

In a wide variety of cellular systems, including the myometrium, the extent to which gap junctions develop between cells is regulated by specific intracellular and extracellular signals.

Control of cell-to-cell communication can be achieved through alterations in the number and size of the gap junctions, i.e., by changing the number of cell-to-cell channels physically present in the tissue. The dramatic increase of gap junctions in the myometrium at term is an example of this mechanism.

Alternatively, cell coupling also may be regulated by controlling the functioning of the gap junctions present, a process that involves control over the permeability or conductance characteristics of the individual cell-to-cell channels within the junctions. On the basis of recent studies, it appears that both mechanisms may operate to control communication between myometrial muscle cells in response to specific hormonal signals.

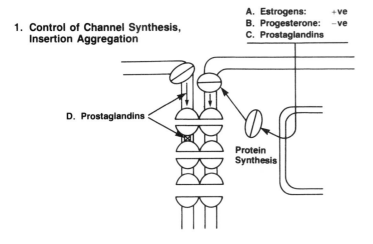

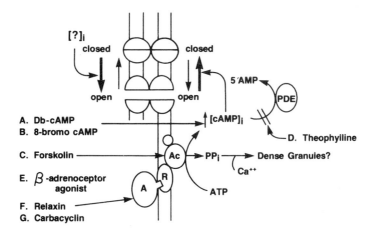

Figure 26. A schematic representation of the different levels for control of cell-to-cell communication between smooth muscle cells in the myometrium. Possible roles are indicated (1) for steroids and prostaglandins in controlling the synthesis, insertion, and/or aggregation of connexons into gap junctions and (2) for control of gap junction channel kinetics and/or permeability. Agents (2A–D) may elevate intracellular levels of cAMP ($[cAMP]_i$) directly (2A,B) or indirectly by either stimulating (2C,E,F,G) its synthesis by adenylate cyclase (Ac) or inhibiting (2D) its degradation by phosphodiesterase (PDE). Stimulation of the agonist–receptor–adenylate cyclase (A–R–Ac) complex is shown to result in the conversion of ATP into cAMP and pyrophosphate (PP_i). The latter may interact with calcium ions (Ca^{2+}) in the fixative solution, possibly giving rise to the electron-dense granules noted on the cytoplasmic surface of myometrial gap junctions. The hypothetical activation of the channels by an as yet unidentified agent (?) also is indicated. From Cole and Garfield (1986b).

There is evidence for hormonal or intracellular control of (1) structural coupling, possibly by regulation of the gene(s) for the gap junction protein or a protein required for the assembly of the proteins into functional connexons and gap junctions, and (2) the permeability of the junctional channels. It has also been suggested that coupling in the myometrium may be controlled by agents that regulate the degradation of the junctions. The view that myometrial gap junctions may be controlled at multiple levels is shown diagrammatically in Fig. 26.

3.4.1. Control of Gap Junction Size and Frequency

Experiments carried out in several different laboratories suggest that the changes in levels of steroid hormones and prostaglandins that precede or are associated with labor and have long been recognized to regulate parturition (Csapo, 1981; Liggins, 1979; Challis and Lye, 1986) are responsible for controlling the development of gap junctions between myometrial cells (Bergman, 1968; Garfield *et al.*, 1977, 1978, 1979, 1980a,b, 1982; Dahl and Berger, 1978; Burden *et al.*, 1979; Merk *et al.*, 1980; Puri and Garfield, 1982; Wathes and Porter, 1982; Mackenzie *et al.*, 1983; Burghardt *et al.*, 1984a,b; Mackenzie and Garfield, 1985, 1986a,b; Saito *et al.*, 1985).

Alterations in steroid hormones, as indicated by changing plasma and tissue levels prior to labor, appear to elevate the synthesis of myometrial gap junctions through a genomic mechanism (Garfield *et al.*, 1980a,b, 1988; Puri and Garfield, 1982; Mackenzie and Garfield, 1985). The possibility that progesterone suppresses synthesis of gap junctions is indicated by the following observations: (1) progesterone levels normally decline in rats and rabbits prior to the development of large numbers of gap junctions and the initiation of labor (Fig. 27); (2) if progesterone levels are maintained experimentally by injections of the hormone, animals neither develop gap junctions nor go into labor (Garfield *et al.*, 1977, 1978); (3) ovariectomy leads to premature progesterone withdrawal, gap junction development, and labor, but progesterone treatment after ovariectomy prevents all three events (Garfield *et al.*, 1982); (4) treatment of animals with antiprogesterones induces the premature formation of gap junctions, and this effect can be blocked by simultaneous treatment with progesterone receptor agonists (Garfield and Baulieu, 1987; Garfield *et al.*, 1988); (5) progesterone treatment suppresses gap junction formation between myometrial cells *in vitro*, provided estrogen is present (Garfield *et al.*, 1980a). These observations prompted Garfield *et al.* (1977, 1978) to suggest that progesterone inhibits labor and maintains pregnancy by suppressing gap junction formation and electrical coupling in the myometrium. Moreover, it was suggested that this control over gap junction development might be the basis for the progesterone block hypothesis advanced by Csapo (1981).

It is not evident how the inhibitory effects of progesterone on gap junction development are manifest. Puri and Garfield (1982) contend that this steroid could act at one or more of the following sites: (1) inhibition of protein (i.e., connexon) synthesis either directly or indirectly through inhibition of the estrogen–genome interaction; (2) a direct plasma membrane effect; or (3) an indirect inhibition mediated by progesterone effects on prostaglandin synthesis. Experiments employing antiprogesterones and progesterone receptor agonists imply that the receptor–genome mechanism is the most likely factor (Garfield and Baulieu, 1987; Garfield *et al.*, 1988).

Estrogens promote the synthesis of gap junctions in the myometrium and other tissues that possess steroid receptors (Bergman, 1968; Dahl and Berger, 1978; Garfield *et al.*, 1980a; Mackenzie *et al.*, 1983; Burghardt *et al.*, 1984a,b; Mackenzie and Garfield, 1985, 1986a). The evidence supporting the involvement of estrogens in the regulation of myometrial gap junction development is as follows: (1) estrogen levels rise prior to the formation of gap junctions and labor (Fig. 27); (2) injections of estrogens into pregnant animals will initiate premature appearance of gap junctions and labor (Mackenzie and Garfield, 1986a); (3) estrogen injections will induce the formation of gap junctions between myometrial cells in

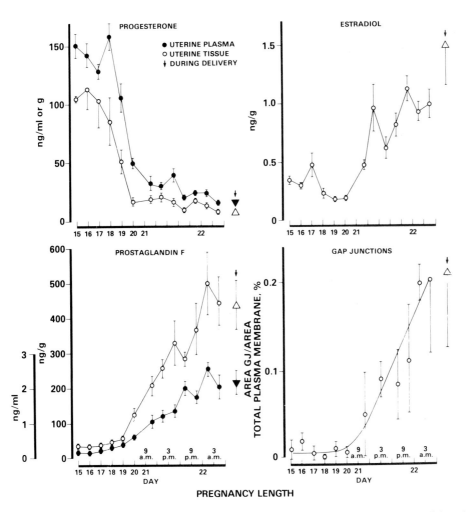

Figure 27. The temporal profile of changes (means ± S.E.) in the levels of progesterone, estradiol, and prostaglandin F in uterine venous plasma (solid circles) and uterine tissues (open circles) as well as gap junctions during the latter days of pregnancy and during delivery (triangles). Note that the time scale is expanded from day 21 to delivery. Each point is three or four samples. From Puri and Garfield (1982).

immature, mature, and ovariectomized rats (Bergman, 1968; Dahl and Berger, 1978; Mackenzie *et al.,* 1983; Burghardt *et al.,* 1984a; Mackenzie and Garfield, 1985, 1986b); (4) antiestrogens, such as tamoxifen, prevent the estrogens from stimulating an increase in gap junctions (Burghardt *et al.,* 1984b; Mackenzie and Garfield 1985, 1986b); (5) myometrial mRNA extracted from animals given injections of estrogens will initiate gap junction formation between cells in culture (Dahl *et al.,* 1980, 1987).

It seems most likely that estrogen elevates gap junctions in the myometrium by interacting with its cytoplasmic and nuclear receptors to stimulate the portion of the genome responsible for coding for the connexon protein or a protein required for the insertion or formation of gap junctions in the plasma membrane. Progesterone could act to block this genomic activation. Steroid receptors have been implicated in the control of gap junctions in the rat uterus (Saito *et al.,* 1985), and the ability of estrogen to control protein synthesis in this manner is well recognized (Gorski and Gannon, 1976). Protein synthesis inhibitors effectively block the synthesis of gap junctions in myometrial tissues *in vivo* and *in vitro* in response to estrogen stimulation. This finding supports the view that protein synthesis is an essential intermediate step in the elaboration of myometrial gap junctions. The exact mechanism by which the steroids influence junction formation will likely become evident very soon through the use of molecular biological techniques for monitoring the expression of the gap junction gene and synthesis of its mRNA.

The ability of prostaglandin synthesis inhibitors, such as indomethacin and meclofenamate, to alter the area of gap junctions between myometrial cells indicates that prostaglandins and/or leukotrienes also are involved in the regulation of structural coupling. The manner in which prostaglandins influence gap junctions is apparently quite complex; under certain circumstances they appear to inhibit junction formation (Garfield et al., 1980a,b), and under others they are stimulatory (Mackenzie et al., 1983; Mackenzie and Garfield, 1985). Considerable further study is required to identify the metabolite(s) of arachidonic acid and their mode(s) of action in the control of myometrial gap junctions. Among the possibilities are an inhibitory prostaglandin that suppresses gap junction development until term, a lipoxygenase product that stimulates junction formation, and a prostaglandin that influences the steroid receptors (Mackenzie et al., 1983).

Most studies concerning the regulation of the presence of gap junctions in myometrium have stressed the role of various agents in the control of the formation of the cell–cell contacts. However, the processes that control the degradation of junctions may also be important. Degradation was previously thought to involve the aggregation of small contacts into very large junctions (Fig. 28) prior to the formation of annular gap junctions (Fig. 29). The latter result from the withdrawal of a large junction into the cytoplasm of one of the cells by endocytosis and are followed by destruction via lysosomal activity (Garfield et al., 1980b). This pathway and its potential involvement in the control of myometrial junctions should be studied, particularly with regard to the possibility that it is subject to the influence of prostaglandins.

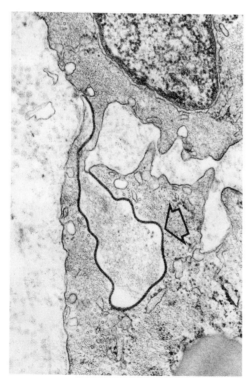

Figure 28. Transverse section of an extremely large gap junction (arrow) present at an invagination of one cell into another (×36,100). From Garfield *et al.* (1980b), with permission.

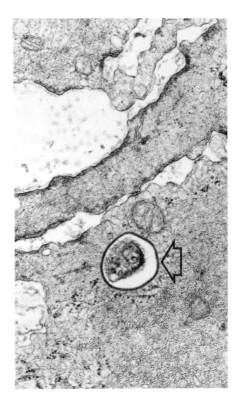

Figure 29. Transverse section of an annular gap junction (arrow) within the cytoplasm of a myometrial smooth muscle cell ($\times 36,100$). From Garfield *et al.* (1980b), with permission.

3.4.2. Control of Gap Junction Channel Properties

There is considerable evidence that the kinetic and conductance/permeability properties of gap junction channels can be modulated by experimental manipulations (Peracchia, 1980; Loewenstein, 1981; Spray *et al.,* 1984; Spray and Bennett, 1985). However, the potential significance of these experiments to smooth muscle physiology is not recognized generally, and few studies have sought to ascertain whether intercellular communication can be manipulated in the absence of any change in gap junction size or numbers.

The aforementioned 2-deoxyglucose diffusion technique was recently employed to assess the effects on coupling in myometrial tissues of several agents that elevate the intracellular levels of cyclic adenosine monophosphate (cAMP) (Cole and Garfield, 1986b). The diffusivity of the tracer in parturient tissues was found to decrease in a concentration-dependent manner after exposure to dibutyryl or 8-bromo-cAMP. Similarly, inhibition of cAMP degradation by phosphodiesterase with theophylline, or stimulation of its synthesis by adenylate cyclase with forskolin, also reduced the apparent diffusion coefficient of the tracer in parturient myometrium. Elevated intracellular levels of cAMP therefore may reduce cell-to-cell coupling in the myometrium. Recent data suggest that elevated levels of cytoplasmic Ca^{2+} ion also may reduce metabolite communication (Cole and Garfield, 1988).

The possibility of a cAMP control of coupling was explored further using agents that are relevant to the control of labor and delivery and interact with specific membrane receptors to elevate intracellular levels of cAMP. Included in this group were relaxin, some prostaglandins (e.g., E_2 and prostacyclin or its stable synthetic analogue carbacylin), and β-adrenoceptor agonists (e.g., isoproterenol). Each of these agonists was found to decrease cell-to-cell exchange of radiolabeled 2-deoxyglucose. A related prostaglandin, $F_{2\alpha}$, which does not elevate intracellular cAMP, had no effect on the tracer movement.

The influence of additional metabolites of arachidonic acid to those previously mentioned was explored using indomethacin and 5,8,11,14-eicosatetraynoic acid (ETYA). Indomethacin prevents synthesis of prostaglandins by inhibiting cyclooxygenase activity, and it had no effect on tracer diffusion. In contrast, ETYA suppresses lipoxygenase metabolism of arachidonic acid (as well as inhibiting cyclooxygenase) and was found to depress the diffusion of 2-deoxyglucose in parturient myometrium. These findings imply that an eicosanoid product of the arachidonic acid cascade may be involved in promoting cell-to-cell coupling in the myometrium.

Examination of the tissues used in the aforementioned experiments failed to demonstrate any change in the extent of junctional contact between the myometrial cells. Thus, it seems likely that elevated levels of cAMP, Ca^{2+}, and several physiologically relevant agonists may influence coupling in the myometrium by altering the kinetic properties or permeability/conductance of the gap junction cell-to-cell channels. A decrease in the mean open time, the pore size of the channels, or both would reduce the intercellular movement of 2-deoxyglucose. The results also support the idea that there is an endogenous mechanism for regulating junctional communication in the myometrium that involves circulating and local hormones and alterations in intracellular cAMP levels. Control of coupling may result from the combined effects of stimulatory and inhibitory agents. The influence of inhibitory factors, such as relaxin and prostacyclin, may predominate during gestation but be offset during labor by stimulatory agents such as eicosanoids.

Structural studies of tissues treated with forskolin and other agents that stimulate adenylate cyclase activity also revealed the presence of many large electron-dense deposits on the cytoplasmic face of the junctions (Fig. 30). Similar deposits were rare or absent in control or dibutyryl-cAMP-treated tissues. Relationships among these deposits, activation of adenylate cyclase, and uncoupling of the myometrial cells remain to be explored. Identical deposits in

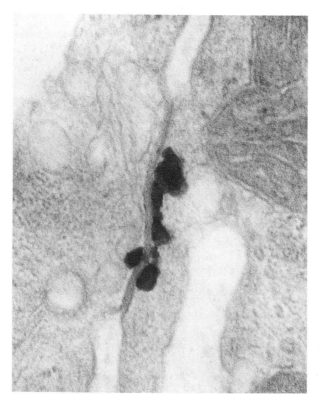

Figure 30. High magnification of a transversely sectioned gap junction with large electron-dense granules in longitudinal myometrial tissue from a parturient rat treated with forskolin (1.0 μM). The tissue was prepared by routine methods (i.e., no special staining) (×140,000). From Cole and Garfield (1986b), with permission.

other tissues have been suggested to be sites of calcium phosphate precipitation, perhaps resulting from the liberation of pyrophosphate by adenylate cyclase and subsequent interaction of this ion with calcium in the fixative (Larsen, 1977b). It is possible, therefore, that their presence in myometrial cells may reflect the localization of adenylate cyclase near the junctional membrane (Fig. 26).

3.5. Significance of Gap Junctions and Their Modulation to Pregnancy and Parturition

Labor in animals and humans is marked by the development of intense, synchronous, and coordinated contractile activity in the smooth muscle layers of the uterus from a state of relative quiescence and asynchrony (Csapo, 1981). This transition is believed to result from changes in plasma and tissue levels of steroids and other agents (Fuchs, 1978; Liggins 1979; Thorburn and Challis, 1979; Csapo, 1981). Our studies imply that the hormonally induced increase and appropriate function of myometrial gap junctions is of fundamental importance to this transition.

Uterine contractions are triggered by action potentials that propagate over large areas of the uterine wall from sites of spontaneous generation within localized pacemaker regions. Because gap junctions participate in the spread of this activity, their absence will impair propagation, promote uterine quiescence and asynchrony, and render the myometrium incapable of generating sufficient intrauterine pressure for delivery of the fetus(es). In contrast, the presence of many open channels would promote propagation of excitation into a greater number of myometrial cells, leading to a more coordinated and rapid development of tension by the uterus, labor, and the termination of pregnancy.

The concept that there may be several levels of control of myometrial junctional communication is summarized in Fig. 26. Coupling is shown to be dependent on the presence of gap junctions and functional, open cell-to-cell channels. It is evident from studies on rats that maintenance of the fetuses within the uterus during pregnancy is accomplished partially by hormonal depression of gap junction formation. It also seems likely that coupling by the few junctions present may be suppressed by control of kinetic or permeability characteristics of the cell-to-cell channels. This latter mechanism is probably most important during late pregnancy, when large numbers of junctions are present between myometrial cells.

With regard to the latter mechanism, it is significant that the myometrium of the rat displays very marked quiescence during the final 24–36 hr before the initiation of labor despite the presence of numerous large gap junctions. If functional, these structures would be expected to improve coupling and promote the onset of labor. However, circulating levels of relaxin peak at this time (Downing and Sherwood, 1985a,b), leading to myometrial quiescence during this period as well as intermittent quiescence and the prevention of sustained high levels of contractile activity during labor (Porter et al., 1979; Downing and Sherwood, 1985a,b).

On the basis of the effect of relaxin on 2-deoxyglucose diffusion, the control of relaxin over myometrial activity may be partly through its influence over junctional kinetics, permeability, or both (Fig. 26). A similar alteration in permeability or kinetics of the gap junction may contribute to the ability of exogenously applied relaxin and β-adrenoceptor agonists to inhibit term and preterm labor in animals and humans. It is pertinent also to recall that the adrenergic innervation of the uteri of most species degenerates during pregnancy and is absent during parturition.

In contrast to the case of the rat, in which gap junctions are sparse until just prior to labor, greater numbers are present throughout pregnancy, and their development occurs over a prolonged period before labor in species such as the guinea pig, sheep, and human (Garfield et al., 1979, 1982; Garfield and Hayashi, 1981). In this case, control of junctional permeability may be of greater importance and may represent the primary mechanism for inhibiting coupling during gestation and promoting enhanced communication at term.

It is clear that an understanding of the mechanisms regulating myometrial gap junctions will lead to effective procedures to initiate or inhibit labor. Moreover, it is possible that conditions of abnormal uterine contractility, such as dysfunctional labor, premature labor, or dysmenorrhea, may be fostered by a failure of the endogenous control mechanisms for regulating the presence and functional properties of myometrial gap junctions. Knowledge of these mechanisms will provide an understanding of such conditions and perhaps offer a rational approach to the development of specific drug therapies.

4. Contractile Mechanism of Myometrial Smooth Muscle Cells

The ability of myometrial smooth muscle to shorten, as with other smooth, cardiac, and skeletal muscles, is thought to depend on the cyclic interaction of actin-based thin filaments with cross bridges on myosin-containing thick filaments, i.e., the sliding filament hypothesis originally proposed by H. E. Huxley (see Huxley, 1988) for skeletal muscle. However, smooth muscle has contractile properties distinct from the other muscle types. For example, it does not have the highly organized sarcomeric structure of striated muscle, it shortens at a considerably slower velocity and to a far greater extent, and it can generate far greater force per cross-sectional area with less myosin than can skeletal muscle (see Bagby, 1983).

Thus, although the contractile apparatus of smooth muscle appears to have some fundamental similarities to that of other types of muscle, it must have important structural and biochemical differences that contribute to its unique character. This section deals with the ultrastructure of the thick and thin filaments, the manner in which they may be arranged into contractile units and oriented within the smooth muscle cell, their interaction with the cytoskeleton and plasma membrane, and the apparatus for transmission of force between cells. The specifics concerning the biochemistry of the filaments and their interactions are dealt with in Chapter 13 by Huszar and Walsh. For greater detail than can be presented here, the reader should consult the excellent review articles by Small and Sobieszek (1980), Bagby (1983), A. V. Somlyo (1980), and Gabella (1984).

4.1. Thin Filaments

Thin filaments (Figs. 31 and 32) were recognized in the earliest electron microscopic studies, even when the thick filaments were not preserved (for reasons described in Section 4.2). The thin filaments in fixed and living samples of intact smooth muscle tissues, or in isolated filament preparations, basically align in parallel with the long axis of the cells (Pease and Molinari, 1960; Hanson and Lowy, 1963; Elliott and Lowy, 1968; Ashton et al., 1975; Bagby, 1983). However, they are arranged in a much more variable fashion than in skeletal muscle. The ratio of thin to thick filaments is also more variable in smooth muscle. For example, values as widely disparate as 1 : 8 in chicken gizzard (Nonomura, 1976) and 1 : 15 in vascular muscle of rabbits (Devine and Somlyo, 1971) have been reported. For this reason Gabella (1984) believes that there are likely to be substantial differences in the arrangement and content of actin filaments among different species and types of smooth muscle.

Three different patterns of thin filament arrangement have been described for smooth muscle, but the functional significance if any remains to be ascertained (see Bagby, 1983). In regions where thin filaments are associated with thick filaments, they tend to be organized into (1) rosettes or hexagonal arrays around the thick filaments (Rice et al., 1970; A. V. Somlyo,

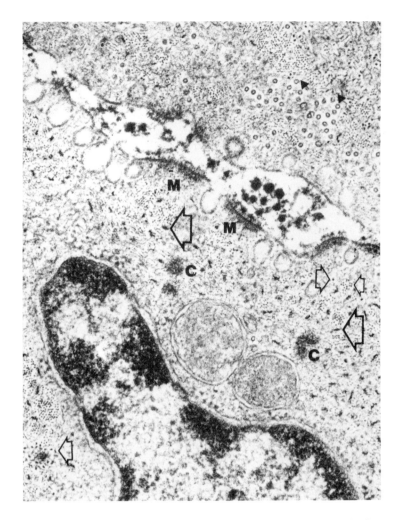

Figure 31. Transverse section of a smooth muscle cell in rat myometrium illustrating the three varieties of filaments: myosin thick filaments (large arrows), intermediate filaments (medium arrows), and thin filaments (small arrows). Microtubules (arrowheads), cytoplasmic- (C) and membrane-associated (M) dense bodies and bands are also evident. Note the filamentous material in the extracellular space at the dense band and the cluster of intermediate filaments around the dense body in the lower left corner (×61,000). From Verhoeff and Garfield (1986), with permission.

1980; A. V. Somlyo *et al.*, 1981) or (2) with two or more rows of thin filaments between thick filaments (Small, 1977; Small and Sobieszek, 1980); (3) in areas where no there is no apparent interaction with myosin, bundles consisting of a few to a hundred thin filaments are observed (Rice *et al.*, 1970; Ashton *et al.*, 1975), frequently showing square lattice (Bagby, 1983) or hexagonal arrays that maintain an 11-nm interfilamentous spacing (Rice *et al.*, 1970; A. P. Somlyo *et al.*, 1973). This latter observation gives credence to the conclusion of Elliott and Lowy (1968) that the 11.5-µm spacing within the equatorial reflections of living taenia coli studied by x-ray diffraction resulted from an orderly arrangement of thin filaments. There is also a suggestion that the thin-filament bundles may branch and divide, suggesting a complex three-dimensional arrangement of the filaments within the cytoplasm (Gabella, 1984).

The width of thin filaments is reported by most investigators to be between 6 and 8 nm

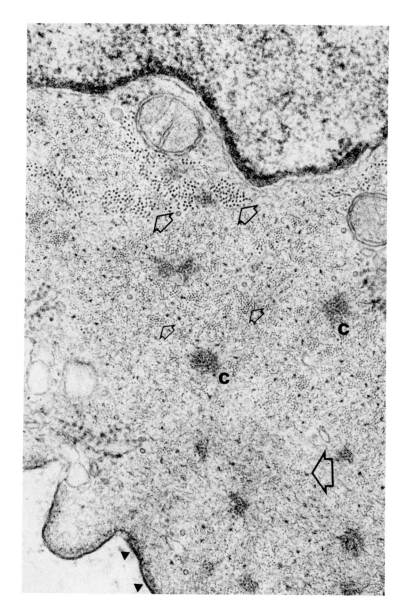

Figure 32. Transverse section of a myometrial cell from nonpregnant human uterus, showing filaments and dense bodies (C). Thick filaments (large arrows), intermediate filaments (medium arrows), and thin filaments (small arrows), intermediate filaments (medium arrows), and thin filaments (small arrows) are indicated. Note the dense bands on the plasma membrane (arrowheads) (×75,000). From Garfield and Hayashi (1981), with permission.

(see Bagby, 1983), but their *in vivo* length is rather uncertain and has never been defined adequately in any smooth muscle. They have been traced in serial ultrathin sections for at least 0.5 μm (Ashton *et al.*, 1975), and reassembled actin filaments *in vitro* of greater than 4 μm in length have been reported (Marston and Smith, 1984). This lack of information about the length of the thin filaments is unfortunate, because very different models for the interaction with thick filaments can be proposed on the basis of different thin filament lengths (Murphy, 1979; Bagby, 1983).

Thin filaments appear to consist of a double helix of actin monomers. A single turn of the helix requires 74 nm, and the monomers repeat every 5.9 nm, which is similar to the F-actin filaments of skeletal muscle (Pease and Molinari, 1960; Hanson and Lowy, 1963; Elliott and Lowy, 1968; Ashton et al., 1975; Marston and Smith, 1985). X-ray diffraction studies also indicate the presence of an extra mass of material that moves toward the center of the grooves between the actin helices when the muscle contracts. This mass is thought to represent tropomyosin (Vibert et al., 1972). Needham and Schoenberg (1967) originally proposed that the content of tropomyosin was greater in smooth muscle than in skeletal muscle; their estimates of the ratio of tropomyosin to actomyosin were 1:14 and 1:17, respectively. For this reason they believed that the thin filaments of the two muscles might differ structurally. However, more recent studies report the same molar ratio (1:7) of actin to tropomyosin (Cohen and Murphy, 1978; Marston and Lehman, 1985), and the observed weight ratio of actin:tropomyosin of 3.5–3.8 in several smooth muscles is not very different from that of rabbit skeletal muscle, which is 4.4 (Murphy et al., 1977; Driska and Murphy, 1978).

Recent studies employing treatment with the detergent saponin have provided exquisite, unobscured views of the contractile apparatus in deep-etched, rotary-shadowed samples of smooth muscle prepared by quick freezing (Bond and Somlyo, 1982; A. V. Somlyo and Franzini-Armstrong, 1985). The structure of the thin filaments and their association with dense bodies revealed in these studies confirm and extend previous observations obtained from thin-sectioned materials.

Saponin permeabilized the cell membrane, permitting direct access of large molecules such as proteins or antibodies to the contractile apparatus in the cell interior. It also results in the washout of soluble proteins that normally would compromise the subsequent visual study of the contractile filaments (Heuser and Kirshner, 1980; Hirokawa and Tilney, 1982; Bond and Somlyo, 1982; A. V. Somlyo and Franzini-Armstrong, 1985). Decorating the thin filaments with myosin subfragment 1 (S$_1$) gives a "ropelike structure" that displays a double helix and appropriate 74-nm repeat (Bond and Somlyo, 1982; A. V. Somlyo and Franzini-Armstrong, 1985). An intermediate periodicity consistent with subfragment binding to the underlying seven actin monomeres per turn was also evident (A. V. Somlyo and Franzini-Armstrong, 1985).

That the thin filaments have a distinct polarity is also evident from these and previous experiments in which the filaments have been decorated with heavy meromyosin or myosin subfragments (Ishikawa et al., 1969; Bond and Somlyo, 1982; A. V. Somlyo and Franzini-Armstrong, 1985). The directions of arrowheads on subfragment-decorated thin filaments emerging on opposite sides of dense bodies within the cell interior are clearly and consistently opposite and away from the dense body (Bond and Somlyo, 1982; A. V. Somlyo and Franzini-Armstrong, 1985). Thus, the thin filaments are of the appropriate polarity for generation of force with the thick filaments. Moreover, such an arrangement supports the idea that there may be some form of organization of dense bodies, thin filaments, and thick filaments into a structured contractile unit (see Section 4.5).

4.2. Thick Filaments

Structural studies of thick filaments have been fraught with difficulties, because these components of smooth muscle cells have proved to be extremely difficult to prepare for electron microscopic study, and efforts to isolate them by homogenization of fresh or glyceri-nated tissue generally have failed. Electron micrographs obtained in the initial structural studies of smooth muscle generally failed to demonstrate the presence of thick filaments despite the fact that the cells appeared to be well preserved and to contain large numbers of thin and intermediate filaments (see reviews by Burnstock, 1970; and Shoenberg and Needham, 1976). Subsequent studies suggested that thick filaments were present only in tissues fixed while in a contracted state (Kelly and Rice, 1968; Rice *et al.*, 1970), a finding that led to the hypothesis that myosin molecules formed filaments only during the shortening process. Later, considerable controversy arose over whether the filaments are ribbon-shaped (Sobieszek and Small, 1973), as opposed to polygonal or round (Ashton *et al.*, 1975), when cut in transverse section. However, all of these problems are now recognized to have resulted from inadequate fixation.

Details of the difficulties associated with preservation of thick filaments and much of the historical background of the development of our understanding of thick filaments in smooth muscle are covered in detail in the chapter by Shoenberg (1978) in the previous edition of this book and in a more recent review by Bagby (1983). Although we have a good idea of the dimensions of the thick filaments in smooth muscle, their fine structure, especially the orientation of the cross bridges along the surface of the filaments, remains a matter of controversy.

Regular arrays of round to polygonal thick filaments (Figs. 31 and 32) have been described in a wide variety of smooth muscle cells (Ashton *et al.*, 1975; Small and Sobieszek, 1980; Bagby, 1983) in the relaxed and contracted states following fixation in aldehyde solutions and in samples of smooth muscle tissues studied by electron microscopy following rapid freezing and freeze-substitution (A. V. Somlyo *et al.*, 1981). Ashton *et al.* (1975) used stereo paired micrographs taken in a high-voltage electron microscope to follow single thick filaments and ascertain their dimensions. Highly accurate measurements of filaments were obtained; their length was measured to be 2.2 ± 0.2 μm, and their diameter 14.6 ± 0.2 nm at the widest point and 0.13 nm at the ends (Ashton *et al.*, 1975). These authors contend that the thick filament structure is similar in smooth and skeletal muscle; that is, the filament is bipolar with a central bare zone. However, unequivocal evidence for this concept was not obtained in their study, and as noted in the following discussion, it is possible that the structure of the thick filament is quite different from that in skeletal muscle.

Native and synthetically prepared filaments have been examined in an attempt to discern the details of orientation and polarity of the cross bridges and to learn whether a central bare zone is present. Although isolation of thick filaments from smooth muscle has proved to be extremely difficult, Small (1977; see also Small and Sobieszek, 1980) has produced an extremely acceptable preparation of thin and thick filaments. Tissues that had been treated with Triton to demembranate the cells were gently fragmented to yield a contractile filament preparation analogous to the myofibril models of skeletal muscle. The length of the thick filaments was relatively uniform, with most between 2 and 3 μm, but some measured over 8 μm (Small, 1977). Most important, they were found to be rod-shaped, as had been described for thick filaments in the intact tissue (Ashton *et al.*, 1975). A central bare zone was not observed; instead, the cross bridges appeared to have a continuous distribution along the length of the filaments with a 14-nm periodicity. This configuration, of course, suggests a structure different from that of the bipolar thick filaments of skeletal muscle cells.

Thick filaments have been grown *in vitro* in several different laboratories (e.g., Sobieszek, 1972; Small, 1977; Craig and Megerman, 1977; Hinssen *et al.*, 1978; Shoenberg and Stewart, 1980). In almost all cases, the only filaments that were found to display a central bare zone were also very short and considerably shorter than the filaments measured in the intact tissue. Longer filaments were consistently found to have a continuous distribution of cross bridges with a 14-nm periodicity and no central bare region. It has been suggested that this type of arrangement indicates that individual myosin molecules align in an antiparallel fashion, giving the so-called "side-polar filaments" in which all the bridges on one side of the filament are oriented in the same direction (Craig and Megerman, 1977). Optical diffraction analysis was used to obtain a cross-bridge organization based on a six-stranded helix with a repeat of 72 nm (Small and Sobieszek, 1980). Hinssen *et al.* (1978) have developed this model further to include the possibility that the cross-bridge heads are of mixed polarity along the filament length.

Whether either model is correct remains to be determined, and although it appears that observations on deep-etched material fixed *in situ* (A. V. Somlyo and Franzini-Armstrong, 1985) will provide an important contribution to the resolution of the fine structure of thick filaments, these data are not yet available. It is apparent that the thick filaments in smooth muscle may be very different from those in skeletal muscle. It follows that the manner in which thin and thick filaments interact in these types of muscles may be very different as well. Most notably, since the polarity of the cross-bridge heads may be the same at one end of the filament as the other, it is possible for the thin filament to move down the entire length of the thick filament in a single direction in smooth muscle. The reconciliation of these different views of thick filament structure must clearly await the presentation of more evidence.

4.3. Cytoplasmic and Membrane-Associated Dense Bodies

Among the most prominent features of myometrial smooth muscle cells when viewed with the electron microscope are the so-called electron-opaque "dense bodies" that either are associated with the plasma membrane (Figs. 11, 31, and 32) or apparently float free in the cytoplasm (Figs. 9, 31, and 32). To differentiate between those in the cytoplasm and those associated with the membrane, the latter are referred to here as dense bands, consistent with Gabella's (1981, 1984) terminology.

Dense bands are large, rather amorphous concentrations of material along the cytoplasmic surface of the plasma membrane in regions between the rows of caveolae (Figs. 11, 31, and 32). In transverse sections they usually measure some 0.1–0.4 μm across, but when sectioned longitudinally, they appear to extend for several micrometers approximately parallel to the long axis of the cell (Gabella, 1977, 1981, 1984). Although the spatial arrangement of the dense bands has not been ascertained, they can be observed at sites all over the surface of the cell, occupying some 30–50% of the cell profile in midregions and approaching 100% in terminal portions (Gabella, 1977, 1981). During partial isotonic contractions the cell surface becomes highly corrugated, and the bands can be seen to form rows between extruded bulges of the cytoplasm and plasma membrane containing caveolae. This arrangement gives the appearance that they are being retracted into the cell (Gabella, 1987a,b).

That the dense bands serve as sites of attachment between thin filaments of the contractile apparatus and the cell membrane is suggested by electron microscopic evidence obtained in many different laboratories (Pease and Molinari, 1960; A. P. Somlyo *et al.*, 1977; Gabella, 1981, 1984). Thin filaments can be seen to penetrate into the dense bands in conventionally sectioned material and in replicas of quick-frozen and deep-etched samples (A. V. Somlyo and Franzini-Armstrong, 1985). In the latter case, the filaments were decorated with myosin S_1 fragments, confirming their actin content and identity as thin filaments. It also was shown that antibodies to α-actinin will bind to the dense bands (Schollenmeyer *et al.*, 1976; Bagby, 1980; Geiger *et al.*, 1980; Small *et al.*, 1986). In skeletal muscle fibers, all thin filaments attach to the Z-line densification, and a major component of this structure is α-actinin. Filamin, another actin-binding protein, and vinculin are also found in the dense bands. These proteins are thought to bind the thin filaments or to stabilize the dense band to the plasma membrane (Davies *et al.*, 1980; Geiger *et al.*, 1980; Small *et al.*, 1986).

In an exhaustive comparison of sectioned and freeze–fractured material fixed at various stages of contraction, Gabella (1976a,b, 1977, 1979a,b) was able to demonstrate clearly that thin filaments insert into the dense bands. Moreover, he showed that during contraction the dense bands that are held by these filaments pull the cell surface inwards, creating troughs between the rows of caveolae. He has suggested, moreover, that the troughs may form a helically arranged system of folds around the cell surface, but details of this pattern have never been presented (Gabella, 1984). This point is important because observations on contraction in single cells (Fisher and Bagby, 1977; Cooke *et al.*, 1987; Warshaw *et al.*, 1987) and in isotonically contracted tissues (Gabella, 1976b) show that shortening occurs in a corkscrewlike fashion, with the ends of the cell rotating as contraction proceeds. A helically arranged system of thin filament attachment sites would be consistent with these observations. The fact that there are dense bodies over the entire length of the cell presumably means that there are sites of thin filament insertion as well. This arrangement is different from that in skeletal muscle, where only the filaments of terminal myofibrils attach to the membrane at the ends of cells. It means that the force generated by the contractile apparatus is distributed over the entire surface of smooth muscle cells.

Cytoplasmic dense bodies are similar to the dense bands in their electron opacity but show no relationship to the plasma membrane (Figs. 9, 32, and 33). In general, they are 0.1 μm in diameter and elongate with their axis parallel to the cell axis (Burnstock, 1970; Gabella, 1977). In some instances, several have been seen to be strung together longitudinally; thus, it is difficult to give a precise measurement of their length (Ashton et al., 1975; A. P. Somlyo et al., 1977).

On the basis of observations that thin filaments enter the dense bodies, it was suggested that the bodies might be analogous to the Z-lines of skeletal muscle (Ashton et al., 1975; Gabella, 1977; Bond and Somlyo, 1982; Cooke et al., 1987). However, this suggestion has been questioned by others who could find no evidence for any relationship between the filaments and dense bodies in sectioned material (see Small and Sobieszek, 1980). As described previously, however, recent studies on rapidly frozen, deep-etched smooth muscle samples clearly showed S_1-decorated thin filaments inserting within dense bodies (A. V. Somlyo and Franzini-Armstrong, 1985). Moreover, the polarity of the arrowheads is opposite on either side of the dense bodies. These data provide strong evidence for a pseudo-Z-line function.

The material forming the dense bodies, like that in the dense bands, appears to be a combination of amorphous and filamentous components (Gabella, 1977, 1981, 1984; Ashton et al., 1975; A. P. Somlyo et al., 1977). Biochemically, the dense bodies and bands appear to be nearly identical as well (Bagby, 1983). Immunolabeling experiments indicate that the dense bodies, like the dense bands described above and the Z-line of skeletal muscle, also contain α-actinin, although they do not appear to contain vinculin (Schollenmeyer et al., 1976; Bagby, 1980; Geiger et al., 1980). Such data provide further support for the concept of a functional similarity between these structures and Z-lines.

Conventional thin-section and the more recent deep-etching studies also demonstrate that intermediate filaments (see below) insert into the dense bands and cytoplasmic dense bodies (Cooke and Fay, 1972; Ashton et al., 1975; Small, 1977; Small and Sobieszek, 1980; A. V. Somlyo and Franzini-Armstrong, 1985). These views are consistent with the idea that the dense bodies and bands serve as cytoskeletal elements as well (Small and Sobieszek, 1980). Indeed, the association of both contractile and cytoskeletal filaments with the dense bands has led to the designation of the latter as attachment plaques by some authors (e.g., Small and Sobieszek, 1980).

4.4. Intermediate Filaments

In addition to thick and thin filaments, smooth muscle cells contain large numbers of a class of filaments the size of which, at 10 nm in diameter, is intermediate between the previously considered filaments. Consequently they have been named intermediate filaments (Figs. 31 and 32) (Lazarides, 1980; Steinert et al., 1984). Although they are similar in size to the thin filaments (8 nm), intermediate filaments are easily differentiated by their electron-lucent core in transverse section (Rice et al., 1970; Small and Squire, 1972). In general, they appear to be distributed in an irregular fashion among the contractile filaments but have been described by some authors as being more numerous in the central regions of smooth muscle cells (e.g., Shoenberg, 1973; A. P. Somlyo et al., 1973) or as changing their location during the contraction–relaxation cycle (Cooke and Fay, 1972). They are particularly evident around dense bands and bodies. In the latter sites it is not unusual to observe a ring of intermediate filaments around the periphery of the structure (Fig. 31) (Shoenberg and Needham, 1976; Small, 1977; A. P. Somlyo et al., 1973; Gabella, 1979a).

Such observations have led to the conclusion that intermediate filaments perform a cytoskeletal role in the structural support and organization of cytoplasmic constituents (Cooke, 1976; Small and Sobieszek, 1980; Bagby, 1983), perhaps including the contractile apparatus (Bagby, 1983). Indeed, if the thick and thin filaments are solubilized by treating smooth muscle samples with EDTA (or EGTA) at neutral pH, the intermediate filaments and dense bodies are left behind, the cell maintains its characteristic shape, and the network shows a tendency to attach to the plasma membrane at the terminal regions of the cells (Cooke and Fay, 1972; Fay and Cooke, 1973; Cooke, 1976; Bagby and Corey, 1981). More recent immunolocalization studies using antibodies against intermediate filament proteins (i.e., skeletin or desmin in visceral muscles and vimentin in vascular muscle) clearly demonstrate a web of filaments within all parts of the interior of cultured smooth muscle cells and confirm that they are particularly numerous around the nucleus (Chamley-Campbell et al., 1979; Small and Sobieszek, 1980). The networks have the same general appearance and distribution as the filament networks in noncontractile cells (Lazarides, 1980; Steinert et al., 1984).

These observations are consistent with the idea that intermediate filaments are cytoskeletal components in smooth muscle, as has been suggested for other contractile and noncontractile cell types (Lazarides, 1980; Steinert et al., 1984). The possible organization of the intermediate filaments and contractile filaments into a skeletal/contractile network is considered in detail in the next section.

4.5. Structural Organization of the Contractile Apparatus and Its Possible Association with the Cytoskeleton

Since the previous edition of this volume was published, several new structural models for the organization of the contractile elements in smooth muscle have been advanced. Despite much debate, however, there is still no consensus concerning the actual arrangement of the thick and thin filaments and their possible interaction with the cytoskeleton. For a detailed discussion of the different models and their limitations, the reader is referred to the excellent review by Bagby (1983).

It is evident that there is no true sarcomere organization of the contractile filaments in smooth muscle. However, evidence is accumulating to suggest that cytoplasmic dense bodies in smooth muscle play the part of Z-lines of skeletal muscle (Ashton et al., 1975; Fay et al., 1983; Cooke et al., 1987) and that the dense bodies and small groups of thick and thin filaments do form quasisarcomeric structures and myofibrils (Small, 1974; Ashton et al., 1975; Bond and Somlyo, 1982; Bagby, 1983). It is evident also that (1) these units may be stabilized within the cytoplasm by a direct interaction between the contractile elements and the cytoskeleton at the cytoplasmic dense bodies (Bagby, 1983) and (2) the cytoplasmic dense bodies and contractile and cytoskeletal filaments undergo marked changes in orientation during contraction (Bozler and Cottrell, 1937; Bagby et al., 1971; Fisher and Bagby, 1977; Fay et al., 1983; Bagby, 1983; Cooke et al., 1987). The contractile filaments change in orientation from predominantly longitudinal to a more oblique and distinctly helical arrangement during cell shortening (Fisher and Bagby, 1977; Small, 1977; Small and Sobieszek, 1980; Bagby, 1983). Reorientation is accompanied by a migration of the dense bodies during contraction (Bagby, 1983; Cooke et al., 1987).

Most models postulate a helical arrangement of the contractile elements in smooth muscle cells (Small, 1977; Fisher and Bagby, 1977; Bagby, 1983). This arrangement is evident from the fact that the cells contract in a corkscrewlike fashion when in isolation (e.g., Warshaw et *al.,* 1987) or in the intact tissue (Gabella, 1976b). Corkscrew shortening has been noted by one of us in single myometrial cells (W. C. Cole and K. M. Sanders, unpublished observation) and is particularly evident in the contracted cells shown in the scanning micrograph in Fig. 33.

A low-pitch helical (i.e., less than 10° and almost longitudinally oriented) arrangement of contractile filaments could be achieved either by attachment of the thin filaments to membrane-associated dense bands that are arranged in a helical fashion around the interior of the cell surface (Small, 1977; Gabella, 1984) or, in the presence of coaxial, longitudinal dense bands (Small *et al.,* 1986), by a low-pitch curved arrangement of all the myofibrils within one end of the cell and a wrapping of the contractile filaments around the axial cytoskeleton elements before attaching to it (Bagby, 1983).

A helical arrangement of the contractile apparatus can explain, at least in part, both the relatively slow velocity of shortening and greater development of force per unit cross-sectional area of smooth muscle cells. A helical arrangement means that there is a greater number of contractile filaments generating force in parallel and that the shortening is a vector process with transverse and longitudinal components. Other biochemical differences between the contractile

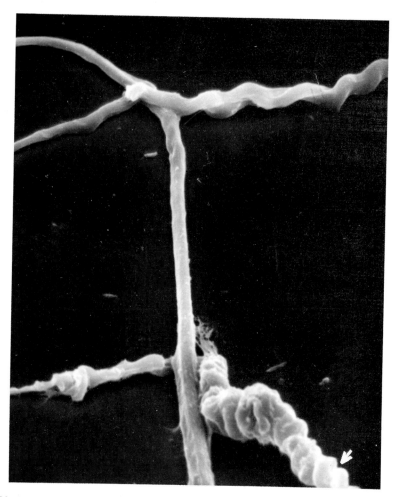

Figure 33. Scanning electron micrograph of three isolated smooth muscle cells in varied states of contraction. That contraction involves a corkscrewlike shortening is evident in the upper partially contracted cell and at the arrow in the lower, completely contracted cell (×1200). Courtesy of Drs. P. Langton and K. Sanders, (unpublished).

apparatus of smooth and skeletal muscle that may contribute to the unique contractile charac-teristics of the former are dealt with in Chapter 13 by Huszar and Walsh.

4.6. Mechanical Transmission in a Multicellular Tissue

The contractile force generated by the interaction between the thick and thin filaments is transmitted to the plasma membrane through the insertion of the thin filaments into the membrane-associated dense bands. α-Actinin and vinculin are thought to function in the linkage of thin filaments to the dense bands and plasma membrane (Geiger *et al.*, 1980; Bond and Somlyo, 1982; A. V. Somlyo and Franzini-Armstrong, 1985). This section briefly covers the crucial mechanisms by which this force is thought to be transmitted across the cell membrane and between cells.

The attachment of thin and intermediate filaments to the dense bodies has been studied in detail in recent deep-etched samples of smooth muscle (A. V. Somlyo and Franzini-Armstrong, 1985), but the mechanism for transmission of force across the membrane still is unresolved. Direct cell-to-cell transmission clearly occurs through the extensive intermediate junctions that structurally link smooth muscle cells (see Section 2.3). Indirect transmission occurs by means of the elastic and collagen fibers that link each cell to the extracellular stroma.

The terminal portions of the intermediate and thin filaments appear to be embedded in a granular material at the membrane surface, which A. V. Somlyo and Franzini-Armstrong (1985) speculate may represent the α-actinin, vinculin, or both shown to be present by biochemical analysis. On the outside of the membrane at sites not involving intermediate junctions, there are numerous small extracellular fibrils that insert into the membrane and attach to collagen fibers (Fig. 31), but there is no evidence of transmembrane structures.

As noted by Gabella (1984), there is no evidence for protein components within the plasma membrane at intermediate junctions or sites of collagen attachment that could function to link intracellular and extracellular filament systems and permit transmission of force. In fact, the membrane under the dense bands characteristically lacks intramembrane protein particles (Devine and Rayns, 1975; Gabella, 1981). Such a lack is in contrast to the situation in desmosomes, where large integral proteins traverse the membrane and are revealed as aggregates of intramembrane proteins by freeze–fracture analysis. Whether their absence is real or the proteins are present but not visualized by freeze–fracture remains to be determined (Gabella, 1984).

5. Conclusion

In this chapter the structure of various components of myometrium has been discussed. Particular attention has been paid to the myometrial smooth muscle cells, their contractile apparatus, and the gap junctions that link the individual cells into a functional syncytium.

We have described the structure of gap junctions and the data that provide evidence for their role in cell-to-cell interactions in the myometrium and their control by hormonal systems. The junctions permit the intercellular exchange of small ions and molecules and in so doing facilitate a synchronization of the electrical, metabolic, and contractile activities in the millions of myometrial muscle cells during labor. The structural development of large numbers of junctions in the myometrium at delivery appears to play a major role in the evolution of uterine contractility at term and during labor. We suggest that this structural event is regulated by the steroid hormones, their receptors, and prostaglandins. The conductance/permeability and kinetic characteristics of the cell-to-cell channels comprising the gap junctions may also be regulated by circulating or locally released agents. Thus, there appear to be several levels at which coordinated uterine activity may be controlled. It is hoped that future efforts will characterize further these mechanisms and develop pharmacological tools for their therapeutic management.

The structural details and possible arrangement of thick, thin, and intermediate filaments in myometrial cells has been presented. It is evident that our understanding of these structures has advanced considerably since publication of the previous edition of this book. We now recognize that there are contractile and cytoskeletal structures arranged in parallel in myometrial cells and that there is a structural linkage between these systems at the dense bands and bodies. The role of the dense bodies and bands as anchoring sites has been established by structural and biochemical evidence. The unique characteristics of the contractile filaments of smooth muscle have been presented and discussed with reference to those of skeletal muscles. Major efforts are underway in several laboratories to ascertain the cross-bridge arrangement on thick filaments, the nature of the interaction between the contractile filaments, and their three-dimensional arrangement within smooth muscle cells. Perhaps by the time the next edition of this book is published we will have a complete understanding of the contractile apparatus of the myometrium.

ACKNOWLEDGMENTS. The authors wish to thank Ms. D. Merrett for her efforts in composing the figures. They also wish to thank Drs. P. Langton, S. Ward, and K. Sanders for supplying the photomicrographs used in Figures 6, 7, and 33. Finally, they thank the Medical Research Council of Canada and the Canadian Heart Foundation for the grants, scholarships, and fellowships that have supported their work on cell-to-cell communication in the myometrium.

6. References

Abe, Y., and Tomita, T., 1968, Cable properties of smooth muscle, *J. Physiol. (Lond.)* **196**:87–102.

Althoff, R. W., and Albert, E. N., 1970, Ultrastructural changes in mouse myometrium during pregnancy, *Am. J. Obstet. Gynecol.* **108**:1224–1233.

Ashton, F. T., Somlyo, A. V., and Somlyo, A. P., 1975, The contractile apparatus of vascular smooth muscle; intermediate high voltage stereoelectron microscopy, *J. Mol. Biol.* **98**:17–29.

Bagby, R. M., 1980, Double immunofluorescent staining of isolated smooth muscle cells, *Histochemistry* **69**:113–130.

Bagby, R. M., 1983, Organization of contractile/cytoskeletal elements, in: *The Biochemistry of Smooth Muscle* (N. L. Stephens, ed.), CRC Press, Boca Raton, FL, pp. 1–84.

Bagby, R. M., and Corey, M. D., 1981, Vertebrate contractile elements attach to an axial cytoskeleton, *Physiologist* **24**:89–95.

Bagby, R. M., Young, A. M., Dotson, R. S., Fisher, B. A., and McKinnon, K., 1971, Contraction of single smooth muscle cells from *Bufo marinus* stomach, *Nature* **234**:351–352.

Batra, S. C., 1973, The role of mitochondrial calcium uptake in contraction and relaxation of the human myometrium, *Biochim. Biophys. Acta* **305**:428–432.

Beams, H. W., and Kessel, R. G., 1968, The Golgi apparatus; structure and function, *Int. Rev. Cytol.* **23**:209–276.

Benedetti, E. L., and Emmelot, P., 1968, Hexagonal array of subunits in tight junctions separated from isolated rat liver plasma membranes, *J. Cell Biol.* **38**:15–22.

Bergman, R. A., 1968, Uterine smooth muscle fibers in castrate and estrogen treated rats, *J. Cell Biol.* **36**:636–648.

Blennerhassett, M. G., Kannan, M. S., and Garfield, R. E., 1987, Regulation of gap junctions in myometrial smooth muscle, *Ann. N.Y. Acad. Sci.* **484**:196–204.

Bo, W. J., Odor, D. L., and Rothrock, M., 1968, The fine structure of uterine smooth muscle of the rat uterus at various time intervals following a single injection of estrogen, *Am. J. Anat.* **123**:369–384.

Bond, M., and Somlyo, A V., 1982, Dense bodies and actin polarity in vertebrate smooth muscle, *J. Cell Biol.* **95**:403–413.

Bond, M., Kitazawa, T., Somlyo, A. V., and Somlyo, A. P., 1984a, Release and recycling of calcium by the sarcoplasmic reticulum in guinea pig portal vein smooth muscle, *J. Physiol. (Lond.)* **355**:677–695.

Bond, M., Somlyo, A. V., and Somlyo, A. P., 1984b, Total cytoplasmic calcium in relaxed and maximally contracted rabbit portal vein smooth muscle, *J. Physiol. (Lond.)* **357**:185–201.

Bozler, E., 1938, Electrical stimulation and conduction of excitation in smooth muscle, *Am. J. Physiol.* **122**:616–635.

Bozler, E., 1940, Influence of estrone on the electrical characteristics and motility of uterine muscle, *Endocrinology* **29**:225–238.

Bozler, E., and Cottrell, C. L., 1937, The birefringence of muscle and its variation during contraction, *J. Cell. Comp. Physiol.* **10**:165–182.

Brandes, D., and Anton, E., 1969, Lysosomes in uterine involution: Intracytoplasmic degragation of myofilaments and collagen, *J. Gerentol.* **24**:55–69.

Buchanan, G. D., and Garfield, R. E., 1984, Myometrial ultrastructure and innervation in *Myotis lucifugus,* the little brown bat, *Anat. Rec.* **210**:463–475.

Burden, H. W., Capps, M. L., and Lawrence, I. E., 1979, Gap junctions in the myometrium of pelvic-neurectomized rats with blocked parturition, *Am. J. Physiol.* **156**:105–111.

Burghardt, R. C., Matheson, R. L., and Gandy, D., 1984a, Gap junction modulation in rat uterus. I. Effects of estrogens on myometrial and serosal cells, *Biol. Reprod.* **30**:239–248.

Burghardt, R. C., Mitchell, P. A., and Kurten, R., 1984b, Gap junction modulation in rat uterus. I. Effects of antiestrogens on myometrial and serosal cells, *Biol. Reprod.* **30**:249–255.

Burnstock, G., 1970, Structure of smooth muscle and its innervation, in: *Smooth Muscle* (E. Bulbring, A. F. Brading, A. W. Jones, and T. Tomita, eds.), Williams & Wilkins, Baltimore, pp. 1–70.

Caspar, D. L. D., Goodenough, D. A., Makowski, L., and Phillips, W. C., 1977, Gap junction structures. I. Correlated electron microscopy and x-ray diffraction, *J. Cell Biol.* **74**:605–611.

Chalcroft, J. P., and Bullivant, S., 1970, An interpretation of liver cell membrane and junction structure based on observation of freeze–fracture replicas of both sides of the structure, *J. Cell Biol.* **47**:49–57.

Challis, J. R. G., and Lye, S. J., 1986, Parturition, in: *Oxford Review of Reproductive Biology* (J. R. Clarke, ed.), Oxford University Press, London, pp. 61–82.

Chamley-Campbell, J., Campbell, G. R., and Ross, R., 1979, The smooth muscle cell in culture, *Physiol. Rev.* **59**:1–61.

Chance, B., 1963, *Energy Linked Functions of Mitochondria,* Academic Press, New York.

Cohen, D. M., and Murphy, R. A., 1978, Differences in cellular contractile protein contents and force generation in porcine smooth muscles, *J. Gen. Physiol.* **72**:369–380.

Cole, W. C., and Garfield, R. E., 1986a, Methods for analysis of myometrial gap junction structure and function, in: *Animal Models in Fetal Medicine,* Vol. 5 (P. W. Nathanielz, ed.), Perinatology Press, New York, pp. 31–65.

Cole, W. C., and Garfield, R. E., 1986b, Evidence for physiological regulation of myometrial gap junction permeability, *Am. J. Physiol.* **251**:C411–420.

Cole, W. C., and Garfield, R. E., 1988, Effects of calcium ionophore, A23187, and calmodulin antagonists on cell-to-cell communication between rat myometrial smooth muscle cells, *Biol. Reprod.* **38**: 55–62.

Cole, W. C., Garfield, R. E., and Kirkaldy, J. S., 1985, Gap junctions and direct intercellular communication between rat uterine smooth muscle cells, *Am. J. Physiol.* **249**:C20–31.

Cooke, P. H., 1976, A filamentous cytoskeleton in vertebrate smooth muscle fibers, *J. Cell Biol.* **68**:539–556.

Cooke, P. H., and Fay, F. S., 1972, Correlation between fiber length, ultrastructure, and the length–tension relationship of mammalian smooth muscle, *J. Cell Biol.* **52**:105–116.

Cooke, P. H., Kargacin G., Craig, R. F., Fogarty, K.E., Hagen, S., and Fay, F. S., 1987, Molecular structure and organization of filaments in single, skinned smooth muscle cells, in: *Regulation and Contraction of Smooth Muscles* (N. L. Stephens, ed.), Alan R. Liss, New York, pp. 1–25.

Craig, R., and Mengerman, J., 1977, Assembly of smooth muscle myosin into side-polar filaments, *J. Cell Biol.* **75**:990–996.

Creed, K., 1979, Functional diversity of smooth muscle, *Br. Med. Bull.* **35**:243–248.

Csapo, A. I., 1962, Smooth muscle as a contractile unit, *Physiol. Rev.* **42** (Suppl. 5):7–33.

Csapo, A. I., 1981, Force of Labor, in: *Principles and Practice of Obstetrics and Perinatology* (L. Iffy and H. A. Kaminetzky, eds.), John Wiley & Sons, New York, pp. 761–799.

Daniel, E. E., Daniel, V. P., Duchon, G., Garfield, R. E., Nichols, M., Malhotra, S. K., and Oki, M., 1976, Is the nexus necessary for cell-to-cell coupling of smooth muscle? *J. Membr. Biol.* **28**:207–239.

Dahl, G. P., and Berger, W., 1978, Nexus formation in the myometrium during parturition and induced by estrogen, *Cell Biol. Int. Rep.* **2**:381–387.

Dahl, G. P., Azarnia, R., and Werner, R., 1980, *De novo* construction of cell-to-cell channels, *In Vitro* **16:**1068–1075.

Dahl, G. P., Levine, R., and Werner, R., 1987, Cell-to-cell channels made from gap junction specific mRNA are gated, *Biophys. J.* **51:**39a.

Davies, P. J., Wallach, D., Willingham, M. C., and Pastan, I., 1980, Filamin–actin interaction, *J. Biol. Chem.* **253:**4036–4041.

Demianczuk, N., Towell, M., and Garfield, R. E., 1984, Myometrial electrophysiologic activity and gap junctions in the pregnant rabbit, *Am. J. Obstet. Gynecol.* **149:**485–493.

Dessouky, A. D., 1968, Electron microscopy studies of the myometrium of the guinea pig: The smooth muscle of the myometrium before and during pregnancy, *Am. J. Obstet. Gynecol.* **100:**1117–1123.

Dessouky, A. D., 1976, Ultrastructural observations of the human uterine smooth muscle cells during gestation, *Am. J. Obstet. Gynecol.* **125:** 1099–1107.

Devine, C. E., and Rayns, D. G., 1975, Freeze–fracture studies of membrane systems in vertebrate muscle: Smooth muscle, *J. Ultrastruct. Res.* **51:**293–306.

Devine, C. E., and Somlyo, A. P., 1971, Thick filaments in vascular smooth muscle, *J. Cell Biol.* **49:**636–649.

Devine, C. E., Somlyo, A.V., and Somlyo, A. P., 1972, Sarcoplasmic reticulum and excitation–contraction coupling in mammalian smooth muscle, *J. Cell Biol.* **52:**690–718.

Dewey, M. M., and Barr, L., 1962, Intercellular connection between smooth muscle cells: The nexus, *Science* **137:**670–672.

Downing, S. J., and Sherwood, O. D., 1985a, The physiological role of relaxin in the pregnant rat. I. The influence of relaxin on parturition, *Endocrinology* **116:**1200–1205.

Downing, S. J., and Sherwood, O. D., 1985b, The physiological role of relaxin in the pregnant rat. II. The influence of relaxin on uterine contractile activity, *Endocrinology* **116:**1205–1211.

Driska, S. P., and Murphy, R. A., 1978, Estimate of cellular force generation in an arterial smooth muscle with high actin : myosin ratio, *Blood Vessels* **15:**26–32.

Elliott, G. F., and Lowy, J., 1968, Organization of actin in a mammalian smooth muscle, *Nature* **219:**156–157.

Fay, F. S., and Cooke, P. H., 1973. Reversible disaggregation of myofilaments in vertebrate smooth musles, *J. Cell Biol.* **56:**399–411.

Fay, F. S., Fujiwara, K., Rees, D. D., and Fogarty, K. E., 1983, Distribution of α-actinin in single isolated smooth muscle cells, *J. Cell Biol.* **96:**783–795.

Fisher, B. A., and Bagby, R. M., 1977, Reorientation of myofilaments during contraction of a vertebrate smooth muscle, *Am. J. Physiol.* **232:**C5–14.

Franzini-Armstrong, C., 1970, Studies of the triad. I. Structure of the junction in frog twitch fibers, *J. Cell Biol.* **47:**488–499.

Frederici, H. H., and DeCloux, R. J., 1968, The early response of immature rat myometrium to estrogenic stimulation, *J. Ultrastruct. Res.* **22:**402–412.

Fuchs, A. R., 1978, Hormonal control of myometrial function during pregnancy and parturition, *Acta Endocrinol. (Kbh.) [Suppl.]* **221:**1–69.

Gabella, G., 1976a, The force generated by a visceral smooth muscle, *J. Physiol. (Lond.)* **262:**199–213.

Gabella, G., 1976b, Quantitative morphological study of smooth muscle cells of taenia coli. Structural changes in smooth muscle cells during isotonic contraction, *Cell Tissue Res.* **170:**161–201.

Gabella, G., 1977, Arrangement of smooth muscle cells and intramuscular septa in the taenia coli, *Cell Tissue Res.* **184:**195–204.

Gabella, G., 1979a, Hypertrophic smooth muscles. IV. Myofilaments, intermediate filaments and some mechanical properties. *Cell Tissue Res.* **201:**27–28.

Gabella, G., 1979b, Smooth muscle cell junctions and structural aspects of contraction, *Br. Med. Bull.* **35:**213–218.

Gabella, G., 1981, Structure of smooth muscles, in: *Smooth Muscle* (E. Bulbring, A. F. Brading, A. W. Jones, and T. Tomita, eds.), Edward Arnold, London, pp. 1–46.

Gabella, G., 1984, Structural apparatus for force transmission in smooth muscles, *Physiol. Rev.* **64:**455–477.

Gabella, G., and Blundell, D., 1978, Effect of stretch and contraction on caveolae of smooth muscle cells, *Cell Tissue Res.* **190:**255–271.

Garfield, R. E., 1984, Myometrial ultrastructure and uterine contractility, in: *Uterine Contractility* (S. Bottari, J. P. Thomas, A. Vokaer, and R. Vokaer, eds.), Masson USA, New York, pp. 81–109.

Garfield, R. E., 1985, Cell-to-cell communication, in: *Calcium and Contractility* (A. K. Grover and E. E. Daniel, eds.) Humana Press, Clifton, NJ, pp. 143–173.

Garfield, R. E., 1986, Structural studies on innervation of nonpregnant rat uterus, *Am. J. Physiol.* **251:**C41–54.

Garfield, R. E., and Baulieu, E. E., 1987, The antiprogesterone steroid RU 486: A short pharmacological and clinical review with emphasis on the interruption of pregnancy, *Baill. Clin. Endocrinol. Metab.* **1:**207–214.

Garfield, R. E., and Daniel, E. E., 1974, The structural basis for electrical coupling (cell-to-cell contacts) in rat myometrium, *Gynecol. Invest.* **5:**284–300.

Garfield, R. E., and Daniel, E. E., 1977a, Relation of membrane vesicles to volume control and Na$^+$ transport in smooth muscle: Effect of metabolic and transport inhibition on fresh tissues, *J. Mechanochem. Cell Motil.* **4:**115–155.

Garfield, R. E., and Daniel, E. E., 1977b, Relation of membrane vesicles to volume control and Na$^+$ transport in smooth muscle: Studies on Na$^+$ rich tissues, *J. Mechanochem. Cell Motil.* **4:**157–176.

Garfield, R. E., and Hayashi, R. H., 1981, Appearance of gap junctions in the myometrium of women during labor, *Am. J. Obstet. Gynecol.* **140:**254–260.

Garfield, R. E., and Somlyo, A. P., 1977, Golgi apparatus and lectin-binding sites: Effects of lasalocid (X537A), *Exp. Cell Res.* **109:**167–177.

Garfield, R. E., and Somlyo, A. P., 1985, Structure of smooth muscle, in: *Calcium and Contractility* (A. K. Grover and E. E. Daniel, eds.), Humana Press, New Jersey, pp. 1–36.

Garfield, R. E., Sims, S. M., and Daniel, E. E., 1977, Gap junctions: Their presence and necessity in myometrium during parturition, *Science* **198:**958–960.

Garfield, R. E., Sims, S. M., Kannan, M. S., and Daniel, E. E., 1978, The possible role of gap junctions in the activation of the myometrium during parturition, *Am. J. Physiol.* **235:**C168–179.

Garfield, R. E., Rabideau, S., Challis, J. R. G., and Daniel, E. E., 1979, Hormonal control of gap junctions in sheep myometrium, *Biol. Reprod.* **21:**999–1007.

Garfield, R. E., Kannan, M. S., and Daniel, E. E., 1980a, Gap junction formation in myometrium: Control by estrogens, progesterone and prostaglandins, *Am. J. Physiol.* **7:**C81–89.

Garfield, R. E., Merrett, D., and Grover, A. K., 1980b, Studies on gap junction formation and regulation in myometrium, *Am. J. Physiol.* **239:**C217–228.

Garfield, R. E., Daniel, E. E., Dukes, M., and Fitzgerald, J. D., 1982, Changes in gap junctions in myometrium of guinea pigs at parturition and abortion, *Can. J. Physiol. Pharmacol.* **60:**335–341.

Garfield, R. E., Gasc, J. M., and Baulieu, E. E., 1987, Effects of the antiprogesterone RU 486 on preterm birth in the rat, *Am. J. Obstet. Gynecol.* **157:** 1281–1285.

Geiger, B., Tokuyasu, K. T., Dutton, A. H., and Singer, S. J., 1980, Vinculin, an intracellular protein localized at specialized sites where microfilament bundles terminate at cell membranes, *Proc. Natl. Acad. Sci. U.S.A.* **77:**4127–4137.

Goodenough, D. A., and Stoeckinius, W., 1972, The isolation of mouse hepatocyte gap junctions. Preliminary chemical characterization and x-ray diffraction, *J. Cell Biol.* **57:**54–67.

Goodford, P. J., 1970, Ion movements in smooth muscle, in: *Membranes and Ion Transport,* Vol. 2 (E. Bittar, ed.), Wiley-Interscience, New York, pp. 33–74.

Goodford, P. J., and Wolowyk, M. W., 1972, Localization of cation interactions in the smooth muscle of the guinea pig taenia coli, *J. Physiol. (Lond.)* **224:**521–535.

Gorski, J., and Gannon, F., 1976, Current models of hormone action: A critique, *Annu. Rev. Physiol.* **38:**425–450.

Hand, A. R., and Oliver, C., 1977, Cytochemical studies on GERL and its role in secretory granule formation in exocrine pancreas, *Histochem. J.* **9:**375–386.

Hanson, J., and Lowy, J., 1963, The structure of F-actin and of actin filaments isolated from muscle. *J. Mol. Biol.* **6:**46–60.

Heuser, J. E., and Kirshner, M. W., 1980, Filament organization revealed in platinum replicas of freeze-dried cytoskeletons, *J. Cell Biol.* **86:**212–234.

Hinssen, H., D'Haese, J., Small, J. V., and Sobieszek, A., 1978, Mode of filament assembly of myosins from muscle and nonmuscle cells, *J. Ultrastruct. Res.* **64:**282–289.

Hirokawa, N., and Tilney, L. G., 1982, Interactions between actin filaments and between actin filaments and membranes in quick-frozen and deeply etched hair cells of the chick ear, *J. Cell Biol.* **95:**149–261.

Huxley, A. F., 1988, Muscular contraction, *Annu. Rev. Physiol.* **50:**1–16.

Ishikawa, H., Bischoff, R., and Holzer, H., 1969, Formation of arrowhead complexes with heavy meromyosin in a variety of cell types, *J. Cell Biol.* **43:**312–328.

Kelly, R. E., and Rice, R. V., 1968, Localization of myosin filaments in smooth muscle, *J. Cell Biol.* **37:**105–116.

Kowarski, D., Shuman, H., Somlyo, A. P., and Somlyo, A. V., 1985, Calcium release by norepinephrine from central sarcoplasmic reticulum in rabbit main pulmonary artery smooth muscle. *J. Physiol. (Lond.)* **366:**153–175.

Kreutziger, G. O., 1968, Freeze-etching of intercellular junctions of mouse liver, in: *26th Proceedings of the Electron Microscopy Society of America,* Claitors Publishing Division, Baton Rouge, LA, p. 138.

Larsen, W. J., 1977a, Structural diversity of gap junctions: A review. *Tissue Cell* **9:**373–394.

Larsen, W. J., 1977b, Gap junctions and hormone action, in: *Transport of Ions and Water in Epithelia* (B. J. Wall, J. L. Oschmanm, and B. Moreton, eds.), Academic Press, London, pp. 333–361.

Larsen, W. J., 1983, Biological implications of gap junction structure, distribution, and composition: A review, *Tissue Cell* **15**:645–671.

Lazarides, E., 1980, Intermediate filaments as mechanical integrators of cellular space, *Nature* **283**:249–256.

Leblond, C. P., and Bennett, G., 1977, Role of the Golgi apparatus in terminal glycosylation, in: *International Cell Biology* (B. R. Brinkley and K. R. Porter, eds.), Rockefeller University Press, New York, pp. 145–157.

Lehninger, A. L., 1965, *Mitochondrion: Molecular Basis for Structure and Function,* Benjamin, New York.

Liggins, G. C., 1979, Initiation of parturition, *Br. Med. Bull.* **35**:45–101.

Loewenstein, W. R., 1981, Junctional intercellular communication; the cell-to-cell membrane channel, *Physiol. Rev.* **61**:829–913.

Mackenzie, L. W., and Garfield, R. E., 1985, Hormonal control of gap junctions in the myometrium, *Am. J. Physiol.* **248**:C296–302.

Mackenzie, L. W., and Garfield, R. E., 1986a, Effects of estradiol-17β and prostaglandins on myometrial gap junctions and pregnancy in the rat, *Can. J. Physiol. Pharmacol.* **64**:462–470.

Mackenzie, L. W., and Garfield, R. E., 1986b, Effects of tamoxifen citrate and cycloheximide on estradiol induction of rat myometrial gap junctions, *Can. J. Physiol. Pharmacol.* **64**:703–711.

Mackenzie, L. W., Puri, C. P., and Garfield, R. E., 1983, Effect of estradiol-17β and prostaglandins on rat myometrial gap junctions, *Prostaglandins* **26**:925–931.

Makowski, L., 1985, Structural domains in gap junctions: Implications for the control of intercellular communication, in: *Gap Junctions* (M. V. L. Bennett and D. C. Spray, eds.), Cold Spring Harbor Laboratory, Cold Spring Harbor, NY, pp. 5–12.

Makowski, L., Caspar, D. L. D., Phillips, W. C., and Goodenough, D. A., 1984, Gap junction structures. V. Structural chemistry inferred from x-ray diffraction measurements on sucrose accessibility and trypsin susceptibility, *J. Mol. Biol.* **174**:449–481.

Marshall, J. M., 1962, Regulation of activity of uterine smooth muscle, *Physiol. Rev.* **42**:213–235.

Marston, S. B., and Lehman, W., 1985, Caldesmon is a Ca^{++}-regulatory protein of native smooth muscle filaments, *Biochem. J.* **231**:517–522.

Marston, S. B., and Smith, C. W. J., 1984, Purification and properties of Ca^{++}-regulated thin filaments and F-actin from sheep aorta smooth muscle, *J. Muscle Res. Cell Motil.* **5**:559–575.

Marston, S. B., and Smith, C. W. J., 1985, The thin filaments of smooth muscle, *J. Muscle Res. Cell Motil.* **6**:669–708.

Merk, F. B., Kwan, P. W. L., and Leav, I., 1980, Gap junctions in the myometrium of hypophysectomized estrogen-treated rats, *Cell Biol. Int. Rep.* **4**:287–294.

Murphy, R. A., 1979, Filament organization and contractile function in vertebrate smooth muscle, *Annu. Rev. Physiol.* **41**:737–748.

Murphy, R. A., Driska, S. P., and Cohen, D. M., 1977, Variation in actin to myosin ratios and cellular force generation in vertebrate smooth muscles, in: *Excitation–Contraction Coupling in Smooth Muscles* (R. Casteels, J. Godfraind, and J. C. Ruegg, eds.), Elsevier/North Holland Amsterdam, pp. 417–424.

Needham, D. M., and Schoenberg, C. F., 1967, The biochemistry of the myometrium, in: *Cellular Biology of the Uterus* (R. M. Wynn, ed.), Appleton-Century-Crofts, New York, pp. 291–352.

Nonomura, J., 1976, Fine structure of myofilaments in chicken gizzard smooth muscle, in: *Recent Progress in Electron Microscopy of Cells and Tissues* (E. Yamada, V. Mazuhira, K. Kurosumi, and T. Nagano, eds.), Georg Thieme, Stuttgart, pp. 40–48.

Novikoff, A. P., and Novikoff, P. M., 1977, Cytochemical contributions to differentiating GERL from the Golgi apparatus, *Histochem. J.* **9**:525–537.

Pease, D. C., and Molinari, S., 1960, Electron microscopy of muscular arteries; pial vessels of the cat and monkey, *J. Ultrastruct. Res.* **3**:447–468.

Peracchia, C., 1980, Structural correlates of gap junction permeation, *Int. Rev. Cytol.* **66**:81–146.

Popescu, L. M., and Diculescu, I., 1975, Calcium in smooth muscle sarcoplasmic reticulum *in situ*. Conventional and x-ray analytic electron microscopy, *J. Cell Biol.* **67**:911–918.

Porter, D. G., Downing, S. J., and Bradshaw, J. M., 1979, Relaxin inhibits spontaneous and prostaglandin-driven myometrial activity in anaesthetized rats, *J. Endocrinol.* **83**:183–189.

Puri, C. P., and Garfield, R. E., 1982, Changes in hormone levels and functional changes in the rat uterus during pregnancy and parturition, *Biol. Reprod.* **27**:967–978.

Revel, J.-P., and Karnovsky, M. J., 1967, Hexagonal array of subunits in intercellular junctions of the mouse heart and liver. *J. Cell Biol.* **33**:C7.

Rice, R. V., Moses, J. A., McManus, G. M., Brady, A. C., and Blasik, L. M., 1970, The organization of contractile filaments in mammalian smooth muscle, *J. Cell Biol.* **47**:183–196.

Ross, R., and Klebanoff, S. J., 1967, Fine structural changes in uterine smooth muscle and fibroblasts in response to estrogen, *J. Cell Biol.* **32**:155–167.

Saito, Y., Sakamoto, H., MacKuskey, N. J., and Naftolin, F., 1985, Gap junctions and myometrial steroid hormone receptors in pregnant and post-partum rats: A possible cellular basis for the progesterone withdrawal hypothesis, *Am. J. Obstet. Gynecol.* **151**:809–821.

Schollenmeyer, J. E., Furcht, L. T., Goll, D. E., Robson, R. M., and Stromer, M. H., 1976, Localization of contractile proteins in smooth muscle cells and in normal and transformed fibroblasts, in: *Cell Motility* (R. Goldman, T. Pollard, and J. Rosenbaum, eds.), Cold Spring Harbor Laboratory, Cold Spring Harbor, NY, pp. 361–368.

Shoenberg, C. F., 1973, The influence of temperature on thick filaments of vertebrate smooth muscle, *Phil. Trans. R. Soc. Lond. [Biol.]* **265**:197–202.

Shoenberg, C. F., 1978, The contractile mechanism and ultrastructure of the myometrium, in: *Cellular Biology of the Uterus* (R. M. Wynn, ed.), pp. 497–544.

Shoenberg, C. F., and Needham, D. M., 1976, A study of the mechanism of contraction in vertebrate smooth muscle, *Biol. Rev.* **51**:53–104.

Shoenberg, C. F., and Stewart, M., 1980, Filament formation in smooth muscle homogenates, *J. Muscle Res. Cell Motil.* **1**:117–127.

Sims, S. M., Garfield, R. E., and Daniel, E. E., 1982, Improved electrical coupling in uterine smooth muscle is associated with increased numbers of gap junctions at parturition, *J. Gen. Physiol.* **80**:353–375.

Sloane, B. F., 1980, Lysosomal apparatus in uterine muscle: Effects of estrogen and ovariectomy, *Biol. Reprod.* **23**:867–876.

Small, J. V., 1974, Contractile units in vertebrate smooth muscle, *Nature* **249**:324–327.

Small, J. V., 1977, Studies on isolated smooth muscle cells: The contractile apparatus, *J. Cell Sci.* **24**:327–349.

Small, J. V., and Sobieszek, A., 1980, The contractile apparatus of smooth muscle, *Int. Rev. Cytol.* **64**:241–306.

Small, J. V., and Squire, J. M., 1972, Structural basis of contraction in vertebrate smooth muscle, *J. Mol. Biol.* **67**:117–149.

Small, J. V., Furst, D. O., and Mey, J. D., 1986, Localization of filamin in smooth muscle, *J. Cell Biol.* **102**:210–220.

Sobieszek, A., 1972, Cross-bridges on self-assembled smooth muscle myosin, *Cold Spring Harbor Symp. Quant. Biol.* **37**:109–112.

Sobieszek, A., and Small, J. V., 1973, The assembly of ribbon-shaped structures in low ionic strength extracts obtained from vertebrate smooth muscle, *Phil. Trans. R. Soc. Lond. [Biol.]* **265**:203–212.

Somlyo, A. P., 1984, Cellular site of calcium regulation, *Nature* **309**:516–517.

Somlyo, A. P., 1985, Excitation–contraction coupling and the ultrastructure of smooth muscle, *Circ. Res.* **57**:497–507.

Somlyo, A. P., Devine, C. E., Somlyo, A. V., and North, S. R., 1971, Sarcoplasmic reticulum and the temperature-dependent contraction of smooth muscle in calcium-free solution, *J. Cell Biol.* **51**:722–741.

Somlyo, A. P., Devine, C. E., Somlyo, A. V., and Rice, R. V., 1973, Filament organization in vertebrate smooth muscle, *Phil. Trans. R. Soc. Lond. [Biol.]* **265**:223–229.

Somlyo, A. P., Somlyo, A. V., Devine, C. E., Peters, D. E., and Hall, T. A., 1974, Electron microscopy and electron probe analysis of mitochondrial cation accumulation in smooth muscle, *J. Cell Biol.* **61**:723–742.

Somlyo, A. P., Garfield, R. E., Chacko, S., and Somlyo, A. V., 1975, Golgi organelle response to the antibotic X537A, *J. Cell Biol.* **66**:425–443.

Somlyo, A. P., Vallieres, I., Garfield, R. E., Shuman, H., Scarpa A., and Somlyo, A. V., 1977, Calcium compartmentalization in vascular smooth muscle: Electron microprobe analysis and studies on isolated mitochondria, in *Biochemistry of Smooth Muscle* (N. L. Stephens, ed.), University Park Press, Baltimore, pp. 563–583.

Somlyo, A. P., Somlyo, A. V., Shuman, H., Sloane, B. F., and Scarpa, A., 1978, Electron probe analysis of calcium compartments in cryosections of smooth and striated muscles, *Ann. N.Y. Acad. Sci.* **307**:523–544.

Somlyo, A. P., Somlyo, A. V., and Shuman, H., 1979, Electron probe analysis of vascular smooth muscle: Composition of mitochondria, nuclei and cytoplasm, *J. Cell Biol.* **81**:316–335.

Somlyo, A. P., Somlyo, A. V., Shuman, H., and Endo, M., 1982, Calcium and monovalent ions in smooth muscle, *Fed. Proc.* **41**:2883–2890.

Somlyo, A. V., 1979, Bridging structures spanning the junctional gap at the triad of striated muscle, *J. Cell Biol.* **80**:743–750.

Somlyo, A. V., 1980, Ultrastructure of smooth muscle, in: *Handbook of Physiology,* Section 2, *The Cardiovascular System,* Vol. II, *Vascular Smooth Muscle* (D. F. Bohr, A. P. Somlyo, and H. V. Sparks, eds.), American Physiological Society, Bethesda, MD, pp. 33–68.

Somlyo, A. V., and Franzini-Armstrong, C., 1985, New views of smooth muscle structure using freezing, deep-etching and rotary shadowing, *Experientia* **41**:841–856.

Somlyo, A. V., and Somlyo, A. P., 1971, Strontium accumulation by sarcoplasmic reticulum and mitochondria in vascular smooth muscle, *Science* **174**:955–958.

Somlyo, A. V., and Somlyo, A. P., 1975, Ultrastructure of smooth muscle, in: *Methods of Pharmacology*, Vol. 3 (E. E. Daniel and D. M. Paton, eds.), Plenum Press, New York, pp. 3–45.

Somlyo, A. V., Vinall, P., and Somlyo, A. P., 1969, Excitation–contraction coupling and electrical events in two types of vascular muscle, *Microvasc. Res.* **1**:354–373.

Somlyo, A. V., Butler, T. M., Bond, M., and Somlyo, A. P., 1981, Myosin filaments have non-phosphorylated light chains in relaxed smooth muscle, *Nature* **294**:567–570.

Somner, J. R., and Johnson, E. A., 1980, Ultrastructure of cardiac muscle, in: *Handbook of Physiology, The Cardiovascular System*, Vol. 1 (R. M. Berne and N. Sperelakis, eds.), American Physiological Society, Washington, pp. 113–186.

Sporrong, B., Alm, P., Owman, C., Sjoberg, N. O., and Thorbert, G., 1978, Ultrastructural evidence for adrenergic nerve degeneration in the guinea pig uterus during pregnancy, *Cell Tissue Res.* **195**:189–193.

Spray, D. C., and Bennett, M. V. L., 1985, Physiology and pharmacology of gap junctions, *Annu. Rev. Physiol.* **47**:281–299.

Spray, D. C., White, R. L., Campos, de Carvalho, A., Harris, A. L., and Bennett, M. V. L., 1984, Gating of gap junctional channels, *Biophys. J.* **45**:219–226.

Steinert, P. M., Jones, J. C. R., and Goldman, R. D., 1984, Intermediate filaments, *J. Cell Biol.* **99**:22s–27s.

Thorbert, G., 1979, Regional changes in structure and function of adrenergic nerves in guinea pig uterus during pregnancy, *Acta Obstet. Gynecol. Scand. [Suppl.]* **79**:5–39.

Thorburn, G. D., and Challis, J. R. G., 1979, Endocrine control of parturition, *Physiol. Rev.* **59**:863–907.

Tomita, T., 1975, Electrical properties of mammalian smooth muscle, *Prog. Biophys. Mol. Biol.* **30**:185–203.

Unwin, P. N. T., and Zampighi, G., 1980, Structure of the junction between communicating cells, *Nature* **283**:545–546.

Vallieres, J., Scarpa, A., and Somlyo, A. P., 1975, Subcellular fractions of smooth muscle; isolation, substrate utilization and Ca^{++} transport by main pulmonary artery and mesenteric vein mitochondria, *Arch. Biochem. Biophys.* **170**:659–669.

Verhoeff, A., and Garfield, R. E., 1986, Ultrastructure of the myometrium and the role of gap junctions in myometrial function, in: *The Physiology and Biochemistry of the Uterus in Pregnancy and Labor* (G. Huszar, ed.), CRC Press, Boca Raton, FL, pp. 73–91.

Verity, M. A., and Bevan, J. A., 1966, A morphopharmacological study of vascular muscle innervation, *Bibl. Anat.* **8**:60–65.

Vibert, P. J., Haselgrove, J. C., Lowy, J., and Poulsen, F. R., 1972, Structural changes in actin containing filaments of muscle, *J. Mol. Biol.* **71**:757–767.

Warshaw, D. M., McBride, W. J., and Work, S. S., 1987, Corkscrew-like shortening in single smooth muscle cells, *Science* **321**:1457–1459.

Wathes, D. C., and Porter, D. G., 1982, Effect of uterine distension and estrogen treatment on gap junction formation in the myometrium of the rat, *J. Reprod. Fertil.* **65**:497–505.

Wikland, M., Lindblom, B., Dahlstrom, A., and Haglid, K. G., 1984, Structural and functional evidence for the denervation of human myometrium during pregnancy, *Obstet. Gynecol.* **64**:503–509.

Wikstrom, M., Akonen, P., and Tuukkainen, T., 1975, The role of mitochondria in uterine contractions, *FEBS Lett.* **56**:77–88.

Uterine Control of Ovarian Function

L. L. ANDERSON and A. I. MUSAH

Regulation of fertile or nonfertile reproductive cycles in mammals depends on interaction of ovarian, uterine, pituitary, and CNS function and exteroceptive stimuli. These cycles can be modified by a variety of actions such as mating, presence of a conceptus or conceptus secretory products, cervical stimulation, endometrial abrasion, and complete or partial absence of the uterus. An essential feature in this regulation is the functional status of the ovary, particularly that of the corpus luteum. It is of particular interest to elucidate the factors that affect the development, maintenance, and regression of the corpus luteum and the role of the uterus in these events. The mammalian uterus has a very profound effect on luteal function. The presence of the uterus alters the process of regression and morphological demise of the corpora lutea. This chapter deals with uterine–ovarian functions in several species and with how uterine–ovarian interactions occur to modify ovarian function during cyclicity and pregnancy.

1. Ovarian Function

Uterine–ovarian interactions have been a very intriguing aspect of reproductive endocrinology. It is not, therefore, surprising that the first demonstration of reproductive cycles in the rat was made by correlating behavioral changes with changes in vaginal cytology and changes in uterine weight and distention (Astwood and Greep, 1938; Schwartz, 1964). The observation that a precise correlation could be made among the changes in the rat lordosis, changes in vaginal cytology, and uterine morphology and weight invariably led to the pursuit of the changes in ovarian morphology that correlated with lordosis, vaginal cytology, and

L. L. ANDERSON and A. I. MUSAH ● Department of Animal Science, Iowa State University, Ames, Iowa 50011.

uterine weight increase. Thus, changes in the ovarian follicle, corpus luteum, and interstitial glands were found to be correlated with sexual behavior, vaginal cytology, and uterine weight (Long and Evans, 1922; Mandl and Zuckerman, 1952).

The corpus luteum (CL) is a transient organ the function of which is primarily secretory. The main secretory products of the CL are progestins (especially progesterone) in most species and peptides such as oxytocin (Fields et al., 1983; Stormshak et al., 1987) and relaxin (Belt et al., 1971; Anderson, 1987). Though luteal cells are morphologically similar among species, their steroidogenic function is by no means identical. The bovine CL secretes primarily progesterone, 20β-hydroxy-4-pregnen-3-one, and pregnenolone. The human CL secretes progesterone, 20α-hydroxy-4-pregnen-3-one, pregnenolone, 17β-hydroxyprogesterone, 4-androstenedione, estrone, and 17β-estradiol (Stormshak et al., 1987). The ovaries of the rabbit and the rat secrete both progesterone and 20α-hydroxypregn-4-ene-3-one (Hilliard et al., 1969; Fajer and Barraclough, 1967; Hashimoto et al., 1968). The 20α-OH-P is considered a catabolite of progesterone with minimal progestational activity. In the rat, the enzyme responsible for conversion of progesterone to 20α-OH-P is 20α-hydroxysteroid dehydrogenase (20α-OH-SDH). This enzyme is found in regressing corpora lutea, whereas functional corpora, follicles, and interstitial tissue lack 20α-OH-SDH activity (Lamprecht et al., 1969; Bast and Melampy, 1972). The bovine and human CL illustrate the extremes of steroidogenic variation. In all species, the rate-limiting step in progesterone biosynthesis is the conversion of 20α-hydroxycholesterol to pregnenolone (3β-hydroxy-5-pregnen-20-one). The enzyme (lyase) required to cleave out six carbon from the side chain of cholesterol is found in the mitochondria of the ovaries, testes, placenta, and adrenal cortex. Some CL possess the capacity for progesterone synthesis de novo by synthesizing cholesterol from acetate or through procuring sterols from high- or low-density lipoproteins.

Progesterone secretion is the main indicator of a functional corpus luteum. In luteal cells the characteristic features of a steroid-secreting cell are large Golgi complexes, few cisternae of granular endoplasmic reticulum, and an extensive network of agranular (smooth) endoplasmic reticulum (Cavazos et al., 1969; Anderson et al., 1969). Protein-synthesizing cells are distinguishable from steroid-secreting cells. Corpora lutea of pregnancy are unique, especially in the sow, in that during the last third of gestation the cells are capable not only of secreting high levels of steroids but also of synthesizing large amounts of the peptide hormone relaxin (Anderson et al., 1983; Fig. 1). Thus, in species in which progesterone secretion is produced from the same cells, the CL acquires the ability to synthesize large quantities of steroids and peptides. The cytosolic features of a peptide-synthesizing cell are prominent granular endoplasmic reticulum with well-developed cisternae (Fawcett et al., 1969).

As pregnancy advances, the internal structure of the mitochondria becomes altered, and the Golgi complexes become more prominent (Fig. 1). In the sow before day 12 of pregnancy, electron-dense granules in luteal cells are rare; however, by day 100–110 (Fig. 1), the granule population becomes maximal (Anderson et al., 1983, Belt et al., 1970, 1971). The granules have been shown to be the storage sites of relaxin (Larkin et al., 1977; P. Fields and Fields, 1985; Ali et al., 1986).

1.1. Corpus Luteum in Rodentia and Lagomorpha

The ovarian follicle, the corpus luteum, and the interstitial gland are the prominent ovarian structures that change during ovarian cyclicity. Of these, the corpus luteum (CL) is the most important organ in terms of interactions with the uterus. The rat corpus luteum is formed from transformed follicular epithelium and ovarian stromal cells (Mossman and Duke, 1973). During the transformation of granulosa to luteal cells, a consistent sequence of lipid changes appears within the cytoplasm of these steroid-producing cells. Histochemical changes include the development of abundant lipoproteins and lipid droplets consisting mainly of phospholipids, which may contribute to steroidogenesis. Diffuse lipoproteins are presumed to

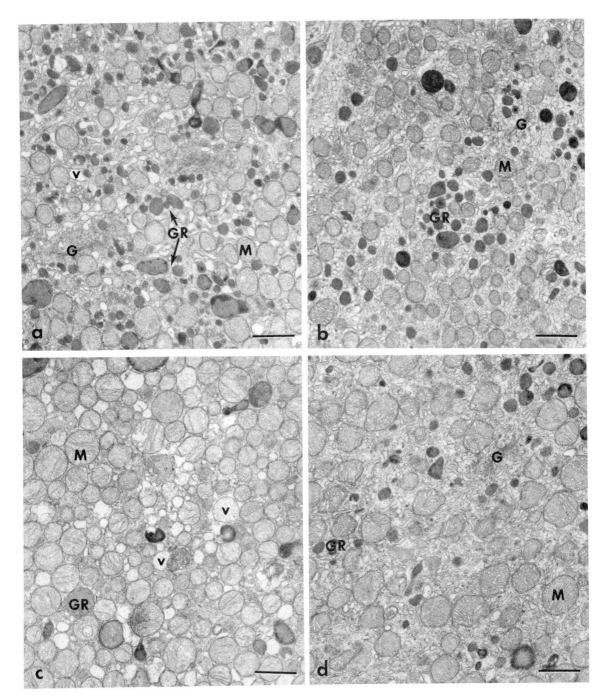

Figure 1. (a) Luteal tissue removed after 100 days of pregnancy contains abundant electron-dense granules (GR). Some vesicles (V) seem to be empty. Golgi apparatus (G) and mitochondria (M) also are prominent. Bar = 1 μm. (b) Luteal tissue removed 100 days after hysterectomy also contains abundant electron-dense granules (GR), Golgi apparatus (G), mitochondria (M), and very small empty vesicles. Bar = 1 μm. (c) After 112 days of pregnancy, small granules are reduced in number, and only a limited number of larger granules (GR) remain. Although mitochondria (M) are structurally unchanged, the number of empty or slightly opaque vesicles (V) has increased. Bar = 1 μm. (d) On day 112 after hysterectomy, granules (GR) are slightly less numerous than on day 100 after hysterectomy. A Golgi apparatus (G) is easily recognized. Mitochondria (M) are larger and somewhat less regular in contour than their day-100 counterparts. Bar = 1 μm. From Anderson *et al.* (1983).

derive from the abundant membranes of smooth reticulum and serve as sites for enzymes involved in steroidogenesis (Armstrong and Flint, 1973). The appearance of increasing numbers of lipid droplets consisting mainly of cholesterol or its esters and triglycerides in the granulosa luteal cells of the rat during proestrus and estrus suggests that they may begin to function in the storage of hormone precursor (Guraya, 1973, 1985); storage of hormone precursor correlates with declining levels of progesterone in ovarian venous blood at this time (Hashimoto et al., 1968) as well as with increased activity of hydrolytic enzymes (Lobel et al., 1961), fragmentation of the Golgi apparatus (McDonald et al., 1969), and appearance of 20α-hydroxysteroid dehydrogenase activity (Balogh, 1964). During the last half of pregnancy and after day 11 of pseudopregnancy in the rat, increasing numbers of lipid droplets consisting of cholesterol and its esters, triglycerides, and some phospholipids in the luteal cells begin to store hormone precursor (Guraya, 1975), and these changes correlate with declining levels of progesterone (Eto et al., 1962; Hashimoto et al., 1968; Wiest et al., 1968; Wiest, 1970). During the last days of pregnancy (days 17–22), there is accumulation of abundant cholesterol- and triglyceride-containing lipid droplets in the luteal cells (Guraya, 1975); progesterone levels are low, while levels of 20α-hydroxypregn-4-en-3-one (20α-OH-P), 20α-hydroxysteroid dehydrogenase (20α-OH-SDH), and relaxin in ovarian tissue increase markedly (Hashimoto et al., 1968; Wiest et al., 1968; Bast and Melampy, 1972; Anderson et al., 1973a).

These changes in histochemical features of the luteal cell, blood progestin levels, and 20α-OH-SDH enzyme activities correlate well with changes in ultrastructural features of the cytoplasmic components of the luteal cell during pregnancy in the rat (Long, 1973). In the rat, ovarian $\triangle^5$-3β-hydroxysteroid dehydrogenase (3β-HSD) activity with dehydroepiandrosterone as substrate shows intense activity in the interstitial gland, corpora lutea, and theca interna of developing follicles throughout pregnancy (Lawrence et al., 1975). With pregnenolone as substrate, the 3β-HSD activity is highest in the interstitial gland at day 14; enzyme activity in the corpus luteum increases at this time, and by day 18 the corpus luteum contains the most intense activity of the ovary.

In the rat, prolactin (PRL) or placental lactogen seems to be necessary for the corpus luteum activity, though under certain conditions the corpus luteum becomes dependent on another hormone (Rothchild, 1981). After day 8 of pseudopregnancy or between days 8 and 12 of pregnancy, the corpus luteum depends on LH as well, and luteolysis occurs in the absence of LH even though circulating levels of PRL maybe adequate (Rothchild, 1981; Ochiai and Rothchild, 1985). During the demise of the corpus luteum, prostaglandins may play a critical role, and PRL may prevent this luteolysis in part by preventing prostaglandin synthesis and/or effect (Rothchild, 1981; Ueda et al., 1985).

In the rabbit, levels of progesterone in the peripheral blood or in ovarian venous blood rise during pregnancy and pseudopregnancy to peak values at days 9 and 11, respectively. The ovaries are the major source of progesterone production during pregnancy (Thau and Lanman, 1974). Peripheral levels of progesterone increase 11-fold by day 7 of pseudopregnancy and 14-fold by day 16 of pregnancy when compared with values obtained during estrus (day 0) (Thau and Lanman, 1975). Serum levels of testosterone in peripheral circulation and in ovarian venous plasma of the nonpregnant rabbit indicate that the ovarian follicle is a source of this steroid and, furthermore, that synthesis and release of this steroid are acutely enhanced by endogenous and exogenous LH (Hilliard et al., 1974). The ovarian interstitial tissue may act as a supplementary source of testosterone, whereas the follicles synthesize estrogen in addition to testosterone (Eaton and Hilliard, 1971).

1.2. Corpus Luteum in Artiodactyla

The sheep, pigs, goats, and cows that make up this mammalian order exhibit a wide range of similarities and differences. The pattern of sexual activity in the ewe varies from monestrus

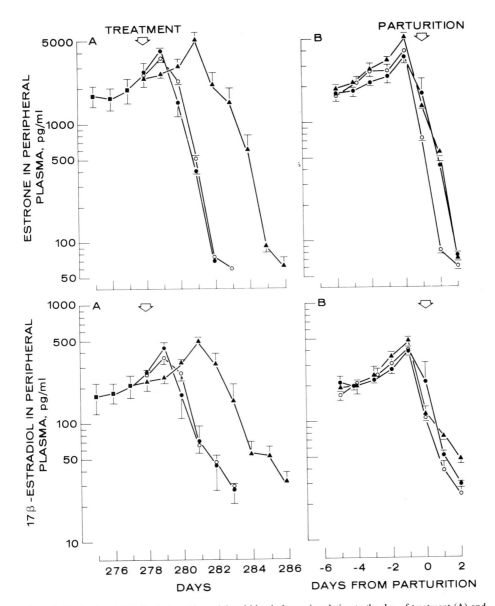

Figure 2. E_1 (top) and 17β-E_2 (bottom) in peripheral blood plasma in relation to the day of treatment (A) and day of parturition (B) in beef heifers receiving (●) relaxin-double (2 × 3000 U 12 hr apart) (*n* = 17), (○) relaxin-single (3000 U) (*n* = 14), and (▲) gel-vehicle controls (*n* = 16). (■) Sequential profiles of E_1 (upper) and 17β-E_2 (lower) in all 47 heifers preceding treatment. Day of treatment is day 0. Values are the means ± S.E. From Musah *et al.* (1986).

in some undomesticated species to seasonal polyestrus in most domesticated breeds. Some tropical breeds are able to breed all year round (Banks, 1964; Robertson, 1977). The sow is polyestrus throughout the year except when interrupted by pregnancy, hysterectomy, or an endocrine dysfunction (Anderson *et al.*, 1969; Musah *et al.*, 1984).

In 3 to 4 days after ovulation, significant quantities of progesterone appear in the ovarian vein and systemic circulation of the ewe (Cunningham *et al.*, 1975). The newly formed ovine CL are the source of progesterone (Short *et al.*, 1963). Progesterone secretion in luteal tissue and peripheral plasma increases to maximal levels by days 10–13 of the estrous cycle and drops to nondetectable amounts by day 16 (Deane *et al.*, 1966; Roche *et al.*, 1970). At midluteal phase, about 3–7 ng/ml P_4 can be measured (Pant *et al.*, 1977) before a decline to less than 1.86 ng/ml on day 13. The decline in progesterone is well correlated with the morphological demise of the CL between days 12 and 13. Structural changes associated with the decline in steroid production include shrinkage of the luteal cells, swelling of mitochondria, accumulation of lipid droplets within the cytoplasm, and decreases in both Δ^5-3β-hydroxysteroid dehydrogenase and diaphorase activities. These degenerative changes, which are evident by day 15, are accompanied by an abundance of lysosomes in the ovine luteal cell (Dingle *et al.*, 1968).

Functional corpora lutea are essential to define the interestrus interval whether relating to the nongravid or gravid state in the pig. During brief 21-day estrous cycles, the corpora lutea develop (>450 mg), and progesterone secretion reaches peak concentrations (e.g., >30 ng/ml in peripheral blood) from days 8 to 12; luteolysis occurs rapidly after day 16 (Hard and Anderson, 1979; Van de Wiel *et al.*, 1981; Fig. 3). A feature unique to this species is its dependence on corpora lutea for their production of progesterone throughout pregnancy; ovariectomy at any time results in abortion within 36 hr (Belt *et al.*, 1971). Pregnancy can be maintained in ovariectomized gilts by exogenous progesterone sufficient to maintain plasma progesterone levels of 4–5 ng/ml (Ellicott and Dziuk, 1973). Removal of the corpora lutea (luteectomy) decreases progesterone and relaxin and increases $PGF_{2\alpha}$ metabolite in maternal plasma and prematurely terminates gestation without causing onset of lactation (Kertiles and Anderson, 1979; Nara *et al.*, 1981a,b). There is a high incidence of stillbirths after ovariectomy or luteectomy in the pig. Removal of follicles, however, does not affect pregnancy or parturition (Nara *et al.*, 1981a,b). Luteolysis after day 13 in this species is associated with an increase in plasma $PGF_{2\alpha}$ and corresponding decreases in progesterone and the proportion of cholesterol bound to the cytochrome P450 side-chain cleavage enzyme ($P450_{scc}$) in luteal tissue (Gleeson *et al.*, 1974; Torday *et al.*, 1980). Prostaglandin $F_{2\alpha}$ administration at this time in hysterectomized gilts causes a similar decrease in progesterone and $P450_{scc}$. These changes in $P450_{scc}$ are consistent with a direct block of LH stimulation by $PGF_{2\alpha}$. In this species hypophysectomy after the preovulatory LH surge is followed by normal development of corpora lutea to day 10 and normal luteal regression after that time (Anderson *et al.*, 1967a).

After the initial LH stimulation at estrus (Fig. 3), porcine corpora lutea do not require pituitary support until after day 10, and they are refractory to $PGF_{2\alpha}$ during that time (Diehl *et al.*, 1974). Thus, once formed porcine corpora lutea do not require luteotropic support up to 10 days. At the time of luteolysis, $PGF_{2\alpha}$, possibly of uterine origin, may cause a decrease in cholesterol available to $P450_{scc}$ and a subsequent decrease in progesterone production. Corpora lutea in cyclic gilts contain little relaxin; this hormone very likely plays no significant role in luteal demise during the estrous cycle. Relaxin levels in luteal tissue remain relatively low during the period of maximal progesterone secretion in cyclic gilts (Fig. 3) (Anderson *et al.*, 1973b; Sherwood and Rutherford, 1981). Human chorionic gonadotropin (hCG) mimics the preovulatory LH surge and delays luteolysis in cyclic gilts and hysterectomized pigs following hypophysectomy (Anderson *et al.*, 1967a; Guthrie and Rexroad, 1981). Exogenous estrogen also delays luteolysis in cyclic gilts and reduces uterine secretion of $PGF_{2\alpha}$ (Gardner *et al.*, 1963; Moeljono *et al.*, 1977). Injection of hCG at midcycle delays luteolysis and causes a transitory increase in plasma estrogen concentrations (Guthrie and Bolt, 1983). The absence of elevated $PGF_{2\alpha}$-metabolite plasma levels, typically observed at the termination of a normal luteal phase, may result from an antagonism by hCG of the action of endogenous $PGF_{2\alpha}$ or possibly a reduction in uterine luteolytic activity caused by increased follicular estrogen production. Exogenous estrogen in nongravid gilts extends luteal function beyond 116 days, and these aging corpora lutea produce relaxin in amounts similar to those in pregnant and hysterectomized gilts (Anderson *et al.*, 1973b).

A major functional difference between ewes, cows, and pigs on one hand and rodents on the other is that of progesterone secretion during the preovulatory period. Since the ovaries of cows, pigs, and sheep contain relatively smaller proportions of interstitial tissue coupled with

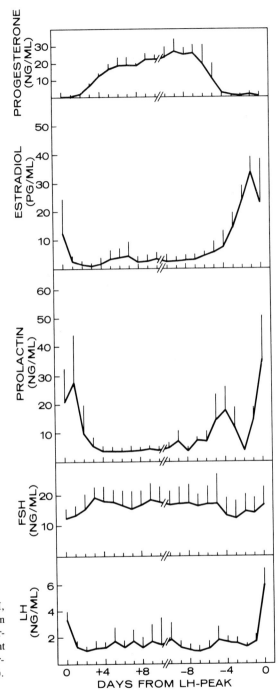

Figure 3. Mean concentrations of LH, FSH, prolactin, estradiol-17β, and progesterone in plasma samples taken daily from four normally cycling pigs. Vertical lines represent positive standard deviations. Data are normalized to the day of the LH peak (day 0). Adapted from Van de Wiel *et al.* (1981).

the differentiation of follicular–thecal cells during atresia, progesterone secretion is almost absent (Hansel *et al.*, 1973). The ovine ovary is also intriguing in another respect; that is, it is almost quiescent during the anestrous period. Small quantities of steroids, particularly estradiol and androstenedione, are released in 5-hr cycles in response to endogenous pulses of LH (Scaramuzzi and Baird, 1977).

1.3. Corpus Luteum in Primates

Primates constitute about 180 species, of which 133 are Old World monkeys, New World monkeys, apes, and man. The remaining 43 species are prosimians. The ovarian cycle and gestation are 28 and 144 days, respectively, for the common marmoset (*Gallithrix jacchus*), 9 and 150 days for the squirrel monkey (*Saimiri sciureus*), 28 and 168 days for the rhesus monkey (*Macaca mulatta*), 33 and 184 days for the baboon (*Papio cynocephalus*), 37 and 235 days for the chimpanzee (*Pan troglodytes*), and 29 and 280 days for man (*Homo sapiens*) (Hearn, 1986).

The menstrual cycle of the rhesus monkey has been well documented and so is used to illustrate ovarian function in primates. The cycle is 28 days, with ovulation occurring midway between menses (Knobil, 1974). The follicular phase is marked by a synchronous rise in estradiol (Knobil, 1974; Czaja *et al.*, 1977) and testosterone (Hess and Resko, 1973) to peak values 4 days before synchronous FSH and LH peaks at midcycle (Hodgen *et al.*, 1976; Dufau *et al.*, 1977). The dominant follicle is the source of estrogen (Goodman *et al.*, 1977).

The luteal phase is marked by a gradual increase in progesterone about 6 hr after the peak release of LH (Weick *et al.*, 1973). A functional CL begins to form 30 hr after the LH surge, and FSH and LH are then at a nadir (Knobil, 1973). The luteolytic factor in primates is estrogen (Karsch and Sutton, 1976) via an intraovarian mechanism. Extrafollicular estrogen production by the primate corpus luteum suppresses the next wave of follicular growth (Baird *et al.*, 1975). Thus, unlike sheep, in which follicular waves proceed through the cycle, a new crop of follicles has to be recruited in the primate.

2. Uterine Function

2.1. Development and Regression of Endometrium and Myometrium

The mammalian uterus functions primarily for gamete transport, provision of a suitable environment for fetal development, and regulation of ovarian function during estrus, menstrual cycles, and pregnancy. Appropriate changes in uterine morphology and environment during the various developmental periods occur in response to changing secretory products of the uterus, ovaries, and conceptus. The development and regression of the endometrium and myometrium are manifestations of the changing role of the uterus.

Uterine response to ovarian hormones may be classified into three distinct categories, which are mediated by different mechanisms. In one group, hormones, especially the estrogen-induced uterine response, involve genomic changes such as increases in RNA, increases in specific enzymes, and protein synthesis. In this category, there is an accompanying biochemical, morphological, and functional differentiation of uterine cells (Tchernitchin, 1983). The second group involves nongenomic changes, such as hormone-induced uterine eosinophilia, edema, vascular permeability, histamine release, and uterine luminal fluid accumulation (Tchernitchin, 1983; Grunert *et al.*, 1984). These responses are mediated by eosinophils, which move from blood to the uterus under hormone induction and then degranulate, thus releasing into the uterine stroma enzymes and other agents that can mediate hormone-induced uterine changes (Tchernitchin, 1983; Tchernitchin *et al.*, 1985). Eosinophil migration to the uterus is dependent on estrogen in blood and not uterine estrogen and, unlike the genomic response, is not blocked by RNA inhibitors (Tchernitchin and Galand, 1982, 1983; Finlay *et al.*, 1983). The third group of hormone-induced uterine changes includes the hormone-induced hyperemia, increased glycogen content, and mitotic response (Hechter *et al.*, 1965; Singhal and LaFreniere, 1972; Galand *et al.*, 1983).

In the rat, DNA synthesis in the uterus has been associated with estrogen secretion by the ovary on the day of proestrus (Shelesnyak and Tic, 1963; Tchernitchin, 1983). During proestrus the increase in uterine DNA reflects not only epithelial proliferation but also stromal and myometrial proliferation (Marcus, 1974). The events of proestrus influence uterine receptivity, particularly as related to induction of a decidual response or induction of implantation of embryos. Incorporation of radio-labeled thymidine into nuclear DNA indicates that the decidual cells are derived from stromal cells (Shelesnyak et al., 1970). The occurrence of stromal mitosis corresponds to the pattern of secretion of estrogen during the estrous cycle (Shaikh, 1971; Shaikh and Abraham, 1969; Galand et al., 1983). During progestation, stromal mitotic activity is more intense than during the estrous cycle, but mitotic activity during the cycle begins when estrogen levels are similar to those found during the progestational estrogen surge (day 4). Portions of the uterus distant from the implanting embryo show mitotic activity similar to that in pseudopregnant animals, whereas segments of the uterine horn adjacent to the implanting embryo exhibit intense mitotic activity. Thus, during pregnancy, stromal mitotic activity occurs in response first to ovarian steroid secretions and later to the presence of implanting blastocysts. The later response is associated with induction of decidualization.

Proliferation and differentiation of endometrial stromal cells play an important part in the decidual reaction and ovum implantation. In the rat, both estrogen and progesterone are required to elicit the full formation of deciduomata. Pretreatment with progesterone for at least 36 hr alters the mitogenic action of estrogen from epithelial to stromal elements of the endometrium (Clark, 1971; Tachi et al., 1971, 1972); a similar shift in mitotic activity occurs during the preimplantation stages of pregnancy. When rats are ovariectomized and adrenalectomized, the nucleoli of endometrial stromal cells become small and compact and consist exclusively of the fibrous component. Daily injections of progesterone for a week induce enlargement of the nucleoli as well as a massive accumulation of a granular component; such changes are accompanied by augmentation of rough-surfaced endoplasmic reticulum and free ribosome clusters in the cytoplasm. Subsequent administration of estradiol intensifies these changes, whereas estradiol without prior progesterone treatment causes the appearance of a small amount of granular component but lacks full nucleolar function. Progesterone seems to promote the elaboration of risobomal precursors by the nucleoli of stromal cells, and this effect may contribute to sensitization of this cell type; however, the mechanism of action of progesterone on cytoplasmic and nucleolar components of these cells is unclear. Stromal cells respond to estradiol by steroid activation of cytoplasmic receptors, nuclear acceptor sites, and transcription and possible translation control mechanisms (Baulieu et al., 1972). Progesterone pretreatment causes a marked increase in the sensitivity of the cells to the stimulatory action of estradiol and may play a part in bringing about the endometrial changes preparatory to implantation of embryos (Tachi et al., 1974).

During postpartum involution of the mammalian uterus, rapid and massive breakdown of tissues occurs. Involution involves resorption of tissue components such as muscle protein, cellular material, and connective tissue. Intracellular digestion of uterine tissues during the process of involution involves certain hydrolases characteristically found in lysosomes. Acid hydrolases (cathepsin, β-glucuronidase, β-galactosidase, acid phosphatase, and deoxyribonuclease II) show quantitative changes typical of catabolic events in the uterus. These hydrolases are localized primarily in the lysosomal fraction of the cell (de Duve et al., 1962; de Duve, 1975).

During postpartum involution in the rat, all of these acid hydrolases except deoxyribonuclease increase two- to fourfold; peak concentrations occur at about the same time that uterine wet weight and collagen have declined to their lowest values (Woessner, 1965). Histochemical evidence suggests that most of the uterine acid phosphatase (Lobel and Deane, 1962) and β-glucuronidase (Hayashi, 1964) are within granules that resemble lysosomes. During the last days of pregnancy, there is a gradual buildup of these acid hydrolases; further increases occur during the postpartum period (Woessner, 1965). Estradiol treatment inhibits the rapid and extensive breakdown of collagen typically found during the postpartum period (Ryan and Woessner, 1972). Injury to the rat uterus immediately after parturition retards involution and collagen breakdown; injury also induces the processes of tissue repair (Woessner and Celio, 1974). During postpartum involution, the rat uterus loses about 85% of its collagen within a 4-day period (Woessner, 1962). When large doses of progesterone (80–150 mg) are given daily, uterine involution is retarded, as indicated by an increase in wet weight of the uterus (30%), an increase in collagen (85%), and a decrease in collagenolytic activity (45%) compared with intact control rats 3 days post-partum (Halme and Woessner, 1975).

Lysosomal enzymes (e.g., acid hydrolases) are stimulated by sex steroids, with the enzymes in turn functioning as regulators of hormonal effects on tissue components (Smith and Henzl, 1969). In endometrial cells, lysosomes are formed and function essentially as they do in other tissues (Smith and Farquhar, 1966). In the endometrium, these processes are initiated by estrogen, and extensive proliferation and differentiation are initiated by progesterone. Endometrial regression occurs when ovarian hormone levels become inadequate and hydrolytic cellular elements emerge. Acid phosphatase, bound in lysosomes and Golgi vesicles, leads to autophagic activity, causing degradation of endometrial intracellular structures within a brief period (Smith and Henzl, 1969). The lysosomes possibly promote tissue damage by releasing their enzymes directly into intracellular cytoplasmic components and intercellular areas. Formation of enlarged lysosomes (autolysosomes) is coincident with reduction in height of epithelial cells. In the earliest stages of regression, changes are noted in the columnar epithelial cells; later, they occur in stromal areas adjacent to the surface and then throughout the entire stromal layer of the endometrium. Dense-body lysosomes seem to be related to release or degradation of secretory material, whereas autophagic bodies serve as sequestering centers for hydrolytic enzymes (Smith and Henzl, 1969). Hydrolytic activities of these enzymes permit physiological change within a cell without causing its death. Autolytic activity in stromal layers results in more active regression of the endometrium than that found in the epithelial layer (Woessner, 1965).

Uterine growth and development in the presence of estrogen are reflected in the deposition and maintenance of collagen bundles and ground substance of stromal layers and synthesis of mucopolysaccharides (Fainstat, 1963; Smith and Henzl, 1969; Grunert et al., 1984). Progesterone does not initiate formation of collagen bundles or support formation of mucopolysaccarides in the endometrium. Prolonged administration of estrogen tends to suppress lysosomal activity. In ovariectomized animals, daily treatment with estradiol-17β is associated with the appearance of thick, multifibrillated collagen fibers throughout the endometrial stroma, whereas during lactation no new collagen bundles appear until the third week. Within 3 weeks after weaning, coarse collagen bundles again permeate the entire endometrial stroma. When progesterone administration is combined with estrogen, lysosomal development in the stromal cells becomes evident and appears to be a prerequisite to rapid endometrial regression (Smith and Henzl, 1969). The combination of estrogen and progesterone is necessary for attaining endometrial proliferation and secretory changes as well as increased mitotic activity and hyperplasia. Ultrastructural features in these cell layers indicate that another action of progesterone is increased lysosomal activity within the cells, possibly altering their physiological functions as well as playing a role in their eventual demise, thus leading to regression of the endometrium.

2.2. Role of the Uterus in Cyclic Periodicity

2.2.1. Pseudopregnancy

Pseudopregnancy can be induced in several species such as the hamster, mouse, rat, rabbit, and ferret by neurogenic stimulation of the uterine cervix (refer to Anderson, 1973). In the hamster, mouse, and rat, the estrus interval is extended several days beyond that of the normal estrous cycle, but the duration of the pseudopregnancy is usually less than that of pregnancy.

Pseudopregnancy lasts about 13.5 days in the rat, and during this period the ovaries secrete progestins. Ovarian venous blood progesterone increases from day 1 to day 6 and declines thereafter to day 13, whereas levels of 20α-OH-P remain similar from day 1 to day 9 and then increase abruptly near the termination of the pseudopregnancy. Peripheral serum levels of progesterone increase from day 1 to day 9 and then decline steadily to day 13 (Pepe and Rothchild, 1974; Bartosik and Szarowski, 1973). Activity of ovarian 20α-OH-SDH declines from day 1 to day 6 and then increases steadily until day 13. Serum levels of prolactin gradually decline throughout pseudopregnancy to the morning of day 13, when they increase sharply. Peripheral levels of LH in serum tend to increase gradually over the later part of pseudopregnancy and then increase abruptly at the onset of proestrus (Bast and Melampy, 1972). A positive correlation exists between serum levels of LH and 20α-OH-SDH in the terminal stages of pseudopregnancy. Progesterone levels in peripheral blood from rats in which the pseudopregnancy was induced by sterile copulation or by electrical stimulation of the uterine cervix show similar changes throughout pseudopregnancy (de Greef and Zeilmaker, 1974).

The *in vitro* release of progesterone by corpora lutea harvested from rats during normal pseudopregnancy is low on the first 2 days and increases rapidly to reach maximal values by day 5; progesterone levels gradually decline after day 8 to low values by days 11–14 (Bartosik *et al.*, 1974). The *in vitro* release of progesterone and 20α-OH-P by the corpora lutea is similar qualitatively to *in vitro* progestin secretion rates (Hashimoto *et al.*, 1968). Luteolysis *in vitro* is characterized by an abrupt and irreversible decrease in progesterone by the luteinized ovary (Bartosik *et al.*, 1974) *In vitro* incorporation of [³H]uridine in rat luteal tissue slices indicates a steady decline of RNA synthesis from day 2 to day 9, with a marked increase from day 10 to day 14. During this later period of pseudopregnancy, the corpora lutea are undergoing progressive luteolysis. The increase in *in vitro* RNA synthesis by these corpora lutea may be interpreted as a new species of RNA to provide the enzyme 20α-OH-SDH for increased conversion of progesterone to 20α-OH-P (Bartosik *et al.*, 1974; Hashimoto and Wiest, 1969).

The duration of pseudopregnancy in the rabbit is about 17 days, and during this period the ovaries secrete progesterone and 20α-OH-P (Strauss *et al.*, 1972). The major source of progesterone in the pseudopregnant rabbit is the corpus luteum, whereas interstitial tissue seems to be the major source of 20α-OH-P. The enzyme 20α-OH-SDH is found in both functional and regressing corpora lutea and in interstitial tissue of the rabbit ovary. The patterns of 20α-OH-P levels in ovarian venous blood and the 20α-OH-SDH activities in whole ovaries increase from low values at day 4 of pseudopregnancy to maximal amounts by days 15–20, a time when there is a marked decline in both luteal weight and progesterone production by the corpora lutea. These events coincide with the termination of the pseudopregnancy. Exogenous estrogen sustains functional corpora lutea in this species (Hilliard *et al.*, 1969) and inhibits *in vitro* 20α-OH-SDH activity in rabbit corpora lutea. Increasing 20α-OH-SDH activity seems to be a specific and sensitive index of luteolysis in this species (Strauss *et al.*, 1972).

2.2.2. Deciduomata

Decidual tissue formation results from proliferation, hypertrophy, and differentiation of the endometrial cells. The phenomenon is common to man, many other primates, and several rodents. Decidual tissue formation occurs at the end of each menstrual cycle in man and primates; on the other hand, the rat must be stimulated to produce a decidual reaction. A complex feedback mechanism exists between decidua and the CL in the rat. Ovarian progesterone is essential for the maintenance of the decidual reaction (Deanesly, 1973; Butterstein and Hirst, 1977; Glasser and McCormack, 1979). Though ovarian progesterone is necessary for decidual tissue, it does not guarantee immortality, since decidual degeneration will eventually occur even in the presence of continual progesterone (Porter, 1974). Decidual tissue in the rat arises from the endometrial stromal cells during the process of implantation. Deciduomata also are produced by traumatization of the endometrium during a sensitive stage of pseudopregnancy or during lactation when adequate levels of endogenous or exogenous estrogen are available to the uterus. Uterine protein and RNA and DNA content increase exponentially during uterine decidualization (Shelesnyak and Tic, 1963). The endometrium concentrates [³H]estradiol to a greater degree than does the myometrium in ovariectomized rats (Alberga and Baulieu, 1968). With initiation of decidualization in the pseudopregnant rat, the myometrium retains four times more [³H]estradiol than does the endometrium (Kimmel *et al.*, 1973). The increases in deciduomal G6PD activity and growth after progesterone treatment may be explained by the estrogen dependence of progesterone-binding components (Feil *et al.*, 1972).

Endometrial sensitivity to an artificial intrauterine decidual stimulus has been ascertained in relation to effects of estrogen priming, progesterone, and nidatory estrogen (Finn and Martin, 1972). After priming by estradiol (100 ng), the uterus is maximally responsive to subsequent treatment with progesterone (400 or 500 ng) and nidatory estradiol (10 ng) for a period of about 3 days beginning the fourth day after the last priming injection. Neither steroid alone induces uterine sensitivity, but when they are administered in combination the uterus becomes maximally sensitive to traumatization within 3 days. Progesterone alone induces a partial uterine sensitivity, which can remain for several days until sensitivity is completed by estrogen (Finn and Martin, 1972).

Decidualization of the endometrium prolongs the life span of rat corpora lutea (Velardo *et al.*, 1953; Melampy *et al.*, 1964), possibly by destroying or inhibiting production of a uterine luteolytic substance or by producing an active luteotropic substance. The uterine traumatization induces deciduomata and extends the duration of pseudopregnancy to that caused by hysterectomy or to that of pregnancy (Melampy *et al.*, 1964; Hashimoto *et al.*, 1968). When the decidual tissue is removed on day 9, it reduces only slightly (19.3 versus 22.2 days) the duration of pseudopregnancy (Pakurar and Rothchild, 1972). Slitting the uterus lengthwise to remove the decidual tissue by curette results in a similar duration of pseudopregnancy. However, slitting nondecidualized uteri on day 9 of pseudopregnancy was found to prolong its duration (19.2 days) as compared with pseudopregnancy in intact controls (13.5 days). Subsequent estrous cycles in rats bearing slit uteri are of normal duration.

In pseudopregnant rats bearing deciduomata (induced on day 5), peripheral serum levels of progesterone were found to reach maximal levels within 72 hr (day 8), a period of maximal decidual tissue growth, and then to decline after day 9 (Rothchild and Gibori, 1975). In pseudopregnant rats subjected to hysterectomy on day 5, daily patterns of serum progesterone levels were compared with those of rats bearing deciduomata. It was found that the latter tend to have higher levels of progesterone in peripheral serum than do those after hysterectomy, an observation that confirms findings of Hashimoto *et al.* (1968) on ovarian venous secretion of progesterone in these experimental preparations.

After induction of deciduomata, progesterone in ovarian venous blood increases to day 9 and then declines to day 21; the pattern of pregn-4-ene-20α-ol-3-one secretion is inverse to that of progesterone during this period (Hashimoto *et al.*, 1968). Peripheral serum levels of progesterone in rats bearing deciduomata increase to peak values by day 9 and gradually decline to day 21 (Pepe and Rothchild, 1974). Ovarian 20α-hydroxysteroid dehydrogenase activity remains low during the major part of the prolonged pseudopregnancy and begins to increase markedly at the terminal stages of that pseudopregnancy (Bast and Melampy, 1972). Elevated prolactin levels in peripheral serum during prolonged pseudopregnancy occur only at day 6 and proestrus day 21 (Bast and Melampy, 1972). A positive correlation exists between peripheral levels of serum LH and serum prolactin and ovarian 20α-hydroxysteroid dehydrogenase activity during pseudopregnancy in rats bearing deciduomata (Bast and Melampy, 1972).

The immediate effect of ovariectomy between days 6 and 9 in rats is decidual degeneration leading to hemorrhagic collapse of the whole conceptus (Deanesly, 1973). It is assumed that decidual degeneration is a direct result of progesterone deficiency; progesterone can maintain pregnancy in the postimplantation rat. During regression of deciduomata, complex proteins and polysaccharides are degraded and resorbed by increased activities of lysosomal enzymes, cathepsin D, and β-glucoronidase (Wood and Barley, 1970). During implantation, there are indications of increased uterine cell growth and metabolism accompanied by cellular differentiation, as well as cellular disintegration and synthesis of new components. Collagen bundle disintegration has been observed histologically at the implantation site, as have cellular hypertrophy and hyperplasia (Fainstat, 1963). The role of lysosomes in cellular degradation is unclear. Lysosomes are mobilized in uterine tissue soon after administration of estrogen (Szego and Seeler, 1973). An investigation of lysosomal enzymes in uterine tissues during early pregnancy in the rat has suggested that uterine cathepsin D activity declines after implantation on day 4, as compared with nonimplantation segments within the same uterus. Levels of β-glucoronidase are lower in implantation sites found in nonimplantation segments, but there is no evident decrease when enzyme activity is expressed per milligram DNA.

3. Uterine–Ovarian and Conceptus Interaction in Regulation of Ovarian Function

3.1. Uterine–Ovarian Function during Pregnancy

3.1.1. Rodentia and Lagomorpha

During the first half of gestation, the adenohypophysis is essential for maintaining pregnancy (Greenwald and Johnson, 1968), whereas placental luteotropins seem to stimulate ovarian function during the second half of gestation (Lyons and Ahmad, 1973). Serum levels of prolactin, LH, and FSH remain below those that characterize the diestrus phase of the estrous cycle (Linkie and Niswender, 1972). Evidence of participation of the uterus in luteotropic action during midpregnancy in the rat has been evaluated by measurement of ovarian venous blood levels of progesterone and 20α-hydroxypregn-4-en-3-one (20α-OH-P) (Sin et al., 1971). During midpregnancy there is a marked rise in progesterone and 20α-OH-P during placentation (Hashimoto et al., 1968), and a corresponding increase in these two progestins occurs after hypophysectomy on day 12 (Sin et al., 1971). The luteotropic effect of the conceptuses was not of pituitary origin. When the hypophysectomized rats are, in addition, hysterectomized, a marked decline results in ovarian venous levels of both progesterone and 20α-OH-P. Fetectomy with the placentas remaining in situ can not produce an increase in these progestin levels similar to that found during normal pregnancy, but the steroid levels are sustained to the same extent as is found in pseudopregnant rats bearing deciduomata. Thus, fetuses are considered essential for the placentas to exert luteotropic action; production of the luteotropins during midpregnancy may result from an interaction of placentas and fetuses.

During the later part of pregnancy, secretion of progesterone declines, and both 20α-OH-P and 20α-OH-SDH increase before parturition (Fajer and Barraclough 1967; Hashimoto et al., 1968; Wiest et al., 1968; Labhsetwar and Watson, 1974). The pattern of progesterone concentration in ovarian venous plasma is characterized by a small peak in early pregnancy and a larger peak in the second half of pregnancy (Ichikawa et al., 1974). The secretion rates of 5α-pregnane compounds are highest at mating, decline markedly to low values by day 3, and remain low through parturition. Only 20α-OH-P increases markedly just preceding parturition. Exogenous LH increases the levels of 5α-pregnane-3,20-dione and 3α-hydroxy-5α-pregnane-20-one throughout all stages of pregnancy. The levels of 20α-hydroxy-5α-pregnane-3-one, 5α-pregnane-3α,20α-diol, and 20α-OH-P remain unresponsive to exogenous LH during the entire gestation.

In pregnant rats, serum progesterone levels consistently are lower in the early morning and steadily increase to reach highest levels at 11 p.m., a finding that suggests a daily rhythm of progesterone secretion (Dohler and Wuttke, 1974). A semicircadian increase in prolactin levels occurs during pregnancy, with highest values during the afternoon and early morning (Butcher *et al.*, 1972; Dohler and Wuttke, 1974), which is out of phase with the rhythm of progesterone secretion. Blood levels of estrogen (Yoshinaga *et al.*, 1969; Shaikh, 1971), LH (Linkie and Niswender, 1972; Bast and Melampy, 1972), and prolactin (Amenomori *et al.*, 1970; Linkie and Niswender, 1972) also increase before parturition. Uterine venous levels of PGF remain constant from day 18 to day 20, when progesterone declines and 20α-OH-P increases (Labhsetwar and Watson, 1974). Prostaglandin levels increase markedly on day 21, coinciding with the increase in estradiol in ovarian venous plasma. Prostaglandin levels in uterine venous blood remain elevated on day 22, then drop within 24 hr after parturition, and continue at a low level during the remainder of the postpartum period (Labhsetwar and Watson, 1974).

Administration of progesterone prolongs pregnancy in the rat (Barrow, 1970), and ovariectomy late in pregnancy prevents parturition (Csapo, 1969). An increased *in vitro* release of prostaglandins from the pregnant uterus in rats occurs on the day of expected delivery, and neither exogenous progesterone nor ovariectomy prevents this release. Ovarian estrogen and progesterone do not seem to affect this release of prostaglandin. During normal pregnancy, *in vitro* prostaglandin release increases from barely detectable levels on day 17 to maximal values by day 22, the expected day of delivery (Harney *et al.*, 1974). Progesterone levels decline (Csapo and Weist, 1969; Hashimoto *et al.*, 1968), estrogen secretion increases (Yoshinaga *et al.*, 1969; Shaikh, 1971), the fetal adrenal glands increase in size (Milkovic *et al.*, 1973), and fetal plasma corticosterone secretion increases (Cohen, 1973). Removal of fetuses with placentas remaining *in situ* on day 16 or 17 reduces prostaglandin F release and spontaneous activity when measured *in vitro* on day 22, the expected day of delivery (Parnham *et al.*, 1975).

In the estrous rabbit, mating induces ovulation 10–12 hr later. Progesterone, 20α-OH-P, and estradiol levels, expressed as units per ovary per hour, increase to peak values during the first 4 hr after mating, seemingly in response to endogenous release of LH (Hilliard and Eaton, 1971). By the time of ovulation, the levels of these steroids are low, and they remain low during the period of 3–4 days required for tubal transport of embryos. When the blastocysts begin implantation between days 7 and 10, progestin and estradiol concentrations gradually increase. Progestin levels continue to increase to peak values between days 12 and 24 and then decline to low values near the time of parturition on day 32 (Hilliard *et al.*, 1973); progesterone in peripheral plasma follows a similar pattern (Baldwin and Stabenfeldt, 1975). Estradiol levels gradually increase to day 28 and decline before parturition.

A progesterone-binding protein (receptor) in the cytoplasmic fraction of the rabbit myometrium was found to undergo a decrease in receptor-site concentration after midpregnancy (Davies *et al.*, 1974). In nonpregnant rabbits, the concentration of progesterone receptor sites in myometrial cytosol was 4.5 pmole/mg protein; this level dropped to 1.3 pmole/mg within 3 days after mating. It remained low and declined (e.g., to 0.6 pmole/mg) after midpregnancy and then showed an increase to 1.9 pmol/mg by day 30 of pregnancy. This pattern of change in myometrial progesterone receptor concentration in pregnant rabbits is qualitatively similar to that observed in the rat (Davies and Ryan, 1973). The concentration of progesterone in the myometrium is related to plasma levels of the steroid, a finding that may indicate equilibration by simple diffusion (Davies *et al.*, 1974). During the first two-thirds of pregnancy, receptor concentration exceeds plasma progesterone, whereas during the last third of pregnancy receptor concentration is less than plasma progesterone.

Myometrial concentrations of progesterone, estrone (E_1), and estradiol-17β (E_2β) during pregnancy in the rabbit are severalfold greater than those found in peripheral plasma, and the levels are, in part, unrelated to the changes that occur in the plasma (Challis *et al.*, 1974). Myometrial concentrations of E_1 and $E_2\beta$ remain severalfold greater than plasma levels throughout gestation, whereas progesterone concentrations in the myometrium closely parallel those found in the plasma. During the last half of pregnancy, myometrial concentrations of $E_2\beta$ increase, the $E_2\beta:E_1$ ratio increases, and the E_1 myometrial:plasma ratio increases. None of these changes is attributed to changes in the peripheral plasma. A decline in peripheral plasma levels of progesterone is a prerequisite for onset of myometrial activity in the rabbit (Challis *et al.*, 1974). A significant increase in plasma prostaglandin F concentration occurs between days 21 and 30 of gestation (Challis *et al.*, 1973), which is coincident with the prepartum decrease in progesterone levels in plasma. Thus, during normal pregnancy, increasing levels of prostaglandin F may be luteolytic and induce the preparturient decline in plasma progesterone concentration.

Progesterone in peripheral plasma of the guinea pig increases markedly between days 15 and 30 of pregnancy, with high levels maintained during the remainder of the gestation (Challis *et al.*, 1971; Evans, 1987). Unconjugated estrogens in the plasma are undetectable before day 25 and increase gradually to maximal levels (e.g., 50 ng/ml) between days 55 and 60 after mating, with a slight decline occurring just preceding parturition. The increase in the progesterone production rate between days 15 and 30 in intact pregnant guinea pigs results mainly from increased ovarian secretion of the steroid. The embryo seems to exert a luteotropic effect on corpora lutea. Placental production of progesterone becomes important later in pregnancy. Guinea pigs ovariectomized during the last half of pregnancy continue their pregnancies to term. Plasma progesterone levels are highest at the end of gestation and are correlated closely with placental development (Heap and Deanesly, 1966). Ovariectomy, adrenalectomy, or both do not affect plasma concentrations of total unconjugated estrogens throughout pregnancy (Illingworth and Challis, 1973). Thus, both progesterone and estrogen are primarily of extraovarian origin, particularly during the second half of gestation.

3.1.2. Artiodactyla

In ungulates a preovulatory increase in the concentration of progesterone in peripheral plasma occurs about 16 hr before the onset of estrus (Ayalon and Shemesh, 1974). The surge is brief, lasting about 4 hr, with subsequent values steadily declining until the onset of estrus. This proestrus rise in plasma progesterone precedes by about 12 hr the peak in plasma estradiol, which occurs about 4 hr before the onset of estrus. In intact heifers, the preovulatory surge of plasma progesterone seems to facilitate the manifestation of estrus and sexual receptivity (Ayalon and Shemesh, 1974). Peripheral blood levels of progesterone are similar between days 3 and 12 in pregnant and nonpregnant heifers, whereas by day 50 of pregnancy the progesterone levels are higher (e.g., 5.0 ng/ml) than those found in nonpregnant heifers (e.g., 0.7 ng/ml) (Hasler *et al.*, 1975). The corpus luteum remains functional throughout pregnancy, with peripheral blood levels of progesterone declining markedly only during the last few days of gestation (Stabenfeldt *et al.*, 1970).

Peripheral plasma levels of estrone increase from about 250–400 pg/ml to about 600 pg/ml between 10 and 13 days; during the last week before parturition the level of estrone is 1000, and it reaches 4000 pg/ml just at parturition (Edqvist and Johansson, 1972; Musah *et al.*, 1987a). Estrone values then drop to less than 300 pg/ml within 5 hr after parturition and continue to decline to less than 25 pg/ml the day after parturition. Estradiol-17β levels are consistently low (80–100 pg/ml) and then increase to 150–400 pg/ml a few days before parturition (Musah *et al.*, 1986, 1987a; Fig. 2). Robertson and King (1974) found similar changes in peripheral plasma levels of E_1 and $E_2\beta$ as well as a marked increase in $E_2\beta$ a few days preceding parturition and a drop to low levels at parturition.

In ewes peripheral plasma levels of progesterone during pregnancy increase steadily from low values (e.g., 1–2 ng/ml) at day 1 to peak levels of ≥9 ng/ml by day 125 and then decline until parturition (Stabenfeldt *et al.*, 1972). In ewes carrying twins, progesterone levels are significantly higher between days 60 and 130. Within 9 days before parturition, progesterone concentrations in ewes carrying single fetuses or twins show a coincident decline to 2 ng/ml by onset of parturition. Concentrations of unconjugated estrone and estradiol-17β begin to rise during the 48 hr preceding delivery and decline to low levels within 12 hr after parturition (Challis, 1971; Chamley *et al.*, 1973). Pregnancy is maintained in ewes ovariectomized after day 50, a fact that implicates placental contribution to steroid production and may explain the steady decline in progesterone levels during the last 2 weeks of pregnancy.

The corpus luteum is required for maintenance of pregnancy in the sow; ovariectomy as late as day 110 results in abortion within a few hours (Belt *et al.*, 1971). Progesterone in peripheral plasma increases to peak values by days 12–20 and then declines to levels of 20–25 ng/ml until the last few days before parturition (Adair *et al.*, 1988; Felder *et al.*, 1986; Fig. 4). With onset of parturition, there is a rapid decline in progesterone to levels that remain low after delivery. Plasma levels of unconjugated estrone and estradiol-17β in peripheral blood are measurable by day 80 and rapidly increase to peak values just before parturition (Anderson *et al.*, 1983; Fig. 5). The fetoplacental unit is the major source of estrogen production, as indicated by similar urinary excretory patterns in intact controls compared with those in sows after ovariectomy, hypophysectomy (Fèvre *et al.*, 1968), or adrenalectomy (Fèvre *et. al.*, 1972).

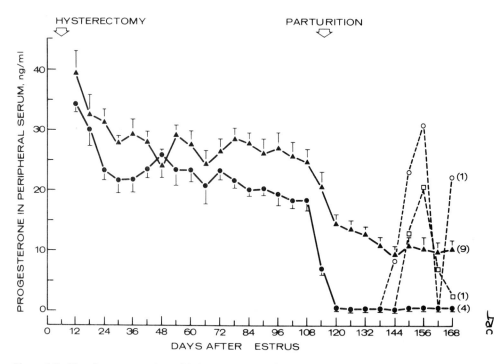

Figure 4. Profiles of progesterone (ng/ml) in hysterectomized (▲) and pregnant/lactating (●) gilts from days 12 to 168. During lactation in the postpartum period, estrous cycles occurred in two gilts (○,□), whereas ovarian function in the other four lactating animals remained quiescent. From Adair *et al.* (1988).

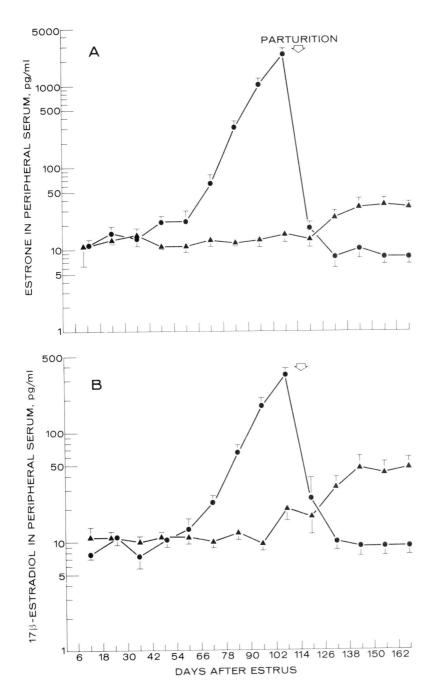

Figure 5. E$_1$ (A) and 17β-E$_2$ (B) concentrations in peripheral blood serum during pregnancy and early lactation (●) compared with those in unmated gilts hysterectomized (▲) on day 6 (day 0 = estrus). The number of gilts in each group is six. Values are the mean ± S.E. From Anderson *et al.* (1983).

3.2. The Role of Uterine–Conceptus Interactions on Ovarian Function

In the cow, ewe, sow, and mare the maintenance of the corpora lutea during the initial phase of pregnancy is highly regulated by the presence of the conceptus and/or conceptus secretory products. Removal of embryos from the uterus before day 13 in the cow, ewe, and sow does not affect the luteal phase; regression occurs and estrus resumes at the regular time characteristic of each species (Rosenfeld, 1980; Ford *et al.*, 1982; Northey and French, 1980). However, if embryos are flushed out after day 12 in sows and ewes and day 16 in cows, the duration of the cycle is extended by the CLs persisting 5 to 6 days longer. Thus, presence of the conceptus or of secretory products of the conceptus such as steroids and proteins may act as an antiluteolysin within the uterine environment.

3.2.1. Rodentia and Lagomorpha

In the rabbit, implantation occurs at the end of the first week after ovulation (Boving, 1961). Prior to implantation there is a gradual elevation in progesterone in peripheral serum. There is evidence that a chorionic gonadotropinlike activity exists in the preimplantation rabbit blastocyst. This CG-like factor is presumed to be associated with the preimplantation elevation in progesterone (Haour and Saxena, 1974; Fuchs and Beling, 1975). The presence of rCG, however, has not been demonstrated by other laboratories (Holt *et al.*, 1976; Sundaram *et al.*, 1975), and Browning *et al.* (1980) did not find any significant change in peripheral serum progesterone between pregnant and pseudopregnant rabbits around the time of implantation. Thus, the role of a rise in progesterone or rCG in the rabbit has not been conclusively demonstrated.

In the rabbit, the placenta does not produce enough progesterone to support pregnancy in the absence of the corpora lutea (Hilliard, 1973; Thau and Lanman, 1974). Ovarian follicular estrogen and antiluteolytic factors of the conceptus are thus essential for the maintenance of luteal function (Keyes *et al.*, 1983; Keyes and Gadsby, 1987). The placental factor essential for luteal maintenance is produced by trophoblastic cells (Holt and Ewing, 1974). Since the placental luteotropic factor requires the simultaneous actions of estrogens, it is not directly luteotropic (Bill and Keyes, 1983; Keyes and Gadsby, 1987). Both intraovarian estrogens and trophoblastic factors play an essential role in providing adequate luteal support during pregnancy. There is also a dependence on estrogen of fetal placental factor for maximum luteotropic support (Gadsby and Keyes, 1984; Keyes and Gadsby, 1987). Fetal placental factors promote luteal function for the third week of gestation by maintaining the levels of estrogen receptors at an adequate level in the corpora lutea of the rabbit (Keyes and Gadsby, 1987).

The rat placenta secretes a luteotropic hormone as early as day 7 of pregnancy. This is a PRL-like substance that arises from the decidua and sustains progesterone activity (Basuray and Gibori, 1980). Decidual luteotropin is detectable in decidual tissue as early as day 6 (24 hr after induction of decidualization), peaks at 9 days, and then begins to decline by day 11. At day 15 decidual luteotropin is undetectable (Gibori *et al.*, 1987). The decline in decidual luteotropin corresponds to the disappearance of luteotropic effects of decidual tissue. By day 11, decidual tissues of both pregnant and pseudopregnant rats are not capable of sustaining luteal cell progesterone production (Rothchild and Gibori, 1975; Gibori *et al.*, 1981; Jayatilak *et al.*, 1984).

Rat placental luteotropin has a molecular weight of about 40–50,000. It is produced basically by the trophoblastic tissue between days 10 and 13 (Linkie and Niswender, 1973; Kelly *et al.*, 1975; de Greef *et al.*, 1977; Robertson *et al.*, 1982). Decidual luteotropin prevents the involution of the CL that occurs after prolactin withdrawal and maintains luteal cell progesterone production (Gibori *et al.*, 1974; Castracane and Rothchild, 1976; Basuray and Gibori, 1980), maintains luteal cell content of LH receptors and adenylate cyclase competency (Gibori et al., 1984), and sustains the capacity of luteal cells to secrete estradiol when stimulated by LH (Gibori et al., 1985).

Prolactinlike proteins (mol. wt. 23,500) have also been identified in rat decidual tissue from day 6 to 12 of gestation (Jayatilak et al., 1985; Herz et al., 1985). The luteotropic role of the decidual PRL-like protein of early gestation is replaced by trophoblastic lactogen at midgestation (Kelly et al., 1975). Rat PRL peaks at day 12 and then declines by day 14. Coincident with the peak in rPRL is an increase in placental androgen and ovarian testosterone production by day 12 (Warshaw et al., 1986). The placenta regulates ovarian androgen between days 12 and 18; placental androgen secretion is independent of hypophyseal factors (Sridaran and Gibori, 1983).

3.2.2. Artiodactyla

Bovine blastocysts are spherical (0.2 mm diameter) on days 8–9, tubular (1.5–3.3 by 0.9–1.7 mm) on days 12–13, and then filamentous (1.5 × 10 mm) on days 13–14; by day 17 to 18 they measure 1.5 × 160 mm, and by day 24 the conceptus occupies both uterine horns (Bazer and First, 1983). A similar pattern of development occurs for porcine and ovine conceptuses (Moor and Rowson, 1966a,b; Bazer and First, 1983). During the period of blastocyst elongation, the bovine conceptus produces limited amounts of progesterone, androstenedione, and estradiol (Shemesh et al., 1979; Eley et al., 1983) as well as 5α-reduced androgens and progestagens (Thatcher et al., 1985). The porcine 10-mm blastocysts are capable of producing estrogen, and that capability increases to day 12, decreases between days 13 and 14, and increases again between days 15 and 25–30 of gestation (Gadsby et al., 1980; Stoner et al., 1981; Fischer et al., 1985). Porcine conceptus estrogen production is the essential signal for establishing pregnancy. The porcine conceptus also produces luteotropin ($M_r \simeq$ 20,000–25,000, pI $\simeq$ 5.6–6.2) and another protein ($M_r \simeq$ 35,000–50,000, pI $\simeq$ 8.0) between days 10.5 and 16–18 (Godkin et al., 1982). The roles of these proteins have not been established.

Ovine blastocysts produce three closely related isoelectric species with a molecular weight of about 18,000 and pI of 5.5–5.8 and named ovine trophoblast protein I (Godkin et al., 1982). The ovine trophoblast protein I (OTP1) is the major protein secreted between days 13 and 21 (Godkin et al., 1982; Hansen et al., 1985). Preliminary evidence suggests that OTP1 may be an interferon-α (Imakawa et al., 1987). Interferons have functions other than being antiviral (Kronenberg, 1985; Friedman et al., 1985). A group of proteins immunologically indistinguishable from OTP1 is produced by the bovine conceptus at an equivalent period (Helmer et al., 1987). The use of cDNA clones to bovine protein (bTP-1) and the inferred primary structure of OTP-1 indicate that it too is an interferon (Imakawa et al., 1987). One may speculate that the IFNs are involved in allograft rejection and inhibition of lymphocyte activation by lectins and autoantigens (Friedman et al., 1985; Kronenberg, 1985), but their role as luteotropins is currently unknown. The OTP1 is produced between days 12 and 21 of gestation; it is produced by the trophoblast and is taken up by surface and upper uterine gland epithelium. It has no lactogenic properties or stimulatory effects on progesterone production by luteal slices or dispersed cells, although there are specific binding sites on luteal membranes, and it is stimulatory to protein secretion by ovine endometrial explants from day 12 in cyclic ewes (Bazer et al., 1986). Purified ovine trophoblast protein I (200 mg/day) is not as effective as total conceptus secretory proteins (2 mg/day) in extending luteal life in cyclic ewes (Godkin et al., 1984).

Subsequent experiments have revealed that ovine conceptus proteins inhibit the ability of estradiol-17β and oxytocin to induce uterine production of prostaglandin F (Bazer et al., 1986; Fairclough et al., 1984). Ovine trophoblast protein I has been shown to decrease cAMP production, although progesterone production is unaffected in luteal cells in culture. The results suggest that these proteins have no direct luteolytic effect on the corpora lutea.

Since uterine PGF production has been shown to be the luteolysin in sheep, it has been proposed that uterine PGF is regulated by estradiol, which induces oxytocin receptors, and that oxytocin–receptor complex stimulates phospholipase A_2, the arachidonic acid circuit, and PGF production (McCracken et al., 1984). Thus, the ovine conceptus protein may affect PGF_2 production and extend luteal function by inhibiting estradiol- and oxytocin-induced $PGF_{2\alpha}$ production. The active substance in maternal recognition of pregnancy in the ewe is undoubtedly OTP1, which, in paracrine fashion, targets the uterine epithelium (Hansen et al., 1985).

3.2.3. Primates

The morphology of and rate of embryonic development vary greatly among the primates. In man and the great apes the trophoblast penetrates the epithelium and invades the stroma. The trophoblast differentiates into the cytotrophoblast and syncytiotrophoblast, and in man both are entirely covered by epithelium by day 11. The primary villi are developed by day 14, and a decidual reaction develops in the endometrium surrounding the conceptus (McLaren, 1985).

Human embryos are attached by day 6–7 (Lenton et al., 1982), chimpanzee by day 7–8 (Reyes et al., 1975), baboon by day 8–10 and rhesus monkey by day 8–10 (Atkinson et al., 1975), and marmoset by day 11–12 (Hearn, 1983). The embryonic signal to the mother is chorionic gonadotropin, which increases in peripheral blood during and after implantation. The preimplantation primate embryo secretes CG, as has been shown in both human (Fishel et al., 1984) and baboon (Pope et al., 1982). When hatched primate blastocysts are incubated in the presence of antisera to hCG-β subunit, embryonic attachment is hindered, and lysis of the blastocysts occurs within 2 days; as a consequence, CG may be essential at a local level for trophoblastic differentiation and implantation (Hearn, 1986). In addition to CG as an embryonic message, preliminary evidence seems to suggest that at least in women an early pregnancy factor (EPF) may be detected within 3 days after fertilization (Morton et al., 1977; Koch and Ellendorff, 1985). The role of these embryonic signals in the regulation of luteal function has yet to be determined.

3.3. Uterine–Ovarian Microcirculation and Ovarian Function

Over the last 20 years much has been learned about the interrelation between the affluent and effluent drainage in and around both uterine and ovarian tissues. The vasculature around these tissues responds to the steroid milieu by altering the contractile properties of its bed. Vascular physiology is the subject of Chapter 5 of this volume; emphasis here is primarily on the uterine–ovarian microcirculatory system as it relates directly to ovarian function. Changes in uterine–ovarian blood flow are of importance to luteal function during the estrous cycle as well as pregnancy; luteal maintenance may be mediated by local vascular transport of a luteotropic or antiluteolytic substance from the gravid uterus to the ovary (Gardner et al., 1963; Mapletoft et al., 1976; Del Campo et al., 1980).

Huckabee et al. (1968) demonstrated that progesterone and estrogen differentially altered blood flow through the nonpregnant ovine uterine vascular bed. Subsequently the temporal changes in uterine–ovarian blood flow were confirmed to be estrogen and progesterone dependent. In most species, especially ewes, cows, and sows, marked increases in uterine blood flow are associated with the onset of behavioral estrus; there is an abrupt decrease thereafter, and the flow is greatly reduced during most of the luteal phase (Ford et al., 1979a,b; Ford, 1982; Fig. 6). The ovarian blood flow during the same period is exactly the opposite of uterine blood flow. The highest flow occurs during the luteal phase, and the lowest is at estrus (Ford, 1982). In the sow and ewe, 90% of the ovarian blood flow is through the corpora lutea (Ford *et al.*, 1979a, 1982). A rhythmicity in uterine blood flow under endogenous hormonal environments has been demonstrated in several species including sows (Dickson *et al.*, 1969), cows (Roman-Ponce *et al.*, 1978; Ford *et al.* 1979b), and ewes (Ford *et al.*, 1979a). The effects of estrogen and progesterone on changing blood flow through the ovary or the uterine vascular bed depend on the estrogen : progesterone ratios. For instance, progesterone reduces the ability of estradiol-17β to stimulate changes in uterine blood flow; the magnitude of such changes is related to their ratios (Caton *et al.*, 1974).

The effects of progesterone and estrogen on blood flow to the ovary and uterus and on luteal integrity may be mediated in part by the effects these hormones have on periarterial sympathetic nerves. Mammalian arterial beds are innervated by adrenergic vasoconstrictors. Blood vessels and smooth muscles of the female reproductive organs also receive these

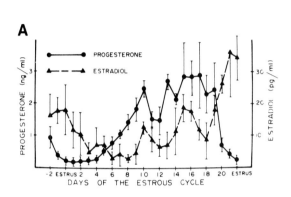

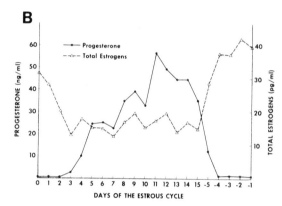

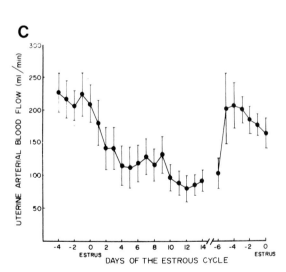

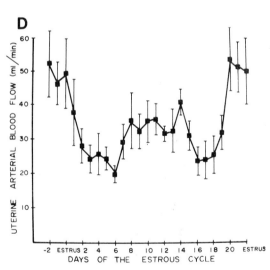

Figure 6. (A) Concentrations of progesterone and estradiol-17β in jugular venous blood throughout the estrous cycle of three nonpregnant cows (day 0 = estrus). Each point represents the mean ± S.E. (B) Concentrations of progesterone and total estrogen (estrone + estradiol-17β) in blood collected from the vena cava of 18 nonpregnant gilts throughout an estrous cycle. Day 0 = first day of estrus. (C) Pattern of blood flow through each uterine artery of six non-pregnant sows throughout an estrous cycle (day 0 = first day of estrus). Each point represents the mean ± S.E. of 12 uterine arteries. (D) Pattern of blood flow to uteri of three nonpregnant cows throughout the estrous cycle (day 0 = estrus). Each point represents the mean ± S.E. of six uterine arteries (three ipsilateral and three contralateral to the ovary containing the corpus luteum). From Ford (1982).

adrenergic vasoconstrictors. Norepinephrine released from adrenergic nerves binds to membrane-bound receptors (α- and β-adrenergic receptors) of smooth muscle cells. The norepinephrine–α-receptor complex stimulates vasoconstriction, whereas the norepinephrine–β-receptor complex mediates vasodilation. The presence of stimulable β receptors in the uterine vascular bed has been confirmed in the cow (Ford and Reynolds, 1981) and ewe (Greiss, 1972). Uterine blood flow in the ewe can be reduced significantly by infusion of relatively low doses of norepinephrine in the uterine artery (Barton *et al.*, 1974). Ladner *et al.* (1970) showed that in the anesthetized ewe stimulation of adrenergic receptors could lead to vasoconstriction in the uterine bed. Steroid hormones may mediate their effect on uterine and ovarian blood flow through the differential effects on catecholamine concentration and catecholamine release from nerve terminal vesicles or by directly altering α- and β-adrenergic receptor population. Estrogens cause vasodilation by reducing norepinephrine levels in uterine periarterial adrenergic nerves (McKercher *et al.*, 1973); progesterone, on the other hand, increases vasoconstriction caused by norepinephrine (Kalsner, 1969).

It is becoming more apparent that periarterial adrenergic vasiconstriction and vasodilation may be modulated by prostaglandins. Uterine prostaglandin $F_{2\alpha}$ ($PGF_{2\alpha}$) plays a critical role in luteolysis and in the regulation of ovarian function in many species. Prostaglandin $F_{2\alpha}$ is associated with norepinephrine release, whereas PGE inhibits norepinephrine release (Kadowitz *et al.*, 1972). During the estrous cycle, high levels of PGF are found in the uteroovarian veins of the sow, ewe, and cow coincident with a fall in peripheral plasma progesterone levels (Thorburn *et al.*, 1972; Gleeson *et al.*, 1974). It has therefore been proposed that the luteolytic action of prostaglandins $F_{2\alpha}$ and analogues (Moeljono *et al.*, 1976; Musah *et al.*, 1987b) mediates in part the ability of $PGF_{2\alpha}$ to reduce ovarian blood flow (Pharriss, 1970). This hypothesis has been supported by the findings that in ewes, ovarian arterial $PGF_{2\alpha}$ infusion reduces blood flow through the ovary and initiates luteolysis (McCracken *et al.*, 1970). Endogenous blood flow to the CL-bearing ovary is relatively reduced during luteal regression in the cow and ewe (Niswender *et al.*, 1975; Ford and Chenault, 1981).

If pregnancy is to be maintained, the luteal phase has to be extended beyond its normal duration encountered during the estrous or menstrual cycles. Over the last few years the role of changes in the levels of blood flow through the uterine vascular bed and ovary has given a clear image of the salient changes in blood flow preceding extended luteal function during pregnancy. A transient increase in uterine blood flow occurs coincident with maternal recognition of pregnancy in cows, ewes, and sows (Greiss and Anderson, 1970; Ford *et al.*, 1979a,b). This increase in uterine blood flow precedes a second rise in uterine blood flow, which occurs coincident with embryonic attachment (Ford *et al.*, 1979b) and occurs simultaneously with a transient increase in ovarian blood flow (Magness *et al.*, 1983; Reynolds *et al.*, 1984). Increased uterine and ovarian blood flows may function to enhance transport of a conceptus luteotropic and/or antiluteolytic substance from gravid uterus to CL-bearing ovary by a local vascular system (Mapletoft *et al.*, 1976; Del Campo *et al.*, 1980). In support of this hypothesis is the observation that progesterone in peripheral blood is elevated at the time of maternal recognition of pregnancy and is associated with an increase in uterine blood flow (Magness *et al.*, 1983; Reynolds *et al.*, 1984). Thus, ovarian vasodilation may prevent luteolysis by maintaining luteal blood flow and thereby luteal morphology and function.

4. Luteolytic Actions of the Uterus: Effects of Hysterectomy on Ovarian Function

The effects of hysterectomy on ovarian function, particularly luteal function, in several species have been reported by numerous investigators. Recent reviews include those of Anderson *et al.* (1969) and Anderson (1973). In the hamster, mouse, and rat, hysterectomy seems not to alter the brief cyclic intervals; pseudopregnancy, however, is increased to a duration similar to that of pregnancy. In the estrus rabbit, uterine removal does not alter occurrence of ovulation but extends the duration of pseudopregnancy. Cyclic periodicity is interrupted after hysterectomy in the guinea pig, ewe, sow, and heifer, and corpora lutea are maintained for a period equal to or exceeding that of pregnancy. When the corpora eventually fail, estrus and ovulation occur, and the newly formed corpora lutea in these animals are maintained again for an equally prolonged period. Likewise, subsequent prolonged pseudopregnancies can be induced after hysterectomy in animals that experience brief estrous cycles. If the animals are subjected to hysterectomy too late in the estrous cycle or pseudopregnancy, the duration of that cycle or pseudopregnancy is not extended, but subsequent cycles or pseudopregnancies are prolonged. In species such as the ground squirrel, ferret, dog, opossum, rhesus monkey, and human, ovarian function and estrous or menstrual cycle continue uninterrupted after hysterectomy (Anderson, 1973).

4.1. The Uterus and Luteal Function in Rodentia and Lagomorpha

In the rat there is a very close anatomic and functional relationship between the ovaries and the uterus (Donovan 1978). In this species a significant portion of the blood supply to the ovaries comes from the uterine horn. Hysterectomy in the rat markedly increases the total RNA production in the anterior pituitary (Biro, 1980, Biro *et al.*, 1987). The role of the increased RNA production is unknown, but the uteri of decidualized or pregnant animals tend to hasten the dependency of the rat corpus luteum on LH, whereas hysterectomy and prolactin delay the onset of the LH dependency (Nanes *et al.*, 1980; Garris and Rothchild, 1980: Sanchez-Criado and Rothchild, 1986).

In adult rats hysterectomized on day 8 of pseudopregnancy, progesterone decreased from 88 ng/ml on day 8 to 44 ng/ml on day 15. In these rats LH antiserum (LHAS) administered on day 10 resulted in a drastic decrease in progesterone to less than 10 ng/ml by day 15 (Sanchez-Criado and Rothchild, 1986). Administration of LHAS to decidua-bearing rats on day 10 induced a rapid and permanent luteolysis.

Quite unlike other species in which the uterus has a significant role in luteal demise through uterine secretion of PGs, the uterus of the nongravid rabbit does not appear to have such a function. Hysterectomy does not prevent the major decline in serum P_4 concentration at the end of pseudopregnancy (Miller and Keyes, 1976). Neither the pituitary, nonluteal ovarian tissue, nor local uterine factors appear to play a critical role in rabbit luteal regression. Luteal regression is not dependent on E_2 withdrawal, since serum E_1 levels increase toward the end of gestation (Browning *et al.*, 1980) and neither nonphysiological nor physiological doses of estrogens (Bill and Keyes, 1983) alter the course of luteal demise. Though the endogenous uterine PG does not appear to mediate luteal demise, exogenous $PGF_{2\alpha}$ causes luteal demise (Carlson and Gole, 1978; Laudanski *et al.*, 1979; Kehl and Carlson, 1981). Thus, the role of endogenous luteal PGF in luteal demise is unknown.

Maintenance of luteal progesterone production is vital for the reproductive function of the guinea pig. Progesterone is derived from the corpus luteum and the placenta during pregnancy (Evans, 1987). Luteal progesterone secretion is essential for the first 30 days of pregnancy, after which placental progesterone production becomes fully competent to sustain the level of progesterone required to maintain pregnancy (Evans, 1987). Though the placenta is fully competent by day 30, the corpus luteum is still active until late pregnancy. Peripheral progesterone levels are elevated if hysterectomy is performed on day 5 after an estrous cycle (Evans, 1987; Fig. 7). The demise of the corpus luteum during the estrous cycle is thought to be mediated in part by $PGF_{2\alpha}$ of uterine origin. Administration of PG to hysterectomized guinea pigs results in a brief, abrupt decrease in progesterone levels, but the decrease does not

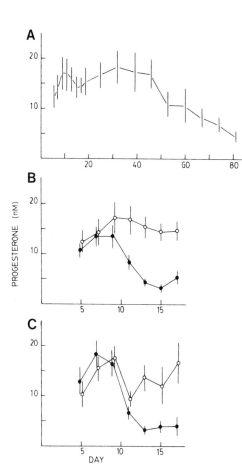

Figure 7. (A) The mean progesterone levels (±S.E.) in guinea pigs (*n* = 5) that were hysterectomized on day 5. (B) Progesterone levels (mean ± S.E.) in guinea pigs hysterectomized on day 5 (○, *n* = 5) compared with intact controls (●, *n* = 7). (C) Progesterone levels (mean ± S.E.) in guinea pigs that were given injections of PGF$_{2\alpha}$ on days 9 and 10 in the presence (●, *n* = 5) and absence (○, *n* = 6) of the uterus. From Evans (1987).

persist; the corpus luteum at this stage is capable of resisting the effects of PGF (Evans, 1987; Fig. 7).

4.2. The Uterus and Luteal Function in Artiodactyla

The functional life of the corpus luteum of the estrous cycle in the ewe can be prolonged in a variety of ways: by pregnancy (Moor and Rowson, 1966a,b), hysterectomy (Lewis and Bolt, 1987), exogenous estrogen (Denamur and Mauleon, 1963), and exogenous LH (Karsch *et al.*, 1969). The effects of pregnancy and hysterectomy may be attributed to removal of a uterine luteolytic stimulus. In ewes, hysterectomy alters the duration of the luteal phase, the PGFm profile, and levels of progesterone in peripheral plasma (Lewis and Bolt, 1983, 1987). Hysterectomy also enhances progesterone production in ewes (Lewis and Bolt, 1987), an observation made earlier in pigs (Adair *et al.*, 1988; Anderson *et al.*, 1983; Musah *et al.*, 1984; Fig. 4).

In the presence of a uterus, progesterone secretion from the ovine corpus luteum is not maintained (Denamur *et al.*, 1970). Functional corpora lutea, as indicated by progesterone in ovarian venous blood, are maintained after hypophyseal stalk transection by daily injections of estradiol benzoate. Luteal function also is prolonged after hypophyseal stalk transection combined with hysterectomy, but progesterone secretion is slightly lower than that found in ewes given estrogen. These experimental results are interpreted to mean that estrogen, like hysterectomy, prolongs the life of cyclic corpora lutea in the ewe, but it can also extend luteal function when the pituitary gland is separated from the brain (Denamur *et al.*, 1970). Implantation of small amounts of estrogen directly in the ovine corpus luteum fails to sustain a luteotropic effect. Estrogen, like hysterectomy, prolongs the life span of ovine corpora lutea even in animals that have undergone hypophyseal stalk transection. The luteotropic role of estrogen in this species may be to inhibit or override the production of uterine luteolysin. Prolonging the life of corpora lutea in ewes during pregnancy by the infusion of LH or by hysterectomy also may occur through inhibition of a uterine luteolytic effect. Removal of the uterus, even as late as day 15 in the ewe, can arrest luteolysis, whereas pregnancy, estrogen treatment, or infusions of LH must be initiated several days earlier to produce luteotropic effects (Karsch *et al.*, 1969; Kann and Denamur, 1973).

Hysterectomy of sexually mature gilts prolongs the duration of the luteal phase (Kraeling *et al.*, 1981; Adair *et al.*, 1988; Anderson *et al.*, 1982; Musah *et al.*, 1984). Pigs hysterectomized during the early phase of the estrous cycle develop fully functional corpora lutea by day 14. Functional corpora lutea are essential to define the interestrus interval whether relating to the nongravid or gravid state in the pig. A feature of the pig that is also shared with the ewe and the guinea pig is the ability of hysterectomy to enhance progesterone production (Adair *et al.*, 1988; Evans, 1987; Lewis and Bolt, 1987). After hysterectomy, circulating peripheral plasma progesterone is consistently greater than during the corresponding stages throughout pregnancy (Fig. 4) (Adair *et al.*, 1988; Lewis and Bolt, 1987). After hysterectomy, peripheral blood levels of estrone and estradiol-17β remain consistently low (<20 pg/ml) from day 12 to day 114 (Fig. 5), in marked contrast to those found during pregnancy (Anderson *et al.*, 1983). Exogenous estradiol-17β between days 45 and 108 decreases progesterone secretion by aging corpora lutea in hysterectomized gilts compared with that in sesame-oil-treated controls (Fig. 8; Musah *et al.*, 1984). This decreased level of progesterone secretion is similar to that found during the second half of normal pregnancy (Adair *et al.*, 1988; Anderson *et al.*, 1983; Musah *et al.*, 1984). Progesterone secretion in hysterectomized gilts is greater than that during pregnancy at a time when circulating estrone and estradiol-17β levels are low in the former and

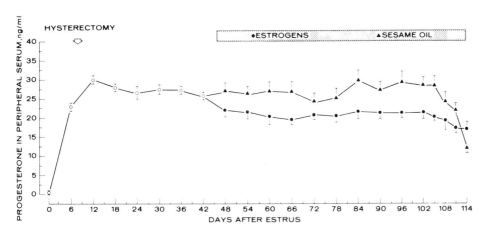

Figure 8. Progesterone concentrations in peripheral blood serum of hysterectomized Yorkshire gilts. Sequential profiles of progesterone in 16 gilts before hormone or oil treatment (○); sesame oil injected i.m. in 7 animals (▲); estrogen injected i.m. in nine gilts (●). Values are the mean ± S.E. From Musah *et al.* (1984).

peak in the latter (Adair *et al.*, 1988; Anderson *et al.*, 1983). Uterine or conceptus metabolism of progesterone to estrogens may account in part for the lower concentrations of progesterone in pregnant than in hysterectomized gilts.

The mechanisms by which estrogen decreases progesterone secretion in hysterectomized gilts may relate to the high secretion rates of estrone and estradiol-17β during the latter half of gestation. Administration of exogenous estrogen to hysterectomized gilts in dosages designed to mimic peripheral blood levels of endogenous estrogen in the pig during pregnancy consistently depressed progesterone levels in hysterectomized gilts to levels comparable with those of pregnant gilts (Musah *et al.*, 1984). Continual administration of estrogen to hysterectomized gilts beyond day 114 does not confer immortality on the corpora lutea. Although ovulation is suppressed and follicular growth is inhibited, the existing corpora lutea eventually regress at about day 165 (Musah *et al.*, 1984).

Luteotrophic support by adenohypophyseal hormones is required for sustaining luteal function in hysterectomized pigs. Hypophysectomy between days 4 and 90 results in immediate termination of pregnancy (Kraeling and Davis, 1974). After hypophyseal stalk transection of hysterectomized pigs, the previously maintained corpora lutea regress (Anderson *et al.*, 1967b); however, if the stalk transection is delayed until day 50, only partial luteal regression occurs, and it can be prevented by daily injections of estradiol benzoate; if the stalk transection is delayed until day 70, no further estrogen treatment is required for luteal maintenance. Hypophyseal stalk transection of pregnant pigs at day 50 results in abortion within a few days, but pregnancy is maintained when the stalk transection is delayed until day 70 or 90. Luteotrophic support of young corpora lutea is primarily through luteinizing hormone (LH) (Anderson *et al.*, 1967b), whereas in older corpora lutea, prolactin may play a prominent role (Fig. 9; Felder *et al.*, 1988). Administration of pLH and pPRL to hysterectomized gilts from day 110 to 120 showed that pPRL could maintain progesterone secretion from existing corpora without contribution from luteinized follicles or new corpora lutea (Fig. 9; Felder *et al.*, 1988).

In heifers, hysterectomy results in an extension of the life of the corpus luteum to a period equivalent to or exceeding that of pregnancy (Anderson, 1973). Adenohypophyseal hormones required for luteotrophic support after hysterectomy implicate LH and prolactin. When the hypophyseal stalk is transected in previously hysterectomized heifers, the adenohypophysis sustains the corpus luteum for at least 48 days, as indicated by maintenance of peripheral blood levels of progesterone (Anderson, 1968; Anderson *et al.*, 1969). Other *in vivo* and *in vitro* experimental evidence is interpreted as suggesting luteotrophic action by LH in the cow (Donaldson and Hansel, 1965). Probable luteotrophic action of LH is inferred from partial luteolytic effects of LH antiserum in hysterectomized animals, whereas prolactin antiserum does not alter luteal function in hysterectomized cows (Hoffman *et al.*, 1974). These data support the contention that LH is probably a dominant luteotrophic factor in cattle.

4.3. The Uterus and Luteal Function in Primates

Continuation of ovarian cycles after hysterectomy in the rhesus monkey indicates no dependence of cyclic periodicity on a uterine luteolytic stimulus (Knobil, 1973, 1974). Endogenous levels of LH remain low during the luteal phase of the menstrual cycle and are interpreted as providing a permissive rather than a controlling influence on luteal function (Knobil, 1973, 1974). Exogenous estradiol benzoate induces premature luteal regression (Dierschke *et al.*, 1973), whereas endogenous estrogens are produced within the corpus luteum and may lead to its own regression, thus playing a role in cyclic periodicity (Knobil, 1973). Luteal function soon after conception depends on chorionic gonadotropic stimulation, with the corpus luteum being sustained throughout the gestation.

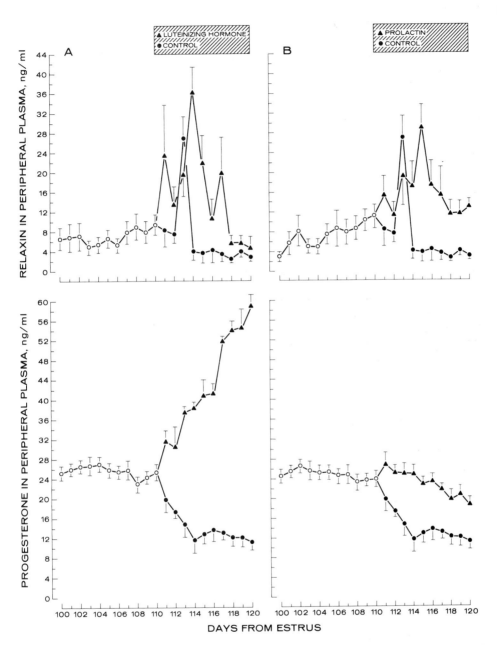

Figure 9. Relaxin (upper panel) and progesterone (lower panel) concentrations in peripheral plasma of unmated hysterectomized gilts from days 100 to 120. Sequential profiles of relaxin and progesterone are shown before hormone or saline treatment (○) in 14 gilts in A and in 15 gilts in B, in hysterectomized controls given i.m. and i.v. injections of saline (●: A, *n* = 9; B, *n* = 9), in hysterectomized gilts given three i.m. injections of pLH at a total dose of 3.2 mg/day on days 110–120 (▲: A, *n* = 5), and in hysterectomized animals given four i.v. injections of pPRL at a total dose of 2.0 mg/day on days 110–120 (▲: B, *n* = 6). Values are the mean ± S.E. From Felder *et al.* (1988).

Steroids such as estrogens and progestins have been the focal point in the assessment of luteal integrity. Since these steroids have been directly and indirectly discussed through this chapter, the emphasis here is on other hormones of ovarian or uterine origin that affect luteal function.

5.1. Prostanoids and Leukotrienes

Prostanoids and leukotrienes are products of arachidonic acid, which is released from phospholipids by phospholipases (Oates, 1982). Depending on tissue and hormonal stimuli, arachidonic acid is utilized in several different ways to produce prostaglandins (PG), prostacyclin I_2 (PGI_2), and thromboxane (TXA_2) via the cyclooxygenase pathway or to produce leukotrienes through the 5-lipoxygenase pathway. Prostaglandins are synthesized in the plasma membranes of cells from a 20-carbon unsaturated hydroxy acid group in four main series: A, B, E, and F according to differences in the five-carbon ring structure. The two most important prostaglandins are PGE and PGF ($PGF_{2\alpha}$). These two differ from each other by the presence of a hydroxyl or keto group, respectively, on carbon 5 within the cyclopentane ring.

A major physiological role of PGE_2 and $PGF_{2\alpha}$ is control of vascular smooth muscle activity. Pharmacological doses of certain PGs (e.g., from the E and F series) as well as synthetic analogues produce marked responses of reproductive organs in both sexes. Of particular interest is the capability of administered prostaglandins to induce premature luteolysis for regulation of sexual cycles (McCracken *et al.*, 1972a,b; Mauleon and Ortavant, 1975), to affect ovulatory processes, and to terminate pregnancy. Evidence of possible roles of endogenous prostaglandins in regulation of cyclic ovarian function and interaction with uterine physiological events exists for certain animals (e.g., ewe; McCracken *et al.*, 1972a,b, 1973; Goding, 1974). Prostaglandin $F_{2\alpha}$ can induce both functional and morphological demise of the corpus luteum. Functional demise of the corpus luteum is reversible on hysterectomy in species in which luteal function is extended (except nonhuman primates and women), on neutralization of $PGF_{2\alpha}$ with antibodies, on treatment with inhibitors of prostaglandin synthesis such as indomethacin, or in the presence of a conceptus at the appropriate time of the cycle. Functional demise results from the acute effects of $PGF_{2\alpha}$ on progesterone production, whereas morphological demise results from a prolonged exposure of luteal cells to $PGF_{2\alpha}$.

A newly emerging concept in regard to luteal function suggests that prostacyclin (PGI_2) plays a luteotrophic role, whereas the products of the lipoxygenase pathways of arachidonic acid metabolism such as 5-hydroxyeicosatetraenoic acid (5-HPETE) play luteolytic roles (Hansel and Dowd, 1986). This concept is supported by the recent finding that injection of PGI_2 directly into the bovine corpus luteum on day 10 of the estrous cycle causes a marked increase in jugular vein progesterone concentration within 5 min. Similarly, corpora lutea from day 5 synthesize more PGI_2 than do luteal tissue from any other day. The cyclooxygenase pathway is required for normal early CL development, so that administration of the PG synthetase inhibitor indomethacin, which blocks the synthesis of $PGF_{2\alpha}$, PGE_2, PGI_2, and PGA_2, on day 4, 5, or 6 inhibits luteal development, shortens the life span of the CL, and decreases the length of the estrous cycle (Milvae and Hansel, 1985; Milvae, 1986).

Products of the 5-lipoxygenase pathway of arachidonic acid metabolism were subsequently shown to have a luteolytic effect. The products of the lipoxygenase pathway induced a dose-dependent reduction in synthesis of progesterone and PGI_2 but not of $PGF_{2\alpha}$ (Milvae *et al.*, 1986). Similarly, 5-HPETE could also produce the same effect on dispersed bovine luteal cells. The role of this lipoxygenase pathway in luteal regression was confirmed from *in vivo* studies in which heifers were given intrauterine infusion of nordihydroguaiaretic acid (NDGH), an inhibitor of the lipoxygenase pathway, twice daily on days 14 through 18 of the estrous cycle (Milvae *et al.*, 1986). The treatment delayed luteolysis and lengthened the estrous cycle (Milvae *et al.*, 1986).

In the ewe, preliminary evidence suggests that $PGF_{2\alpha}$ released from the uterus may reach the ovary containing the corpus luteum by a countercurrent mechanism (McCracken *et al.*, 1984). Ligation of the uterine artery and vein, but not of the artery alone, inhibits luteal regression (Kiracofe *et al.*, 1966), and separation of the structures between the ovary and the uterus also results in prolonged maintenance of luteal function (Inskeep and Butcher, 1966). When the uterine vein remains intact, ovarian cycles continue, a fact that suggests that a luteolytic substance is transported from the uterus through the uterine vein (Baird and Land, 1973). Endogenous levels of $PGF_{2\alpha}$ in ovine endometrium undergo a significant increase by day 14 of the estrous cycle relative to earlier stages (days 3–11) (Wilson *et al.*, 1972a,b). Prostaglandin $F_{2\alpha}$ also increases significantly in uterine venous blood by late stages (day 15) of the estrous cycle (Bland *et al.*, 1971; Thorburn *et al.*, 1972). Uterine venous plasma collected from donor ewes around the time of luteal regression during the estrous cycle (day 15) depresses progesterone secretion when the plasma is infused into the ovarian arteries of ewes bearing an ovarian autotransplant (Baird *et al.*, 1973). The luteolytic activity of uterine venous plasma collected at days 14–16 is greater than that of plasma obtained at days 9–11. Also, $PGF_{2\alpha}$ concentrations are higher in plasma samples collected during the last days of the cycle than in those from day 9 to day 11.

A single injection of estradiol-17β given during the late luteal phase of the estrous cycle in ewes induces premature luteolysis (Hawk and Bolt, 1970); this effect is abolished by hysterectomy. Endogenous estrogens in the ewe may play a role in the synthesis or release of a uterine luteolysin. Infusion of physiological amounts of estradiol-17β directly into the arterial supply of the ovine uterus results in a marked release of $PGF_{2\alpha}$, whereas systemic infusion of the same amount of the steroid does not stimulate $PGF_{2\alpha}$ release (Barcikowski *et al.*, 1974). Local infusion of estrogen into the uterus late in the estrous cycle induces $PGF_{2\alpha}$ release. The production of $PGF_{2\alpha}$ in the ewe is regulated by estradiol and oxytocin. Pulse surges of luteal oxytocin occur during ovine luteolysis (Flint and Sheldrick, 1986). Significant increases in uteroovarian venous $PGF_{2\alpha}$ precede the pulses of oxytocin on day 15 of the cycle (Moore *et al.*, 1986).

Levels of $PGF_{2\alpha}$ in blood and uterine tissue vary with the stage of the estrous cycle in the rat. Estrogens induce uterine hyperemia and hypertrophy; similar uterine vasodilation results when PGE_1 is administered to the rat (Clark *et al.*, 1973). Indomethacin, a potent antiinflammatory agent, also is a potent inhibitor of prostaglandin synthetase (Lerner *et al.*, 1975). Estrogens (e.g., diethylstilbestrol) and nonsteroidal antiinflammatory agents are capable of inhibiting prostaglandin synthetase. Under *in vitro* conditions, there is a gradual increase in $PGF_{2\alpha}$ output from low levels at day 17 of pregnancy in the rat to maximal levels by day 22, the day of expected delivery (Harney *et al.*, 1974). When fetuses are surgically removed on day 16 or 17 from only one uterine horn, fetuses in the remaining uterine horn as well as placentas from the intact and fetectomized uterine horn are delivered normally (Parnham *et al.*, 1975). Removal of fetuses from one or both horns reduces PGF output and spontaneous uterine activity *in vitro*, a finding that is interpreted as indicating that the presence of viable fetuses exerts some control over prostaglandin synthesis. Quiescent uteri respond to exogenous $PGF_{2\alpha}$ by restoration of rhythmic contractions.

Infusion of prostaglandin $F_{2\alpha}$ at selected stages after mating terminates pregnancy in the rat (Nutting and Cammarata, 1969; Fuchs and Mok, 1973, 1974). The $PGF_{2\alpha}$ is particularly effective in terminating pregnancy when given at days 9–12 or days 18–20; pregnancy is interrupted at these stages at levels of 125 μg or more. Prostaglandin E_1 and PGE_2 are much less effective than $PGF_{2\alpha}$ in terminating pregnancy in this species.

Intravenous infusion of prostaglandin $F_{2\alpha}$ over a brief period in pseudopregnant rabbits causes no consistent changes in vascular resistance of the corpora lutea, whereas there is a pronounced vasodilation in the interstitial tissue (Janson *et al.*, 1975). Luteal blood is the predominant part of the total ovarian flow, and interstitial vasodilation causes only negligible changes in blood flow to the whole ovary. The experimental results do not support the hypothesis of a prostaglandin-induced reduction in luteal blood flow preceding luteolysis.

The porcine endometrium acts as an endocrine gland during the estrous cycle. The endometrium produces $PGF_{2\alpha}$, which is released into the uterine venous drainage for transport to the CL, where it induces luteolysis to ensure that cyclicity is maintained. There is no evidence for an increase in endocrine secretion of PGF or PGF metabolites in the uteroovarian vein or peripheral plasma. This finding contrasts sharply with the situation in the cow and ewe (Fincher et al., 1984). The role of uterine $PGF_{2\alpha}$ may be via changes in uterine blood flow, vascular permeability, fluid and electrolyte transport, cellular proliferation, steroid bio-synthesis, and immune protection of the conceptus (Bazer et al., 1982). The role of $PGF_{2\alpha}$ in natural luteolysis in the pig is not conclusive. The bovine corpus luteum seems capable of converting arachidonic acid to prostaglandin. Prostaglandin F levels in bovine endometrium and uterine venous blood rise at the time the corpus luteum begins to regress and plasma progesterone levels fall (Shemesh and Hansel, 1975). By the time the signs of estrous behavior are detected, the PGF levels already have begun to decline. The rise and fall of PGF before onset of estrus correspond with the elevation and decline in peripheral plasma testosterone (Shemesh and Hansel, 1974) and estradiol (Hansel et al., 1973), which occur 3 days preceding estrus. In the pig, an intramuscular injection of either 10 or 20 mg $PGF_{2\alpha}$ during the luteal phase of the estrous cycle induces luteal regression, but the animals do not return to estrus or ovulate before day 16 (Douglas and Ginther, 1975); lower levels of $PGF_{2\alpha}$ (2 or 5 mg) given during the midluteal phase fail to cause luteolysis (Diehl and Day, 1974).

In heifers, the introduction of prostaglandin $F_{2\alpha}$ into the uterine horn ipsilateral to the corpus luteum induces premature luteolysis (Liehr et al., 1972; Louis et al., 1974) provided that it is given after day 4 of the estrous cycle (Rowson et al., 1972). A single intrauterine administration of 350 µg of a $PGF_{2\alpha}$ analogue (ICI 79939) effectively induces luteolysis; intramuscular injection of 800 µg and 200 µg on two consecutive days also results in precise synchronization of estrus in heifers (Tervit et al., 1973). In heifers, the increase in luteinizing hormone 6 hr after injection of $PGF_{2\alpha}$ seems related to effects of progesterone withdrawal rather than to the direct action of $PGF_{2\alpha}$ on the hypothalamic–hypophyseal axis. Evidence from several trials indicates that an intramuscular injection of $PGF_{2\alpha}$ (e.g., 30 mg) beginning day 4 of the estrous cycle effectively induces premature luteolysis, with estrus and ovulation occurring within 2–4 days after treatment (Inskeep, 1973; Lauderdale et al., 1974).

5.2. Relaxin

Relaxin plays a critical role in suppressing uterine motility during pregnancy and in remodeling connective tissue in preparation for imminent parturition (Porter, 1984; Anderson 1987). The initial studies on fine structure of porcine corpora lutea throughout pregnancy and after hysterectomy revealed marked changes in granular endoplasmic reticulum and striking numbers of electron-dense membrane-limited granules (Belt et al., 1970, 1971; Fig. 1). These features were virtually absent during the 21-day estrous cycle (Cavazos et al., 1969). Fluores-cent light microscopy and peroxidase–antiperoxidase immunohistochemistry confirmed that the relaxin was localized in luteal cells of late pregnant pigs (Larkin et al., 1977, 1983). P. Fields and Fields (1985) observed increasing numbers of gold-labeled granules from days 17–25 of pregnancy and maximal numbers of them at day 106 of pregnancy and day 110 of pseudopregnancy in the pig. Relaxin levels in luteal tissue are low during the porcine estrous cycle (Anderson et al., 1973a), though not completely absent as ascertained by the avidin–biotin immunoperoxidase method and an antiserum to porcine relaxin (Ali et al., 1986). An extraluteal source of relaxin includes ovarian follicles from prepuberal gilts and pregnant and nonpregnant sows with normal or polycystic ovaries (Anderson, 1987; Matsumoto and Cham-ley, 1980).

Porcine follicular fluid contains high-molecular-weight forms of relaxin or prorelaxins (e.g., 42,000, 27,500, 19,000, and 10,000 daltons) in addition to a protein of molecular weight approximately 6000 (Kwok *et al.,* 1978; Matsumoto and Chamley, 1980). Porcine follicular cells can produce relaxin *in vitro,* and the preovulatory theca cells have been identified as a source of the hormone (Bryant-Greenwood *et al.,* 1980; Evans *et al.,* 1983). Relaxin has been found in other species including rat, human, cattle, rabbit, cat, guinea pig, and sheep (Anderson, 1987). In the rat, the appearance and disappearance of the granules during pregnancy parallel not only ovarian relaxin bioactivity and immunoactivity but also peripheral serum levels of relaxin immunoactivity (Sherwood *et al.,* 1980; Sherwood and Rutherford, 1981). With the use of a radiolabeled cDNA probe for rat relaxin and histochemical techniques, relaxin mRNA was observed within the corpus luteum of pregnancy but not in other parts of the ovary (Hudson *et al.,* 1981). Relaxin was undetectable in rat uteri, placenta, and metrial glands by biological and immunologic methods (Anderson *et al.,* 1975; Sherwood *et al.,* 1980).

The placenta is a major source of relaxin in the rabbit. This initially was suggested by elevated blood levels of bioactive relaxin in ovariectomized does with their pregnancy maintained by progesterone. Relaxin has been isolated and purified from rabbit placental tissue, and it yielded a molecular weight of approximately 7200, but its amino acid sequence is not yet known (Eldridge and Fields, 1985). At the light microscopic level, immunohistochemical staining with guinea pig antiporcine relaxin serum indicated that relaxin was located in the syncytiotrophoblast of the placental labyrinth at days 23 and 30 but not at day 16 of pregnancy. Examination of the fine structure of the rabbit syncytiotrophoblast revealed membrane-bound granules (150–400 nm in diameter) near the Golgi complexes and in close association with the cell membrane (Eldridge and Fields, 1986). These granules labeled positively for relaxin after treatment with guinea pig antirabbit relaxin serum and goat antiguinea pig immunoglobulin G colloidal gold. These results provide evidence that relaxin is synthesized and secreted by the syncytiotrophoblasts of the rabbit placenta. Furthermore the subcellular site of storage for relaxin is the electron-dense membrane-bound granules in this species (Eldridge and Fields, 1986). In contrast, the rabbit ovary contains little immunohistochemical staining for relaxin.

In cattle, low concentrations of immunoreactive relaxin were found in corpora lutea during late pregnancy (M. Fields *et al.,* 1980). Also during late pregnancy, relaxin levels in peripheral blood are low (<200 pg/ml) a week preceding parturition and increase to peak concentrations (>800 pg/ml) on the day of parturition in beef heifers (Anderson *et al.,* 1982; Musah *et al.,* 1987a). Although there is evidence for relaxin in the bovine corpus luteum, its presence in membrane-bound granules has not been confirmed (M. Fields *et al.,* 1980, 1985). In heifers, endogenous relaxin in peripheral plasma ranged from undetectable levels (<180 pg/ml) to 1 ng/ml (Musah *et al.,* 1987a). Administration of porcine relaxin to late pregnant heifers is associated with marked shifts in progesterone, estrone, and estradiol-17β secretion, reflecting premature parturition induced by relaxin in cattle (Musah *et al.,* 1986). Progesterone plasma levels decreased soon after relaxin treatment, whereas estrone and estradiol-17β concentrations peaked earlier than found in gel-vehicle control heifers. Recent evidence suggests that exogenous relaxin has a dual effect on oxytocin and progesterone. Low levels inhibit oxytocin and maintain progesterone, whereas high levels of relaxin induce spike release and acute depression of progesterone (Musah *et al.,* 1987c). The decrease in progesterone secretion may be complete, thereby leading to parturition, or incomplete and followed by a rebound (Musah *et al.,* 1986, 1987a). The mechanisms by which exogenous porcine relaxin mediates luteolysis in beef heifers are unknown.

Relaxin concentrations in peripheral blood serum are low in hysterectomized gilts on day 6 and similar to those in pregnant animals (Anderson *et al.,* 1983). During the period from days 6 to 114, every-sixth-day bleeding revealed a steady increase in relaxin concentrations from day 6 to peak levels on day 114 in both groups of hysterectomized and pregnant gilts. From days 18 to 114 serum relaxin levels in hysterectomized gilts remain consistently higher than those in pregnant gilts. After parturition relaxin is low and remains low from days 120 to

168 in lactating dams. Maximal plasma concentrations of relaxin occur about 15 hr before parturition, and they are associated with elevated endogenous plasma $PGF_{2\alpha}$ and termination of luteal function (Belt *et al.*, 1971; Sherwood *et al.*, 1978, 1979; Nara and First, 1981a,b). In pigs, whether hysterectomized or pregnant, a prepartum relaxin surge occurs at a precise time a few hours before parturition (Fig. 10; Felder *et al.*, 1986, 1988; Anderson *et al.*, 1983) and is associated with a decline in circulating progesterone, which seems to be initiated by an increase in $PGF_{2\alpha}$ before parturition. Parturition can be induced in this species by dex-amethasone, prostaglandin $F_{2\alpha}$, or prostaglandin E_2 (Coggins and First, 1977). A non-luteolytic dose (50 μg) of $PGF_{2\alpha}$ that is based on maintenance of progesterone blood levels in late pregnant gilts causes peak relaxin concentrations in peripheral blood within 10 min (Nara *et al.*, 1982). Thus, $PGF_{2\alpha}$ can cause relaxin release from porcine corpora lutea independent of a luteolytic effect. Whether $PGF_{2\alpha}$ acts through separate mechanisms for relaxin release and luteolysis or whether these two events may be affected in a similar manner in the luteal cell has not been established.

Parturition can be delayed by maintaining high endogenous blood levels of progesterone with injected progesterone or endogenous progesterone from induced corpora lutea (Coggins *et al.*, 1977). Although injected progesterone delays parturition, the prepartum relaxin surge occurs at the normal time (day 113) (Sherwood *et al.*, 1978). Thus, the surge in relaxin levels in pigs experiencing progesterone-delayed parturition is not sufficient by itself to initiate parturition within 24 hr. Furthermore, relaxin blood levels are markedly increased approx-imately 1 hr after administration of a luteolytic dosage (5 mg) of $PGF_{2\alpha}$ (Sherwood *et al.*, 1979). The prepartum surge in plasma relaxin occurs coincident with an increase in $PGF_{2\alpha}$ and a decrease in progesterone when parturition is advanced, is delayed, or occurs at the expected time (Nara and First, 1981b). Prevention of prostaglandin synthesis by indomethacin prevents release of relaxin as well as luteolysis, whereas simultaneous treatment with $PGF_{2\alpha}$ induces luteolysis and relaxin release (Nara and First, 1981a,b). Although indomethacin prevents relaxin release, after such drug treatment a prepartum relaxin surge occurs just preceding the delayed parturition (Sherwood *et al.*, 1979). These results were interpreted to indicate that release of relaxin depends on and is a result of luteolysis.

5.3. Oxytocin

Oxytocin is a neuropeptide as well as a luteal peptide. As a neuropeptide, it is produced by cells of the supraoptic and paraventricular nuclei of the hypothalamus and is transported by axonal flow to be stored at axon terminals in the pars nervosa. Oxytocin is also produced by luteal cells, and this peptide is immunologically indistinguishable from neural oxytocin. Luteal oxytocin increases uterine smooth muscle contraction, stimulates strips of uterine tissue *in vitro,* and increases intramammary pressure in an almost similar manner to pituitary oxytocin (Wathes and Swann, 1982; Wathes *et al.*, 1983b). Bovine, human, and ovine oxytocin extracts are eluded by Sephadex G50 and reverse-phase HPLC at the same position as pituitary oxytocin (Stormshak *et al.*, 1987). The first conclusive demonstration of the presence of oxytocin in luteal tissue can be attributed to the detection of a mRNA for oxytocin-neurophysin prohormone, subsequent cloning of the cDNA, and sequencing (Ivell and Richter, 1984; Ivell *et al.*, 1985). It is now clear that the corpus luteum of the cow (P. Fields *et al.*, 1983; Wathes *et al.*, 1983a,b; Abdelgadir *et al.*, 1986), ewe (Wathes and Swann, 1982), woman (Wathes *et al.*, 1982; Khan-Dawood and Dawood, 1983), rhesus monkey (Khan-Dawood *et al.*, 1984), and rabbit (Khan-Dawood and Dawood, 1986) contain oxytocin. In the cow, there is evidence that oxytocin-neurophysins are associated with luteal granules (M. Fields and Fields, 1986; Wathes *et al.*, 1983a; Schams *et al.*, 1983; Ivell *et al.*, 1985).

Armstrong and Hansel (1959) first demonstrated that administration of pharmacological doses of oxytocin could indeed shorten the estrous cycle in heifers. This observation indicated for the first time that oxytocin had reproductive functions in addition to those associated with

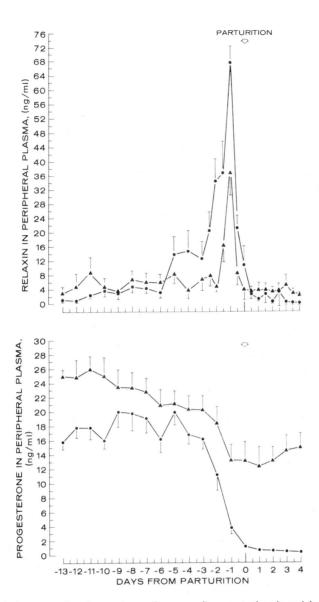

Figure 10. Relaxin (upper panel) and progesterone (lower panel) concentrations in peripheral plasma during pregnancy and lactation (●; $n = 7$) compared with those in unmated gilts hysterectomized (▲; $n = 9$) on day 6 after estrus. Day 0 is the day of parturition (114 days) in pregnant animals and the day after peak relaxin levels (113 days) in hysterectomized and pregnant animals. Relaxin in peripheral plasma from 0800 and 2000 hr bleedings are included from days 110 to 120. Values are the mean ± S.E. From Felder *et al.* (1986).

lactation and expulsive contractions. The effect of oxytocin in cyclic heifers was shown to be dependent on a functional uterus or factor since hysterectomy obliterated the oxytocin-induced shortening of the estrous cycle (Dobowolski, 1973; Hatjiminaoglou *et al.*, 1979). Subsequent work showed that uterine oxytocin receptor levels increased at the end of the estrous cycle (Roberts *et al.*, 1976) and that oxytocin could stimulate uterine secretion of the luteolysin $PGF_{2\alpha}$ (Mitchell *et al.*, 1975; Roberts *et al.*, 1976). In the cow, both oxytocin and $PGF_{2\alpha}$ are luteolytic, but oxytocin-induced luteolysis is thought to be mediated by the release of PGs (Summerlee *et al.*, 1984; Mitchell *et al.*, 1975). In sheep, oxytocin similarly stimulates endometrial prostaglandin secretion (Roberts *et al.*, 1976) and is itself stimulated by $PGF_{2\alpha}$

(Flint and Sheldrick, 1986). Based on these observations, the current hypothesis is that $PGF_{2\alpha}$, relaxin, and oxytocin may exert a positive feedback effect on each other (Musah *et al.*, 1986, 1987a). Relaxin effects the central release of oxytocin in rats (Summerlee *et al.*, 1984). Peripheral blood levels of oxytocin in response to exogenous relaxin in late pregnant beef heifers show a biphasic release of oxytocin. Low levels of relaxin during late pregnancy inhibit oxytocin release, but a surge in pharmacological doses of relaxin tends to stimulate oxytocin release (Musah *et al.*, 1987b). It is, however, not known whether both responses are mediated via neurohypophyseal or luteal release of oxytocin or both.

Oxytocin-neurophysin is released synchronously with $PGF_{2\alpha}$ during luteal regression. In the cow and ewe oxytocin is detectable in the follicular fluid and granulosa cells during or shortly after the LH surge (Kruip *et al.*, 1985; Wathes *et al.*, 1986), and luteal oxytocin-specific mRNA transcription increases and is maximal by ovulation and decreases thereafter (Ivell *et al.*, 1985). Oxytocin receptor population more than concentration determines the biological action. For instance, the myometrium and mammary gland, which are sensitive to oxytocin during labor, are relatively insensitive at other times. Uterine receptors for oxytocin in pregnant rats remain low throughout pregnancy and increase markedly only at the onset of parturition. The paucity of oxytocin receptors before term may explain the inability of oxytocin to induce parturition more than a few hours before delivery.

5.4. Other Hormones Affecting Uterine Ovarian Function: ACTH

The hypothalamic–pituitary axis of mammals is activated during pregnancy and parturition. For most of pregnancy, circulating levels of immunoreactive corticotropin-releasing factor (irCRF) and immunoreactive adrenocroticotropic hormone (irACTH) and cortisol concentrations are elevated; they then increase further during prepartum labor before decreasing precipitously after parturition (Goland *et al.*, 1986). Earlier evidence suggests that the placenta contains biologically active CRF and ACTH (Shibasaki *et al.*, 1982). Further evidence showed that irCRF is located in the cytotrophoblast of the human placenta (Petraglia *et al.*, 1987). With use of a monolayer of primary culture of human placental cells, it was shown that CRF stimulates secretion of peptides containing the ACTH sequence in a dose-dependent manner, as it does in the pituitary (Petraglia *et al.*, 1987). This effect is reversed by CRF antagonist and mimicked by dibutyryl cAMP and forskolin. Glucocorticoids that suppress pituitary ACTH have no effect on irACTH release by the placenta (Petraglia *et al.*, 1987). Furthermore, oxytocin and prostaglandin stimulate irACTH and irCRF secretion from cultured human placental cells (Petraglia *et al.*, 1987). Prostaglandins participate in the regulation of placental hormonogenesis, and those produced by the placenta increase adenylate cyclase activity and intracellular concentration of cAMP in the human placenta. Placental ACTH has both a paracrine activity by locally stimulating placental progesterone and estradiol production (Barnea *et al.*, 1986) and an endocrine effect by supplementing maternal and fetal adrenal steroidogenesis (Osathanondh and Tulchinsky, 1980).

6. Mechanisms of Uterine–Ovarian Interactions in Regulating Ovarian Function

6.1. Morphology and Function of Placental and Luteal Cells

6.1.1. Placental Morphology and Function

The organization of fetal membranes, i.e., the relationships among the yolk sac, amnion, chorion, and allantois, as well as the degree of trophoblastic invasion of maternal uterine tissue determine placental type and form the basis for placental classification. The many functions of the placenta include the transport of water and nutrients and removal of waste products, exchange of gases, and removal of secretory products. Myometrial, endometrial, allantoic, chorionic, and amniotic cells are important in the synthesis and secretion of hormones that regulate ovarian function. These tissues have been shown to produce steroids and peptide hormones (Power and Challis, 1983; Olson *et al.*, 1984; Petraglia *et al.*, 1987). Fatty acids are an essential requirement of the placenta for the synthesis of phospholipids, sphingolipids, and triacylglycerol. These lipids are essential for cellular structure, energy storage, membrane biosynthesis, signal transduction, and biosynthesis of secretory products such as steroid hormones. In order to meet the fatty acid requirements, either fetal membranes synthesize fatty acids or they are derived from the dam (Jones and Rolph, 1985). Placental synthesis of fatty acid is poor (Hummel *et al.*, 1976); thus, the maternal contribution is very significant. It is possible for placental lipoprotein lipase on the maternal side to release fatty acids from lipoprotein-carried triacylglycerol in the guinea pig (Thomas *et al.*, 1984), thus providing a direct mechanism for obtaining fatty acid adjacent to the fetal membranes without having to go through maternal and fetal circulations. In the rabbit the placenta takes up serum phospholipids, but these compounds have not been shown to leave the placenta and enter the fetus. Trophoblastic cells also take up LDL by a receptor-mediated endocytosis; the LDL provides the cholesterol for intracellular progesterone synthesis (Winkel *et al.*, 1980).

There is a tissue specificity of steroid metabolic and enzymatic activity in intrauterine tissue and fetal membranes. Power and Challis (1983) showed earlier that ovine fetal membranes could produce progesterone from pregnenolone and that this production could be inhibited by steroids such as estrone and estradiol. Fetal membranes also are a major source of prostaglandin biosynthesis (Olson *et al.*, 1984). The subcellular fractions of the endometrium and myometrium in some species have been shown to contain the activities of 5α-reductase, 20α-hydroxysteroid dehydrogenase, estrone sulfatase, and 17β-hydrogenase (Dwyer and Robertson, 1980). Consequently, these tissues are completely equipped with the enzymatic requirements for steroid biosynthesis from a host of intermediate steroids.

Ovine intrauterine tissue and fetal membranes can produce progesterone from 20α-dihydroprogesterone. The activity of 3β-HSD for progesterone production, however, is predominant in the chorion and the endometrium (Power and Challis, 1987). As a substrate, 20α-dihydroprogesterone is better than pregnenolone for progesterone production by the fetal membranes and intrauterine tissue of women and sheep *in vitro* (Power and Challis, 1986). Similarly, progesterone can be metabolized to 20α-dihydroprogesterone in the human and ovine chorion (Marcus *et al.*, 1979; Power and Challis; 1986), and such conversion of progesterone to dihydroprogesterone is inhibited by excess dihydroprogesterone (Power and Challis, 1986). Dispersed chorion and decidual cells from women after spontaneous induction of labor have shown an increased capability for converting estrone sulfate to estrone (Mitchell *et al.*, 1984). Earlier studies also support the presence of the enzymes estrone sulfatase and sulfatransferase in the ovine endometrium (Dwyer and Robertson, 1980).

6.1.2. Luteal Cell Morphology and Function

Lemon and Loir (1977), Ursely and Leymarie (1979), and Koos and Hansel (1981) all demonstrated the existence of morphological size classes in the luteal cells of the pig, cow, and sheep after dispersing the corpus luteum. The different luteal cells were classified according to size. Cells greater than 25 μm in diameter are called large luteal cells, and those cells with a diameter of 10–20 μm are designated as small luteal cells. There is, however, another class of small luteal cells; these are generally less than 10 μm in diameter and are nonsteroidogenic. The steroidogenic small luteal cells possess acentric, cup-shaped nuclei with heterochromatin lining their nuclear envelope. Small luteal cells also have both rough and smooth endoplasmic reticulum and pleomorphic mitochondria that contain tubular cristae (Hansel and Dowd, 1986). In small luteal cells the tubular cristae of the pleomorphic mitochondria are arranged in an arc opposite the nucleus and contain a central region, usually with a pair of centrioles and large Golgi complex (Hansel and Dowd, 1986). Large luteal cells have round central nuclei with dispersed chromatin and a distinct nucleolus, two types of mitochondria, extensive smooth endoplasmic reticulum, a highly convoluted cell surface, and small (0.3-μm) electron-dense granules (Hansel and Dowd, 1986).

Using highly specific labeled monoclonal antibodies to theca and granulosa cell surface antigens, Alila and Hansel (1984) provided new insight into the origin of the large and small luteal cells: large cells of early cyclic CL expressed granulosa cell antigens, whereas small cells express thecal cell antigens. However, they showed that small cells (theca-derived) appear to develop into large cells as the CL ages. At 100 days of gestation, no granulosa-derived large cells were present in the bovine CL (Alila and Hansel, 1984).

Since small and large cells are derived from different cellular components, these cell types would be expected to be controlled by different mechanisms. Additionally, since large cells of the early luteal phase are different developmentally from large cells at later stages, the mechanism of luteal regulation of large cells will change with age. Large luteal cells produce more progesterone, whereas small luteal cells are six times more sensitive to LH (Koos and Hansel, 1981). It is not surprising that the small ovine luteal cells also contain most of the receptors for LH (33,260/small cells versus 3074/large cells) whereas the large cells contain most of the $PGF_{2\alpha}$ receptors (8143/large versus 2115/small) (Fitz et al., 1982).

The large luteal cells contribute the major progesterone, whereas the smaller cells secrete small quantities of progesterone in the absence of gonadotropic stimulation. Culture of both large and small luteal cells results in higher progesterone production than produced by each individual cell subpopulation (Lemon and Mauleon, 1982). Furthermore, superfusate from the small cell type caused increased P_4 production by the large cell types. It has also been shown recently by reverse hemolytic plaque assay for porcine relaxin that 50% of the large porcine luteal cells were capable of secreting relaxin, whereas the small luteal cells died (Taylor et al., 1988). This finding is consistent with the cellular organization of the various cell types (Hansel and Dowd, 1986). Current research findings indicate that the small theca-derived luteal cells respond to elements of the cAMP system (LH) and that elevated intracellular Ca^{2+} inhibits LH-stimulated progesterone synthesis (Hansel and Dowd, 1986). An influx of extracellular Ca^{2+} inhibits the activation of adenylate cyclase of rat luteal cells (Gore and Behrman, 1984).

6.2. Cellular and Biochemical Basis of Uterine–Ovarian Interactions

If estrous cyclicity is to be maintained, regulatory processes must exist that ensure that luteal function is maintained for an exact period and then ends. During both the estrous cycle and pregnancy, maintenance and termination of luteal function are both essential aspects for regulating reproductive cycles. Luteinizing hormone is the main luteotropic hormone in the cow and ewe (Bazer and First, 1983). Porcine corpora lutea prior to day 14 are autonomous and require only basal LH support until day 40–50 of gestation, after which prolactin assumes an essential role in CL maintenance. Recently the possible luteotropic role of prolactin in the pig has been enhanced by evidence provided from hysterectomy, hypophysectomy, and hypophyseal stalk transection (Felder et al., 1988; Li et al., 1987, 1988).

The mechanism by which hormones induce cellular changes are as diverse as the hormones themselves. Some physiological functions may be affected by two or more distinct hormones acting through very different mechanisms to accomplish the same response. In many cases, a hormone may affect several physiological properties differently and by very different mechanisms. In all cases of hormone interaction, the physiological changes are mediated by means of interactions between the hormone and highly specific receptors. Steroid hormones generally alter the cellular processes they affect mainly through changes in gene expression and induction of synthesis of new gene products. Effects of LH are manifested on luteal steroidogenic cells by increasing the action of adenylate cyclase and cyclic adenosine mono-phosphate (cAMP) (Marsh, 1971, 1976; Marsh and LeMarie, 1974). Gonadotropic-releasing hormone (GnRH) is thus luteotropic by virtue of its ability to induce the release of LH.

Mechanisms of LH-induced luteal stimulation may be summarized as follows: (1) LH binds to its plasma-membrane-bound receptors; (2) adenylate cyclase is activated with the result of formation of cAMP; (3) specific protein kinase activation occurs, followed by (4) phosphorylation of steroidogenic enzymes and protein synthesis; (5) internalization of portions of LH–receptor complex and its degradation; (6) LH receptor recycling via secretory granules, which are then incorporated into plasma membranes, thereby returning the LH receptors to their usual concentration (Marsh and LeMarie, 1974).

The whole concept of luteal regulation with LH as the central dogma has been completely reworked. Much has been learned about the role of other hormones in luteal integrity. The current hypotheses have been elaborately reviewed by Hansel and Dowd (1986). The central theme of luteal function heretofore included three key tenets; (1) LH is the main luteotropic factor of pituitary origin; (2) the uterus in most species plays a crucial role in luteolysis (Brunner et al., 1969; Anderson et al., 1969; Anderson, 1973; Musah et al., 1984); (3) prostaglandins, especially $PGF_{2\alpha}$ of uterine origin as the main luteolysin, reach the ipsilateral CL-bearing ovary by a venous–arterial transfer mechanism (Hansel et al., 1973), especially in the ewe (McCracken et al., 1984).

Luteal regulation, however, has proved to be more complex. Just as the hormones, neurotransmitters, and other biologically active compounds that affect uterine ovarian func-tions are numerous and diverse, so are the mechanisms by which these responses are mediated. In one instance, signal transduction is accomplished by stimulation of adenylate cyclase. Examples include norepinephrine, LH, relaxin, ACTH, PTH, and prostaglandin. This mecha-nism involves a hormone-dependent, receptor-induced dissociation of an oligomeric (i.e., three-subunit) protein, GTP-binding or "N" protein, complex into a component that in the presence of GTP binds to and activates adenylate cyclase (Cuatrecasas, 1986). On hydrolysis and thus removal of the GTP, the α subunit dissociates spontaneously, and the enzyme activity returns to basal value.

Phospholipids have been shown to be important in intracellular messenger systems in-volved in the action of hormones and neurotransmitters (Farese, 1983; Cuatrecasas, 1986). Hansel and Dowd (1986) in particular have described the emerging role of Ca^{2+}–poly-phosphoinositol–protein kinase C second messenger system in addition to the LH–cAMP system as a mechanism involved in regulating progesterone biosynthesis. In this system, signal transduction occurs by two routes: protein kinase C activation and Ca^{2+} mobilization (Nishizuka, 1984). Substrate phosphorylation by protein kinase C, an enzyme that requires calcium and phospholipid, is activated by diacylglycerol or phorbol esters and phosphorylates serine and threonine residues (Kawahara et al., 1980; Takai et al., 1981). In this system, stimuli or hormone–receptor complexes activate rapidly (within seconds). A phos-phodiesterase or phospholipase C is specific for phosphatidylinositol-4,5-bisphosphate (Ber-ridge and Irvine, 1984; Nishizuka, 1984). There is a resultant production of diacylglycerol, which can stimulate protein kinase C and then convert to phosphatidic acid. Phosphatidic acid may on its own stimulate phospholipases of the A variety. The other product of phos-phodiesterase hydrolysis is inositol trisphosphate (IP_3), which is an extremely potent and selective agent for the release of calcium from the endoplasmic reticulum; IP_3 is a second messenger in physiological responses that require mobilization of calcium and reactivation of calcium-dependent processes (Berridge and Irvine, 1984).

The Ca^{2+}–polyphosphoinositol–protein kinase C second messenger system has been demonstrated to operate in both pigs and cattle to modulate progesterone secretion (Clark et al., 1983; Davis and Clark 1983; Noland and Dimino, 1986). Bovine placental cells from both fetal cotyledon and maternal caruncles secrete progesterone by a calcium-dependent and cyclic–nucleotide-independent mechanism (Shemesh et al., 1984). Veldhuis et al. (1987)

have also reported that in bovine luteal cells, maitotoxin, a putative activator of calcium channels, transiently increases luteal calcium content without altering cAMP generation and elicits concomitant release of both a steroid (progesterone) and a nonsteroid (relaxin). Protein kinase C may be activated in ovarian tissue by a number of processes: intracellular production of diacylglycerol, phorbol esters, and calcium-activated neutral proteases (Kishimoto *et al.*, 1980). Protein kinase C also affects the synthesis of progesterone in cultured dispersed bovine luteal cells (Hansel and Dowd, 1986; Brunsuig *et al.*, 1986). Further experimentation has revealed that steroidogenesis in the small theca-derived cells is controlled primarily by cAMP-dependent mechanisms and that elevated intracellular Ca^{2+} inhibits progesterone synthesis in these cells (Hansel and Dowd, 1986).

ACKNOWLEDGMENTS. This work was supported in part by the U.S. Department of Agriculture, ARS, CSRS, OGPS Competitive Grants 85-CRCR-1-1862 and 86-CRCR-1-2130. Journal Paper No. J-13096 of the Iowa Agriculture and Home Economics Experiment Station, Ames, Projects No. 2444, 2754, and 2797.

7. *References*

Abdelgadir, S. E., Swanson, L. V., Oldfield, J. E., and Stormshak, F., 1986, *In vitro* release of oxytocin from bovine corpora lutea by prostaglandin $F_{2\alpha}$, *Biol. Reprod.* **37**:550–555.

Adair, V., Stromer, M. H., and Anderson, L. L., 1988, Progesterone secretion and mitochondrial size of aging porcine corpora lutea, *Anat. Rec.* (in press).

Alberga, A., and Baulieu, E., 1968, Binding of estradiol in castrated rat endometrium *in vivo* and *in vitro*, *Mol. Pharmacol.* **4**:311–323.

Ali, M. S., McMurtry, J. P., Bagnell, C. A., and Bryant-Greenwood, G. D., 1986, Immunocytochemical localization of relaxin in corpora lutea of sows throughout the estrous cycle, *Biol. Reprod.* **34**:139–143.

Alila, H. W., and Hansel, W., 1984, Origin of different cell types in the bovine corpus luteum as characterized by specific monoclonal antibodies, *Biol. Reprod.* **31**:1015–1025.

Amenomori, U., Chen, C. L., and Meites, J., 1970, Serum prolactin levels in rats during different reproductive states, *Endocrinology* **86**:506–510.

Anderson, L. L., 1968, Hypophysial influences on ovarian function in the cow, *VI Cong. Int. Reprod. Anim. Insem. Artif. Paris* **1**:645–647.

Anderson, L. L., 1973, Effects of hysterectomy and other factors on luteal function, in: *Handbook of Physiology, Endocrinology,* Section 7, Vol. 2, Part 2 (R. O. Greep and E. B. Astwood, ed.), American Physiological Society, Washington, pp. 69–86.

Anderson, L. L., 1987, Regulation of relaxin secretion and its role in pregnancy, *Adv. Exp. Med. Biol.* **219**:421–466.

Anderson, L. L., Melampy, R. M., and Chen, C. L., 1967a, Uterus and duration of pseudopregnancy in the rat, *Arch. Anat. Microsc. Morphol. Exp.* **56**:373–384.

Anderson, L. L., Dyck, G. W., Mori, H., Hendricks, D. M., and Melampy, R. M., 1967b, Ovarian function in pigs following hypophysial stalk transection or hypophysectomy, *Am. J. Physiol.* **212**:1188–1194.

Anderson, L. L., Bland, K. P., and Melampy, R. M., 1969, Comparative aspects of uterine-luteal relationships, *Recent Prog. Horm. Res.* **25**:57–104.

Anderson, L. L., Bast, J. D., and Melampy, R. M., 1973a, Relaxin in ovarian tissue during different reproductive stages in the rat, *J. Endocrinol.* **59**:371–372.

Anderson, L. L., Ford, J. J., Melampy, R. M., and Cox, D. F., 1973b, Relaxin in porcine corpora lutea during pregnancy and after hysterectomy. *Am. J. Physiol.* **225**:1215–1219.

Anderson, L. L., Perezgrovas, R., O'Byrne, E. M., and Steinetz, B. G., 1982, Biological actions of relaxin in pigs and beef cattle, *Ann. N.Y. Acad. Sci.* **380**:131–150.

Anderson, L. L., Adair, V., Stromer, M. H., and McDonald, W. G., 1983, Relaxin production and release after hysterectomy in the pig, *Endocrinology* **113**:677–686.

Anderson, M. L., Long, J. A., and Hayashida, T., 1975, Immunofluorescence studies on the localization of relaxin in the corpus luteum of the pregnant rat, *Biol. Reprod.* **13**:499–504.

Armstrong, D. T., and Hansel, W. J., 1959, Alteration of the bovine estrous cycle with oxytocin, *J. Dairy Sci.* **42**:533–542.

Armstrong, D. T., and Flint, A. P. F., 1973, Isolation and properties of cholesterol ester-storage granules from ovarian tissues, *Biochem. J.* **134**:399–406.

Astwood, E. B., and Greep, R. O., 1938, A corpus luteum-stimulating substance in the rat placenta, *Proc. Soc. Exp. Biol. Med.* **38**:713–716.

Atkinson, L. E., Hotchkiss, J., Fritz, G. R., Surve, A. H., Neill, J. D., and Knobil, E., 1975, Circulating levels of steroids and chorionic gonadotropin during pregnancy in the rhesus monkey, with special attention to the rescue of the corpus luteum in early pregnancy, *Biol. Reprod.* **12**:335–345.

Ayalon, N., and Shemesh, M., 1974, Pro-oestrous surge in plasma progesterone in the cow, *J. Reprod. Fertil.* **36**:239–243.

Baird, D. T., and Land, R. B., 1973, Division of the uterine vein and function of the adjacent ovary in the ewe, *J. Reprod. Fertil.* **33**:393–397.

Baird, D. T., Collett, R. A., Fraser, I. S., Kelly, R. W., Land, R. B., and Wheeler, A. G., 1973, Progesterone secretion from the ovary in the ewe following infusion of uterine venous plasma, *J. Reprod. Fertil.* **35**:13–22.

Baird, D. T., Baker, T. G., McNatty, K. P., and Neal, P., 1975, Relationship between the secretion of the corpus luteum and the length of the follicular phase of the ovarian cycle, *J. Reprod. Fertil.* **45**:611–619.

Baldwin, D. M., and Stabenfeldt, G. H., 1975, Endocrine changes in the pig during late pregnancy, parturition, and lactation, *Biol. Reprod.* **12**:508–515.

Balogh, K., 1964, A histochemical method for the demonstration of 20α-hydroxysteroid dehydrogenase activity in rat ovaries, *J. Histochem. Cytochem.* **12**:670–673.

Banks, E., 1964, Some aspects of sexual behavior in domestic sheep. *Ovis aries, Behaviour* 23:249–279.

Barcikowski, B., Carlson, J. C., Wilson, L., and McCracken, J. A., 1974, The effect of endogenous and exogenous estradiol-17β on the release of prostaglandin $F_{2\alpha}$ from the ovine uterus, *Endocrinology* **95**:1340–1349.

Barnea, E. R., Lavy, G., Fakih, H., and DeCherney, A. H., 1986, The role of ACTH in placental steroidogenesis, *Placenta* **7**:307–313.

Barrow, M. V., 1970, Dissociation of phenomena associated with birth in Long–Evans rats, *Biol. Neonate* **15**:61–64.

Barton, M. D., Killam, A. P., and Meschia, G., 1974, Response of ovine uterine blood flow to epinephrine and norepinephrine, *Proc. Soc. Exp. Biol. Med.* **145**:996–1003.

Bartosik, D., and Szarowski, D. H., 1973, Progravid phase of the rat reproductive cycle: Day to day changes in peripheral plasma progestin concentrations, *Endocrinology* **92**:949–952.

Bartosik, D., Zaccheo, V., Taylor, R. J., and Azarowski, D. H., 1974, Progravid phase of the rat reproductive cycle: Daily changes in the *in vitro* RNA synthesis and progestin secretion by isolated corpora lutea, *Endocrinology* **94**:45–48.

Bast, J. D., and Melampy, R. M., 1972, Luteinizing hormone, prolactin and ovarian 20α-hydroxysteroid dehydrogenase levels during pregnancy and pseudopregnancy in the rat, *Endocrinology* **91**:1499–1505.

Basuray, R., and Gibori, G., 1980, Luteotropic action of the decidual tissue in the pregnant rat, *Biol. Reprod.* **23**:507–512.

Baulieu, E. E., Wira, C. R., Milgrom, E., and Raynaud-Jammet, C., 1972, Ribonucleic acid synthesis and oestradiol action in the uterus, in: *Gene Transcription in Reproductive Tissue* (E. Diczfalusy, ed.), Karolinska Institutet, Stockholm, pp. 396–419.

Bazer, F. W., and First, N. L., 1983, Pregnancy and parturition, *J. Anim. Sci.* **57**(Suppl. 2):425–460.

Bazer, F. W., Geisert, R. D., Thatcher, W. W., and Roberts, R. M., 1982, The establishment and maintenance of pregnancy, in: *Control of Pig Reproduction* (J. A. Cole and G. R. Foxcroft, ed.), Butterworth Scientific, London, pp. 227–252.

Bazer, F. W., Vallet, J. L., Roberts, R. M., Sharp, D. C., and Thatcher, W. W., 1986, Role of conceptus secretory products in establishment of pregnancy, *J. Reprod. Fertil.* **76**:841–850.

Belt, W. D., Cavazos, L. F., Anderson, L. L., and Kraeling, R. R., 1970, Fine structure and progesterone levels in the corpus luteum of the pig during pregnancy and after hysterectomy, *Biol. Reprod.* **2**:98–113.

Belt, W. D., Anderson, L. L., Cavazos, L. F., and Melampy, R. M., 1971, Cytoplasmic granules and relaxin levels in porcine corpora lutea, *Endocrinology* **89**:1–10.

Berridge, M. J., and Irvine, R. F., 1984, Inositol triphosphate, a novel second messenger in cellular signal transduction, *Nature* **312**:315–321.

Bill, C. H., and Keyes, P. L., 1983, 17β-Estradiol maintains normal function of corpora lutea throughout pseudopregnancy in hypophysectomized rabbits, *Biol. Reprod.* **28**:608–617.

Biro, J., 1980, Regulation of pituitary milieu and metabolism in female rats, *J. Steroid Biochem.* **12**:351–354.

Biro, J. C., Ritzen, M. E., and Eneroth, P., 1987, Effects of hysterectomy and uterine extracts on the gonadotropic hormones and weight of endocrine organs of female rats, *Exp. Clin. Endocrinol.* **84**:23–30.

Bland, K. P., Horton, E. W., and Poyser, N. L., 1971, Levels of prostaglandin $F_{2\alpha}$ in the uterine venous blood of sheep during the oestrous cycle, *Life Sci.* **10**:509–517.

Boving, B. G., 1961, Anatomical analyses of rabbit trophoblast invasion, *Contrib. Embryol. Carnegie Inst. Wash.* **37:**925–926.

Browning, J. Y., Keyes, P. L., and Wolf, R. C., 1980, Comparison of serum progesterone, 20α-dihydroprogesterone, and estradiol-17β in pregnant and pseudopregnant rabbits: Evidence for postimplantation recognition of pregnancy, *Biol. Reprod.* **23:**1014–1019.

Brunner, M. A., Donaldson, L. E., and Hansel, W., 1969, Exogenous hormones and luteal function in hysterectomized and intact heifers, *J. Dairy Sci.* **52:**1849–1854.

Brunsuig, B., Mukhopadhyay, A. K., Budnik, L. T., Bohnet, H. G., and Leidenberger, F. A., 1986, Phorbol ester stimulates progesterone production by isolated bovine luteal cells, *Endocrinology* **118:**743–749.

Bryant-Greenwood, G. D., Jeffrey, R., Ralph, M. M., and Seamark, R. F., 1980, Relaxin production by the porcine ovarian graafian follicle *in vitro*, *Biol. Reprod.* **23:**792–800.

Butcher, R. L., Fugo, N. W., and Collins, W. E., 1972, Semicircadian rhythm in plasma levels of prolactin during early gestation in the rat, *Endocrinology* **90:**1125–1127.

Butterstein, G. M., and Hirst, J. A., 1977, Serum progesterone and fetal morphology following ovariectomy and adrenalectomy in the pregnant rat, *Biol. Reprod.* **16:**654–660.

Carlson, J. C., and Gole, J. W. D., 1978, CL regression in the pseudopregnant rabbit and the effects of treatment with prostaglandin F$_{2\alpha}$ and arachidonic acid, *J. Reprod. Fertil.* **53:**381–387.

Castracane, V. D., and Rothchild, I., 1976, Luteotropic action of decidual tissue in the rat: Comparison of jugular and uterine vein progesterone level and the effect of ligation of the utero–ovarian connections, *Biol. Reprod.* **15:**497–503.

Caton, D., Abrams, R. M., Clapp, J. R., and Barron, D. H., 1974, The effect of exogenous progesterone on the rate of blood flow of the uterus of ovariectomized sheep, *Q. J. Exp. Physiol.* **59:**225–231.

Cavazos, L. F., Anderson, L. L., Belt, W. D.; Hendricks, D. M., Kraeling, R. R., and Malempy, R. M., 1969, Fine structure and progesterone levels in the corpus luteum of the pig during the estrous cycle, *Biol. Reprod.* **1:**83–106.

Challis, J. R. G., 1971, Sharp increase in free circulating oestrogens immediately before parturition in sheep, *Nature* **229:**208.

Challis, J. R. G., Heap, R. B., and Illingworth, D. V., 1971, Concentrations of oestrogen and progesterone in the plasma of nonpregnant, pregnant, and lactating guinea pigs, *J. Endocrinol.* **51:**333–345.

Challis, J. R. G., Davies, I. J., and Ryan, K. J., 1973, The concentration of progesterone, estrone, and estradiol-17β in the plasma of pregnant rabbits, *Endocrinology* **93:**971–976.

Challis, J. R. G., Davies, I. J., and Ryan, K. J., 1974, The concentration of progesterone, estrone, and estradiol-17β in the myometrium of the pregnant rabbit and their relationship to the peripheral plasma steroid concentrations, *Endocrinology* **95:**160–164.

Chamley, W. A., Buckmaster, J. M., Cerini, M. E., Cumming, I. A., Goding, J. R., Obst, J. M., Williams, A., and Winfield, C., 1973, Changes in the levels of progesterone, corticosteroids, estrone, estradiol-17β, luteinizing hormone, and prolactin in the peripheral plasma of the ewe during late pregnancy and at parturition, *Biol. Reprod.* **9:**30–35.

Clark, B. F., 1971, The effects of oestrogen and progesterone on uterine cell division and epithelial morphology in spayed, adrenalectomized rats, *J. Endocrinol.* **50:**527–528.

Clark, K. E., Ryan, M. J., and Brody, M. J., 1973, Effects of prostaglandins E$_1$ and F$_{2\alpha}$ on uterine hemodynamics and motility, *Adv. Biosci.* **9:**779–782.

Clark, M. R., Davis, T. S., and Lemaire, W. T., 1983, Calcium- and lipid-dependent protein phosphosylation in the human ovary, *J. Clin. Endocrinol. Metab.* **57:**872–874.

Coggins, E. G., and First, N. L., 1977, Effect of dexamethasone, methallibure and fetal decapitation on porcine gestation, *J. Anim. Sci.* **44:**1041–1049.

Coggins, E. G., Van Horn, D., and First, N. L., 1977, Influence of prostaglandin F$_{2\alpha}$, dexamethasone, progesterone and induced CL on porcine parturition, *J. Anim. Sci.* **46:**754–762.

Cohen, A., 1973, Plasma corticosterone concentration in the foetal rat, *Horm. Metab. Res.* **5:**66.

Csapo, A., 1969, The four direct regulatory factors of myometrial function, in: *Progesterone: Its Regulatory Effect on the Myometrium* (G. E. W. Wolstenholme and J. A. Knight, ed.), Churchill, London, pp. 13–55.

Csapo, A., and Wiest, W., 1969, An examination of the quantitative relationship between progesterone and the maintenance of pregnancy, *Endocrinology* **85:**735–746.

Cuatrecasas, P., 1986, Hormone receptors, membrane phospholipids, and protein kinases, *Harvey Lect.* **80:**89–128.

Cunningham, N. F., Symons, A. M., and Saba, N., 1975, Levels of progesterone, LH and FSH in the plasma of sheep during the oestrous cycle, *J. Reprod. Fertil.* **45:**177–180.

Czaja, J. A., Robinson, J. A., Eisele, S. G., Scheffler, G., and Goy, R. W., 1977, Relationship between sexual skin colour of female rhesus monkeys and midcycle plasma levels of oestradiol and progesterone, *J. Reprod. Fertil.* **49:**147–150.

Davies, I. J., and Ryan, K. J., 1973, Modulation of progesterone concentration in the myometrium of the pregnant rat by changes in cytoplasmic receptor protein activity, *Endocrinology* **92**:394–401.

Davies, I. J., Challis, J. R. G., and Ryan, K. J., 1974, Progesterone receptors in the myometrium of pregnant rabbits, *Endocrinology* **95**:165–173.

Davis, J. S. and Clark, M. R., 1983, Activation of protein kinase in bovine corpus luteum by phosphoslipid and calcium, *Biochem. J.* **214**:569–574.

Deane, H. W., Hay, M. F., Moor, R. M., Rowson, L. E. A., and Short, R. V., 1966, The corpus luteum of the sheep: Relationship between morphology and function during the oestrous cycle, *Acta Endocrinol. (Kbh.)* **51**:245–263.

Deanesly, R., 1973, Termination of early pregnancy in rats after ovariectomy is due to immediate collapse of the progesterone-dependent decidua, *J. Reprod. Fertil.* **35**:183–186.

deDuve, C., 1975, Exploring cells with a centrifuge, *Science* **189**:186–194.

de Duve, C., Wattiaux, R., and Baudhuin, P., 1962, Distribution of enzymes between subcellular fractions in animal tissues, *Adv. Enzymol.* **24**:291–358.

de Greef, W. J., and Zeilmaker, G. H., 1974, Blood progesterone levels in pseudopregnant rats: Effects of partial removal of luteal tissue, *Endocrinology* **95**:565–571.

de Greef, W. J., Dullaart, J., and Zeilmaker, G. H., 1977, Serum concentration of progesterone, luteinizing hormone, follicle stimulating hormone and prolactin in pseudopregnant rats: Effect of decidualization, *Endocrinology* **101**:1054–1063.

Del Campo, M. R., Mapletoft, R. J., Rowe, R. F., Cirtser, J. K., and Ginther, O. J., 1980, Unilateral uteroovarian relationship in pregnant cattle and role of uterine vein, *Theriogenology* **14**:185–193.

Denamur, R., and Mauleon, P., 1963, Controle endocrinien de la persistance du corps jaune chez le ovins, *C.R. Acad. Sci. (Paris)* **257**:527–530.

Denamur, R., Martinet, J., and Short, R. V., 1970, Mode of action of oestrogen in maintaining the functional life of corpora lutea in sheep, *J. Reprod. Fertil.* **23**:109–116.

Dickson, W. M., Bosc, M. J., and Locatelli, A., 1969, Effect of estrogen and progesterone on uterine blood flow in castrate sows, *Am. J. Physiol.* **217**:1431–1434.

Diehl, J. R., and Day, B. N., 1974, Effect of prostaglandin $F_{2\alpha}$ on luteal function in swine, *J. Anim. Sci.* **39**:392–396.

Diehl, J. R., Godki, R. A., Killian, D. B., and Day, B. N., 1974, Induction of parturition in swine with prostaglandin $F_{2\alpha}$, *J. Anim. Sci.* **38**:1229–1234.

Dierschke, D. J., Yamaji, T., Karsch, F. J., Weick, R. F., Weiss, G., and Knobil, E., 1973, Blockade by progesterone of estrogen induced LH and FSH release in the rhesus monkey, *Endocrinology* **92**:1496–1501.

Dingle, J. T., Hay, M. F., and Moor, R. M., 1968, Lysosomal function in the corpus luteum of the sheep, *J. Endocrinol.* **40**:325–336.

Dobowolski, W., 1973, Wplyw oksytocyny na cykl plciowy owcy w sezonie rozplodu i ciszy seksualnej, *Pol. Arch. Weter.* **16**:649–654.

Dohler, K. D., and Wuttke, W., 1974, Total blockade of phasic pituitary prolactin release in rats: Effect on serum LH and progesterone during the estrous cycle and pregnancy, *Endocrinology* **94**:1595–1600.

Donaldson, L. E., and Hansel, W., 1965, Prolongation of life span of the bovine corpus luteum by single injections of bovine luteinizing hormone, *J. Dairy Sci.* **48**:903–904.

Donovan, B. T., 1978, Uterine–ovarian interactions, *Uppsala J. Med. Sci.* **22**:71–72 (Suppl. 1).

Douglas, R. H., and Ginther, O. J., 1975, Effects of prostaglandin $F_{2\alpha}$ on estrous cycle or corpus luteum in mares and gilts, *J. Anim. Sci.* **40**:518–522.

Dufau, M. L., Hodgen, G. D., Goodman, A. L., and Catt, K. J., 1977, Bioassay of circulating luteinizing hormone in the rhesus monkey: Comparison with radioimmunoassay during physiological changes, *Endocrinology* **100**:1557–1565.

Dwyer, R. J., and Robertson, H. A., 1980, Oestrogen sulphatase and sulphotransferase activities in the endometrium of the sow and ewe during pregnancy, *J. Reprod. Fert.* **60**:187–191.

Eaton, L. W., Jr., and Hilliard, J., 1971, Estradiol-17β, progesterone, and 20α-hydroxypregn-4-en-3-one in rabbit ovarian venous plasma. I. Steroid secretion from paired ovaries with and without corpora lutea; effect of LH, *Endocrinology* **89**:105–111.

Edqvist, L. E., and Johansson, E. D. B., 1972, Radioimmunoassay of oesterone and oestradiol in human and bovine peripheral plasma, *Acta Endocrinol. (Kbh.)* **71**:716–730.

Eldridge, R. K., and Fields, P. A., 1985, Rabbit placental relaxin: Purification and immunohistochemical localization, *Endocrinology* **117**:2512–2519.

Eldridge, R. K., and Fields, P. A., 1986, Rabbit placental relaxin: Ultrastructural localization in secretory granules of the syncytiotrophoblast using rabbit placental relaxin antiserum, *Endocrinology* **119**:606–615.

Eley, R. M., Thatcher, W. W., Bazer, F. W., and Fields, M., 1983, Steroid metabolism by the bovine uterus, endometrium and conceptus, *Biol. Reprod.* **28**:804–816.

Ellicott, A. R., and Dziuk, P. J., 1973, Minimum daily dose of progesterone and plasma concentration for maintenance of pregnancy in ovariectomized gilts, *Biol. Reprod.* **9**:300–304.

Eto, T., Masuda, H., Suzuki, T., and Hosi, T., 1962, Progesterone and pregn-4-ene-20α-ol-3-one in rat ovarian venous blood at different stages of reproductive cycle, *Jpn. J. Anim. Reprod.* **8**:34–40.

Evans, J. J., 1987, The effects of prostaglandin F_2 alpha administration on progesterone after hysterectomy of guinea-pigs, *Prostaglandins* **33**:561–567.

Evans, G., Wathes, D. C., King, G. J., Armstrong, D. T., and Porter, D. G., 1983, Changes in relaxin production by the theca during the preovulatory period in the pig, *J. Reprod. Fertil.* **69**:677–683.

Fainstat, T., 1963, Extracellular studies of uterus. I. Disappearance of the discrete collagen bundles in endometrial stroma during various reproductive states in the rat, *Am. J. Anat.* **112**:337–370.

Fairclough, R. J., Moore, L. G. Peterson, A. J., and Watkin, W. B., 1984, Effect of oxytocin on plasma concentrations of 13,14-dihydro-15-keto prostaglandin and the oxytocin associated neurophysin during the estrous cycle and early pregnancy in the ewe, *Biol. Reprod.* **31**:36–43.

Fajer, A. B., and Barraclough, C. A., 1967, Ovarian secretion of progesterone and 20α-hydroxypregn-4-en-3-one during pseudopregnancy and pregnancy in rats, *Endocrinology* **81**:617–622.

Farese, R. V., 1983, The phosphatidate–phosphoinositide cycle: An intracellular messenger system in the action of hormones and neurotransmitter, *Metabolism* **32**:628–641.

Fawcett, D. W., Long, J. A., and Jones, A. L., 1969, The ultrastructure of endocrine organs, *Recent Prog. Horm. Res.* **25**:315–380.

Feil, P. K., Glasser, S. R., Toft, D. O., and O'Malley, B. W., 1972, Progesterone binding in the mouse and rat uterus, *Endocrinology* **91**:738–746.

Felder, K. J., Molina, J. R., Benoit, A. M., and Anderson, L. L., 1986, Precise timing for peak relaxin and decreased progesterone secretion after hysterectomy in the pig, *Endocrinology* **119**:1502–1509.

Felder, K. J., Klindt, J., Bolt, D. J., and Anderson, L. L., 1988, Relaxin and progesterone secretion as affected by luteinizing hormone and prolactin after hysterectomy in the pig, *Endocrinology* **122**:1751–1760.

Fèvre, J., Leglise, P. C., and Rombauts, P., 1968, Du role de l'hypophyse et des ovaires dans la biosynthese des oestrogenes au cours de la gestation chez la truie, *Ann. Biol. Anim. Biochim. Biophys.* **8**:225–233.

Fèvre, J., Leglise, P. C., and Revnaud, O., 1972, Role de surrenales maternelles dans la production d'oestrogenes par la truie gravide, *Ann. Biol. Anim. Biochim. Biophys.* **12**:559–567.

Fields, M. J., and Fields, P.A., 1986, Luteal neurophysin in the nonpregnant cow and ewe: Immunocytochemical localization in membrane-bounded secretory granules of the large luteal cell, *Endocrinology* **118**:1723–1725.

Fields, M. J., Fields, P. A., Castro-Hernandez, A., and Larkin L. M., 1980, Evidence for relaxin in corpora lutea of late pregnant cows, *Endocrinology* **107**:869–876.

Fields, M. J., Dubois, W., and Fields, P. A., 1985, Dynamic features of luteal secretory granules: Ultrastructural changes during the course of pregnancy in the cow, *Endocrinology* **117**:1675–1682.

Fields, P. A., and Fields, M. J., 1985, Ultrastructural localization of relaxin in the corpus luteum of the nonpregnant, pseudopregnant, and pregnant pig, *Biol. Reprod.* **32**:1169–1179.

Fields, P. A., Eldridge, R. K., Fuchs, A. R., Roberts, R. F., and Fields, M. J., 1983, Human placental and bovine corpora luteal oxytocin, *Endocrinology* **112**:1544–1546.

Fincher, K. B., Hansen, P. J., Thatcher, W. W., Rober, R. M., and Bazer, F. W., 1984, Ovine conceptus secretory proteins suppress induction of prostglandin $F_{2\alpha}$ release by estradiol and oxytocin, *J. Reprod. Fertil.* **76**:426–437.

Finlay, T. H., Katz, J., Kirsch, L., Levitz, M., Nathoo, S. W., and Seiler, S., 1983, Estrogen-stimulated uptake of plasminogen by the mouse uterus, *Endocrinology* **112**:856–861.

Finn. C. A., and Martin, L., 1972, Endocrine control of the timing of endometrial sensitivity to a decidual stimulus, *Biol. Reprod.* **7**:82–86.

Fischer, H. E., Bazer, F. W., and Fields, M. J., 1985, Steroid metabolism by endometrial and conceptus tissue during early pregnancy and pseudopregnancy in swine, *J. Reprod. Fertil.* **75**:69–78.

Fishel, S. B., Edwards, R. G., and Evans, C., 1984, Human chorionic gonadotrophin secreted by preimplantation embryos cultured *in vitro, Science* **223**:816–818.

Fitz, T. A., Mayan, M. H., Sawyer, H. R., and Niswender, G. D., 1982, Characterization of two steroidogenic cell types in the ovine corpus luteum, *Biol. Reprod.* **27**:703–711.

Flint, A. P. F., and Sheldrick, E. L., 1986, Ovarian oxytocin and the maternal recognition of pregnancy, *J. Reprod. Fertil.* **76**:831–839.

Ford, S. P., 1982, Control of uterine and ovarian blood flow throughout the estrous cycle and pregnancy of the ewe, sow and cow, *J. Anim. Sci.* **55**(Suppl. II):32–42.

Ford, S. P., and Chenault, J. R., 1981, Blood flow to the corpus luteum-bearing ovary and ipsilateral uterine horn of cows during the oestrous cycle and early pregnancy, *J. Reprod. Fertil.* **62**:555–562.

Ford, S. P., and Reynolds, L. P., 1981, Interaction of estradiol-17β and adrenergic antagonists in controlling uterine arterial blood flow of cows, *J. Anim. Sci.* **53**(Suppl. 1):317.

Ford, S. P., Christenson, R. K., and Chenault, J. R., 1979a, Patterns of blood flow to the uterus and ovaries of ewes during the period of luteal regression, *J. Anim. Sci.* **49**:1510–1516.

Ford, S. P., Chenault, J. R., and Echternkamp, S. E., 1979b, Uterine blood flow of cows during the oestrous cycle and early pregnancy: Effect of conceptus on the uterine blood supply, *J. Reprod. Fertil.* **56**:53–62.

Ford, S. P., Christenson, R. K., and Ford, J. J., 1982, Uterine blood flow and uterine arterial, venous and luminal concentrations of oestrogens on days 11, 13, and 15 post-oestrus in pregnant and nonpregnant sows, *J. Reprod. Fertil.* **64**:185–190.

Friedman, R. M., Merigan, R., and Sreevalsan, T., 1985, Interferons as cell growth inhibitors and anitumor factors, *UCLA Symp. Mol. Cell Biol.* **50**:1–541.

Fuchs, A. R., and Beling, C., 1975, Evidence for early ovarian recognition of blastocysts in rabbits, *Endocrinology* **95**:1054–1058.

Fuchs, A. R., and Mok, E., 1973, Prostaglandin effects on rat pregnancy. II. Interruption of pregnancy, *Fertil. Steril.* **24**:275–283.

Fuchs, A. R., and Mok, E., 1974, Histochemical study of the effects of prostaglandin $F_{2\alpha}$ and E_2 on the corpus luteum of pregnant rats, *Biol. Reprod.* **10**:24–38.

Gadsby, J. E., and Keyes, P. L., 1984, Control of corpus luteum function in the pregnant rabbit: Role of the placenta ("placental luteotropin") in regulating responsiveness of corpora lutea to estrogen, *Biol. Reprod.* **31**:16–24.

Gadsby, J. E., Heap, R. B., and Burton, R. D., 1980, Oestrogen production by blastocyst and early embryonic tissue of various species, *J. Reprod. Fertil.* **60**:409–417.

Galand, P., Mairesse, N., Roorijck, J., and Flandroy, L., 1983, Differential blockade of estrogen-induced uterine responses by the antiestrogen nafoxidine, *J. Steroid Biochem.* **19**:1259–1263.

Gardner, M. L., First, N. L., and Casida, L. E., 1963, Effect of exogenous estrogens on corpus luteum maintenance in gilts, *J. Anim. Sci.* **22**:132–134.

Garris, D. R., and Rothchild, I., 1980, Temporal aspects of the involvement of the uterus and prolactin in the establishment of luteinizing hormone dependent progesterone secretion in the rat, *Endocrinology* **107**:1112–1116.

Gibori, G., Rothchild, I., Pepe, G. J., Morishige, W. K., and Lam, P., 1974, Luteotrophic action of decidual tissue in the rat, *Endocrinology* **95**: 1113–1118.

Gibori, G., Basuray, R., and McReynolds, B., 1981, Luteotropic role of the decidual tissue in the rat: Dependency on intraluteal estradiol, *Endocrinology* **108**:2060–2066.

Gibori, G., Kalison, B., Basuray, R., Rao, M. C., and Hunzicker-Dunn, M., 1984, Endocrine role of the decidual tissue: Decidual luteotropin regulation of luteal adenyl cyclase activity, luteinizing hormone receptors, and steroidogenesis, *Endocrinology* **115**:1157–1163.

Gibori, G., Kalison, B., Warshaw, M. L., Basuray, R., and Glaser, L. A., 1985, Differential action of decidual luteotropin on luteal and follicular production of testosterone and estradiol, *Endocrinology* **116**:1784–1791.

Gibori, G., Jayatilak, P. G., Khan, I., Rigby, B., Puryear, T., Nelson, S., and Herz, T., 1987, Decidual luteotropin secretion and action. Its role in pregnancy maintenance in the rat, *Adv. Exp. Med. Biol.* **219**:379–397.

Glasser, S. R., and McCormack, S. A., 1979, Functional development of rat trophoblast and decidual cells during establishment of the hemochorial placenta, *Adv. Biosci.* **25**:165–197.

Gleeson, A. R., Thorburn, G. D., and Cox, R. I., 1974, Prostaglandin F concentration in the utero–ovarian venous plasma of the sow during late luteal phase of the estrous cycle, *Prostaglandins* **5**:521–530.

Goding, J. R., 1974, The demonstration that $PGF_{2\alpha}$ is the uterine luteolysin in the ewe, *J. Reprod. Fertil.* **38**:261–271.

Godkin, J. D., Bazer, F. W., Moffatt, J., Sessions, F., and Roberts, R. M., 1982, Purification and properties of a major, low molecular weight protein released by the trophoblast of sheep blastocysts on day 13–21, *J. Reprod. Fertil.* **65**:141–150.

Godkin, J. D., Bazer, F. W., Thatcher, W. W., and Roberts, R. M., 1984, Proteins released by cultured day 15–16 conceptuses prolong luteal maintenance when introduced into the uterine lumen of cyclic ewes, *J. Reprod. Fertil.* **71**:57–64.

Goland, R. S., Wardlaw, S.L., Stark, R. I., Brown, L. S., and Frantz, A. G., 1986, High levels of corticotropin-releasing hormone immunoactivity in maternal and fetal plasma during pregnancy, *J. Clin. Endocr. Metab.* **63**:1199–1203.

Goodman, A. L., Nixon, W. E., Johnson, D. K., and Hodgen, G. D., 1977, Regulation of folliculogenesis in the cycling rhesus monkey: Selection of the dominant follicle, *Endocrinology* **100**:155–161.

Gore, S. D., and Behrman, H. R., 1984, Alteration of transmembrane sodium and potassium gradients inhibits the action of luteinizing hormone in the luteal cell, *Endocrinology* **114**:2020–2031.

Greenwald, G. S., and Johnson, D. C., 1968, Gonadotropic requirements for the maintenance of pregnancy in the hypophysectomized rat, *Endocrinology* **83**:1052–1064.

Greiss, F. C., Jr., 1972, Differential reactivity of the myoendometrial and placenta vasculatures: Adrenergic responses, *Am. J. Obstet. Gynecol.* **112**:20–30.

Greiss, F. C., Jr., and Anderson, S. G., 1970, Uterine blood flow during early ovine pregnancy, *Am. J. Obstet. Gynecol.* **106**:30–38.

Grunert, G., Porcia, M., Neumann, G., Sepulveda, A., and Tchernitchin, A. N., 1984, Progesterone interaction with eosinophils and with responses already induced by oestrogen in the uterus, *J. Endocrinol.* **102**:295–303.

Guraya, S. S., 1973, Interstitial gland tissue of mammalian ovary, *Acta Endocrinol. (Kbh.) [Suppl.]* **171**:1–27.

Guraya, S. S., 1975, Histochemical observations on the lipid changes in rat corpora lutea during reproductive states after treatment with exogenous hormones, *J. Reprod. Fertil.* **43**:67–75.

Guthrie, H. D., and Bolt, D. J., 1983, Changes in plasma estrogen, luteinizing hormone, follicle-stimulating hormone and 13,14-dihydro-15-keto-prostaglandin $F_{2\alpha}$ during blockade of luteolysis in pigs after human chorionic gonadotropin treatment, *J. Anim. Sci.* **57**:993–1000.

Guthrie, H. D., and Rexroad, Jr., C. E., 1981, Endometrial prostaglandin F release *in vitro* and plasma 13,14-dihydro-15-keto-prostaglandin $F_{2\alpha}$ in pigs with luteolysis blocked by pregnancy, estradiol benzoate or human chorionic gonadotropin, *J. Anim. Sci.* **52**:330–339.

Halme, J., and Woessner, J. F., Jr., 1975, Effect of progesterone on collagen breakdown and tissue collagenolytic activity in the involuting rat uterus, *J. Endocrinol.* **66**:357–362.

Hansel, W., and Dowd, P. T., 1986, New concepts of the control of the corpus luteum function, *J. Reprod. Fertil.* **78**:755–768.

Hansel, W., Concannon, P. W., and Lukaszewska, J. H., 1973, Corpora lutea of the large domestic animals, *Biol. Reprod.* **8**:222–245.

Hansen, P. J., Anthony, R. V., Bazer, F. W., Baumbach, G. A., and Roberts, R. M., 1985, *In vitro* synthesis and secretion of ovine trophoblast protein-1 during the period of maternal recognition of pregnancy, *Endocrinology* **117**:1424–1430.

Haour, F., and Saxena, B. B., 1974, Detection of a gonadotropin in rabbit blastocyst before implantation, *Science* **185**:444–445.

Hard, D. L., and Anderson, L. L., 1979, Maternal starvation on progesterone secretion, litter size, and growth in the pig, *Am. J. Physiol.* **237**:73–78.

Harney, P. J., Sneddon, J. M., and Williams, K. I., 1974, The influence of ovarian hormones upon the motility and prostaglandin production of the pregnant rat uterus *in vitro*, *J. Endocrinol.* **60**:343–351.

Hashimoto, I., and Wiest, W. G., 1969, Luteotrophic and luteolytic mechanisms in rat corpora lutea, *Endocrinology* **84**:886–892.

Hashimoto, I., Hendricks, D. M., Anderson, L. L., and Melampy, R. M., 1968, Progesterone and pregn-4-en 20α-ol-3-one in ovarian venous blood during various reproductive states in the rat, *Endocrinology* **82**:333–341.

Hasler, J. F., Bowen, R. A., and Seidel, G. E., Jr., 1975, Progesterone in pregnant vs. nonpregnant cows, *J. Anim. Sci.* **41**:356.

Hatjiminaoglou, I., Alifakiotis, T., and Zeras, N., 1979, The effect of exogenous oxytocin in estrous cycle length and corpus luteum lysis in ewes, *Ann. Biol. Anim. Biochim. Biophys.* **19**:355–365.

Hawk, H. W., and Bolt, D. J., 1970, Luteolytic effect of estradiol-17β when administered after midcycle in the ewe, *Biol. Reprod.* **2**:275–278.

Hayashi, M., 1964, Distribution of β-glucuronidase activity in rat tissues employing the naphthol AS-BI glucuronidase hexazonium pararosanilin method, *J. Histochem. Cytochem.* **12**:659–669.

Heap, R. B., and Deanesly, R., 1966, Progesterone in systemic blood and placentae of intact and ovariectomized pregnant guinea pigs, *J. Endocrinol.* **34**:417–423.

Hearn, J. P., 1983, The common marmoset (*Callithrix jacchus*), in: *Reproduction in New World Primates* (J. P. Hearn, ed.), MTP Press, Lancaster, pp. 181–215.

Hearn, J. P., 1986, The embryo–maternal dialogue during early pregnancy in primates, *J. Reprod. Fertil.* **76**:809–819.

Hechter, O., Yoshinaga, K., Cohn, C., Dodd, P., and Halkerston, I. D. K., 1965, *In vitro* stimulatory effects of nucleotides and nucleosides on biosynthesis process in castrate rat uterus, *Fed. Proc.* **24**:384.

Helmer, S. D., Hansen, P. J., Anthony, R. V., Thatcher, W. W., Bazer, F. W., and Roberts, R. M., 1987,

Identification of bovine trophoblast protein-1, a secretory protein immunologically related to ovine trophoblast protein-1, *J. Reprod. Fertil.* **79**:83–91.

Herz, Z., Khan, I., Jayatilak, P. G., and Gibori, G., 1985, Evidence for the synthesis and secretion of decidual luteotropin, a prolactin-like hormone produced by rat decidual cells, *Endocrinology* **118**:2203–2209.

Hess, D. L., and Resko, J. A., 1973, The effects of progesterone on the patterns of testosterone and estradiol concentrations in the systemic plasma of the remale rhesus monkey during the intermenstrual period, *Endocrinology* **92**:446–453.

Hilliard, J., 1973, Corpus luteum function in guinea pigs, hamsters, rats, mice and rabbits, *Biol. Reprod.* **8**:203–221.

Hilliard, J., and Eaton, L. M., Jr., 1971, Estradiol-17β, progesterone and 20α-hydroxypregn-4-en-3-one in rabbit ovarian venous plasma, II. From mating through implantation, *Endocrinology* **89**:522–527.

Hilliard, J., Spies, H. G., and Sawyer, C. H., 1969, Hormonal factors regulating ovarian cholesterol mobilization and progestin secretion in intact and hypophysectomized rabbits, in: *The Gonads* (K. McKerns, ed.), Appelton-Century-Crofts, New York, pp. 55–92.

Hilliard, J., Scaramuzzi, R. J., Penardi, R., and Sawyer, C. H., 1973, Progesterone, estradiol, and testosterone levels in ovarian venous blood of pregnant rabbits, *Endocrinology* **93**:1235–1238.

Hilliard, J., Scaramuzzi, R. J., Pang, C. N., Penardi, R., and Sawyer, C. H., 1974, Testosterone secretion by rabbit ovary *in vivo*, *Endocrinology* **94**:267–271.

Hodgen, G. D., Wilks, J. W., Vaitukaitis, J. L., Chen, H. C., Papkogg, H., and Ross, G. T., 1976, A new radioimmunoassay for follicle-stimulating hormone in macaques: Ovulatory menstrual cycles, *Endocrinology* **99**:137–145.

Hoffman, B., Schams, D., Bopp, R., Ender, M. L., Giminez, T., and Karg, H., 1974, Luteotropic factors in the cow: Evidence for LH rather than prolactin, *J. Reprod. Fertil.* **40**:77–85.

Holt, J. A., and Ewing, L. L., 1974, Acute dependence of ovarian progesterone output on the presence of placentas in 21-day pregnant rabbits, *Endocrinology* **94**:1438–1444.

Holt, J. A., Heise, W. F., Wilson, S. M., and Keyes, P. L., 1976, Lack of gonadotropic activity in the rabbit blastocyst prior to implantation, *Endocrinology* **98**:904–909.

Huckabee, W. E., Crenshaw, C., Curet, L. B., and Barron, D. H., 1968, Blood flow and oxygen consumption of the uterus of the nonpregnant ewe, *Q.J. Exp. Physiol.* **53**:349–356.

Hudson, P., Haley, J., Cronk, M., Shine, J., and Niall, H., 1981, Molecular cloning and characterization of cDNA sequences coding for rat relaxin, *Nature* **291**:127–131.

Hummel, L., Schwartze, A., Schirrmeister, W., and Wagner, H., 1976, Maternal plasma triglycerides as a source of fetal fatty acids, *Acta Biol. Med. Ger.* **35**:1635–1641.

Ichikawa, S., Sawada, T., Nakamura, Y., and Morioka, H., 1974, Ovarian secretion of pregnane compounds during the estrous cycle and pregnancy in rats, *Endocrinology* **94**:1615–1620.

Illingworth, D. V., and Challis, J. R. G., 1973, Concentrations of oestrogens and progesterone in the plasma of ovariectomized norgestrel-treated pregnant guinea pigs, *J. Reprod. Fertil.* **34**:289–296.

Imakawa, K., Anthony, R. V., Kazemi, M., Marotti, K. R., Polites, H. A., and Roberts, R. M., 1987, Interferon-like sequence of ovine trophoblast protein secreted by embryonic trophectoderm, *Nature* **330**:377–379.

Inskeep, E. K., 1973, Potential uses of prostaglandins in control of reproductive cycles of domestic animals, *J. Anim. Sci.* **36**:1149–1157.

Inskeep, E. K., and Butcher, R. L., 1966, Local component of utero–ovarian relationships in the ewe, *J. Anim. Sci.* **25**:1164–1171.

Ivell, R., and Richter, D., 1984, The gene for the hypothalamic peptide hormone oxytocin is highly expressed in the bovine corpus luteum: Biosynthesis, structure and sequence analysis, *EMBO J.* **3**:2351–2354.

Ivell, R., Brackett, K. H. Y., Fields, M. J., and Richter, D., 1985, Ovulation triggers oxytocin gene expression in the bovine ovary, *FEBS Lett.* **190**:263–267.

Janson, P. O., Albrecht, I., and Ahren, K., 1975, Effects of prostaglandin $F_{2\alpha}$ on ovarian blood flow and vascular resistance in the pseudopregnant rabbit, *Acta Endocrinol. (Kbh.)* **79**:337–350.

Jayatilak, P. G., Glaser, L. A., Warshaw, M. L., Herz, Z., Grueber, J. R., and Gibori, G., 1984, Relationship between luteinizing hormone and decidual luteotropin in the maintenance of luteal steroidogenesis, *Biol. Reprod.* **31**:556–564.

Jayatilak, P. G., Glaser, L. A., Basuray, R., Kelly, P. A., and Gibori, G., 1985, Identification and partial characterization of a prolactin-like hormone produced by the rat decidual tissue, *Proc. Natl. Acad. Sci. U.S.A.* **82**:217–221.

Jones, C. T., and Rolph, T. P., 1985, Metabolism during fetal life, a functional assessment of metabolic development, *Physiol. Rev.* **65**:357–430.

Kadowitz, P. J., Sweet, C. S., and Brody, M. J., 1972, Enhancement of sympathetic neurotransmission by prostaglandin $F_{2\alpha}$ in the cutaneous vascular bed of the dog, *Eur. J. Pharmacol.* **18**:189–194.

Kalsner, S., 1969, Steroid potentiation of responses to sympathomimetic amines in aortic strips, *Br. J. Pharmacol.* **36:**582–593.

Kann, G., and Denamur, R., 1973, Changes in plasma levels of prolactin and LH induced by luteolytic or luteotrophic treatment in intact cycling sheep after section of the pituitary stalk, *Acta Endocrinol. (Kbh)* **73:**625–634.

Karsch, F. J., and Sutton, G. P., 1976, An intra-ovarian site for the luteolytic action of estrogen in the rhesus monkey, *Endocrinology* **99:**553–561.

Karsch, F. J., Noveroske, J. W., Roche, J. F., and Nalbandov, A. V., 1969, Response to infused LH depends on age of ovine corpora lutea, *J. Anim. Sci.* **29:**192.

Kawahara, Y., Takai, Y., Minakuchi, R., Sano, K., and Nishizuka, Y., 1980, Phospholipid turnover as a possible transmembrane signal for protein phosphorylation during human platelet activation by thrombin, *Biochem. Biophys. Res. Commun.* **97:**309–317.

Kehl, S. J., and Carlson, J. C., 1981, Assessment of the luteolytic potency of various prostaglandins in the pseudopregnant rabbit, *J. Reprod. Fertil.* **62:**117–122.

Kelly, P. A., Shiu, R. P. C., Robertson, M. C., and Friesen, H. G., 1975, Characterization of rat chorionic mammotropin, *Endocrinology* **96:**1187–1195.

Kertiles, L. P., and Anderson, L. L., 1979, Effect of relaxin on cervical dilatation, parturition and lactation in the pig, *Biol. Reprod.* **21:**57–68.

Keyes, P. L., and Gadsby, J. E., 1987, Role of estrogen and the placenta in the maintenance of the rabbit corpus luteum, *Adv. Exp. Med. Biol.* **219:**367–378.

Keyes, P. L., Gadsby, J. E., Yuh, K.-C. M., and Bill, C. H., 1983, The corpus luteum, *Int. Rev. Physiol.* **4:**57–97.

Khan-Dawood, F. S., and Dawood, M. Y., 1983, Human ovaries contain immunoreactive oxytocin, *J. Clin. Endocrinol. Metab.* **57:**1129–1132.

Khan-Dawood, F. S., and Dawood, M. Y., 1986, Paracrine regulation of luteal function, *J. Mol. Cell. Endocrinol.* **15:**171–184.

Khan-Dawood, F. S., Marut, E. L., and Dawood, M. Y., 1984, Oxytocin in the corpus luteum of the cynomolgus monkey *(Macaca fascicularis), Endocrinology* **115:**570–574.

Kimmel, G. L., Moulton, B. G. C., and Leavitt, W. W., 1973, Uptake and retention of ^{3}H-oestradiol by myometrium and deciduomal tissue in the pseudopregnant rat, *J. Endocrinol.* **56:**335–336.

Kiracofe, G. H., Menzies, C. S., Gier, H. T., and Spies, H. G., 1966, Effect of uterine extracts and uterine or ovarian blood vessel ligation on ovarian function of ewes, *J. Anim. Sci.* **25:**1159–1163.

Kishimoto, A., Takai, Y., Mori, T., Kikkawa, U., and Nishizuka, Y., 1980, Activation of calcium and phospholipid-dependent protein kinase by diacylglycerol, its possible relation to phosphatidylinositol turnover, *J. Chem.* **255:**2273–2276.

Knobil, E., 1973, On the regulation of the primate corpus luteum, *Biol. Reprod.* **8:**246–258.

Knobil, E., 1974, On the control of gonadotropin secretion in the rhesus monkey, *Recent Prog. Horm. Res.* **30:**1–46.

Koch, E., and Ellendorff, F., 1985, Prospects and limitations of the rosette inhibition test to detect activity of early pregnancy factor in the pig, *J. Reprod. Fertil.* **74:**29–38.

Koos, R., and Hansel, W., 1981, The large and small cells of the bovine corpus luteum: Ultra-structural and functional differences, in: *Dynamics of Ovarian Function* (N. B. Schwartz and M. Hunziker-Dunn, ed.), Raven Press, New York, pp. 197–203.

Kraeling, R. R., and Davis, B. J., 1974, Termination of pregnancy by hypophysectomy in the pig, *J. Reprod. Fertil.* **36:**215–217.

Kraeling, R. R., Rampacek, A. B., and Kiser, T. E., 1981, Corpus luteum function after indomethacin treatment during the estrous cycle and following hysterectomy in the gilt, *Biol. Reprod.* **25:**511–518.

Kronenberg, L. H., 1985, Interferons: Manufacture and applications in medicine, in: *Biotechnology: Applications and Research* (P. Cheresmisinoff and R. Ouellette, ed.), Technomic, Lancaster, PA, pp. 451–462.

Kruip, T. A. M., Vulklings, H. G. B., Schams, D., Jonis, J., and Klarenbeek, A., 1985, Immunocytochemical demonstration of oxytocin in bovine ovarian tissues, *Acta Endocrinol. (Kbh.)* **109:**537–542.

Kwok, S. C. M., Chamley, W. A., and Bryant-Greenwood, G. D., 1978, High molecular weight forms of relaxin in pregnant sow ovaries, *Biochem. Biophys. Res. Commun.* **82:**997–1005.

Labhsetwar, A. P., and Watson, D. J., 1974, Temporal relationships between secreting patterns of gonadotropins, estrogens, progestins, and prostaglandin-F in periparturient rats, *Biol. Reprod.* **10:**103–110.

Ladner, C. C., Brinkman, R. III, Weston, P., and Assali, N. S., 1970, Dynamics of uterine circulation in pregnant and nonpregnant sheep, *Am. J. Physiol.* **218:**257–263.

Lamprecht, S. A., Lindner, H. R., and Strauss, J. F. III, 1969, Induction of 20α-hydroxysteroid dehydrogenase in rat corpora lutea by pharmacological blockade of pituitary prolactin secretion, *Biochim. Biophys. Acta* **187:**133–143.

Larkin, L. H., Fields, P. A., and Oliver, R. M., 1977, Production of antisera against electrophoretically separated relaxin and immunofluorescent localization of relaxin in the porcine corpus luteum, *Endocrinology* **101**:679–685.

Larkin, L. H., Pardo, R. J., and Renegar, R. H., 1983, Sources of relaxin and morphology of relaxin containing cells, in: *Biology of Relaxin and Its Role in the Human* (M. Bigazzi, F. C. Greenwood, and F. Gasparri, eds.), Excerpta Medica, Amsterdam, pp. 191–205.

Laudanski, T., Batra, S., and Akerlund, M., 1979, Prostaglandin-induced luteolysis in pregnant and pseudopregnant rabbits and the resultant effects on the myometrial activity, *J. Reprod. Fertil.* **56**:141–148.

Lauderdale, J. W., Sequin, B. E., Stellflug, J. N., Chenault, J. R., Thatcher, W. W., Vincent, C. K., and Loyancano, A. F., 1974, Fertility of cattle following PGF$_{2\alpha}$ injection, *J. Anim. Sci.* **38**:964–967.

Lawrence, I. E., Jr., Burden, H. W., and Joyner, R. S., 1975, Studies on the noradrenergic innervation and Δ^5-3β-hydroxysteroid dehydrogenase activity in the interstitial gland of the rat ovary during pregnancy, *Anat. Rec.* **181**:406–407.

Lemon, M., and Loir, M., 1977, Steroid release *in vitro* by two luteal cell types in the corpus luteum of the pregnant sow, *J. Endocrinol.* **72**:351–359.

Lemon, M., and Mauleon, P., 1982, Interaction between two cell types in the corpus luteum of the pregnant sow, *J. Endocrinol.* **72**:351–359.

Lenton, E. A., Neal, L. M., and Sulaiman, R., 1982, Plasma concentrations of human chorionic gonadotrophin from the time of implantation until the second week of pregnancy, *Fertil. Steril.* **37**:773–778.

Lerner, L. J., Carminati, P., and Schiatti, P., 1975, Correlation of anti-inflammatory activity with inhibition of prostaglandin synthesis activity of nonsteroidal anti-estrogens and estrogens, *Proc. Soc. Exp. Biol. Med.* **148**:329–332.

Lewis, G. S., and Bolt, J. D., 1983, Effects of suckling on postpartum changes in 13,14-dihydro-15-keto-PGF$_{2\alpha}$ and progesterone and induced release of gonadotropin in autumn lambing ewes, *J. Anim. Sci.* **57**:673–678.

Lewis, G. S., and Bolt, J. D., 1987, Effects of suckling, progestagen-impregnated pessaries or hysterectomy on ovarian function in antumn lambing postpartum ewes, *J. Anim. Sci.* **64**:216–225.

Li, Y., Molina, J. R., Klindt, J., Bolt, D. J., and Anderson, L. L., 1987, Prolactin maintains progesterone secretion by aging corpora lutea in hypophysectomized pigs, *J. Anim. Sci.* **65** (Suppl. 1):367.

Li, Y., Molina, J. R., Klindt, J., Bolt, D. J., and Anderson, L. L., 1989, Prolactin maintains relaxin and progesterone secretion by aging corpora lutea after hypophysial stalk transduction or hypophysectomy in the pig, *Endocrinology* **122**(Suppl. 1):296.

Liehr, R. A., Marion, G. B., and Olson, H. H., 1972, Effects of prostaglandin on cattle estrus cycles, *J. Anim. Sci.* **35**:247.

Linkie, D. M., and Niswender, G. D., 1972, Serum levels of prolactin, luteinizing hormone, and follicle-stimulating hormone during pregnancy in the rat, *Endocrinology* **90**:632–637.

Linkie, D. M., and Niswender, G. D., 1973, Characterization of rat placental luteotrophin, *Biol. Reprod.* **8**:48–57.

Lobel, B. L., and Deane, H. W., 1962, Enzymic activity associated with postpartum involution of the uterus and with its regression after hormone withdrawal in the rat, *Endocrinology* **70**:567–578.

Lobel, R., Rosenbaum, R. M., and Deane, H. W., 1961, Enzymic correlates of physiological regression follicles and corpora lutea in the ovaries of normal rats, *Endocrinology* **68**:232–247.

Long, J. A., 1973, Corpus luteum of pregnancy in the rat—ultrastructural and cytochemical observations, *Biol. Reprod.* **8**:87–99.

Long, J. A., and Evans, H. M., 1922, The oestrous cycle in the rat and its associated phenomena, *Mem. Univ. Calif.* **6**:1–147.

Louis, T. M., Hafs, H. D., and Morrow, D. A., 1974, Intrauterine administration of prostaglandin F$_{2\alpha}$ in cows: Progesterone, estrogen, LH, estrus, and ovulation, *J. Anim. Sci.* **38**:347–353.

Lyons, W. R., and Ahmad, N., 1973, Hormonal maintenance of pregnancy in hypophysectomized rats, *Proc. Soc. Exp. Biol. Med.* **142**:198–202.

Magness, R. R., Christenson, R. K., and Ford, S. P., 1983, Ovarian blood flow throughout the estrous cycle and early pregnancy in sows, *Biol. Reprod.* **28**:1090–1096.

Mandl, A. M., and Zuckerman, S., 1952, Cyclical changes in the number of medium and large follicles in the adult rat ovary, *J. Endocrinol.* **8**:341–346.

Mapletoft, R. J., Lapin, D. R., and Ginther, O. J., 1976, The ovarian artery as the final component of the local luteotropic pathway between a gravid uterine horn and ovary in ewes, *Biol. Reprod.* **15**:414–421.

Marcus, G. J., 1974, Mitosis in the rat uterus during the estrous cycle, early pregnancy, and early pseudopregnancy, *Biol. Reprod.* **10**:447–452.

Marcus, G., Lucis, R., and Ainsworth, L., 1979, Metabolism of progesterone by chorionic cells of the early sheep conceptus *in vitro, Steroids* **34**:807–815.

Marsh, J. M., 1971, The effect of prostaglandins on the adenyl cyclase of the bovine corpus luteum, *Ann. N.Y. Acad. Sci.* **180:**416–425.

Marsh, J. M., 1976, The role of cyclic AMP in gonadal steroidogenesis, *Biol. Reprod.* **14:**30–53.

Marsh, J. M., and Le Marie, W. J., 1974, Cyclic AMP accumulation and steroidogenesis in the human corpus luteum: Effect of gonadotropins and prostaglandins, *J. Clin. Endocrinol. Metab.* **38:**99–106.

Matsumoto, D., and Chamley, W. A., 1980, Identification of relaxins in porcine follicular fluid and in the ovary of the immature sow, *J. Reprod. Fertil.* **58:**369–375.

Mauleon, P., and Ortavant, R., 1975, Colloque: Control of sexual cycles in domestic animals, *Ann. Biol. Anim. Biochim. Biophys.* **15:**131–498.

McCracken, J. A., Glew, M. E., and Scaramuzzi, R. J., 1970, Corpus luteum regression induced by prostaglandin $F_{2\alpha}$, *J. Clin. Endocrinol. Metab.* **30:**544–548.

McCracken, J. A., Carlson, J. C., Glew, M. E., Goding, J. R., Baird, D. T., Green, K., and Samuelsson, B., 1972a, Prostaglandin $F_{2\alpha}$ identified as a luteolytic hormone in sheep, *Nature (New Biol.)* **238:**129–134.

McCracken, J. A., Barcikowski, B., Carlson, J. C., Green, K., and Samuelsson, B., 1972b, The physiological role of prostaglandin $F_{2\alpha}$ in corpus luteum regression, *Adv. Biosci.* **9:**599–624.

McCracken, J. A., Baird, D. T., Carlson, J. C., Goding, J. R., and Barcikowski, B., 1973, The role of prostaglandins in luteal regression, *J. Reprod. Fertil. Suppl.* **18:**133–142.

McCracken, J. A., Schramm, W., and Okuliez, W. C., 1984, Hormone receptor control of pulsatile secretion of $PGF_{2\alpha}$ from the ovine uterus during luteolysis and its abrogation in early pregnancy, *Anim. Reprod. Sci.* **7:**31–55.

McDonald, D. M., Seiki, J., Prizant, M., and Goldfien, A., 1969, Ovarian secretion of progesterone in relation to the Golgi apparatus in lutein cells during the estrous cycle of the rat, *Endocrinology* **85:**236–243.

McKercher, T. C., Van Orden, L. S. III, Bhatnagar, R. K., and Burke, J. P., 1973, Estrogen-induced biogenic amine reduction in rat uterus, *J. Pharmacol. Exp. Ther.* **185:**514–522.

McLaren, A., 1985, The control of implantation, in: *In Vitro Fertilisation and Donor Insemination* (W. Thompson, D. N. Joyce, and J. R. Newton, eds.), Royal College of Obstetricians and Gynaecologist, London, pp. 13–22.

Melampy, R. M., Anderson, L. L., and Kragt, C. L., 1964, Uterus and life span of rat corpora lutea, *Endocrinology* **74:**501–504.

Milkovic, S., Milkovic, K., and Paunovic, J., 1973, The initiation of fetal adrenocorticotrophic activity in the rat, *Endocrinology* **92:**380–384.

Miller, J. B., and Keyes, P. L., 1976, A mechanism for regression of the rabbit corpus luteum: Uterine-induced loss of luteal responsiveness to 17β-estradiol, *Biol. Reprod.* **15:**511–518.

Milvae, R. A., 1986, Role of luteal prostaglandins in the control of bovine corpus luteum functions, *J. Anim. Sci.* **62**(Suppl. 2):72–78.

Milvae, R. A., and Hansel, W., 1985, Inhibition of bovine luteal function by indomethacin, *J. Anim. Sci.* **60:**528–531.

Milvae, R. A., Alila, H. W., and Hansel, W., 1986, Involvement of lipoxygenase products of arachidonic acid metabolism in bovine luteal function, *Biol. Reprod.* **35:**1210–1215.

Mitchell, B. F., Cross, J., Hobkirk, R., and Challis, J. R. G., 1984, Formation of unconjugated estrogens from estrone sulphate by dispersed cells from human fetal membranes and decidua, *J. Clin. Endocrinol. Metab.* **58:**845–849.

Mitchell, M. D., Flint, A. P. F., and Turnbull, A. C., 1975, Stimulation by oxytocin of prostaglandin F levels in uterine venous effluent in pregnant and puerperal sheep, *Prostaglandins* **9:**47–56.

Moeljono, M. P., Bazer, F. W., and Thatcher, W. W., 1976, A study of prostaglandin $F_{2\alpha}$ as the luteolysin in swine: I. Effect of prostaglandin F in hysterectomized gilts, *Prostaglandins* **11:**737–743.

Moeljono, M. P. E., Thatcher, W. W., Bazer, F. W., Frank, M., Owens, L. J., and Wilcox, C. J., 1977, A study of prostaglandin $F_{2\alpha}$ as the luteolysin in swine: II. Characterization and comparison of prostaglandin F, estrogens and progestin concentrations in utero–ovarian vein plasma of nonpregnant and pregnant gilts, *Prostaglandins* **14:**543–555.

Moor, R. M., and Rowson, L. E. A., 1966a, Local uterine mechanisms affecting luteal function in the sheep, *J. Reprod. Fertil.* **11:**307–310.

Moor, R. M., and Rowson, L. E. A., 1966b, The corpus luteum of the sheep: Effect of the removal of embryo on luteal function, *J. Endocrinol.* **34:**497–502.

Moore, L. G., Watkins, W. B., Choy, V. C., and Elliot, R. L., 1986, Evidence for the pulsatile release of $PGF_{2\alpha}$ inducing the release of ovarian oxytocin during luteolysis in the ewe, *J. Reprod. Fertil.* **76:**159–166.

Morton, H., Rolfe, B., Clunie, G. J. A., Anderson, M. J., and Morrison, J., 1977, An early pregnancy factor detected in human serum by the rosette inhibition test, *Lancet* **1:**394–397.

Mossman, H. W., and Duke, K. L., 1973, Some comparative aspects of the mammalian ovary, in: *Handbook of*

Physiology, Endocrinology Section 7, Vol. 2, Part 2 (R. O. Greep and E. B. Astwood, eds.), American Physiological Society, Washington, D.C., pp. 389–402.

Musah, A. I., Ford, J. J., and Anderson, L. L., 1984, Progesterone secretion as affected by 17β-estradiol after hysterectomy in the pig, *Endocrinology* **115:**1876–1882.

Musah, A. I., Schwabe, C., Willham, R. L., and Anderson, L. L., 1986, Relaxin on induction of parturition in beef heifers, *Endocrinology* **118:**1476–1482.

Musah, A. I., Schwabe, C., and Anderson, L. L., 1987a, Acute decrease in progesterone and increase in estrogen secretion caused by relaxin during late pregnancy in beef heifers, *Endocrinology* **120:**317–324.

Musah, A. I., Schwabe, C., and Anderson, L. L., 1987b, Porcine relaxin induced spike release of oxytocin in late pregnant beef heifers, *Biol. Reprod.* **36:**(Suppl. 1):149.

Musah, A. I., Schwabe, C., Willham, R. L., and Anderson, L. L., 1987c, Induction of parturition, progesterone secretion and delivery of placenta in beef heifers given relaxin with cloprostenol or dexamethasone, *Biol. Reprod.* **37:**797–803.

Nanes, M. S., Garris, D. R., and Rothchild, I., 1980, Prolactin and hysterectomy delay rather than prevent the critical need for LH (LH dependency) in the luteotrophic process of the rat, *Proc. Soc. Exp. Biol. Med.* **164:**299–302.

Nara, B. S., and First, N. L., 1981a, Effect of indomethacin on dexamethasone-induced parturition in swine, *J. Anim. Sci.* **52:**788–793.

Nara, B. S., and First, N. L., 1981b, Effect of indomethacin and prostaglandin $F_{2\alpha}$ on parturition in swine, *J. Anim. Sci.* **51:**1360–1370.

Nara, B. S., Ball, G. D., Rutherford, J. E., Sherwood, O. D., and First, N. L., 1982, Release of relaxin by a nonluteolytic dose of prostaglandin $F_{2\alpha}$ in pregnant swine, *Biol. Reprod.* **27:**1190–1195.

Nishizuka, Y., 1984, Turnover of inositol phospholipids and signal transduction, *Science* **225:**1365–1367.

Niswender, G. D., Moore, R. T., Akbar, A. M., Nett, T. M., and Diekman, M. A., 1975, Flow of blood to the ovaries of ewes throughout the estrous cycle, *Biol. Reprod.* **13:**381–388.

Noland, T. A., Jr., and Dimino, M. J., 1986, Characteristics and distribution of protein kinase C in ovarian tissue, *Biol. Reprod.* **35:**863–872.

Northey, D. L., and French, L. R., 1980, Effect of embryo removal and intrauterine infusion of embryonic homogenates on the lifespan of the bovine corpus luteum, *J. Anim. Sci.* **50:**298–302.

Nutting, E. F., and Cammarata, P. S., 1969, Effects of prostaglandins on fertility in female rats, *Nature* **222:**287–288.

Oates, T. A., 1982, The 1982 Nobel Prize in Physiology or Medicine, *Science* **218:**765–768.

Ochiai, K., and Rothchild, I., 1985, The patterns of progesterone secretion in hypophysectomized rats bearing pituitary implants: Effects of hysterectomy, estrogen and indomethacin, *Endocrinology* **116:**765–771.

Olson, D. M., Lye, S. J., Skinner, K., and Challis, J. R. G., 1984, Early changes in prostaglandin concentrations in ovine maternal and fetal plasma, amniotic fluid and from dispersed cells of intrauterine tissues before the onset of ACTH-induced pre-term labour, *J. Reprod. Fertil.* **71:**45–55.

Osathanondh, R., and Tulchinsky, D., 1980, Placental polypeptide hormones, in: *Maternal–Fetal Endocrinology* (D. Tulchinsky and K. J. Ryan, ed.), W. B. Saunders, Philadelphia, pp. 17–42.

Pakurar, A. S., and Rothchild, I., 1972, Prolongation of pseudopregnancy in the rat by slitting the uterus, *J. Endocrinol.* **55:**441–447.

Pant, H. S., Hopkinson, C. R. N., and Fitzpatrick, R. J., 1977, Concentration of oestradiol, progesterone, luteinizing hormone and follicle-stimulating hormone in the jugular venous plasma of ewes during the oestrous cycle, *J. Endocrinol.* **73:**247–251.

Parnham, M. J., Sneddon, J. M., and Williams, K. I., 1975, Evidence for a possible foetal control of prostaglandin release from the pregnant rat uterus *in vitro*, *J. Endocrinol.* **65:**429–437.

Pepe, G. J., and Rothchild, I., 1974, A comparative study of serum progesterone levels in pregnancy and in various types of pseudopregnancy in the rat, *Endocrinology* **95:**275–279.

Petraglia, F., Sawchenko, P. E., Risier, T., and Vale, W., 1987, Evidence for local stimulation of ACTH secretion by corticotropin-releasing factor in the human placenta, *Nature* **328:**717–719.

Pharriss, B. B., 1970, Vascular control of luteal steroidogenesis, *J. Reprod. Fertil.* (Suppl. 10):97–103.

Pope, C. E., Pope, V. Z., and Beck, L. R., 1982, Development of baboon preimplantation embryos to postimplanation stages *in vitro*, *Biol. Reprod.* **27:**915–923.

Porter, D. G., 1974, Inhibition of myometrial activity in the pregnant rabbit: Evidence for a "new" factor, *Biol. Reprod.* **10:**54–61.

Porter, D. G., 1984, Relaxin: A multipurpose hormone, in: *Endocrinology International Congress Series* No. 655 (F. Labrie and L. Proulx, eds.), Elsevier, New York, pp. 522–526.

Power, S. G. A., and Challis, J. R. G., 1983, Activity of 3α-hydroxysteroid dehydrogenase 5.4-en isomerase in chorioallantois and amnion from pregnant sheep, *J. Endocrinol.* **97:**347–356.

Power, S. G. A., and Challis, J. R. G., 1987, Steroid production by dispersed cells from fetal membranes and intrauterine tissues of sheep, *J. Reprod. Fertil.* **81**:65–76.

Power, W. A., and Challis, J. R. G., 1986, Influence of 20α-dihydroprogesterone on progesterone output by human chorion explants, *Gynecol. Obstet. Invest.* **22**:73–78.

Reyes, F. I., Winter, J. S. D., Faiman, C., and Hobson, W. C., 1975, Serial serum levels of gonadotropins, prolactin and sex steroids in the nonpregnant and pregnant chimpanzee, *Endocrinology* **96**:1447–1455.

Reynolds, L. P., Magness, R. R., and Ford, S. P., 1984, Uterine blood flow during early pregnancy in ewes: Interaction between the conceptus and the ovary bearing the corpus luteum, *J. Anim. Sci.* **58**:423–429.

Roberts, J. S., McCracken, J. A., Gavagan, J. E., and Soloff, M. S., 1976, Oxytocin stimulated release of prostaglandin F$_{2\alpha}$ from ovine endometrium *in vitro:* Correlation with oestrus cycle and oxytocin receptor binding, *Endocrinology* **99**:1107–1114.

Robertson, H. A., 1977, Reproduction in the ewe and goat, in: *Reproduction in Domestic Animals,* third edition (H. H. Cole and P. T. Cupps, eds.), New York, Academic Press, pp. 477–498.

Robertson, H. A., and King, G. J., 1974, Plasma concentrations of progesterone, oestrone, oestradiol-17β and of oestrone sulphate in the pig at implantation, during development and at parturition, *J. Reprod. Fertil.* **40**:133–141.

Robertson, M. C., Gillespie, B., and Friesen, H. G., 1982, Characterization of the two forms of rat placental lactogen (rPL): rPL-I and r PL-II, *Endocrinology* **111**:1862–1866.

Roche, J. F., Foster, D. L., Karsch, F. J., Cook, B., and Dziuk, P. J., 1970, Levels of luteinizing hormone in sera and pituitaries of ewes during the estrous cycle and anestrus, *Endocrinology* **86**:568–572.

Roman-Ponce, H., Thatcher, W. W., Caton, D., Barron, D. H., and Wilcox, C. J., 1978, Thermal stress effects on uterine blood flow in dairy cows, *J. Anim. Sci.* **46**:175–180.

Rosenfeld, C. R., 1980, Responses of reproductive and nonreproductive tissues to 17β-estradiol during ovine puerperium, *Am. J. Physiol.* **239**:E333–E339.

Rothchild, I., 1981, The regulation of the mammalian corpus luteum, *Recent Prog. Horm. Res.* **37**:183–298.

Rothchild, I., and Gibori, G., 1975, The luteotrophic effect of decidual tissue: The stimulating effect of decidualization on serum progesterone level of pseudopregnant rats, *Endocrinology* **97**:838–842.

Rowson, L. E. A., Tervit, H. R., and Brand, A., 1972, The use of prostaglandins for synchronization of oestrus in cattle, *J. Reprod. Fertil.* **29**:145.

Ryan, J. N., and Woessner, J. F., Jr., 1972, Oestradiol inhibits collagen breakdown in the involuting rat uterus, *Biochem. J.* **127**:705–713.

Sanchez-Criado, J., and Rothchild, I., 1986, The relationship between the effects of hysterectomy, decidual tissue, prolactin or luteinizing hormone (LH) and the ability of indomethacin to prevent luteolysis in rat bearing LH-dependent corpora lutea, *Endocrinology* **119**:1750–1756.

Scaramuzzi, R. J., and Baird, D. T., 1977, Pulsatile release of luteinizing hormone and the secretion of ovarian steroids in sheep during anestrus, *Endocrinology* **101**:1801–1806.

Schams, D., Walters, D. L., Schallenberger, E., Butterman, B., and Karg, H., 1983, Ovarian oxytocin in the cow, *Acta Endocrinol. (Kbh.) [Suppl.]* **253**:147.

Schwartz, N. B., 1964, Acute effects of ovariectomy on pituitary LH, uterine weight, and vaginal cornification, *Am. J. Physiol.* **207**:1251–1259.

Shaikh, A. A., 1971, Estrone and estradiol levels in ovarian venous blood from rats during the estrous cycle and pregnancy, *Biol. Reprod.* **5**:297–307.

Shaikh, A. A., and Abraham, G. E., 1969, Measurement of estrogen surge during pseudopregnancy in rats by radioimmunoassay, *Biol. Reprod.* **1**:378–380.

Shelesnyak, M. C., and Tic, L., 1963, Studies on the mechanism of nidation. IV. Synthetic processes in the decidualizing uterus, *Acta Endocrinol. (Kbh.)* **42**:465–472.

Shelesnyak, M. C., Marcus, G. J., and Lindner, H. R., 1970, Determinants of the decidual reaction, in: *Ovo-implantation, Human Gonadotropins, and Prolactin* (P. O. Hubinont, F. Leroy, C. Robyn, and P. Leleux, eds.), Karger, Basel, pp. 118–129.

Shemesh, M., and Hansel, W., 1974, Measurement of bovine plasma testosterone by radioimmunoassay (RIA) and by a rapid competitive protein binding (CPB) assay, *J. Anim. Sci.* **39**:720–724.

Shemesh, M., and Hansel, W., 1975, Levels of prostaglandin F (PGF) in bovine endometrium, uterine venous, ovarian arterial, and jugular plasma during the estrous cycle, *Proc. Soc. Exp. Biol. Med.* **148**:123–126.

Shemesh, M., Milaguir, F., Ayalon, N., and Hansel, W., 1979, Steroidogenesis and prostaglandin synthesis by cultured bovine blastocysts, *J. Reprod. Fertil.* **56**:181–185.

Shemesh, M., Hansel, W., and Strauss, J. F., III, 1984, Calcium-dependent, cyclic nucleotide-independent steroidogenesis in the bovine placenta, *Proc. Natl. Acad. Sci. U.S.A.* **81**:6403–6407.

Sherwood, O. D., and Rutherford, J. E., 1981, Relaxin immunoactivity levels in ovarian extracts obtained from rats during various reproductive states and from adult cycling pigs, *Endocrinology* **108**:1171–1177.

Sherwood, O. D., Wilson, M. E., Edgerton, L. A., and Chang, C. C., 1978, Serum relaxin concentrations in pigs with parturition delayed by progesterone administration, *Endocrinology* **102**:471–475.

Sherwood, O. D., Nara, B. S., Crnekovic, V. E., and First, N. L., 1979, Relaxin concentrations in pig plasma after the administration of indomethacin and prostaglandin $F_{2\alpha}$ during late pregnancy, *Endocrinology* **104**:1716–1721.

Sherwood, O. D., Crnekovic, V. E., Gordon, W. L., and Rutherford, J. E., 1980, Radioimmunoassay of relaxin throughout pregnancy and during parturition in the rat, *Endocrinology* **107**:691–698.

Shibasaki, T., Odagiri, E., Shizume, K., and Ling, J., 1982, Corticotropin-releasing factor-like activity in human placental extracts, *J. Clin. Endocrinol. Metab.* **55**:384–386.

Short, R. V., McDonald, M. E., and Rowson, L. E. A., 1963, Steroids in the ovarian venous blood of ewes before and after gonadotrophic stimulation, *J. Endocrinol.* **26**:155–169.

Sin, J. G., Eto, T., Hashimoto, I., and Suzuki, Y., 1971, Participation of pregnant uterus upon the gestagen secretion during midpregnancy in the rat, *Endocrinol. Jpn.* **18**:495–500.

Singhal, R., and LaFreniere, R. T., 1972, Metabolic control mechanisms in mammalian system, XV. Studies on the role of adenosine 3′, 5′-monophosphate in estrogen action on the uterus, *J. Pharmacol. Exp. Ther.* **180**:86–97.

Smith, R. E., and Farquhar, M. G., 1966, Lysosome function in the regulation of the secretory process in cells of the anterior pituitary gland, *J. Cell Biol.* **31**:319–347.

Smith, R. E., and Henzl, M. R., 1969, Role of mucopolysaccharides and lysosomal hydrolases in endometrial regression following withdrawal of estradiol and chlormadinone acetate, I. Epithelium and stroma, *Endocrinology* **85**:50–66.

Sridaran, R., and Gibori, G., 1983, Control of placental and ovarian secretion of testosterone in the pregnant rat, in: *Factors Regulating Ovarian Function* (G. S. Greenwald and P. F. Terranova, eds.), Raven Press, New York, pp. 87–91.

Stabenfeldt, G. H., Osburn, B. I., and Ewing, L. L., 1970, Peripheral plasma progesterone levels in the cow during pregnancy and parturition, *Am. J. Physiol.* **218**:571–575.

Stabenfeldt, G. H., Drost, M., and Franti, C., 1972, Peripheral plasma progesterone levels in the ewe during pregnancy and parturition, *Endocrinology* **90**:114–150.

Stoner, C. S., Geisert, R. D., Bazer, F. W., and Thatcher, W. W., 1981, Characterization of estrogen patterns in early pregnancy and cyclic gilts, *J. Anim. Sci.* **53**(Suppl. 1):308.

Stormshak, F., Zelinsk-Wosten, M. B., and Abdelgadir, S. E., 1987, Comparative aspects of the regulation of the corpus luteum function in various species, *Adv. Exp. Med. Biol.* **219**:327–360.

Strauss, J. F., Foley, B., and Stambaugh, R., 1972, 20α-Hydroxysteroid dehydrogenase activity in the rabbit ovary, *Biol. Reprod.* **6**:78–86.

Summerlee, A. J. S., O'Byrne, K. T., Paisley, A. C., Breeze, M. F., and Porter, D. G., 1984, Relaxin affects the central control of oxytocin release, *Nature* **309**:372–374.

Sundaram, K., Connell, K. G., and Passantino, T., 1975, Implication of absence of hCG-like gonadotrophin in the blastocyst for control of corpus luteum function in the pregnant rabbit, *Nature* **256**:739–741.

Szego, C. M., and Seeler, B. M., 1973, Hormone induced activation of target-specific lysosomes: Acute translocation to the nucleus after administration of gonadal hormones *in vivo*, *J. Endocrinol.* **56**:347–360.

Tachi, C., Tachi, S., and Lindner, H. R., 1971, Studies on estradiol-binding in mammalian tissues, *Adv. Biosci.* **7**:40–43.

Tachi, C., Tachi, S., and Lindner, H. R., 1972, Modification by progesterone of oestradiol-induced cell proliferation, RNA synthesis, and oestradiol distribution in the rat uterus, *J. Reprod. Fertil.* **31**:59–76.

Tachi, C., Tachi, S., and Lindner, H. R., 1974, Effect of ovarian hormones upon nucleolar ultrastructure in endometrial stromal cells of the rat, *Biol. Reprod.* **10**:404–413.

Takai, Y., Kaibuchi, K., Matsubara, T., and Nishizuka, Y., 1981, Inhibitory action of guanosine 3′,5′-monophosphate on thrombin-induced phosphatidylinositol turnover and protein phosphorylation in human platelets, *Biochem. Biophys. Res. Commun.* **101**:61–67.

Taylor, M. J., Clark, C. L., and Frawley, L. S., 1988, Analysis of relaxin release by reverse hemotylic plaque assay: Influence of gestational age and $PGF_{2\alpha}$, *Endocrinology* **120**:2085–2091.

Tchernitchin, A. N., 1983, Eosinophil-medicated non-genomic parameters of estrogen stimulation: A separate group of responses mediated by an independent mechanism, *J. Steroid Biochem.* **19**:95–100.

Tchernitchin, A. N., and Galand, P., 1982, Dissociation of separate mechanisms of estrogen action by actinomycin D, *Experientia* **38**:511–513.

Tchernitchin, A. N., and Galand, P., 1983, Oestrogen levels in the blood, not in the uterus, determine uterine eosinophilia and oedema, *J. Endocrinol.* **99**:123–130.

Tchernitchin, A. N., Mena, M. A., Rodriguez, A., and Maturana, M., 1985, Radioautographic localization of estrogen receptors in the uterus: A tool for the study of classical and nontraditional mechanisms of hormone action, in: *Localization of Putative Steroid Receptors,* Vol. 1. (L. P. Pertschuk and S. H. Lee, eds.), CRC Press, Boca Raton, FL, pp. 5–37.

Tervit, H. R., Rowson, L. E. A., and Brand, A., 1973, Synchronization of oestrus in cattle using a prostaglandin $F_{2\alpha}$ analogue (ICI 79939), *J. Reprod. Fertil.* **34:**179–181.

Thatcher, W. W., Knickerbocker, J. J., Bartol, F. F., Bazer, F. W., and Drost, M., 1985, Maternal recognition of pregnancy in relation to the survival of transferred embryos: Endocrine aspects, *Theriogenology* **23:**129–144.

Thau, R. B., and Lanman, J. T., 1974, Evaluation of progesterone synthesis in rabbit placentas, *Endocrinology* **94:**925–926.

Thau, R. B., and Lanman, J. T., 1975, Metabolic clearance rates (MCR) and production rates (PR) of plasma progesterone in pregnant and pseudopregnant rabbits, *Endocrinology* **97:**454–457.

Thomas, C. R., Lowy, C., St. Hillaire, R. J., and Brunzell, F. D., 1984, Studies on the placental hydrolysis and transfer of lipids to the fetal guinea pig, in: *Fetal Nutrition, Metabolism and Immunology, the Role of the Placenta* (R. K. Miller and H. A. Thiede, eds.), Plenum Press, New York, pp. 135–148.

Thorburn, G. D., Cox, R. I., Currie, W. B., Restall, B. J., and Schneider, W., 1972, Prostaglandin F concentration in the utero–ovarian venous plasma of the ewe during the oestrous cycle, *J. Endocrinol.* **53:**325–326.

Torday, J. S., Jefcoate, C. R., and First, N. L., 1980, Effect of prostaglandin $F_{2\alpha}$ on steroidogenesis by porcine corpora lutea, *J. Reprod. Fertil.* **58:**301–310.

Ueda, K., Ochiai, K., and Rothchild, I., 1985, A luteotropic action of prolactin: Suppression of intraluteal progesterone production or effect? *Endocrinology* **116:**772–778.

Ursely, J., and Leymarie, P., 1979, Varying response to luteinizing hormone of two luteal cell types isolated from the bovine corpus luteum, *J. Endocrinol.* **83:**303–310.

Van de Wiel, D. F. M., Erkens, J., Koops, W., Vos, E., and Van Landeghem, A. A. J., 1981, Perestrous, and mid-luteal time courses of circulating LH, FSH, prolactin, estradiol-17β and progesterone in the domestic pig, *Biol. Reprod.* **24:**223–233.

Velardo, J. T., Olsen, A. G., Hisaw, F. L., and Dawson, A. B., 1953, The influence of decidual tissue upon pseudopregnancy, *Endocrinology* **53:**216–220.

Veldhuis, T. D., Yoshid, K., DuBois, W., and Fields, M. T., 1987, Maitotoxin stimulates steroid and peptide secretion by swine luteal tissue, *Am. J. Physiol.* **252:**E8–12.

Warshaw, M. L., Johnson, D. C., Khan, I., Eckstein, B., and Gibori, G., 1986, Placental secretion of androgens in the rat, *Endocrinology* **119:**2642–2648.

Wathes, D. C., and Swann, R. W., 1982, Is oxytocin an ovarian hormone? *Nature* **297:**225–227.

Wathes, D. C., Swann, R. W., Pickering, B. T., Porter, D. G., Hull, M. G. R., and Driefe, J. O., 1982, Neurohypophysial hormones in the human ovary, *Lancet* **2:**410–412.

Wathes, D. C., Swann, R. W., Birkett, S. D., Porter, D. G., and Pickering, B. T., 1983a, Characterization of oxytocin, vasopressin and neurophysin from the bovine corpus luteum, *Endocrinology* **113:**693–698.

Wathes, D. C., Swann, R. W., Hull, M. G. R., Drief, J. O., Porter, D. G., and Pickering, B. T., 1983b, Gonadal sources of the posterior pituitary hormones, *Prog. Brain Res.* **60:**513–520.

Wathes, D. C., Swann, R. W., Porter, D. G., and Pickering R. I., 1986, Oxytocin as an ovarian hormone, in: *Current Topics in Neuroendocrinology,* Vol. 6 (D. Ganten and D. Pfaff, eds.), Springer-Verlag, Berlin, Heidelberg, pp. 129–152.

Weick, R. E., Dierschke, D. J., Karsch, F. J., Butler, W. R., Hotchkiss, J., and Knobil, E., 1973, Periovulatory time courses of circulating gonadotropic and ovarian hormones in the rhesus monkey, *Endocrinology* **93:**1140–1147.

Wiest, W. G., 1970, Progesterone and 20α-hydroxypregn-4-en-3-one in plasma, ovaries, and uteri during pregnancy in the rat, *Endocrinology* **87:**43–48.

Wiest, W. G., Kidwell, W. R., and Balogh, K., Jr., 1968, Progesterone catabolism in the ovary; a regulatory mechanism for progestational potency during pregnancy, *Endocrinology* **82:**844–859.

Wilson, L., Jr., Butcher, R. L., Cenedella, R. J., and Inskeep, E. K., 1972a, Effects of progesterone on endometrial prostaglandins in sheep, *Prostaglandins* **1:**183–190.

Wilson, L., Jr., Cenedella, R. J., Butcher, R. L., and Inskeep, E. K., 1972b, Levels of prostaglandins in the uterine endometrium during the ovine estrous cycle, *J. Anim. Sci.* **34:**93–99.

Winkel, C. A., Snyder, J. M., MacDonald, P. C., and Simpson, E. R., 1980, Regulation of cholesterol and progesterone synthesis in human placental cells in culture by serum lipoproteins, *Endocrinology* **106:**1054–1060.

Woessner, J. F., Jr., 1962, Catabolism of collagen and non-collagen protein in the rat uterus during postpartum involution, *Biochem. J.* 83:304–314.

Woessner, J. F., Jr., 1965, Acid hydroxylases of the rat uterus in relation to pregnancy, postpartum involution, and collagen breakdown, *Biochem. J.* **97:**855–866.

Woessner, J. R., Jr., and Celio, J. R., 1974, Effect of injury on collagen resorption in the involuting rat uterus, *Proc. Soc. Exp. Biol. Med.* **147:**475–478.

Wood, J. C., and Barley, V. L., 1970, Biochemical changes in forming and regressing deciduoma in the rat uterus, *J. Reprod. Fertil.* **23:**469–475.

Yoshinaga, K., Hawkins, R. A., and Stocker, J. L., 1969, Estrogen secretion by the rat ovary *in vivo* during the estrous cycle and pregnancy, *Endocrinology* **85:**103–112.

17

Endocrine Control of Parturition

MELVYN S. SOLOFF

1. Problems in Understanding Basic Mechanisms of Parturition

In their introduction to the previous edition, Thorburn *et al.* (1977) stated: ''We now recognize that in late pregnancy a train of events is initiated that ultimately results in the delivery of the fetus. However, we still do not know exactly how and where the train starts, or exactly how it exerts its ultimate action on the myometrial cell.'' Little has changed in the last decade to increase our understanding of these events. Although the initiation of parturition is generally understood, the precise trigger for labor is still unknown. In addition, labor is complicated by different mechanisms in different species. For example, the onset of labor in rats and rabbits is rapid: uterine contractions become intense immediately before delivery, and the newborn are expelled rapidly. In humans, monkeys, and guinea pigs, labor develops slowly and is protracted. Schofield (1968) suggested that in species with a large fetus relative to the mother, a more protracted delivery may be an advantage. In the human and monkey, uterine motility evolves gradually during the last trimester of pregnancy, and actual labor often precedes delivery by many hours. It is possible that different mechanisms are at play in rapid-onset and protracted-onset types of labor.

Generally, attempts to explain the initiation of labor have focused on labor-associated changes in the circulating concentrations of hormones in both fetus and mother. They illuminated the importance of the fetal production of cortisol in the initiation of labor in sheep, cows, and goats. In other species, however, the important factor may be the changes in receptor levels for specific hormones. Examples of both agonist and receptor regulation of myometrial activity are cited in Sections 3 and 4.

Many investigators believe that the maintenance of the pregnant uterus results from a balance between factors promoting and inhibiting the termination of pregnancy, such as the balance between oxytocic agents and progesterone. Reduction in progesterone reduces the quiescent state of the uterine musculature, resulting in labor contractions.

MELVYN S. SOLOFF ● Department of Biochemistry, Medical College of Ohio, Toledo, Ohio 43699.

559

In the rat and rabbit, the concentration of progesterone decreases in the maternal peripheral plasma before labor, and delivery is usually preceded by an increase in the concentration of circulating estrogen. Gestation can be abruptly terminated by administration of agents that block the synthesis of progesterone. The administration of progesterone prevents the effects of these agents and prolongs gestation in otherwise untreated animals.

Withdrawal of progesterone from the systemic maternal circulation is not required in primates and guinea pigs for the initiation of parturition. In these species, maternal plasma progesterone levels remain elevated until delivery of the placenta. Labor cannot be prolonged by administration of progesterone. Therefore, although progesterone withdrawal may be important in some species, it does not readily explain the onset of labor in others.

To add to the complexity, parturition may be triggered by several initiating agents. Triggering of the expulsion of the newborn requires the interplay of multiple endocrine factors that prepare uterine cells to respond to the appropriate uterotonic stimuli. In some cases, it is difficult to distinguish between the action of an agent in the development of the response and in the response itself.

Despite the present lack of understanding of the precise sequence of molecular events leading to labor contractions, however, there are some features of parturition common to all species, suggesting that mechanisms involved in labor initiation may be basically the same. These include roles for estrogens and prostaglandins. In addition, the sensitivity of the uterine musculature to oxytocin is greatest at the time of labor in all species studied, suggesting an important role for this peptide. These common features of parturition are discussed in the sections that follow.

2. Preparation of the Uterus for Labor: Estrogen

Estrogens are vital for the preparation of the uterus for parturition, but it is not clear whether increases in blood estrogen levels at the end of gestation serve as a trigger for the initiation of labor. Estrogen treatment results in hyperplasia and hypertrophy of uterine cells and in stimulation of the synthesis of contractile proteins, metabolic enzymes, and ATP (Marshall, 1974). Estrogens also contribute to the sharp rise in glycogen content of the rat myometrium just before labor (Chew and Rinard, 1979). In addition, estrogens elicit heterologous up-regulation of hormone and growth factor receptors in the myometrium. These include receptors for oxytocin, α-adrenergic agonists, serotonin (Ichida, 1983), angiotensin II (Schirar et al., 1980), and epidermal growth factor (Mukku and Stancel, 1985). Estrogens also stimulate the biosynthesis of prostaglandins; they regulate myometrial levels of calcium and modify the phosphorylation of specific proteins in the myometrium at the time of labor, so that putative second messenger pathways also are stimulated. Changes in the phosphorylation of specific myometrial proteins at the time of labor in the rat (Fig. 1) can be mimicked in nonpregnant animals by administration of estrogen (Joseph et al., 1982). Estrogen also induces oxytocin-inhibited (Ca^{2+}, Mg^{2+})-ATPase activity in rat myometrium (Soloff and Sweet, 1982).

Estrogens regulate membrane components involved in the permeability of Na^+, K^+, and Cl^-, which are responsible for the resting membrane potential and electrical excitability of myometrial cells (Marshall, 1974). Injection of poly(A)$^+$ RNA from estrogen-treated rat uteri into frog oocytes resulted in the expression of a very slow-activating votage-dependent postassium current (Boyle et al., 1987). The mRNA expressing the channel was rapidly and reversibly induced by estrogen, as indicated by its appearance and disappearance during the estrous cycle, its reappearance at the end of pregnancy when the uterus is estrogen dominated, and its induction by estrogen treatment in ovariectomized rats. Garfield and colleagues (1980) have shown that estrogens appear to promote synchronous uterine contractility by stimulating

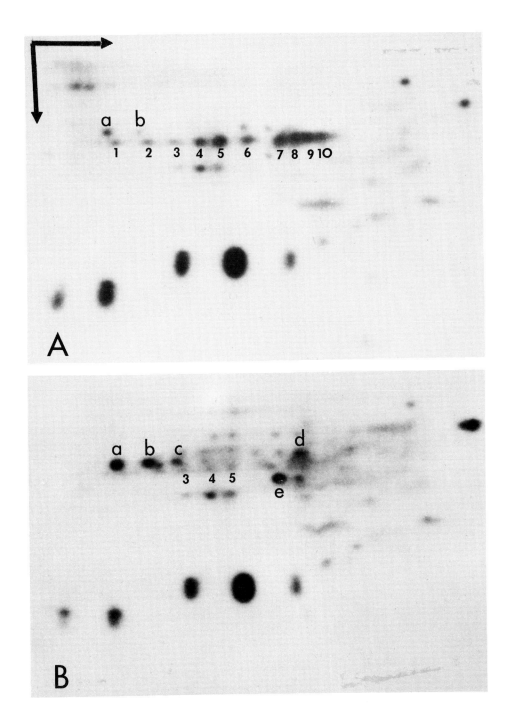

Figure 1. Changes in the phosphorylation of specific rat myometrial proteins during labor, as demonstrated by two-dimensional gel electrophoresis. (A) Day 19 of pregnancy. (B) Labor. Myometrial minces were incubated with $^{32}P_i$ for 60 min, and the proteins were analyzed for incorporation of radioactivity after electrophoresis by fluorography. Labor-specific phosphoproteins are indicated by a–e. From Joseph *et al.* (1982).

the formation of gap junctions between adjacent myometrial cells. The estrogen up-regulation of progesterone receptors (Vu Hai *et al.*, 1977) may explain why many of the physiological effects of progesterone are dependent on previous exposure to estrogen.

Estrogens also are involved in cervical maturation: collagen breakdown in the cervix is caused by increasing collagenase synthesis and activation. Overall, estrogen actions on the myometrium include metabolic, membrane, and structural changes that promote spontaneous contractility and enhance myometrial responsiveness to many agonists.

As an example of the importance of estrogens in primates, suppression of adrenal estrogen precursor formation in rhesus monkeys prolonged pregnancy (Novy, 1983). Treatment of monkeys for about the last 65 days of pregnancy (gestation length about 167 days) with dexamethasone caused adrenal atrophy, reduced basal levels of maternal estradiol (but not progesterone), and abolished the prepartum estrogen surge. More than 70% of the fetuses were born after day 175 of gestation. However, large doses of estradiol benzoate administered systemically to pregnant rhesus monkeys did not cause premature labor unless the fetuses were dead (Walsh *et al.*, 1979a). Such findings indicate that estrogens are important in primates for the development of the ability of the uterus to contract at the end of gestation, but they do not play a role in triggering labor. In other species, however, the administration of estrogen near the end of gestation is a very effective means of inducing premature labor (see Thorburn and Challis, 1979, for references), perhaps by estrogen-induced increases in the concentration of oxytocin receptors and the number of myometrial gap junctions.

2.1. Possible Regulation of Estrogen Action at the Receptor Level

The concentrations of estrogen receptors in both the nuclear fraction and the cytosol of rat myometrium increased abruptly, were maximal near the time of labor, and fell abruptly after parturition (Fig. 2). Because estrogen up-regulates its own receptor concentration (Pavlik and Coulson, 1976), it is likely that the occurrence of estrogen dominance in the rat before parturition is enhanced by increases in both circulating estrogen concentrations and receptor number. In contrast to the rat, no significant labor-related changes in estrogen receptor concentrations appeared in human uteri (Giannopoulos *et al.*, 1980). In humans increased plasma estrogen concentrations may be sufficient to bring about estrogen dominance at the end of gestation.

2.2. The Role of Estrogens in Humans

The importance of estrogens in human pregnancy is controversial. Pinto *et al.* (1967), using a double-blind design, gave intravenous infusions of either estradiol or vehicle to equal numbers of women at term. Those given estradiol went into spontaneous labor significantly sooner or required significantly lower doses of intravenous oxytocin for labor induction. Estrogen administration seemed to facilitate the onset of labor (Järvinen *et al.*, 1965). However, Klopper and Dennis (1962) found no effect of estrogen on the length of labor.

2.3. Identification of Active Estrogens in Humans

Darne and co-workers (1987) suggested that estriol is more active in the human than is usually assumed. Estriol was considered to be a weak or impeded estrogen because there was no sustained uterine growth following a single injection of estriol compared with a similar dose of estradiol. Repeated doses of estriol, rather than a single injection, produced a full uterine

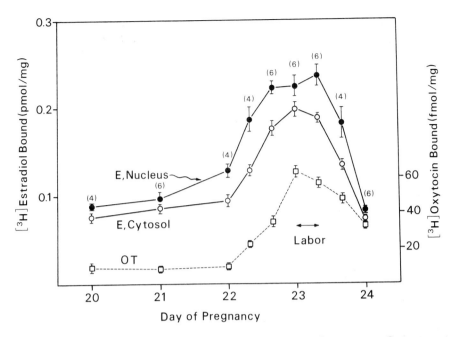

Figure 2. Increases in the concentration of estrogen receptors in the nuclear (●) and cytosol (○) fractions of rat myometrium preceding labor. Each point is the mean ± S.E., with the number of rats shown in parentheses. Oxytocin (OT) receptor concentrations in the myometrium are also shown. From Alexandrova and Soloff (1980a).

growth response similar to that to estradiol (Clark and Markaverich, 1984). The apparent weakness of estriol could be explained partly by its shorter half-life in plasma and its shorter occupancy of uterine estrogen receptors.

Both human endometrium and myometrium have the ability to accumulate tritium-labeled estriol and estradiol with equal facility following continuous infusion of subphysiological doses before hysterectomy (Wiegerinck *et al.*, 1983). Estriol is as effective as estradiol in stimulating $PGF_{2\alpha}$ production by human endometrial cells in culture (Schatz *et al.*, 1984). Darne and co-workers (1987) found that the ratio of estriol to progesterone in the saliva of women was maximal near the time of labor. These workers suggested that a fine balance is maintained between free progesterone and free estriol and estradiol throughout pregnancy until a few weeks before delivery. The surge in the estriol : progesterone ratio secondary to the rise in estriol levels than overcomes the myometrial stabilizing effect of progesterone and provokes the changes in the uterus (such as an increase in the number of oxytocin receptors and gap junctions, an increase in the synthesis and release of prostaglandins, and an increase in the levels of free intracellular calcium) that are necessary for normal labor.

2.4. *Control of Estrogen Levels*

The endocrine mechanisms regulating parturition in ruminants or laboratory animals and primates differ in several respects. The primate fetus contributes estrogens by adrenal production of estrogen precursors (i.e., androstenedione and dehydroepiandrosterone sulfate), which are converted to estrogens by the placenta (Diczfalusy, 1974; Walsh *et al.*, 1980). The fetus thus provides a mechanism for the endocrine control of parturition.

It has not been possible to demonstrate that the human fetus is involved in the initiation of labor. The human fetal pituitary–adrenal axis, however, plays an indirect role by the secretion of estrogen precursors by the fetal zone of the fetal adrenal, thereby increasing the plasma concentration of estrogen in mother and fetus. In women, there is a gradual but steady increase in plasma estradiol-17β and estrone sulfate concentrations from 36 weeks of gestation. In normal rhesus monkeys, estradiol and estrone concentrations increase gradually and significantly in maternal blood during the 7 to 10 days preceding spontaneous vaginal delivery (Novy, 1983). Progesterone does not decrease before parturition and may increase.

The stimulus for the rise in fetal and maternal estrogens before parturition is unknown, but a functioning fetal adrenal in monkeys is required because the prepartum estrogen trends are absent when the fetus is dead or functionally hypophysectomized (Walsh et al., 1979a). In addition, the administration of ACTH, but not other peptides, to the fetus results in augmented fetal dehydroepiandrosterone sulfate, androstenedione, progesterone, and estrogen concentrations (Walsh et al., 1979b). Continuous infusion of ACTH to the fetus also produced elevated estrogen levels in the amniotic fluid (Novy, 1983). It remains to be shown in rhesus monkeys, however, that levels of ACTH rise in fetal plasma before parturition.

3. Uterine Quiescence

3.1. Progesterone

The inhibitory effect of progesterone on myometrial activity has been referred to as "progesterone block" (Csapo, 1956). It is characterized by a dose-dependent suppression of the amplitude of myometrial contractions, reduction in the rate of rise of pressure during intrauterine pressure cycles, and loss of reactivity to oxytocic agents (Csapo 1956; Schofield 1957; Csapo and Takeda, 1965). Marshall (1959) found that progesterone treatment of estrogen-primed ovariectomized rats increased the membrane potential in single uterine fibers and caused the dissociation of contractile activity of the whole uterus from spike discharges. These results suggested to Kao (1976) that local groups of myometrial cells became electrically independent following progesterone treatment. This suggestion is supported by later observations that progesterone treatment caused a sharp reduction in the number of myometrial gap junctions (Garfield et al., 1980). The progesterone-induced impairment in the spread of excitation explains the reduced amplitude and rate of intrauterine pressure cycles. Many of the effects of progesterone also may be related to its antagonism of estrogen actions, possibly at the level of estrogen receptors (Pavlik and Coulson, 1976; Clark et al., 1977).

In part because of the ability of progesterone to maintain myometrial activity in a blocked state, Csapo proposed that the decline of circulating progesterone levels in species like the rat and rabbit results in increased excitability of the myometrium by lowering the threshold for excitation by endogenous oxytocic agents (Csapo, 1975). In the rat, ovariectomy (progesterone withdrawal) in late pregnancy resulted in premature labor, which was prevented by the administration of exogenous progesterone (Csapo and Wiest, 1969). The importance of progesterone withdrawal in the termination of gestation in rodents is further evident from observations that several pregnancy-interceptive agents operating by different mechanisms all reduce circulating progesterone concentrations (Creange et al., 1978; Raziano et al., 1972; Glasser et al., 1972; Warnock and Csapo, 1975; Csapo and Resch, 1979; Fuchs et al., 1974; Strauss et al., 1975). The effects of these agents, which include inhibitors of progesterone synthesis, luteolytic prostaglandins, antisera to progesterone, and a progesterone antagonist, were reversed by the administration of progesterone. Only partial restoration of progesterone levels was required to block the ability of $PGF_{2\alpha}$ to induce premature labor in rats (Fuchs et al., 1974; Alexandrova and Soloff, 1980b). The reduction of plasma progesterone to as little as 20% of the initial levels by $PGF_{2\alpha}$ treatment was compatible with undisturbed gestation, whereas a drop to 15% of the initial levels was associated with the termination of pregnancy (Fuchs *et al.*, 1974).

A fall in plasma progesterone concentrations near the end of gestation does not occur in all species (e.g., guinea pig and human). Progesterone also does not inhibit myometrial activity in the guinea pig (Zarrow *et al.*, 1963; Schofield, 1964). Csapo (1975) argued that measurement of blood levels of progesterone in species in which the steroid is produced by the placenta may not reflect the concentrations seen at uterine target cells because progesterone presumably is transported to the uterus locally. Infusion of progesterone into the maternal circulation may not increase the amounts available locally. Despite the lack of a preparturitional fall in blood progesterone levels in humans and the absence of any effect of progesterone administration on the length of gestation, an important role for progesterone is illustrated by the ability of a progesterone antagonist, RU486, to initate labor in humans. RU486, which inhibits progesterone action by competing for receptor sites, induced labor and delivery in women with dead fetuses at about 24 weeks of pregnancy (Cabrol *et al.*, 1985). Although RU486 also antagonizes the effects of glucocorticoids, the dose used minimized this effect. These findings suggest that progesterone might play an important role in labor in humans, as in other species. The actions of progesterone in humans may not be regulated by levels of the steroid in the blood but by changing levels of its receptors.

The production and metabolism of progesterone and estrogen by intrauterine tissues have been studied with the idea that they act on uterine cells in a paracrine fashion. Human amnion, chorion, and decidua converted pregnenolone to progesterone (Gibb *et al.*, 1978; Mitchell *et al.*, 1982). The conversion by either dispersed cells from chorion and decidua or explants maintained in culture was lower in tissues obtained at spontaneous labor than in tissues obtained at term but before labor (elective cesarean section) (Challis and Vaughan, 1987; Mitchell *et al.*, 1987). Because there was no increased rate of progesterone metabolism by human fetal membranes (Milewich *et al.*, 1977), the reduced rate of synthesis may bring about "local progesterone withdrawal." The reduced conversion of pregnenolone to progesterone by human fetal membranes *in vitro* during spontaneous labor may be the result of estrone or estradiol inhibition. Both estrogens are increased locally at the end of term (Mitchell *et al.*, 1982).

3.1.1. Mechanisms of Progesterone Withdrawal

In the cow, rabbit, goat, and rat, the major source of progesterone in peripheral plasma is the corpus luteum (for a review see Thorburn and Challis, 1979), and a mechanism exists for the reduction of luteal production of progesterone. In the goat and sheep, the fetus appears to control partutition through adrenal cortisol output (Thorburn and Challis, 1979). Cortisol-stimulated production of uterine prostaglandins may result in a luteolytic effect with a resultant decrease in progesterone concentrations.

In rats near term, there was an increase in ovarian 20α-hydroxysteroid dehydrogenase and in the corresponding conversion of progesterone to 20α-dihydroxyprogesterone (Wiest *et al.*, 1968). The drop in progesterone levels in the blood was accompanied by an increase in 20α-dihydroxyprogesterone, which has greatly reduced progestational potency (Wiest *et al.*, 1968). Prostaglandin F_α-induced luteolysis in pregnant rats appears to be mediated by an increase in ovarian 20α-hydroxysteroid dehydrogenase activity and a significant drop in plasma progesterone concentrations (Strauss and Stambaugh, 1974). There is strong evidence indicating that $PGF_{2\alpha}$ from the uterus is the physiological mediator of luteolysis in the rat. Prostaglandin $F_{2\alpha}$ is luteolytic in pseudopregnant rabbits, causing a decline in corpus luteum weight and progesterone secretion (Scott and Rennie, 1970; Gutknecht *et al.*, 1972). The administration of the prostaglandin synthesis inhibitor indomethacin prolonged the activity of the corpus luteum in pseudopregnant rabbits (O'Grady *et al.*, 1972). The decline in luteal progesterone secretion in late pregnancy in the rabbit may be determined by the withdrawal of luteotropic support by estrogens. In the rabbit, estrogens are luteotrophic (Hilliard, 1973); administration of the antiestrogen tamoxifen to pregnant rabbits produced a rapid fall in plasma progesterone and caused premature labor (Furr *et al.*, 1976). The sharp decline in progesterone output by the corpus luteum of the rabbit in late pregnancy may result from a combination of increased luteolytic and diminished luteotrophic activities.

Progesterone withdrawal is not limited to species that depend on the corpus luteum for its production. In sheep, progesterone production after day 50 of pregnancy is primarily by the placenta, but plasma progesterone concentrations declined in a variable fashion over the last 5–15 days of pregnancy, following the increase in fetal plasma cortisol (for reviews see Thorburn and Challis, 1979; Liggins *et al.*, 1973). Premature parturition induced by the administration of either ACTH or glucocorticoids to the fetus was preceded by a fall in maternal progesterone concentrations. In sheep, the fall in progesterone concentration is accompanied by a rise in the concentration of the progesterone metabolite $17\alpha,20\alpha$-dihydroxyprogesterone.

Taylor *et al.* (1982) used an inhibitor of 3β-hydroxysteroid dehydrogenase activity to induce progesterone withdrawal in sheep during late pregnancy. They found that a decrease in plasma progesterone preceded premature delivery in most animals. The major site of action of progesterone in pregnant sheep has been suggested to be the maternal component (decidua) rather than the myometrium (Liggins *et al.*, 1973).

3.1.2. Changes in the Balance between Estrogen and Progesterone

Initiation of labor in sheep, goats, and cows is linked to maturation of the fetal hypothalamopituitary–adrenal axis, which results in an increase in fetal cortisol production (for reviews see Liggins *et al.*, 1973; Thorburn and Challis, 1979). Cortisol appears to induce 17-OH hydroxylase activity, resulting in suppression of either placental (sheep) or ovarian (goat) progesterone production and a concomitant stimulation in estrogen secretion. The net result is a hormonal environment favorable to the stimulation of uterine contractions and the termination of gestation, including increased $PGF_{2\alpha}$ production by uterine tissues. Elevations in plasma glucocorticoid, either by direct administration or by administration of ACTH to pregnant sheep, results in premature labor and hormone changes similar to those observed before spontaneous parturition. Glucocorticoids, however, do not appear to be directly involved in the initiation of labor in most other species studied. Maternal plasma cortisol levels essentially remain unchanged in primates during pregnancy, and glucocorticoids administered to monkeys do not induce premature labor (Novy, 1983). Treatment of women in the last trimester of pregnancy with a synthetic corticosteroid for prevention of idiopathic respiratory syndrome likewise did not influence the timing of the onset or the duration of labor (Gennser *et al.*, 1977). Murphy (1982) measured cortisol levels in umbilical cord serum arising from the fetus. She found a steady rise in fetal cortisol levels with increasing gestational age in late pregnancy, regardless of whether labor occurred. The sharp increase in the concentration of cortisol in monkeys on the day of vaginal delivery (Novy, 1983) has been attributed to maternal or fetal stress associated with parturition.

3.2. Relaxin

One of the effects of relaxin in a number of species, when administered either *in vivo* or *in vitro,* is the inhibition of spontaneous uterine contractions (for reviews see Schwabe *et al.*, 1978; Bryant-Greenwood 1982). Relaxin added to a muscle bath reduced the amplitude of contractions of rat uterine strips (Sawyer *et al.*, 1953). *In vivo,* relaxin decreased the frequency of contractions (Porter *et al.*, 1979). Extracts of human corpora lutea of pregnancy inhibited the spontaneous activity of myometrial strips from nonpregnant women (Szlachter *et al.*, 1980), suggesting that relaxin may also have some significance in the human.

Relaxin may be biologically important in preventing premature uterine contractions. Relaxin administered to estrogen-treated ovariectomized rats abolished myometrial activity that was induced by infusions of either oxytocin or $PGF_{2\alpha}$ (Porter *et al.*, 1981). Apparently this phenomenon can be observed only *in vivo*, because the addition of oxytocin or prostaglandins to rat myometrial strips overcame the inhbitory effects of relaxin *in vitro* (Chamley *et al.*, 1977). The *in vivo* and *in vitro* differences of the overriding effects of uterotonic agents on the inhibitory activity of relaxin may be more apparent than real and result from differences in the concentrations of uterotonic agents that are effective *in vivo* and *in vitro*. The effect of relaxin is highly dependent on the uterine response to the dose of oxytocin or $PGF_{2\alpha}$. Sanborn (1986) pointed out that concentrations of oxytocin and $PGF_{2\alpha}$ that promoted only phasic contractions *in vitro* were antagonized by relaxin, whereas relaxin was ineffective as an antagonist at higher concentrations of these uterotonic agents, which caused stronger, tonic uterine contractions.

Relaxin may be important in keeping the myometrium quiescent. The quiescence seen in several species shortly before parturition corresponds temporally with high levels of relaxin in the circulation (Downing and Sherwood, 1985b). Downing and Sherwood (1985b) showed that increasingly prolonged periods of myometrial quiescence that occur in the intact rat during the course of pregnancy, until about 3 hr prepartum, could be mimicked by the administration of porcine relaxin, estradiol, and progesterone to ovariectomized pregnant rats. Without relaxin, there was a significant increase in myometrial activity from day 12 through the remainder of pregnancy. The animals treated with estradiol, progesterone, and relaxin exhibited a pattern of myometrial activity during labor that was similar to that of intact controls.

Relaxin may also contribute to myometrial quiescence by inhibiting oxytocin release. In anesthetized lactating rats, intravenous injections of porcine relaxin suppressed the onset of reflex milk ejection, which is dependent on circulating oxytocin concentrations (Summerlee *et al.*, 1984). Mammary sensitivity to exogenous oxytocin was reduced by relaxin treatment, but not sufficiently to explain the effects observed after relaxin administration. Because injection of relaxin into the cerebral ventricles disturbed the pattern of reflex milk ejection without affecting the response of the mammary gland to oxytocin, the authors suggested that relaxin has a central action on the release of oxytocin. Additional studies showed that inhibition of oxytocin release also occurred after chronic infusion of porcine relaxin into conscious lactating rats (Jones and Summerlee, 1987).

The effects of relaxin on uterine smooth muscle are apparent only after estrogen priming (for a review see Schwabe *et al.*, 1978). Estrogens up-regulate the concentration of relaxin receptors in the myometrium (Mercado-Simmen *et al.*, 1980). The concentration of relaxin receptors in rat myometrial plasma membrane fractions was high at proestrus and estrus and nondectectable for the rest of the cycle (Mercado-Simmen *et al.*, 1980). On the basis of these findings, relaxin receptor levels should be suppressed throughout most of pregnancy, during progesterone domination, and rise sharply near term with the sudden onset of estrogen domination. Instead, receptor levels began to rise at about 15 days, peaked at 17 days, and declined thereafter (Mercado-Simmen *et al.*, 1980). These findings indicate that other factors also may be involved in regulation of relaxin receptor concentrations. Relaxin may down-regulate its own receptor (Mercado-Simmen *et al.*, 1980). The relationship between uterine quiescence and relaxin receptor concentration is uncertain because uterine quiescence is greatest at times when relaxin receptor concentrations are declining.

Relaxin, administered either *in vitro* or *in vivo*, produced small but significant increases in rat uterine cAMP levels (Sanborn *et al.*, 1980; Cheah and Sherwood, 1980; Judson *et al.*, 1980). The increases in intracellular cAMP concentrations are postulated to result in myometrial cell relaxation, by analogy with the mechanism of isoproterenol-induced relaxation.

As with other smooth muscle cells, elevation of intracellular Ca^{2+} concentrations initiates contractions of the myometrial cell by the following mechanism. Increased Ca^{2+} binding to calmodulin results in a Ca^{2+}_4-calmodulin complex that binds to and activates myosin light chain kinase, which catalyzes the phosphorylation of the 20-kDa light-chain subunit of myosin. Myosin phosphorylation results in stimulation of actin-activated ATPase and actin–myosin interactions.

Adelstein and colleagues (1978) observed that avian smooth muscle myosin light chain kinase was phosphorylated by cAMP-dependent protein kinase, resulting in a tenfold increase in the concentration of Ca^{2+}–calmodulin required for half-maximal activation of myosin light chain kinase. Myosin light chain kinase phosphorylated by cAMP-dependent protein kinase requires higher concentrations of cytoplasmic Ca^{2+} for activation. This decrease in sensitivity to Ca^{2+} can result in relaxation or inhibition of contraction and may explain why elevation of intracellular levels of cAMP relaxes uterine smooth muscle. There are, however, observations that are not consistent with the regulation of smooth muscle contractility by cAMP levels: (1) the rate of dissociation of Ca^{2+}–calmodulin from myosin light chain kinase is much slower than the relaxation produced by agents that increase cAMP (Kamm and Stull, 1985); (2) isoproterenol-induced increases in cAMP levels in myometrial cells in culture occurred more than five times faster than relaxin-induced increases (Hsu *et al.*, 1985); (3) cAMP levels were unchanged under conditions of inhibition of contractile activity by relaxin. These finding suggest either that very small changes in cAMP concentrations are effective in mediating relaxin action or that cAMP is not a mediator. The role of cAMP in uterine relaxation is further complicated by the observation that prostaglandins, which stimulate uterine contractions, also caused an elevation in myometrial cell cAMP levels (Vesin *et al.*, 1978). Nishikori *et al.* (1983) showed that relaxin added to the medium bathing myometrial strips from estrogen-primed, $PGF_{2\alpha}$-treated rats decreased the ratio of phosphorylated to nonphosphorylated 20-kDa myosin light chain. Relaxin also decreased myosin light chain kinase activity. The decreases in both the relative amount of phosphorylated light chain and kinase activity paralleled relaxin inhibition of contractile activity with respect to both time and dose.

3.3. Adrenergic Agents

The myometrial response to sympathetic stimulation shifts from contraction in the non-pregnant state to relaxation late in pregnancy. It is now clear that these effects occur through selective activation of α- and β-adrenergic activities, respectively (Ahlquist, 1966). The shift during pregnancy appears to be the result of changing levels of estrogen and progesterone. Estrogen administration enhanced the contractile response of immature rabbit uterus to hypogastric nerve stimulation *in vitro,* whereas progesterone given to estrogen-primed rabbits inhibited spontaneous uterine contractions (Miller and Marshall, 1965). The shift from α to β responses appeared to result in part from modifications of adrenergic receptor concentrations. In the rabbit, the α-adrenergic receptor concentration increased threefold after administration of estrogen, and the estrogen effect was inhibited by progesterone (Roberts *et al.*, 1981; Williams and Lefkowitz, 1977). Estrogen administration had no effect on the number of β-adrenergic receptors. The importance of α-adrenergic receptor regulation in determining an α-adrenergic response, however, is not clear. In the rabbit the increase in α-adrenergic receptor caused by estrogen administration consisted only of an increase in the α_2 subtype, whereas uterine contractions appear to be mediated by the α_1 subtype (Hoffman *et al.*, 1981). In the rat, estrogen administration caused an increase only in the number of myometrial β-adrenergic receptors (Krall *et al.*, 1978). Thus, the mechanisms of steroid regulation of the response to α-adrenergic agents still require clarification.

It also does not appear that β-adrenergic dominance under the influence of progesterone can be explained by receptor changes. Neither the absolute concentration of β receptors nor the ratio of α to β receptors appears to account for the predominance of a β-adrenergic response (Roberts *et al.*, 1981). Progesterone also did not appear to affect the coupling between β receptors and guanosyl nucleotide regulatory proteins because the affinity of the receptors for isoproterenol was not affected by progesterone treatment.

The role of adrenergic stimulation of the uterus during pregnancy is not known. Pregnancy lowers the norepinephrine content, tyrosine hydroxylase activity, axonal uptake of [^{3}H]norepinephrine, and the number of adrenergic nerves in the myometrium (Thorbert, 1978). Complete nerve degeneration occurs by the end of gestation (Thorbert et al., 1979). Progesterone, when elevated for extended periods as in pregnancy, also induces a functional sympathetic denervation of the myometrium (Bell and Malcolm, 1978). Consequently, neural activity has no influence on myometrial function at the time of parturition.

β_2-Adrenergic agonists are among the more useful agents in the treatment of premature labor in humans (see Falck Larsen et al., 1986). The β-mimetic drug ritodrine inhibited preterm labor in the initial stage, resulting in a gain of a few days to a few weeks in length of gestation (Falck Larsen et al., 1986). The ability of β-mimetic therapy to prolong gestation significantly in preterm labor, however, is equivocal (Spellacy et al., 1979; Falck Larsen et al., 1980). Myometrial relaxation followed by desensitization with return of myometrial contractions results from continuous exposure to β-adrenergic agonists both in vivo and in vitro (Andersson et al., 1980). Selective β_2 agonists inhibit myometrial contractibility by activation of receptor-mediated adenylate cyclase, leading to increased cAMP content (Andersson et al., 1980; Harden 1983). The mechanism of desensitization is not completely understood. Downregulation of β receptors, decrease in adenylate cyclase activity, and modifications in interactions of receptor or adenylate cyclase with G proteins may be involved (Harden, 1983).

4. Activators of Uterine Activity

4.1. Prostaglandins

Prostaglandins are produced by nearly all mammalian cells except erythrocytes. Prostaglandins are not stored but are released immediately after synthesis. They act locally and are metabolized by the same cells that produce them or by neighboring cells, and they enter the systemic circulation only as inactive products. Those primary prostaglandins that escape local metabolism are broken down to inactive metabolites after a single pass through the lungs, which have high concentrations of 15-hydroxyprostaglandin dehydrogenase and 13,14-dehydroprostaglandin reductase.

Prostaglandins play an important role in parturition. Following the discovery of prostaglandins in amniotic fluid and in the circulation of women in labor (Karim and Devlin, 1967), Karim proposed that $PGF_{2\alpha}$ was involved in spontaneous labor (Karim, 1971). Prostaglandin$_{2\alpha}$ is used for labor induction and for the induction of abortion between the ninth and 22nd weeks of pregnancy (for references see Karim, 1971).

Because treatment of women with PGE_2 or $PGF_{2\alpha}$ stimulates uterine contractions at any stage of gestation, many investigators assumed that endogenous prostaglandins were involved in the initiation of labor. Indeed, gestation could be extended in a number of species by drugs that block prostaglandin synthesis (Aiken, 1972; Chester et al., 1972; Lewis and Schulman, 1983; Waltman et al., 1973; Novy et al., 1974; Zuckerman et al., 1974; Wiqvist, et al., 1975). Stimuli known to cause prostaglandin release, such as cervical manipulation, stripping of the chorion laeve from the contiguous decidua, and infections of the membranes, usually result in labor near term (Mitchell et al., 1977).

Substantial increases in the concentration of prostaglandins or their metabolites in amniotic fluid (Keirse and Turnbull, 1973; Keirse et al., 1977) and in the maternal circulation (Gréen et al., 1974; Lackritz et al., 1978) during advanced labor have suggested a causal relationship between prostaglandin release and uterine activity. However, *in vivo* production and concentrations of prostaglandins in the intrauterine environment have been difficult to evaluate because of the presence of prostaglandin-synthesizing and -metabolizing enzymes. For example, cellular trauma caused by handling tissues is a major stimulus of prostaglandin production (Piper and Vane, 1971). Abnormally high rates of prostaglandin release may, therefore, be observed for some time after removal of a tissue. The effect of handling was minimized by use of cells separated from tissues and maintained in culture, cultured organ explants, or perifused tissues. Prostaglandin production usually stabilizes at a lower level after an initial burst. Unfortunately, modification of the natural milieu and the interjection of a time interval between obtaining the tissues and making the measurements may alter the characteristics of the response.

Prostaglandin E_2 and $PGF_{2\alpha}$ are produced in largest amounts by uterine and intrauterine tissues during human parturition. The measurement of these prostaglandins in peripheral plasma also is hampered by their low concentrations, rapid clearance from the bloodstream, and the contribution of platelets to prostaglandin production. Estimates of $PGF_{2\alpha}$ levels have been obtained more reliably by measurement of the stable metabolite, PGFM (13,14-dihydro-15 keto $PGF_{2\alpha}$) (Levine and Gutierrez-Cernosek, 1973; Cornette *et al.*, 1974; Samuelsson *et al.*, 1975). The estimate of PGE_2 in peripheral maternal plasma has become more reliable with the development of assays for the stable metabolite, bicyclo-PGEM (11-deoxy-13,14-dehydro-15-keto-13-11β-16ξ-cyclo-PGE_2) (Fitzpatrick *et al.*, 1980; Granström *et al.*, 1980; Bothwell *et al.*, 1982).

Prostaglandin-synthesizing and -degrading enzyme activities are absent in amniotic fluid (Keirse and Turnbull, 1975). Measurement of prostaglandin levels in amniotic fluid, therefore, has been one of the most popular approaches to ascertaining changes in the initiation and progression of labor. Contributing to prostaglandin levels in amniotic fluid are the amnion, which produces primarily PGE_2 (Mitchell *et al.*, 1978; Okazaki *et al.*, 1981; Casey *et al.*, 1984), prostaglandins and metabolites from fetal urine, presumably arising from fetal kidneys (Casey *et al.*, 1983a), and prostaglandins and metabolites produced by other uterine and intrauterine tissues.

Investigators have also measured the rates of production of a variety of prostanoids by intrauterine tissues *in vitro*, both before and after establishment of labor. The rate of production of PGE_2 by amnion homogenates or cultured cells was greater when taken at or after labor than in late gestation in the absence of labor (Okazaki *et al.*, 1981a; Olson *et al.*, 1983a). Likewise, the concentration of prostaglandins in the first voided urine of human babies was greater in infants born after spontaneous labor than in those delivered by cesarean section in the absence of labor (Casey *et al.*, 1983a). These findings were consistent with the rise in amniotic fluid PGE_2 and $PGF_{2\alpha}$ levels during term labor (Keirse and Turnbull, 1973; Keirse *et al.*, 1977).

In favor of a labor-initiating role for prostaglandins are the findings that there was a sharp prelabor rise in $PGF_{2\alpha}$ and PGFM in ewe uterine venous blood (Liggins *et al.*, 1973) and peripheral circulation (Mitchell *et al.*, 1976a), respectively. In rhesus monkey amniotic fluid, levels of PGF and its metabolite began to rise a few days before parturition (Mitchell *et al.*, 1976b). It is not clear, however, whether prostaglandin levels increase in humans before labor. Although some investigators have suggested that $PGF_{2\alpha}$ levels in human amniotic fluid rose before the onset of labor (Keirse *et al.* 1977), the results of most studies have shown that there was a marked rise in plasma PGFM levels only during or after labor (Gréen *et al.*, 1974; Lackritz *et al.*, 1978; Fuchs *et al.*, 1983b; Sellers *et al.*, 1982). Fuchs *et al.* (1983b) reported that plasma PGFM levels did not increase in women until cervical dilatation was about 6 cm, both in patients with intact membranes and in those with ruptured membranes. These observations suggest that prostaglandins may be released only as a consequence of labor in humans.

Other observations suggest that endogenous prostaglandins are not associated with labor initiation in humans. Many women with premature rupture of the membranes and increased prostaglandin metabolite levels in their circulation did not go into labor spontaneously but required oxytocin stimulation (Husslein *et al.*, 1981). The same was true in some women after artificial rupture of membranes (Husslein *et al.*, 1983). Padayachi *et al.* (1986) showed that oxytocin administration to patients with comparable levels of cervical dilation and with delayed labor initiated uterine contractions and permitted normal vaginal delivery without materially affecting PGF or PGFM levels in amniotic fluid. Only after efficient uterine contractions had continued for several hours was there an increase in prostaglandins in amniotic fluid. On the other hand, Husslein *et al.* (1981) and Fuchs *et al.* (1983b) found that induction of labor by oxytocin was associated with a rise in circulating levels of PGFM. When there was no increase in PGFM levels, induction of labor with oxytocin was unsuccessful. Taken together, the findings suggest that $PGF_{2\alpha}$ does not play a role in initiating labor but may be related to events associated with labor. Release of $PGF_{2\alpha}$ from extraamniotic sites, probably the decidua, may be more relevant with regard to these events than prostaglandins produced by the amnion. In the human, endogenous prostaglandins may support the initiation of parturition by oxytocin and other factors or maintain labor once it has begun.

4.1.1. Sites of Prostaglandin Action

Because prostaglandins are uterotonic, endogenously released prostanoids have been assumed to act directly on uterine myometrial cells to elicit labor contractions. Their actions on myometrial cells, however, may not be primary. Intravenous infusion of prostaglandins into women stimulated uterine activity only after a latency period of 15–20 min (Embrey, 1969), and the uterotonic effect persisted for 30–60 min after the infusion was stopped. In addition, blood levels of prostaglandins attained during infusion for the induction of labor are too low to promote uterine contractions directly.

4.1.2. Induced Labor in Humans

Nagata and co-workers (1987) compared PGFM levels in the circulation of women with induced and spontaneous labor. Although prostaglandin levels increased only during or after delivery in spontaneous labor, there was a significant elevation when labor was induced by amniotomy. These findings suggest that $PGF_{2\alpha}$ may play different roles in induced and spontaneous labor. In bacterial sepsis, Bejar *et al.* (1981) showed that many bacteria associated with intrauterine infections, chorioamnionitis, urinary tract infections, and early neonatal sepsis have substantial phospholipase activities, some of which were several times greater than phospholipase A_2 activities in amnion and chorion. These workers postulated that premature labor associated with endocervical or intrauterine infections could arise from bacterially induced release of prostaglandins.

4.1.3. Sites of Prostaglandin Synthesis in Labor

4.1.3a. Myometrium. Because virtually all cells are capable of prostaglandin synthesis, the question of the sources of prostaglandins involved in myometrial contractions has not been completely resolved. If prostaglandins are to affect myometrial contractility, they should arise from or very near to myometrial cells. There is little evidence to suggest that the myometrium itself is the source of prostaglandins that are involved in labor. Whereas the endometrium and decidua synthesize predominantly $PGF_{2\alpha}$ and PGE_2 in almost equal amounts (Okazaki *et al.*, 1981), the myometrium produces primarily prostacyclin (PGI_2) (Williams *et al.*, 1978; Abel and Kelly, 1979; Omini *et al.*, 1979). Prostacyclin administered either *in vivo* (Lumsden and Baird, 1986) or *in vitro* (Omini *et al.*, 1979) relaxed uterine smooth muscle or induced an initial excitatory response followed in the majority of experiments by transient inhibition (Wikland *et al.*, 1983). The inhibitory effects of PGI$_2$ have not been universally observed, however. Using strips of pregnant rat uterus, Williams *et al.* (1979) found that PGI$_2$ stimulated uterine contractions, and threshold concentrations caused a threefold potentiation of threshold doses of oxytocin. Protacyclin may not be a physiological activator of uterine contractions because the uterotonic potency of PGI$_2$ is about one-eighth that of PGF$_{2\alpha}$ and $\frac{1}{30}$ that of PGE$_2$. Others have found that PGI$_2$ had no effect on human uterine contractility *in vivo* (Wilhelmsson *et al.*, 1981).

Specific binding sites for [^{3}H]PGI$_2$ have been demonstrated by autoradiography in the myometrium but not the endometrium of nonpregnant human uteri (Chegini and Rao, 1988). Prostaglandin E$_2$, PGF$_{2\alpha}$ and leukotriene C$_4$, which bind to nonpregnant human uterus (Hofmann *et al.*, 1983), had no effect on PGI$_2$ binding, suggesting that there are separate receptor sites for the different eicosanoids (Chegini and Rao, 1988). The biological significance of prostacyclins and their binding sites in the myometrium remains to be established. Prostacyclin formation in human myometrium may modulate the stimulatory activities of prostaglandins and other hormones during pregnancy (Omini *et al.*, 1979). Prostacyclin abolished spontaneous electrical and mechanical activity *in vivo* in sheep within minutes of administration; however, it did not block the response of the myometrium to oxytocin or PGF$_{2\alpha}$ (Lye and Challis, 1982). Prostacyclin also did not block the contractile activities of PGF$_{2\alpha}$ and oxytocin on human myometrial strips (Wikland *et al.*, 1983).

The fetal membranes, notably the amnion, or decidua may be the source of prostaglandins involved in labor. Implicit in the argument for extramyometrial production of activator prostaglandins is the existence of some mechanism for transport of prostaglandins to the myometrium without inactivation.

4.1.3b. Amnion. Amniotic fluid is surrounded by tissues that do not metabolize prostaglandins (Keirse and Turnbull, 1973). Keirse *et al.* (1977) showed that in women concentrations of PGF and PGFM in amniotic fluid were higher at the onset of labor than in late pregnancy and increased significantly with advancing cervical dilatation. Similar findings were made in rhesus monkeys. The mean concentrations of PGF and PGFM in amniotic fluid of rhesus monkeys increased about fourfold during the last 5 days of pregnancy (Mitchell *et al.*, 1976b).

Some investigators have suggested that the amnion is the major site of increased prostaglandin production at the time of labor (Casey and MacDonald, 1984). These conclusions were based in part on the large capacity for prostaglandin synthesis by amnion cells (Kinoshita *et al.*, 1977; Willman and Collins, 1978; Mitchell *et al.*, 1978; Okazaki *et al.*, 1981), and the production rates of PGE by dispersed amnion cells were significantly higher after spontaneous labor at term than at elective cesarean section (Okazaki *et al.*, 1981; Olson *et al.*, 1983a; Manzai and Liggins, 1984). Other studies, however, have shown no statistically significant difference in amniotic PGE production rates before and after labor at term (Mitchell *et al.*, 1978). Reddi *et al.* (1984) showed that multiparous patients with comparable levels of cervical dilatation and with delayed labor had very low concentrations of PGF$_{2\alpha}$ in the amniotic fluid, suggesting that the delay might be associated with low levels of prostaglandin. Oxytocin administration restored uterine contractions to normal and permitted normal vaginal delivery but did not materially affect the low level of PGF and its metabolite PGFM in amniotic fluid (Reddi *et al.*, 1984; Padayachi *et al.*, 1986). Only after efficient uterine contractions had occurred for several hours was there an increase in prostaglandins. Results such as these question whether prostaglandin levels in amniotic fluid reflect the events leading up to the initiation of labor contractions.

4.1.3c. Decidua. Peripheral blood levels of PGFM increased slightly in late human pregnancy and greatly during labor or immediately post-partum (Greén *et al.*, 1974). It is not certain which cells were the source of PGF, but it is likely that they arose from the decidua.

Collagenase-dispersed decidual cells exhibited higher rates of PGE_2, $PGF_{2\alpha}$ and PGFM production when the tissue was taken from patients in spontaneous labor than at the time of elective cesarean section when the patients were not in labor (Skinner and Challis, 1985).

4.1.3d. Transport of Prostaglandins from Fetal Membranes to Myometrium. The increase in fetal membrane production of prostaglandins has led to speculation that the availability of prostanoids to the myometrium increases about the time of the onset of labor. Intraamniotic injection of prostaglandins is known to induce labor in a number of circumstances (Karim, 1971), presumably by simulating the physiological conditions associated with spontaneous labor.

In decidua, PGE_2 originating from the amnion may be converted to $PGF_{2\alpha}$ through 9-ketoreductase activity or may stimulate further arachidonate metabolism. Prostaglandin E_2 or $PGF_{2\alpha}$ from decidua may then reach the myometrium. An objection to the importance of amniotic PGE_2 acting on the myometrium is that human chorion contains high 15-prostaglandin dehydrogenase and $\Delta^{13,14}$-reductase activities and exhibits a high rate of prostaglandin metabolism (Keirse and Turnbull, 1975; Okazaki et al., 1981). Nakla et al. (1986), however, showed that $[^3H]PGE_2$ was able to traverse full-thickness human fetal membranes (amnion, chorion, and decidua) partitioning two chambers in vitro. After the introduction of $[^3H]PGE_2$ on the amnion side, about half of the radioactivity recovered on the decidual side was identified as $[^3H]PGE_2$. The rate of transport was significantly higher in tissues collected at spontaneous onset of labor than in tissues taken at elective cesarean section at term. These authors conclude that PGE_2 produced by human amnion at term may escape metabolism in the chorion and reach the decidua, myometrium, or both.

In contrast, McCoshen et al. (1987), using a dual-compartment perfusion chamber, found that the release of endogenous PGE_2 on the decidual side of fetal membranes diminished after spontaneous labor despite an increased release from the fetal (amnion) surface. In support of these in vitro findings, they found that the PGE_2 content of chorion–decidua taken at the time of vaginal deliveries was one-quarter that from tissues taken during non-labor-associated cesarean deliveries. From these results, there is little likelihood that PGE_2 arising from amnion cells plays a role in initiating uterine contractions, emphasizing the importance of decidual prostaglandins as the source of myometrial activating agents.

4.1.3e. Amnion versus Decidua. The site of origin of prostaglandins involved in labor is still being resolved. Because little or no $PGF_{2\alpha}$ is produced by fetal membranes, and levels of PGFM increase in the amniotic fluid and maternal circulation around the time of parturition, many investigators have concluded that the decidua is the major site of prostaglandin production involved in parturition. In support of this view, Brennecke et al. (1985) found that levels of the stable metabolite of PGE_2 were not significantly altered in human maternal peripheral plasma during the second or third trimesters or labor. These findings contrasted with levels of PGFM, which were increased severalfold during labor. The presence of $PGF_{2\alpha}$ and PGFM in amniotic fluid during labor appears to result from its influx from extraamniotic sources because a significant fraction of PGE_2 applied to the vagina reached the amniotic fluid compartment unchanged after a lag period of a few hours (MacKenzie and Mitchell, 1981). It seems unlikely that $PGF_{2\alpha}$ in decidual tissue could be synthesized from PGE_2 arising from the amnion, because the degradation of PGE_2 by 15-ketoprostaglandin dehydrogenase appears to be favored over the conversion to $PGF_{2\alpha}$ by 15-ketoprostaglandin dehydrogenase (Niesert et al., 1986).

Whether prostaglandins in amniotic fluid play any part in the mechanisms of the onset and progression of labor is unknown. The concentrations of PGE (Keirse and Turnbull, 1973) and PGF and PGFM (Keirse et al., 1977) increased in amniotic fluid in proportion to cervical dilatation. Although the increases in PGF and PGFM began before the apparent onset of spontaneous labor, the increase in prostaglandin concentrations in amniotic fluid reflects the progression of labor and probably not the initiation. Indeed, prostaglandins can be released as a result of intrauterine pressure and stretching or manipulation of the uterus (Poyser *et al.*, 1971). In agreement with these results, cervical dilatation at either weeks 9 to 12 or 37 to 42 of pregnancy resulted in a rapid, 13-fold elevation in PGF, but not PGE, concentrations in human amniotic fluid (Nieder and Augustin, 1983). Regardless of the biological significance of prostaglandins in amniotic fluid, their concentrations are an index of important changes during labor, since abnormally low levels of prostaglandins are found in the amniotic fluid of women with clinically delayed labor (Keirse *et al.*, 1977; Reddi *et al.*, 1984). There is no strong evidence, however, to suggest that the participation of the decidua or amnion in labor need exclude the other.

4.1.4. *Uterotonic Effects of Prostaglandins and Myometrial Prostaglandin Receptors*

Because prostaglandins stimulate myometrial contractions, increased levels of prostaglandins arriving at the myometrium were assumed to stimulate labor. There are observations, however, that suggest that the effects of endogenously released prostaglandins on the myometrium are indirect. Prostaglandin-induced contractions of the isolated uterus of the rat are characterized by a rapid onset and rapid recovery after washing (Johnson *et al.*, 1974). *In vivo*, however, there is a lag of about 48 hr between the administration of $PGF_{2\alpha}$ and induction of labor (Alexandrova and Soloff, 1980b). Prostaglandin $F_{2\alpha}$ does not induce labor when given to rats after day 21 of gestation, a time when oxytocin is very effective (Fuchs, 1972). In addition, PGE_2 and $PGF_{2\alpha}$ are almost equipotent uterotonic agents in the rat, but only $PGF_{2\alpha}$ terminated gestation when administered on day 18 (Fuchs *et al.*, 1974).

The effects of $PGF_{2\alpha}$ on the myometrium in the rat appear to result, at least in part, from its luteolytic activity (Pharriss and Wyngarden, 1969; Fuchs *et al.*, 1974; Strauss *et al.*, 1975). The simultaneous administration of progestin and $PGF_{2\alpha}$ prevented $PGF_{2\alpha}$-induced premature labor (Strauss *et al.*, 1975; Alexandrova and Soloff 1980b). Although evidence suggests that $PGF_{2\alpha}$ inhibits progesterone secretion in nonprimates (Horton and Poyser, 1976), similar effects could not be demonstrated in humans between 7 and 20 weeks of pregnancy (Speroff *et al.*, 1972).

The action of prostaglandin is mediated by specific receptors located on the plasma membranes of target cells. Specific binding sites for PGEs with apparent K_d values in the nanomolar range have been demonstrated in crude myometrial membrane preparations (Schillinger and Prior, 1976; Crankshaw *et al.*, 1979; Bauknecht *et al.*, 1981). Uterine binding sites were found autoradiographically in longitudinal and circular smooth muscle, stromal cells, glandular epithelium, arterioles, and erythrocytes within the lumen of the arterioles (Chegini *et al.*, 1986; Chegini and Rao, 1988). Prostaglandin $F_{2\alpha}$ binding by human myometrial plasma membranes, however, was associated with relatively low-affinity sites (K_d in the micromolar range), suggesting that there are separate receptors for PGE and PGF (Schillinger and Prior, 1976). Although PGE_2 is several times as potent as $PGF_{2\alpha}$ in stimulating contractions of human myometrium (Embrey, 1969; Schillinger and Prior, 1976), the affinity of binding sites for PGE_2 was over 1000 times that for $PGF_{2\alpha}$. Prostaglandin $F_{2\alpha}$ may undergo modification before binding, but the lack of correlation between uterotonic potency and binding creates doubt about the physiological significance of the binding sites. Other investigators, however, have found that the affinity of myometrial membranes from pregnant women for $PGF_{2\alpha}$ was about 0.3 nM (Fukai *et al.*, 1984). Unlike myometrial receptors for other uterotonic agents, the number of PGE_2 binding sites was reduced to one-third after nonpregnant patients were treated with estradiol. The reduced binding capacity may result from occupation of the sites by endogenous PGEs, the production of which is stimulated by estrogen (Abel and Baird, 1980).

The relationship between the affinities of a series of prostaglandin analogues and their relative potencies as uterotonic agonists remains to be established. The mechanisms of prostaglandin–receptor interaction and subsequent steps are poorly understood. Regulation of prostaglandin action at the receptor level during pregnancy and parturition has not been investigated. Fukai *et al.* (1984) found that the concentration of high-affinity binding sites (K_d about 0.3 nM) for [³H]PGF$_{2\alpha}$ on human myometrial membranes remained unchanged throughout pregnancy and labor. The myometrial PGF$_{2\alpha}$ binding capacity was about 3 to 5% that of oxytocin, which increased substantially as gestation advanced (Fukai *et al.*, 1984).

4.1.5. *Control of Prostaglandin Synthesis*

The control of prostaglandin release during labor remains unknown. Changes in prostaglandin output are not related to a decrease in prostaglandin metabolism. The capacity to produce prostaglandins from endogenous substrates exists long before labor begins. The increased production of prostaglandins may result from a change in the balance of stimulatory to inhibitory factors modulating prostaglandin biosynthesis.

4.1.5a. Stimulatory Factors. Stimulatory factors have been found in fetal urine (Strickland *et al.*, 1983; Casey *et al.*, 1983b), amniotic fluid (Rehnström *et al.*, 1983; Mitchell *et al.*, 1984), and the cytosol fractions of placenta and decidua (Saeed and Mitchell, 1982).

Casey and co-workers (1983b) found a protein or protein-associated material in human fetal urine that caused a ten- to 600-fold increase in PGE$_2$ synthesis by human amnion cells maintained in monolayer culture. Fetal urine did not cause a similar increase in PGE$_2$ production by cells derived from human myometrium or endometrium. The activity was also present in adult urine. Strickland *et al.* (1983) found a material in neonatal urine that stimulated the *in vitro* conversion of arachidonic acid to PGE$_2$ by a microsome-enriched preparation from bovine seminal vesicles. Stimulation was greater in urine of babies delivered after labor than by cesarean section before the onset of labor. These workers postulated that the resulting stimulation of prostaglandin synthesis by fetal membranes could serve as the signal for the initiation of parturition.

Rehnström et al. (1983) examined the influence of amniotic fluid on the synthesis of prostanoids by tissue slices of human amnion, decidua, and myometrium. They found that amniotic fluid taken at term, either before or after the onset of labor, stimulated prostaglandin synthesis by decidua and myometrium but not by amnion. Amniotic fluid taken at midtrimester was without activity. The stimulating effect could not be explained by free arachidonic acid in amniotic fluid. Arachidonate, which is known to increase in late pregnancy, would have stimulated prostaglandin synthesis by amnion. Other investigators (López Bernal *et al.*, 1987) showed that the addition of arachidonic acid to dispersed amnion cells resulted in a two- to threefold increase in PGE output, whether the cells were obtained at term either before or after labor. The absence of a significant stimulatory effect of amniotic fluid on amnion (Rehnström *et al.*, 1983) suggests that factors arising in amniotic fluid, presumably from the fetus, must reach the decidua and myometrium to be effective.

Arachidonic acid. Regulation of prostaglandin synthesis may be by arachidonic acid availability and the activities of enzymes involved in the conversion of arachidonic acid to prostaglandins (prostaglandin synthetase). Prostaglandins are formed from polyunsaturated fatty acids released from phospholipids in the plasma membranes of cells. An early step in the formation of prostaglandins is the formation of arachidonic acid from its esterified form in phospholipids, primarily phosphatidylethanolamine and phosphatidylinositol, through the activities of phospholipases A$_2$ and C, respectively. The activities of these enzymes increase during pregnancy, although not in association with labor *per se* (Okazaki *et al.*, 1981). Phospholipase A$_2$ is specific for phosphatidylethanolamine containing arachidonic acid in the *sn*-2 position. From arachidonic acid, a cyclopentane ring is formed, and oxygen atoms are introduced by prostaglandin synthetase to yield PGE$_2$ and PGF$_{2\alpha}$, the two prostaglandins of importance in parturition.

A rate-limiting step in the synthesis of prostaglandins is phospholipase-mediated cleavage of arachidonic acid from phospholipid stores, because the pool of free arachidonic acid in most mammalian cells is very small (Irvine, 1982). The binding of agonists to cell surface receptors is associated with phospholipase activation and increased production of prostaglandins (Samuelsson et al., 1978; Hong and Deykin, 1981; Majerus, 1983). At least part of the increase in the production of prostaglandins after stimulation, however, results from increased prostaglandin synthetase activity, measured by the conversion of exogenous arachidonic acid to prostaglandins (see Habernicht et al., 1985, for additional references).

It is not clear whether arachidonate is the limiting, and thus regulated, step of prostaglandin synthesis in fetal membranes and uterine tissues in parturition. In support of a rate-limiting role is the eightfold increase in concentration of nonesterified arachidonic acid in amniotic fluid during labor (MacDonald et al., 1974). Because arachidonic acid increased much more than other fatty acids, the mobilization of arachidonic acid may be associated with labor. Although the specific activity of phospholipase C in fetal membranes and decidua did not change with the onset of labor in humans (Di Renzo et al., 1981), the tacit assumption is that an increase in arachidonate levels results in synthesis of more prostaglandins. In support of this argument, the instillation of arachidonic acid into the amniotic sac resulted in abortion in midpregnancy (MacDonald et al., 1974), whereas oleate instillation had no effect. Arachidonic acid increased PGE output significantly by amnion cells, whether the amnion was obtained from patients in spontaneous term labor, spontaneous preterm labor, induced labor, or at term but not in labor (Lopez Bernal et al., 1987). These findings support the hypothesis that substrate availability is an important determinant of the rate of PGE synthesis.

Others, however, have shown that human amniotic fluid and uterine tissues contain a great excess of arachidonic acid compared with PGE and PGF. Arachidonic acid in both esterified and free forms accounted for between 7% and 25% of the fatty acid content (Keirse, 1983). Extraamniotic instillation of arachidonic acid into pregnant rhesus monkeys was ineffective in elevating prostaglandin concentrations in either amniotic fluid or peripheral plasma or in inducing labor prematurely (Robinson et al., 1978), suggesting that the formation of arachidonate is not limiting. In contrast, the extraamniotic administration of PGE_2 resulted in increased concentrations of PGE, PGF, and PGFM in amniotic fluid, and labor was induced prematurely. The basis for the discrepancy in results between the human and rhesus monkey is not known.

Arachidonic acid itself affects the secretion of placental lactogen, prolactin, and insulin from the placenta (Zeitler and Handwerger, 1985), cloned rat anterior pituitary cells (Kolesnick et al., 1984), and pancreatic β-cells (Metz et al., 1987), respectively, independent of both lipoxygenase and cyclooxygenase pathways. Arachidonic acid's effects on placental cells might be mediated by activation of phospholipase C because addition of arachidonic acid to the medium caused the production of inositol phosphates in the cells (Zeitler and Handwerger, 1985). Arachidonic acid also stimulates guanylate cyclase (Gerzer et al., 1986) and protein kinase C (McPhail et al., 1984) and causes the release of calcium from intracellular stores (Wolf et al., 1986).

Estrogen. The effects of estrogen on prostaglandin synthesis have been studied for the most part with uterine tissues from nonpregnant subjects. Estradiol treatment increases the uterine content and/or release of $PGF_{2\alpha}$ in several species (Blatchley et al., 1971; Caldwell et al., 1972; Ham et al., 1975; see Horton and Poyser, 1976, for additional references). Estrogen, added to human endometrial explants in organ culture, stimulated the output of $PGF_{2\alpha}$ (Abel and Baird, 1980; Leaver and Richmond, 1984; Schatz et al., 1984). The effects of estrogen on human endometrium were primarily on glandular epithelium and not on stromal cells (Schatz et al., 1987).

The parallel rise in the concentration of estrone and PGFM in amniotic fluid of rhesus monkeys before spontaneous vaginal delivery (Mitchell et al., 1976b) led to speculation that the increasing estrogen concentrations in amniotic fluid promote production of prostaglandins by decidual tissue. Intrafetal infusion of ACTH to rhesus monkeys at about 130 days of gestation stimulated increases in the concentrations of estrogens and prostaglandins, particularly PGE, in amniotic fluid (Novy, 1983).

Estrogen-induced increases in prostaglandin production appear to be associated with the prostaglandin synthase complex and not with the availability of arachidonic acid for prostaglandin synthesis. Administration of estrogen to guinea pigs (Wlodawer *et al.*, 1976) and rats (Ham *et al.*, 1975) increased the conversion of exogenous arachidonic acid to $PGF_{2\alpha}$ by uterine microsomes. Estrogen may have a general effect not limited to reproductive tissues. Estrogen increased the concentration of fatty acid cyclooxygenase, measured immunologically, in cultures of rat aortic smooth muscle cells (Chang *et al.*, 1983). Estrogen administration affected neither the uptake of [^{3}H]arachidonic acid by human glandular epithelial cells in cultures nor the rate of metabolism of [^{3}H]$PGF_{2\alpha}$ added to the cells (Schatz *et al.*, 1987).

Progesterone. Progesterone sometimes supported estrogen-induced increases in prostaglandin output, but in other studies progesterone antagonized the effects of estrogen (Abel and Baird, 1980). Isoxazol, an inhibitor of 3β-hydroxysteroid dehydrogenase, given to rats in late pregnancy decreased plasma progesterone and resulted in premature delivery (Csapo and Resch, 1979). At the same time, plasma estradiol and PGF levels increased. These increases were blocked by progesterone and isoxazol. Similar findings have been reported in pregnant sheep. Inhibition of 3β-hydoxysteroid dehydrogenase activity in pregnant sheep decreased placental progesterone output and led to a rapid rise in PGFM concentrations in peripheral blood and to premature delivery in most animals (Taylor *et al.*, 1982).

Khan-Dawood and Dawood (1984) found that term human decidua and myometrium had nuclear receptors for both estradiol and progesterone. Placenta, amnion, and chorion had only nuclear estrogen receptors, indicating that progesterone's effects on prostaglandin generation are more likely to be exerted on decidua than on amnion.

Calcium. Free calcium was suggested to be a major factor influencing prostaglandin output by fetal membranes (Bleasdale *et al.*, 1983). The calcium ionophore A23187 increased $PGF_{2\alpha}$ output by guinea pig (Leaver and Seawright, 1982) and human (Leaver and Richmond, 1984) endometrial explants. Because the addition of arachidonic acid also stimulated prostaglandin output, increases in intracellular ionized calcium concentrations may result in liberation of arachidonic acid from phospholipid stores. Indeed, both phospholipases A_2 and C were stimulated by Ca^{2+} *in vitro,* as was diacylglycerol lipase, which catalyzes the conversion of diacylglycerol to monoacylglycerol and frees arachidonic acid (Fig. 3). In contrast, Ca^{2+} inhibited enzymes involved in reducing arachidonic acid levels, such as diacylglycerol kinase, catalyzing the conversion of diacylglycerol to the glycerophospholipid precursor phosphatidic acid (Bleasdale *et al.*, 1983). The action of this kinase inhibits the release of arachidonic acid from diacylglycerols by recycling the diacylglycerols to phospholipids.

The effects of Ca^{2+} were clear, but they occurred at concentrations 1000 times greater than intracellular levels. Therefore, the role of intracellular changes in free calcium ion concentrations in modifying phospholipase activity is not clear. Calcium may activate protein kinase C, resulting in phosphorylation of lipocortin and the subsequent release from inhibition of phospholipase A_2 activity (see Section 4.1.5b). Phorbol 12-myristate 13-acetate (TPA), an activator of protein kinase C, stimulated $PGF_{2\alpha}$ synthesis by cultured human endometrial cells (Skinner *et al.*, 1984). However, TPA had no effect on $PGF_{2\alpha}$ production by guinea pig endometrium (Riley and Poyser, 1987), indicating that species differences exist. In guinea pig endometrium, calmodulin inhibitors prevented the stimulation of phospholipase A_2 (Riley and Poyser, 1987). The ouput of $PGF_{2\alpha}$ from guinea pig endometrium was reduced significantly by the use of Ca^{2+}-depleted medium, calcium chelator (EGTA), and an intracellular Ca^{2+} antagonist (Riley and Poyser, 1987). Calcium channel blockers also inhibited $PGF_{2\alpha}$ output. These findings indicate that extracellular Ca^{2+} is required for the high output of $PGF_{2\alpha}$ from the guinea pig uterus after day 11 of the estrous cycle

The removal of Ca^{2+} from the incubation medium reduced the output of PGE and PGF

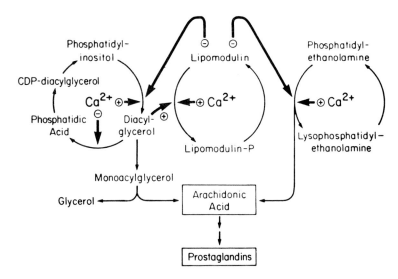

Figure 3. Proposed regulation of arachidonic acid metabolism in human fetal membranes by Ca^{2+}. From Bleasdale *et al.* (1983).

by collagenase-dispersed human amnion cells (Olson *et al.*, 1983b). Prostaglandin release also was inhibited by addition of methoxyverapamil (D-600), a calcium channel blocker. Conversely, addition of the calcium ionophore A23187 to cells was stimulatory. These results suggest that prostaglandin output by the human amnion is dependent on the entry of Ca^{2+} from amniotic fluid.

Platelet-activating factor. Billah and Johnston (1983) reported that platelet-activating factor (1-O-alkyl-2-acetyl-3-glycerophosphocholine; PAF) was present in amniotic fluid obtained from about 50% of women after active labor but was absent in fluid obtained before labor. The PAF was shown to increase cytosolic Ca^{2+} concentrations in a number of systems (see Billah *et al.*, 1985, for references). Billah *et al.* (1985) reasoned that PAF in amniotic fluid might stimulate prostaglandin synthesis by amnion cells in a calcium-dependent manner because the enzymes involved in arachidonic formation are Ca^{2+} dependent. They found that addition of PAF to amnionic tissue disks resulted in almost a threefold increase in the release of PGE_2 into the incubation medium. A similar stimulation was seen after the addition of Ca^{2+} and the calcium ionophore A23187.

Nishihara and colleagues (1984) found that PAF induced contractions of the rat isolated uterus. Similar findings were obtained with guinea pig (Montrucchio *et al.*, 1986) and human (Tetta *et al.*, 1986) myometrial strips. The response to PAF was distinct from that to oxytocin. Cyclooxygenase and lipoxygenase inhibitors blocked the PAF effect (Montrucchio *et al.*, 1986; Tetta *et al.*, 1986). In addition, desensitization to PAF but not to oxytocin occurred with a second dose. The relationship between PAF activation of prostaglandin production in amniotic fluid and its direct effects on stimulation of uterine contractions remain to be determined.

Oxytocin. Oxytocin stimulates the production of prostaglandins by endometrial and decidual tissues. This topic is elaborated on in Section 4.2.

Catecholamines and cAMP. Isoproterenol added to human amnionic disks maintained *in vitro* caused a sustained release of arachidonic acid and PGE_2 (Di Renzo *et al.*, 1984a). The effects of isoproterenol appeared to be the result of β-adrenergic activation, because dibutyryl cAMP stimulated the release of PGE_2. Similar results were obtained with other activators of adenylate cyclase including cholera toxin, forskolin, and several β agonists (Warrick *et al.*,

1985). These agents increased both cAMP production and the release of PGE and PGF from cells isolated from amnion and decidua obtained from women following spontaneous labor (Warrick *et al.*, 1985). The mechanisms of cAMP stimulation of prostaglandin synthesis are not known. It has been suggested that the catalytic subunit of cAMP-dependent protein kinase can inhibit protein kinase C-dependent phosphorylation of lipocortin in thymocytes (Hirata *et al.*, 1984). Apparently cAMP acts by different mechanisms on amnion cells, because inhibition of lipocortin phosphorylation represses prostaglandin synthesis rather than stimulates it.

During late pregnancy, the concentration of catecholamines in amniotic fluid increases (Divers *et al.*, 1981). β-Adrenoreceptors of the β_2 subtype were associated with amnionic cells and increased threefold between midtrimester and late gestation (Di Renzo *et al.*, 1984b). Increases in both agonists and receptors suggest that there would be an increased responsiveness of amnionic cells to catecholamines, resulting in increased PGE production.

Physical stimulation and tissue damage. Amniotic fluid concentrations of PGF and PGFM were significantly higher in samples obtained by amniotomy (surgical rupture of the fetal membranes) than by amniocentesis (Mitchell *et al.*, 1975b). Similarly, amniotomy or vaginal examination with sweeping of the fetal membranes caused increases in circulating PGFM levels in women studied after the 37th week of pregnancy (Mitchell *et al.*, 1977). Because labor often can be induced near term by sweeping or rupture of the membranes, some investigators consider fetal membranes to be the site of prostaglandin release. Labor usually starts, however, with intact membranes.

4.1.5b. Inhibitory Factors. *Endogenous inhibitors of prostaglandin synthesis.* Several lines of evidence suggest that prostaglandin production is tonically inhibited during pregnancy, leading some investigators to postulate that the mechanism of parturition includes withdrawal of this inhibition. Maathuis and Kelly (1978) showed that the concentration of prostaglandins in human decidual tissue obtained at 3 to 10 weeks of gestation was lower than that measured in the endometrium at any stage in the normal menstrual cycle. During the proliferative stages, the concentration of PGF in the endometrium was correlated with plasma estradiol levels. The endometrial concentration of PGE did not show any cyclic variation. The reduced level of prostaglandins in the endometrium in early pregnancy suggested that the conceptus blocked the synthesis or increased catabolism of prostaglandins. Subsequent studies showed that decidual $PGF_{2\alpha}$ and PGE concentrations in women with ectopic pregnancies were comparable to those from women with intrauterine pregnancies of the same gestational age (Abel *et al.*, 1980). Such findings suggest that suppression of endometrial prostaglandin synthesis during pregnancy may be regulated systemically instead of through a local action of the conceptus.

Saeed *et al.* (1977) demonstrated that plasma from several mammalian species inhibited the conversion of arachidonic acid to prostaglandins by homogenates of bovine seminal vesicles. This activity was ascribed to endogenous inhibitors of prostaglandin synthesis (EIPS) in Cohn fraction IV-4 of human plasma; EIPS activity also was found in human amniotic fluid (Saeed *et al.*, 1982). Inhibitory activity was greater in amniotic fluid taken in early pregnancy than in fluid taken at term but before the onset of labor. There was a further significant reduction in inhibitory activity in amniotic fluid collected during labor. These results suggested that the onset of labor was associated with the local withdrawal of inhibition of prostaglandin synthesis. It is possible that part of the inhibition was by albumin, because inhibition of prostaglandin synthesis in early and term gestation was proportional to the concentration of albumin in amniotic fluid (Saeed *et al.*, 1982). There was no correlation, however, in amniotic fluid obtained after labor.

Manzai and Liggins (1984) reported that dispersed amnionic cells released substances into the incubation medium that reduced by about 30% the output of PGE and PGF by human endometrial cells. The inhibitory activity was associated only with cells obtained from women near term before labor, not from women in spontaneous labor. Romero *et al.* (1987) reported the presence of soluble products from human decidua that inhibited prostaglandin production by human amnion.

Brennecke *et al.* (1984) measured human maternal plasma EIPS levels during pregnancy, labor, and the puerperium. In contrast to amniotic fluid, they found no significant trends in maternal plasma levels of EIPS in relation to pregnancy and parturition. In other studies, a small but significant increase in EIPS activity was found in plasmas from women in the third trimester and at term, but this level was not maintained in labor (Fig. 4). Maternal peripheral plasma EIPS activity could not be responsible for the striking suppression of endometrial prostaglandin synthesis in early pregnancy, since there was no significant increase in plasma EIPS levels compared with values in nonpregnant women (Brennecke *et al.*, 1982). These results do not support a role for maternal plasma EIPS in the control of prostaglandin production during human pregnancy or parturition. The mechanisms that so effectively inhibit decidual prostaglandin synthesis in human pregnancy remains to be clarified.

Lipocortin. Lipocortins, a family of steroid-inducible proteins that inhibit phospholipase A_2 activity and the formation of arachidonic acid, have been isolated from various tissues and cells, including lung (Flower and Blackwell, 1979), thymocytes (Hirata *et al.*, 1984), and platelets (Touqui *et al.*, 1986). Using the amino acid sequence obtained from purified rat lipocortin, Wallner *et al.* (1986) cloned human lipocortin cDNA and expressed the gene in *E. coli.* Lipocortin produced in this way was a potent inhibitor of phospholipase A_2 activity.

Enhanced phosphorylation of lipocortin by calcium-stimulated protein kinases suppressed lipocortin inhibition of PLA_2 activity in thymocytes treated with mitogens (Hirata *et al.*, 1984) and in platelets treated with thrombin or phorbol esters (Touqui *et al.*, 1986). Lipocortins may inhibit prostaglandin production by uterine and intrauterine tissues during pregnancy, but definitive studies remain to be carried out.

4.2. Oxytocin

Oxytocin was considered to be the sole physiological initiator of labor because (1) it is the most potent natural substance stimulating labor, (2) the frequency and amplitude of oxytocin-

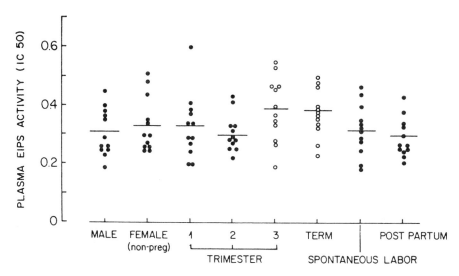

Figure 4. EIPS activities in plasmas from human subjects. The third-trimester and term groups (○) had significantly different ($P < 0.05$) activities from the first- and second-trimester and postpartum groups. From Mitchell *et al.* (1983).

induced uterine contractions are identical with those occurring during spontaneous labor, and (3) labor contractions could be induced by electrical stimulation of the posterior pituitary gland, increasing oxytocin concentrations in the blood.

Early attempts to ablate oxytocin-producing cells gave mixed results. In retrospect, the wide distribution of oxytocin-containing neurons in the magnocellular system explains why production of lesions of the posterior pituitary gland did not entirely eliminate oxytocin. Interruption of the hypothalamoneurohypophyseal tract by precise surgical lesions in the hypothalamus caused prolonged unproductive labor with a high incidence of maternal and fetal deaths in cats and guinea pigs (Dey et al., 1941; Fisher et al., 1938).

With the development of sensitive radioimmunoassays for oxytocin, its role in labor initiation was reassessed based on the inability to show a consistent rise in oxytocin concentrations in the peripheral maternal circulation preceding labor. Furthermore, uterine activity did not reflect oxytocin concentrations in the blood. Some proposed that maternal oxytocin levels are less significant than myometrial oxytocin concentrations arising from the fetal circulation (Fuchs and Fuchs, 1984). This concept has not been widely accepted.

During the expulsive stage of labor, there is a substantial rise in oxytocin concentrations in the maternal circulation (Leake et al., 1981), leading to the conclusion that, although oxytocin may not initiate labor, the release of oxytocin during labor results in more forceful uterine contractions, facilitating delivery of the baby and placenta. The stimulation of oxytocin release during the expulsive phase of labor has been attributed to the Ferguson reflex following cervical and vaginal distension by the emerging baby (Ferguson, 1941).

Oxytocin was displaced as a candidate for the initiator of labor by the almost universal acceptance of the importance of prostaglandins. Present evidence suggests that oxytocin is involved in labor initiation, perhaps alone but probably in conjunction with prostaglandins. This conclusion is based on the following observations. First, the myometrium of all species that have been studied is most sensitive to oxytocin either near or at the time of labor. The sensitivity changes appear to result, at least in part, from increases in myometrial oxytocin receptor concentrations. Second, oxytocin receptors have been demonstrated in endometrium and decidua, and oxytocin is capable of stimulating prostaglandin synthesis in these tissues. The elevation of prostaglandin levels makes the myometrium more sensitive to oxytocin. Third, an oxytocin antagonist inhibits uterine contractions of premature labor. Teleologically, oxytocin must be important to the organism inasmuch as no oxytocin-deficient states have yet been described.

4.2.1. Sensitivity of the Myometrium to Oxytocin

In all species that have been studied, maximal myometrial sensitivity to oxytocin occurs at or near the time of labor (Fig. 5). More than 100 mU of oxytocin infused per minute is needed to elicit uterine contractions in nonpregnant women, whereas 16 mU/min is sufficient to elicit contractions at 20 weeks of pregnancy, 2 mU/min at 32 weeks, and 1 mU/min at term (Caldeyro-Barcia and Sereno, 1961). Theobald (1959) suggested that labor commences when the uterus becomes sufficiently sensitive to circulating oxytocin. However, this suggestion was largely ignored, and plasma oxytocin levels were given greater emphasis.

Support for Theobald's notion has come from Takahashi et al. (1980), who performed weekly oxytocin challenge tests on a group of high-risk patients. They found retrospectively that women who would give birth prematurely responded to lower doses of oxytocin than did those at the same time of gestation who would go to full term. Women with gestational length beyond term required the highest doses of oxytocin. At delivery, irrespective of the length of gestation, the uteri of preterm, postterm, and normal-term patients had similar sensitivities to oxytocin.

The enhanced uterine sensitivity to oxytocin appears to be largely a consequence of an increase in the effective concentration of oxytocin receptors on myometrial plasma mem-

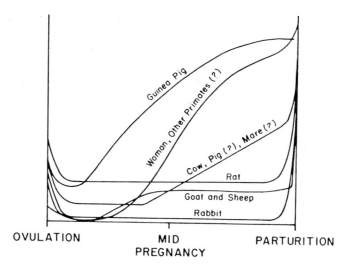

Figure 5. Changes in uterine sensitivity to oxytocin in various species, based on publications by different authors. From Fuchs (1985).

branes. In the rat, exogenous oxytocin initiates parturition only 1 day or less before the time of labor (Fuchs and Poblete, 1970), when there is a sharp rise in the concentration of myometrial oxytocin receptors (Fig. 2). The concentration of receptors is highest at labor and then falls abruptly to preterm levels 1 or 2 days after parturition (Alexandrova and Soloff, 1980a; Soloff *et al.,* 1979). When labor is induced 2 or 3 days early with $PGF_{2\alpha}$ there is a premature rise in oxytocin receptor concentrations in the myometrium (Alexandrova and Soloff, 1980b). If labor is delayed by 1 or 2 days by pharmacological amounts of LHRH, there is a similar delay in the increase in myometrial oxytocin receptor concentrations (Bercu *et al.,* 1980).

Therefore, an increased oxytocin concentration in the blood may not be necessary to stimulate myometrial cells; an increase in the number of oxytocin receptors allows myometrial cells to respond to basal levels of oxytocin.

4.2.2. *Oxytocin Receptors*

4.2.2a. Relationship between Oxytocin Receptor Concentration and Sensitivity. The relationship between the concentration of myometrial oxytocin receptors and the sensitivity of the myometrium to oxytocin *in vivo* was studied in individual pregnant rats (Fuchs *et al.,* 1983a). The animals, with intrauterine balloons to monitor uterine contractions, were given intravenous infusions on days 20, 21, 22, or 23 of gestation of increasing concentrations of oxytocin. After the threshold dose of oxytocin was ascertained, oxytocin receptor concentrations in myometrial plasma membranes were measured. A significant correlation was found between the concentration of oxytocin receptors and the sensitivity of the uterus to oxytocin.

Parturition in the rat is followed by a sharp decline in the concentration of myometrial oxytocin receptors. The marked reduction in uterine sensitivity to increased concentrations of oxytocin in the blood resulting from milk-ejection stimuli results from down-regulation of receptors. In the absence of other changes, a reduction in membrane receptors decreases target cell sensitivity in tissues containing abundant spare receptors and decreases target cell response when receptor concentration is limited.

Changes in receptor concentrations in guinea pig (Alexandrova and Soloff, 1980c) and human (Fuchs *et al.,* 1982) myometrial plasma membranes also corresponded to well-established oxytocin sensitivities. In women in labor, the number of myometrial oxytocin receptors per milligram of DNA was more than 150 times greater than that in nonpregnant women (Fuchs *et al.*, 1982, 1984). The timing of the increase in sensitivity corresponds to the time of increase in oxytocin receptor concentrations. Oxytocin receptor concentrations doubled at the onset of labor (cervix dilated less than 4 cm). Women at term or beyond but not responsive to oxytocin had relatively low oxytocin receptor levels. Women in preterm labor had elevated receptor concentrations comparable to those of women in term labor. The concentration of myometrial oxytocin receptors increases abruptly on the last day of gestation in rabbits (Riemer *et al.*, 1986) and corresponds to the time of the increased sensitivity to oxytocin in this species (Caldeyro-Barcia and Sereno, 1961).

An apparent exception to the relationship between receptor number and sensitivity was the observation that estrogen-treated Brattleboro rats had 15% the receptor concentration of myometrial membranes from similarly treated Sprague–Dawley rats (Goren *et al.*, 1980). Despite this difference, the uterine contractile response to oxytocin *in vitro* was the same in both strains. However, Haldar and co-workers (1982) found that uteri from estrogen-treated Brattleboro rats had about 25% the sensitivity to oxytocin as did uteri from Long–Evans rats, a strain more closely related to Brattleboro rats than the Sprague–Dawley strain. Similar results were obtained when oxytocic activity was measured either *in vitro* or *in vivo*.

Crankshaw (1987) surmised that changes in the number of receptor sites for oxytocin in uterine smooth muscle are not important for the changes in oxytocin sensitivity. Using longitudinally cut strips from rat uteri, he found that there was no significant change in the dose of oxytocin giving half-maximal stimulation *in vitro* with advancing gestation. A considerable number of strips responded to oxytocin in early and midgestation, when binding sites for oxytocin are relatively low. Circularly cut muscle strips, however, were essentially refractory to oxytocin until day 21 of pregnancy, suggesting that oxytocin receptor concentrations might be important in regulating the response to oxytocin only in circular smooth muscle. Not only were Crankshaw's findings in disagreement with *in vivo* data (Fuchs and Poblete, 1970), but they also did not concur with the observations of Kuriyama and Suzuki (1976) that the threshold dose of oxytocin required to stimulate electrical activity in longitudinally cut strips of rat myometrium declined sharply at the end of gestation.

Interpretations of experiments with cut muscle strips *in vitro* should be taken with caution. Riemer *et al.* (1986) found a nearly tenfold increase in the concentration of oxytocin receptors in the rabbit myometrium between days 30 and 31 (term) of gestation, along with at least a fourfold oxytocin sensitivity increase *in vitro*. The lesser sensitivity to oxytocin on day 30, however, was apparent only in the presence of meclofenamate, an inhibitor of eicosanoid formation. Because the rabbit myometrium *in vivo* becomes abruptly sensitive to oxytocin only at the end of gestation (Caldeyro-Barcia and Sereno, 1961), the release of prostaglandins *in vitro*, probably as the result of tissue damage, obliterated the shift in oxytocin sensitivity between days 30 and 31. There is evidence to suggest, however, that endogenous prostaglandins, released perhaps in response to oxytocin stimulation, may play an important part in modulating oxytocin action *in vivo*. Notwithstanding the possibility that regulation of sensitivity to oxytocin *in vivo* may occur at sites beyond oxytocin–receptor interaction, data from several species are all consistent with regulation occurring at the receptor level.

4.2.2b.   Topographical Distribution of Oxytocin Receptors.   The localization of oxytocin receptors in the human myometrium corresponds to the directionality of uterine contractions during labor. The concentration of receptors in plama membrane fractions from uterine fundus and corpus were significantly higher than the concentration from the isthmus or ampulla of fallopian tubes (Fuchs *et al.*, 1984, 1985). The lowest concentration of oxytocin binding sites per cell (milligram of DNA) was found in cervical plasma membranes. The topographical distribution of receptor sites appears to follow the relative content of smooth muscle cells (Schwalm and Dubrauszky, 1966). Similar results have been obtained with [3H-

PGE_1 and $[^3H]PGE_2$ binding sites in crude membrane preparations from nonpregnant human myometrium (Hofmann *et al.*, 1983). These findings may explain why during the first stage of labor the work of the fundus exceeds that of any other part of the uterus, while the lower uterine segment is inactive (Reynolds *et al.*, 1948). Parenthetically, the distinct topographical distribution of oxytocin receptors suggests that care be taken in ensuring that myometrial samples are obtained from the same region of the uterus.

4.2.2c. Regulation of Oxytocin Receptor Concentrations. It is not yet clear whether increases in oxytocin binding at the end of gestation are the result of increased numbers of receptors per cell, increased numbers of cells containing oxytocin receptors, or both. This question probably can be answered most directly by autoradiographic techniques, which also could define whether the longitudinal, circular, or both layers of the myometrium undergo changes in receptor number during pregnancy.

The molecular basis for the increase in receptor number is also unclear. Possibilities include the *de novo* synthesis of receptors, unmasking of cryptic receptor sites, activation of existing receptor sites by mechanisms such as phosphorylation/dephosphorylation, conversion of a precursor to an active protein, or the appearance/disappearance of activating/inhibiting substances. Understanding of the mechanisms of up-regulation of oxytocin receptors will be facilitated by their purification or the development of specific antireceptor antibodies.

Factors involved in up- and down-regulation of oxytocin receptors. Parturition in the rat appears to occur as a result of a fall in progesterone and a rise in estrogen levels in the blood. These changes are correlated with increases in the concentration of myometrial oxytocin receptors (Alexandrova and Soloff, 1980a; Soloff *et al.*, 1979). Induction of premature labor (Alexandrova and Soloff, 1980b) or delay of parturition (Bercu *et al.*, 1980) in rats is accompanied by premature or delayed increases, respectively, in both plasma estrogen/progesterone ratios and oxytocin receptor concentrations.

The effects of estrogen and progesterone on oxytocin receptor concentrations in rat myometrium have been demonstrated both *in vivo* (Fuchs *et al.*, 1983d) and *in vitro* (Fig. 6). Estrogen treatment increased oxytocin receptor concentrations about five-fold; this increase was completely blocked by progesterone. On the basis of these findings, changes in oxytocin receptor concentrations may explain why estrogen administered at the appropriate time of gestation causes abortion in the rat and several other species and why progesterone administration prolongs pregnancy.

Estrogen treatment of women at 40 to 42 weeks of pregnancy potentiated the effects of a single dose of oxytocin by increasing the intensity of uterine contractions (Pinto *et al.*, 1964). It is not clear, however, whether these effects were mediated by increases in oxytocin receptor concentrations.

Mechanisms of estrogen and progesterone regulation of oxytocin receptors. Estrogen and progesterone act directly on immature rat uteri in organ culture (Soloff *et al.*, 1983). The protein synthesis inhibitor cycloheximide in the culture medium prevented estrogen-induced increases in oxytocin receptor concentrations. Estrogen, therefore, may induce *de novo* synthesis of oxytocin receptors or the synthesis of substances that enhance oxytocin binding to its receptors. When cycloheximide was added after estrogen-induced up-regulation of oxytocin receptors, receptor concentrations remained elevated for at least several days, indicating that there was little or no turnover of receptors. When progesterone was also added, however, there was a sharp reduction in the amount of oxytocin bound. These results suggest that the down-regulating effects of progesterone are distinct from its antiestrogenic activity, because estrogen action was presumably already antagonized by the presence of cycloheximide. Progesterone, therefore, appears to down-regulate oxytocin receptors by pathways that are not the reverse of up-regulation.

Metal ions. Magnesium directly enhances the contractile activities of oxytocin and analogues in uterine smooth muscle, mammary myoepithelial, and vascular smooth muscle

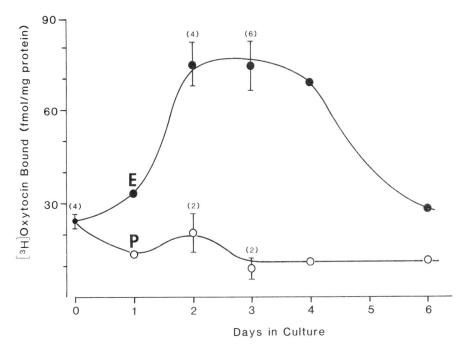

Figure 6. Effects of estradiol (E) and progesterone (P) *in vitro* on the concentration of oxytocin receptors in uterine explants from immature rats. Each point is the mean ± S.E. of *n* replicates. From Soloff *et al.* (1983).

cells (see Soloff and Grzonka, 1986, for references). Other contracting agents are not affected by Mg^{2+}. Certain divalent cations, but not Ca^{2+}, are required for the binding of [^{3}H]oxytocin to both myometrial (Soloff and Grzonka, 1986; Soloff and Swartz, 1974) and mammary gland (Pearlmutter and Soloff, 1979; Soloff and Grzonka, 1986) plasma membranes. The effects of metal ions in potentiating the activities of oxytocin and its analogues are at the receptor level (Soloff and Grzonka, 1986). Metal ions may be important in the up- and down-regulation of oxytocin receptor concentrations and for the coupling between oxytocin receptors and effectors.

4.2.3. *Coupling of Oxytocin–Receptor Occupancy and Contraction*

4.2.3a.   Calcium.   Extracellular Ca^{2+} is involved in the interaction with calmodulin, leading to phosphorylation of myosin light chains and cell contractions. Voltage-clamp studies suggest that an increased Ca^{2+} permeability explains at least some of the inward current during electrical depolarization of the myometrium (Janis and Triggle, 1986). The generation of an action potential, however, does not appear to mediate the effects of many agonists such as acetylcholine (Edman and Schild, 1962) and oxytocin (Marshall, 1974), which cause Ca^{2+}-dependent contractions of the rat myometrium even after K^+-induced depolarization.

4.2.3b.   Calcium Channels.   Dihydropyridine calcium channel blockers inhibit spontaneous uterine contractions and contractions induced by oxytocin, $PGF_{2\alpha}$, and methylergometrine (Forman *et al.*, 1982). There are functionally distinct Ca^{2+} channels in estrogen-dominated myometrium (Sakai *et al.*, 1983). Channels mediating the action of oxytocin transport Mn^{2+} as well as Ca^{2+}, whereas Ca^{2+} channels activated by acetylcholine are specific for Ca^{2+} and impermeable to Mn^{2+} (Sakai *et al.*, 1983).

Nicardipine, a dihydropyridine blocker, protracted delivery of pups when given to parturient rats immediately after birth of the first pup (Csapo *et al.*, 1982). Nifedipine, another dihydropyridine blocker, postponed premature labor in humans for 3 days without serious side effects in either mother or child (Ulmsten *et al.*, 1980).

The characteristics of [^{3}H]nitrendipine and [^{3}H]nimodipine binding to uterine membranes and other smooth muscle membranes are similar. A high-affinity binding site, apparent K_d about 0.1 nM, is present in rat and rabbit myometrium (Grover *et al.*, 1984; Miller and Moore, 1984; Golichowski and Tzeng, 1985; Janis and Triggle, 1986). Neither estrogen treatment of rats nor pregnancy produced any marked change in the affinity (Janis and Triggle, 1986). Similarly, the concentration of binding sites was not significantly changed between day 1 of pregnancy and term (Janis and Triggle, 1986). The appearance of Ca^{2+} channel binding sites therefore does not appear to be linked to the increase of oxytocin receptors near the time of labor. Uterine contractions caused by relatively low concentrations of oxytocin are inhibited more by Ca^{2+} channel blockers than are contractions induced by higher concentrations of oxytocin (Janis and Triggle, 1986). The coupling between agonist receptors and calcium channels has not yet been defined.

4.2.3c. Oxytocin-Inhibited (Ca^{2+}, Mg^{2+})-ATPase. Relaxation of myometrial cells is thought to occur when intracellular free Ca^{2+} concentrations decline. This can be brought about by a switch in sarcolemmal Ca^{2+} channels from an open to a closed state or by an increased rate of efflux of Ca^{2+} from the cytosol. If myometrial cells are similar to other cell types, the efflux of Ca^{2+} is controlled by a plasma-membrane calcium pump, which has been shown in a variety of cells to exhibit (Ca^{2+}, Mg^{2+})-ATPase activity (Gietzen *et al.*, 1980). Oxytocin inhibits (Ca^{2+}, Mg^{2+})-ATPase activity in the plasma membrane fraction of myometrium from the rabbit (Åkerman and Wikström, 1979) and rat (Soloff and Sweet, 1982). By inhibiting the efflux of Ca^{2+}, oxytocin allows a transient rise in intracellular Ca^{2+} concentration to remain elevated longer, sustaining a contractile state. The inhibition of the ATPase by a series of oxytocin analogues corresponded to their ability to inhibit the binding of [^{3}H]oxytocin and to their relative uterotonic potencies (Soloff and Sweet, 1982). Concentrations of oxytocin for half-maximal inhibition of (Ca^{2+}, Mg^{2+})-ATPase activity also corresponded to the apparent K_d for oxytocin binding to its receptor sites (Soloff and Sweet, 1980). Oxytocin receptors and oxytocin-inhibited (Ca^{2+}, Mg^{2+})-ATPase in rat myometrium were induced by estrogen treatment and inhibited by progesterone (Soloff and Sweet, 1980). At the beginning of labor in the rat, the suppressibility of myometrial (Ca^{2+}, Mg^{2+})-ATPase activity was increased about 10,000-fold, as compared to the inhibition on day 18 (Fig. 7). These changes probably are the result of the sudden shift to estrogen domination at the time of labor and reflect sharp increases in both oxytocin receptor concentrations and basal (Ca^{2+}, Mg^{2+})-ATPase activity.

4.2.3d. Phosphoinositol Metabolism. Several studies have suggested that the effects of oxytocin on the myometrium are mediated by polyphosphoinositide hydrolysis. Marc *et al.* (1986), using guinea pig myometrial strips that were prelabeled with [^{3}H]*myo*-inositol, found that both carbachol and oxytocin enhanced the rapid formation of inositol trisphosphate. Similarly, oxytocin and vasopressin stimulated the production of inositol phosphates in human gestational myometrium and decidua (Schrey *et al.*, 1986). These findings, along with those of Carsten and Miller (1985), who showed that inositol trisphosphate caused release of Ca^{2+} from sarcoplasmic reticulum vesicles from the myometrium of pregnant cows, suggest that phosphoinositol formation could mediate the actions of oxytocin in elevating intracellular Ca^{2+} concentrations from intracellular stores as well as from the exterior. Studies on the stimulatory activities of a series of oxytocin analogues remain to be done to show whether the effects of oxytocin on phosphoinositol hydrolysis are mediated by oxytocin and not vasopressin receptors. Vasopressin has been shown to stimulate phosphosinositol degradation in the vasculature (Fox *et al.*, 1987), and it is possible that oxytocin's effects are on vascular cells in the endometrium and myometrium.

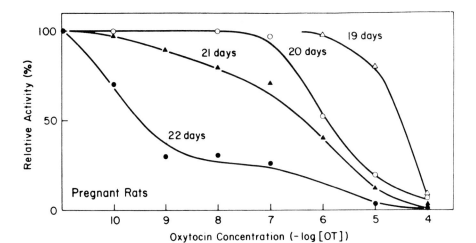

Figure 7. Oxytocin inhibition of Ca^{2+}, Mg^{2+}-ATPase activity of rat myometrial plasma membranes on days 19–22 of pregnancy. From Huszar (1986).

4.2.4. *Stimulation of Endometrial/Decidual Prostaglandin Synthesis by Oxytocin*

Apart from its uterotonic activity, oxytocin stimulates uterine prostaglandin release in several species (Chan, 1977; Mitchell *et al.,* 1975a; Roberts *et al.,* 1975; Sharma and Fitzpatrick, 1974). Oxytocin receptor concentrations in the plasma membrane fraction from homogenates of ewe endometrium increased at estrus, in conjunction with an increased sensitivity to oxytocin of $PGF_{2\alpha}$ release by endometrial explants (Roberts *et al.,* 1976). Several days before and after estrus, both oxytocin receptor concentrations and oxytocin stimulation of $PGF_{2\alpha}$ synthesis were substantially lower. Oxytocin is likely to play a role in luteal regression and to control estrous cyclicity in some species by stimulating the uterine synthesis of prostaglandins, which are luteolytic (McCracken *et al.,* 1972). Oxytocin, administered before or near the time of estrus, shortened the estrous cycle in heifers (Anderson *et al.,* 1965; Armstrong and Hansel, 1959). Immunization against oxytocin delayed luteolysis in sheep (Sheldrick *et al.,* 1980) and goats (Cooke and Homeida, 1985).

Oxytocin stimulated PGF and PGE release from decidual explants of patients at the end of gestation, either before or after the onset of labor (Fuchs *et al.,* 1982). Basal and oxytocin-stimulated prostaglandin production were significantly higher in decidual samples taken from patients after the onset of labor. In contrast to decidua, oxytocin had no effect on prostaglandin production by myometrial samples from the same uteri. An increase in oxytocin-stimulated prostaglandin release also occurred in the rat uterus in late pregnancy (Chan, 1977).

As in myometrium, oxytocin stimulated the formation of inositol trisphosphate in carnucular endometrium from ovariectomized ewes treated with estrogen and progestin (Flint *et al.,* 1986). Flint and co-workers (1986) proposed that stimulation of endometrial prostaglandin synthesis by oxytocin is the result of increased hydrolysis of phosphoinositides to diacylglycerol and inositol phosphates. The hydrolysis of diacylglycerol then releases arachidonic acid to serve as the substrate for the synthesis of prostaglandins.

4.2.5. *Decidual Oxytocin Receptors*

Concentrations of oxytocin receptors in parietal decidua increased during pregnancy and were maximal in early labor (Fuchs *et al.,* 1982, 1984). Decidual receptors had the same affinity for oxytocin as did myometrial receptors, but the binding sites have not yet been further characterized. A relationship between receptor occupancy and stimulation of prostaglandin synthesis also has not been characterized yet, nor have the factors regulating receptor concentrations during pregnancy. Because the increases in decidual and myometrial oxytocin receptor concentrations appear to be parallel, the same factors probably regulate both receptors. It is clear from results in nonpregnant sheep that oxytocin receptor concentrations in the endometrium and the release of $PGF_{2\alpha}$ in response to oxytocin *in vitro* are greatest during estrogen domination (Roberts *et al.*, 1976).

The effects of oxytocin on prostaglandin synthesis appear to be important in labor. Husslein *et al.* (1981) found that oxytocin infusion into women at term led to successful induction of labor only when PGFM levels in the maternal circulation became elevated. These workers also found that the success rate for the induction of labor by amniotomy was associated with the uterine sensitivity to oxytocin (see Husslein *et al.*, 1983). Presumably, prostaglandins released as a result of amniotomy reached the myometrium and potentiated the action of subthreshold levels of oxytocin so that contractile activity was initiated.

4.2.6. Relationship between Oxytocin and Prostaglandins

4.2.6a. Prostaglandin Sensitization of Myometrium to Oxytocin.   Saldana *et al.* (1974) showed that prostaglandin converted the human uterus from an oxytocin-resistant to an oxytocin-sensitive organ. They and others (Perry *et al.*, 1977; Salomy *et al.*, 1975; Seppala *et al.*, 1972) demonstrated shorter injection–abortion intervals in midtrimester patients receiving intravenous oxytocin along with prostaglandin. The mechanism of the sensitization has not been studied to date. Unlike oxytocin, endogenous prostaglandins might not act primarily as uterotonic agents because intravenous infusion of prostaglandins resulted in notably slow stimulation of uterine activity, with a latency period of 15 to 20 min and persistence of the uterotonic effect for 30 to 60 min after the end of the infusion (Embrey, 1969). Oxytocin infusions, on the other hand, result in almost immediate and sustained uterine contractions only for the duration of the infusion.

Other studies have shown that following the addition of PGE to the medium bathing either guinea pig (Clegg and Pickles, 1966) or human myometrial strips (Brummer, 1971), the subsequent response and sensitivity to oxytocin were enhanced. This effect, which did not result from the additive uterotonic properties of PGE and oxytocin, was seen with strips from human uteri taken at midtrimester and at term. Sometimes the enhancement lasted for as long as 90 min after the PGE had been washed out of the bath. Uterine contractions elicited by oxytocin *in vivo* could also be enhanced when patients were pretreated with PGE_2 (Gillespie, 1972). The enhancement, which persisted for 60 to 90 min after the end of the PGE_2 infusion, was distinct from potentiation, which occurred when oxytocin and PGE_2 were administered simultaneously. Brummer (1971) hypothesized that during the process of parturition endogenous prostaglandins, rather than having a direct action on the myometrium, sensitize the uterine smooth muscle to oxytocin. This might explain why the blood levels of prostaglandins attained during infusion for the induction of labor seem to be too low to promote uterine contractions directly.

4.2.6b. Mechanisms of Prostaglandin Enhancement of Oxytocin Action.   The molecular mechanisms of prostaglandin enhancement of myometrial sensitivity to oxytocin are unknown. Prostaglandins and oxytocin, both uterotonic agents, do not act through a common pathway in eliciting uterine contractions because their effects are not additive.

Because of an earlier observation that prostaglandin synthesis inhibitors inhibited the action of oxytocin on the myometrium (Hertelendy, 1973; Vane and Williams, 1972), it was assumed that the actions of oxytocin were mediated by prostaglandins. However, several laboratories showed by different approaches that the stimulation of uterine muscle contraction by oxytocin did not require prostaglandin release (Chan 1980; Dubin *et al.*, 1979; Roberts and McCracken, 1976). Unfortunately, these experiments were not designed to ascertain whether prostaglandins sensitized the uterus to oxytocin. The doses of indomethacin, a prostaglandin synthesis inhibitor used to inhibit the effects of oxytocin in the earlier experiments, might have inhibited calcium uptake rather than prostaglandin synthesis (Northover, 1972). A still untested possibility is that during the period between the infusion of prostaglandin and the effect on the uterus, the number of gap junctions between myometrial cells increases, allowing more cells to respond to a given dose of oxytocin. When a response to a low dose of oxytocin becomes perceptible because of the increased participation of cells, the myometrium would appear to be more sensitive to oxytocin.

Another possibility is that prostaglandins affect the number of oxytocin receptors. Prostaglandin $F_{2\alpha}$ administered to rats on day 18 of pregnancy caused a marked rise in oxytocin receptor concentrations in myometrial membranes 2 days later, in conjunction with premature delivery (Alexandrova and Soloff, 1980b). But the effect of prostaglandin may be indirect and the result of its luteolytic activity, causing a sharp fall in blood progesterone. Exogenous progesterone administration overrides the effects of the prostaglandin. Estrogen-induced increases in oxytocin receptor concentrations in ovariectomized rats are not prostaglandin mediated because concomitant treatment of the rats with indomethacin had no effect (Soloff and Alexandrova, 1981).

Apart from the pharmacological actions of prostaglandins, Chan (1987) suggested that prostaglandins stimulate physiological increases in myometrial oxytocin receptor concentrations during pregnancy. He found that suppression of prostaglandin synthesis with naproxen reduced the sensitivity of the myometrium of the rat to oxytocin in late pregnancy and reduced the concentration of myometrial oxytocin receptors. Simultaneous treatment with $PGF_{2\alpha}$ prevented the effects of naproxen. Although the actions of prostaglandins may be mediated by luteolysis in rats, the same mechanism does not occur in humans, who do not require a corpus luteum for the synthesis of progesterone near the end of gestation. The human does not depend on the demise of the corpus luteum or on progesterone withdrawal as a prerequisite for the initiation of parturition. The addition of 10 μM $PGF_{2\alpha}$ to myometrial plasma membranes of uteri from pregnant women caused about a twofold, significant increase in affinity for oxytocin (Fukai *et al.*, 1984). There was no change in the concentration of oxytocin binding sites. The $PGF_{2\alpha}$ effect was seen only with myometrial membranes obtained from patients at term but before labor and not in the first trimester or at term after labor (Fukai *et al.*, 1984). Whether the effects of $PGF_{2\alpha}$ on oxytocin binding are pharmacological or physiological remains to be established.

The concept that prostaglandins affect oxytocin receptor concentrations may explain the requirement for a latency period between the administration of prostaglandins and a uterotonic response *in vivo*. Latency may be the time required for an effective increase in the number of oxytocin receptors in the myometrium, allowing smooth muscle cells to respond to basal levels of oxytocin in the blood. The latency may also result from the establishment of postreceptor modifications.

4.2.6c. *Prostaglandin-Induced Release of Oxytocin.* Intravenous infusion of PGE_2 or $PGF_{2\alpha}$ increased plasma oxytocin levels in pregnant women (Gillespie *et al.*, 1972). Intramuscular injection of $PGF_{2\alpha}$ also elevated plasma oxytocin concentrations in sows both in the postpartum period and during diestrus (Ellendorff *et al.*, 1979). In addition, prostaglandins stimulated the release of oxytocin from ewe ovaries (Flint and Sheldrick, 1982). Other studies, however, showed that although oxytocin stimulates the release of uterine $PGF_{2\alpha}$ in pregnant and nonpregnant sheep, prostaglandins do not appear to affect plasma oxytocin levels (Hooper *et al.*, 1986). Although prostaglandins may enhance oxytocin action *in vivo* by stimulating an increase in oxytocin levels in the blood, it is not clear how this mechanism would account for the enhancing effects of prostaglandins on oxytocin action *in vitro*.

4.2.7. Oxytocin Antagonists

A recently synthesized competitive inhibitor of the effects of oxytocin on the uterus, 1-deamino-2-D-Tyr-(OEt)-4-Thr-8-Orn-oxytocin, has become available (Åkerlund *et al.*, 1987). Intravenous infusion of 10 to 100 µg/min for 1 to 10 hr in 13 patients exhibiting uncomplicated premature labor resulted in inhibition of uterine activity (Åkerlund *et al.*, 1987). No side effects were observed on either mother or fetus. This preliminary study supports the concept that an increased concentration of uterine oxytocin receptors is important in uncomplicated premature labor.

4.3. Relaxin

Despite the evidence for a role of relaxin in promoting myometrial quiescence, other studies have shown that the administration of relaxin near the end of gestation accelerates the time of delivery. The administration of purified porcine relaxin into the cervical os of primiparous beef heifers about 5 days before term induced premature calving (Musah *et al.*, 1986). Similarly, the administration of porcine relaxin induced labor in 10 of 30 patients 15 hr after vaginal application, whereas no patients in the control group went into labor (MacLennan *et al.*, 1980).

Downing and Sherwood (1985a) made pregnant rats relaxin-deficient by removing the ovaries and replacing estradiol and progesterone by injection. These animals exhibited significantly prolonged gestation, prolonged duration of labor and delivery, and reduced fetal survival compared with animals receiving porcine relaxin or intact controls. The parturitional effects of relaxin might may be the result of better coordination of contractions (Downing *et al.*, 1980). The mechanism of this relaxin effect is not known. Relaxin may stimulate uterine glycogen synthesis. Relaxin administered after large doses of estrogen was shown to increase myometrial glycogen content. Administration of progesterone with relaxin in estrogen-primed animals caused a further increase in uterine glycogen (Kroc *et al.*, 1959). Because of the sharp change in glycogen content in the rat myometrium near the time of labor (Chew and Rinard, 1979), glycogen serves as a likely energy source for uterine contractions in labor.

5. Cervical Distensibility

The histological structure of the cervical stroma undergoes marked changes prior to parturition in most species. This reflects the conversion of the cervix from a closed and rigid to a soft and distensible structure, permitting passage of the term fetus. Abnormalities in the cervical ripening process may result in preterm delivery if they occur too early and may be associated with postterm or prolonged labor if they fail. In the rat, cervical softening begins by day 12 of pregnancy and increases progressively throughout the remainder of pregnancy (Downing and Sherwood, 1985c). In humans, cervical maturation begins at about the 34th week of pregnancy, a time when irregular Braxton–Hicks uterine contractions are also noted.

The biochemical changes in the cervix leading to changes in its mechanical properties have been reviewed by Golichowski (1986) and Stys (1986). The bulk of normal cervix is collagen; the muscle fiber content is less than 10% of cervical bulk (Danforth, 1947). Cervical maturation is characterized by a degradation of collagen and other proteins, resulting in loosening of the compactly arranged collagen fibers, and changes in the composition of the glycosaminoglycan ground substance. A marked increase in hyaluronic acid and its associated high water content causes the soft, swollen appearance of the cervix, whereas loss of collagen and dermatan/chondroitin sulfates increases flexibility and distensibility (Danforth *et al.*, 1974).

5.1. Hormonal Control of Cervical Maturation

Several hormones influence cervical ripening. Some have been used to promote cervical ripening before induction of labor to increase the success rate of induction and to shorten the induction-to-delivery time.

5.1.1. Estrogens

Ripening of the cervix occurs under the influence of estradiol (Pinto *et al.*, 1964). In a double-blind study, Gordon and Calder (1977) showed that extraamniotic instillation of estradiol in primigravid patients near term with unripe cervices increased the Bishop scores significantly and allowed induction of labor with greater success. The involuting uterus and explants of cervical and uterine tissues have served as experimental models for a study of the effects on collagenase activity and collagen breakdown of steroid hormones. Estrogens increase collagenase formation by synthesis and activation of zymogens. The inhibitory effect of progesterone on cervical maturation is well documented. In response to progesterone administration, collagen breakdown was diminished in the uterus of parturient rats (Tansey *et al.*, 1978) and in the guinea pig pubic symphysis ligament (Wahl *et al.*, 1977).

5.1.2. Relaxin

Relaxin is involved in the biochemical and biophysical changes in the uterine cervix that promote cervical dilatation immediately prior to parturition (for reviews see Schwabe *et al.*, 1978; Bryant-Greenwood, 1982). In rats, removal of the ovaries, the source of relaxin, during late pregnancy followed by treatment with progesterone and estrogen resulted in failure of the cervix to exhibit increased extensibility (see Downing and Sherwood, 1985c, for references). When ovariectomized pregnant rats were treated with porcine relaxin in conjunction with estrogen and progesterone, their cervices exhibited similar extensibility and an ability to accommodate to stretch as did cervices from intact pregnant rats of the same stage of late pregnancy (Downing and Sherwood, 1985c). The extensibility of the cervix of estrogen-primed mice also was increased by treatment with porcine relaxin (Fields and Larkin, 1980). In pigs, injection of relaxin induced premature cervical dilatation and reduced the delivery time (Kertiles and Anderson, 1979). In the human near term, MacLennan *et al.* (1980) have presented evidence suggesting that exogenous relaxin facilitates cervical ripening with little change in uterine activity.

Relaxin binding sites have been demonstrated in membrane preparations from the cervices of pigs treated with gonadotropins (Mercado-Simmen *et al.*, 1982). The concentration of [^{125}I]relaxin binding sites fell sharply after ovariectomy and could not be restored by estrogen treatment. In contrast, the number of myometrial membrane binding sites, which also fell after ovariectomy, increased after estrogen treatment. These findings suggest that relaxin receptors concentrations in the cervix are regulated differently from those in the myometrium and that the control of sensitivity to relaxin, as expressed by receptor concentrations, differs in the two tissues. Events occurring after relaxin–receptor interaction are not well understood; cAMP levels increase in the cervices of rats (Cheah and Sherwood, 1980) and pigs (Judson *et al.*, 1980). The consequence of this action is, as yet, unknown.

5.1.3. Prostaglandins

Prostaglandins have been shown to be effective in cervical ripening when administered orally (Pearce, 1977; Valentine, 1977), extraamniotically (Calder *et al.*, 1977), or intravaginally (MacKenzie and Embrey, 1977). Locally administered forms of PGE_2, including intracervical gels and vaginal suppositories, have been found to be effective and safe methods for preinduction of cervical ripening as well as for induction of labor (Ekman *et al.*, 1983).

Evidence suggests that PGE_2 has a local ripening effect on the gravid cervix independent of uterine contractile activity when administered in a fashion that avoided exposure of the extraamniotic space to PGE_2 gel. Intracervical PGE_2 in the first-trimester pregnant woman caused ultrastructural changes characteristic of cervical ripening at term (Theobald *et al.*, 1982). Intracervical administration of PGE_2 in gel to women for cervical priming and induction of labor significantly increased collagenolytic activity in cervical biopsy specimens (Ekman *et al.*, 1986). Others, however, have suggested that enzymatic degradation of collagen does not play a predominent role in prostaglandin-induced cervical ripening (Rath *et al.*, 1987). Instead, changes in glycosaminoglycan content may be more important.

The administration of either PGE_2 or $PGF_{2\alpha}$ to rats on day 18 of pregnancy doubled the extensibility of the cervix by day 19 (Hollingsworth *et al.*, 1980). The administration of progesterone had no effect alone or on the effect of PGE_2 but inhibited the action of $PGF_{2\alpha}$. The effects of $PGF_{2\alpha}$, but not those of PGE_2, also were inhibited by ovariectomy in the rat. These results suggest that PGE_2 and $PGF_{2\alpha}$ act differently in promoting cervical extensibility in the rat. Whereas PGE_2 might act directly on the cervix, the effects of $PGF_{2\alpha}$ appear to be mediated by luteal regression. Prostaglandin $F_{2\alpha}$ infusion into pigs during late pregnancy caused a relaxin surge from the ovaries into the circulation (Sherwood *et al.*, 1969). The administration of indomethacin delayed the release of relaxin before parturition. These findings, along with those of Hollingsworth *et al.*, (1980), suggest that effects of prostaglandins on the cervix might be mediated by relaxin. However, induction of labor in women with $PGF_{2\alpha}$ did not cause a significant elevation in serum relaxin immunoactivity (Hochman *et al.*, 1978), implying that $PGF_{2\alpha}$ acts directly on the cervix. It is possible that the effects of relaxin are mediated by prostaglandins, but definitive experiments to test this relationship have not been carried out.

5.2. Relationship between Cervical Maturation and Myometrial Contractions

Cervical maturation and myometrial contractions can occur independently. Yet, the two processes occur together temporally and appear to be regulated similarly. In patients with prolonged pregnancies, those with unripe cervices were only rarely good candidates for induction of labor (Harris *et al.*, 1983). In a retrospective study by Lange *et al.* (1982), about 1200 patients were analyzed for a correlation between cervical status and inducibility of labor. Cervical dilatation and effacement were the best predictors of the onset of labor. Similar conclusions have been drawn by other investigators (Bouyer *et al.*, 1986).

Some of the similarities in regulation of cervical changes and myometrial activity have been pointed out by Huszar *et al.* (1986). They include the following.

1. Progesterone dominance during pregnancy is associated with a firmly closed cervix and a quiescent myometrium.
2. At term, estrogen or rising estrogen/progesterone ratios have been shown to be important in increased uterine contractility and in cervical ripening.
3. Prostaglandin $F_{2\alpha}$ and other prostanoids have direct stimulatory effects on uterine contractility as well as direct and indirect actions on cervical ripening. Whereas prostaglandins at low levels bring about cervical maturation, administration of PGE_2 and $PGF_{2\alpha}$ in larger amounts will induce myometrial contractions in pregnant women at any stage of gestation.

On the basis of the preceding, the following sequence of events in initiation of labor in humans is proposed. The concentration of oxytocin receptors increases during gestation and doubles before the onset of labor. There is more than a 100-fold increase in the concentration of myometrial oxytocin receptors from the beginning to the end of gestation. This increase is probably caused by increasing estrogen concentrations in the blood, but additional factors may be involved. Although there is little or no change in circulating oxytocin levels, increased receptor levels allow more oxytocin to be bound to myometrial cells. The threshold to oxytocin is then lowered to the point at which the smooth muscle cells contract in response to basal or slightly elevated levels of oxytocin.

Oxytocin also binds to decidual cell receptors, which are up-regulated during pregnancy, stimulating prostaglandin synthesis. Prostaglandins likely enhance the sensitivity of the myometrial response to oxytocin, possibly at the postreceptor level. Part or all of the effects of increased prostaglandin levels may be to increase the number of gap junctions between myometrial cells (Garfield *et al.,* 1980). Cells that do not have oxytocin receptors or cells with unoccupied receptors may be coupled chemically to those that do. As a result, a given concentration of oxytocin elicits a magnified response, which could appear as an increase in sensitivity to oxytocin.

During the expulsive stage of labor, oxytocin levels in the blood increase, and a greater fraction of oxytocin receptor sites is occupied. Myometrial contractions are enhanced, and delivery is facilitated. Following parturition, the concentration of uterine oxytocin receptors falls off rapidly, dampening the response of the uterus to elevated levels of oxytocin in the blood during lactation.

Progesterone and estrogens play a facilitatory role in the initiation of labor. As suggested by Fuchs and Fuchs (1984), oxytocin may be important for the initial phase of labor, whereas increased synthesis of $PGF_{2\alpha}$ would be essential for the progression of labor. Prostaglandin E_2 may play a role in the ripening of the cervix as an essential step for successful parturition. Cervical dilitation appears to operate independently of uterine contractions, but both processes may be governed by some of the same operators. Relaxin serves to prepare the cervix for delivery.

7. Unification of Mechanisms Proposed for Spontaneous Labor Induction

Although different mechanisms of labor initiation operate in different species, physiological processes generally tend to be more similar than different in related species. Accordingly, a unified mechanism for initiation of labor should take into account the various models that have been proposed. The postulate that labor is initiated by increased sensitivity of the myometrium to oxytocin and that this is accomplished by up-regulation of oxytocin receptors is compatible with other hypotheses because of the following observations.

7.1. Prostaglandins

Demonstration of elevated oxytocin receptors in decidual tissues at the end of pregnancy makes it possible to reconcile hypotheses that have excluded either prostaglandins or oxytocin as natural labor initiators. Elevation of prostaglandin levels during labor may be the result of oxytocin stimulation of decidual cells. The role for prostaglandins, whether uterotonic, supportive of the uterotonic effects of oxytocin, or acting instead at other loci, remains to be clarified. Oxytocin, therefore, may be capable of serving a dual function in initiating labor by its effects on both myometrium and endometrium. Whether oxytocin receptors on fetal membranes are capable of stimulating prostaglandin release remains to be clarified.

In species like the rat that depend on the luteal synthesis of progesterone for maintenance of pregnancy, administration of a single dose of $PGF_{2\alpha}$ beyond 15 days of pregnancy results in premature termination of gestation with a corresponding increase in oxytocin receptor concentrations in the myometrium. Because this action of $PGF_{2\alpha}$ can be prevented by simultaneous administration of progesterone, it is likely that the increase in oxytocin receptor concentration is the result of the luteolytic activity of PGF. In species like the human that do not require an intact corpus luteum for maintenance of pregnancy, prostaglandins may induce increases in oxytocin receptor concentration by other mechanisms that remain to be studied or by sensitizing the myometrium to basal levels of oxytocin in the blood.

7.2. Estrogen/Progesterone

Changes in uterine oxytocin receptor concentrations are regulated by estrogen/progesterone concentrations. Estrogen domination of the uterus, which may result from increases in the ratio of estrogen/progesterone concentrations in blood or from increases in estrogen levels alone, is compatible with the progesterone block theory of Csapo (1956). An absence of progesterone withdrawal in species such as the human and guinea pig does not necessarily preclude estrogen stimulation of oxytocin receptor concentrations in the myometrium and possibly the endometrium during pregnancy, particularly the latter stages.

7.3. Fetal ACTH

In the sheep, there is strong evidence that implicates the fetal release of ACTH in initiation of labor. Resultant elevations in glucocorticoids, in turn, likely lower progesterone and increase estrogen levels in the maternal circulation. These changes result in an increase in concentrations of oxytocin receptors. The oxytocin receptor mechanism is compatible with other models that have been suggested for the initiation of labor. The fetus may be involved in coordinating activities leading to labor through its influence on placental production of estrogen and possibly its secretion of neurohypophyseal hormones and other stimulators (or inhibitors) of prostaglandin synthesis. In conclusion, the up- and down-regulation of receptors illustrate that it is important to understand that uterine status cannot necessarily be assessed from circulating hormone levels alone. An understanding of factors involved in initiating labor therefore must take into consideration levels of receptor as well as those of circulating hormones.

ACKNOWLEDGMENTS. I am grateful to Murray Saffran for editorial advice.

8. References

Abel, M. H., and Baird, D. T., 1980, The effect of 17β-estradiol and progesterone on prostaglandin production by human endometrium maintained in organ culture. *Endocrinology* **106:**1599–1606.

Abel, M. H., and Kelly, R. W., 1979, Differential production of prostaglandins within the human uterus, *Prostaglandins* **18:**821–828.

Abel, M. H., Smith, S. K., and Baird, D. T., 1980, Suppression of concentration of endometrial prostaglandin in early intra-uterine and ectopic pregnancy in women, *J. Endocrinol.* **85:**379–386.

Adelstein, R. S., Conti, M. A., Hathaway, D. R., and Klee, C. B., 1978, Phosphorylation of smooth muscle myosin light chain kinase by the catalytic subunit of adenosine 3':5'-monophosphate-dependent protein kinase. *J. Biol. Chem.* **253:**8347–8350.

Ahlquist, R. P., 1966, The adrenergic receptor, *J. Pharm. Sci.* **55:**359–367.

Aiken, J. W., 1972, Aspirin and indomethacin prolong parturition in rats. Evidence that prostaglandins contribute to expulsion of foetus, *Nature* **240:**21–25.

Åkerlund, M., Strömberg, P., Hauksson, A., Andersen, L. F., Lyndrup, J., Trojnar, J., and Melin, P., 1987, Inhibition of uterine contractions of premature labour with an oxytocin analogue, *Br. J. Obstet. Gynaecol.* **94:**1040–1044.

Åkerman, K. E. O., and Wikström, M. K. F., 1979, (Ca^{2+} + Mg^{2+})-stimulated ATPase activity of rabbit myometrium plasma membrane is blocked by oxytocin *FEBS Lett.* **97:**283–287.

Alexandrova, M., and Soloff, M. S., 1980a, Oxytocin receptors and parturition. I. Control of oxytocin receptor concentration in the rat myometrium at term, *Endocrinology* **106:**730–735.

Alexandrova, M., and Soloff, M. S., 1980b, Oxytocin receptors and parturition. III. Increases in estrogen receptor and oxytocin receptor concentrations in the rat myometrium during PGF$_{2\alpha}$-induced abortion, *Endocrinology* **106:**739–743.

Alexandrova, M., and Soloff, M. S., 1980c, Oxytocin receptors and parturition in the guinea pig, *Biol. Reprod.* **22:**1106–1111.

Anderson, L. L., Bowerman, A. M., and Melampy, R. M., 1965, Oxytocin on ovarian function in cycling and hysterectomized heifers, *J. Anim. Sci.* **24:**964–968.

Andersson, R. G. G., Berg, G., Johansson, S.R. M., and Rydén, G., 1980, Effects of non-selective and selective beta-adrenergic agonists on spontaneous contractions and cyclic AMP levels in myometrial strips from pregnant women, *Gynecol. Obstet. Invest.* **11:**286–293.

Armstrong, D. T., and Hansel, W., 1959, Alteration of the bovine estrous cycle with oxytocin, *J. Dairy Sci.* **42:**533–542.

Bauknecht, T., Krahe, B., Rechenbach, U., Zahradnik, H. P., and Breckwoldt, M., 1981, Distribution of prostaglandin E$_2$ and prostaglandin F$_{2\alpha}$ receptors in human myometrium, *Acta Endocrinol. (Kbh.)* **98:**446–450.

Bejar, R., Curbelo, V., Davis, C., and Gluck, L., 1981, Premature labor. II. Bacterial sources of phospholipase, *Obstet. Gynecol.* **57:**479–482.

Bell, C., and Malcolm, S. J., 1978, Observations on the loss of catecholamine fluorescence from intrauterine adrenergic nerves during pregnancy in the guinea pig, *J. Reprod. Fertil.* **53:**51–58.

Bercu, B. B., Hyashi, A., Poth, M., Alexandrova, M., Soloff, M. S., and Donahoe, P. K., 1980, LHRH-induced delay of parturition, *Endocrinology* **107:**504–508.

Billah, M. M., and Johnston, J. M., 1983, Identification of phospholipid platelet-activating factor (1-O-alkyl-2-acetyl-*sn*-glycero-3-phosphocholine) in human amniotic fluid and urine, *Biochem. Biophys. Res. Commun.* **113:**51–58.

Billah, M. M., Di Renzo, G. C., Ban, C., Truong, C. T., Hoffman, D. R., Anceschi, M. M., Bleasdale, J. E., and Johnston, J. M., 1985, Platelet-activating factor metabolism in human amnion and the responses of this tissue to extracellular platelet-activating factor, *Prostaglandins* **30:**841–850.

Blatchley, F. R., Donovan, B. T., Poyser, N. L., Horton, E. W., Thompson, C. J., and Los, M., 1971, Identification of prostaglandin F$_{2\alpha}$ in the utero-ovarian blood of guinea-pig after treatment with estrogen, *Nature* **230:**243–244.

Bleasdale, J. E., Okazaki, T., Sagawa, N., Di Renzo, G. C., Okita, J. R., MacDonald, P. C., and Johnston, J. M., 1983, The mobilization of arachidonic acid for prostaglandin production during parturition, in: *Initiation of Parturition: Prevention of Prematurity* (P. C. MacDonald and J. Porter, eds.), Ross Laboratories, Columbus, OH, pp. 129–137.

Bothwell, W., Verburg, M., Wynalda, M., Daniels, E. G., and Fitzpatrick, F. A., 1982, A radioimmunoassay for the unstable pulmonary metabolite of prostaglandin E$_1$ and E$_2$: An indirect index of their *in vivo* disposition and pharmacokinetics, *J. Pharmacol. Exp. Ther.* **220:**229–235.

Bouyer, J., Papiernik, E., Dreyfus, J., Collin, D., Winisdoerffer, B., and Gueguen, S., 1986, Maturation signs of the cervix and prediction of preterm birth, *Obstet. Gynecol.* **68:**209–214.

Boyle, M. B., MacLusky, N. J., Naftolin, F., and Kaczmarek, L., 1987, Hormonal regulation of potassium channel mRNA in cycling and pregnant myometrium, *Nature* **330:**373–375.

Brennecke, S. P., Lenton, E. A., Turnbull, A. C., and Mitchell, M. D., 1982, Inhibition of prostaglandin synthase by maternal plasma factor(s) in early human pregnancy, *Br. J. Obstet. Gynaecol.* **89:**612–616.

Brennecke, S. P., Humphreys, J., Bryce, R. L., Teasdale, W. P., Turnbull, A. C., and Mitchell, M. D., 1984, Maternal plasma inhibition of prostaglandin synthase during human pregnancy, parturition and the puerperium, *Br. J. Obstet. Gynaecol.* **91:**349–352.

Brennecke, S. P., Castle, B. M., Demers, L. M., and Turnbull, A. C., 1985, Maternal plasma prostaglandin E_2 metabolite levels during human pregnancy and parturition, *Br. J. Obstet. Gynaecol.* **92**:345–349.

Brummer, H. C., 1971, Interaction of E prostaglandins and syntocinon on the pregnant human myometrium, *J. Obstet. Gynaecol. Br. Commonw.* **78**:305–309.

Bryant-Greenwood, G. D., 1982, Relaxin as new hormone, *Endocrine Rev.* **3**:62–90.

Cabrol, D., Bouviér d'Yvoire, M., Mermet, E., Cedard, L., Sureau, C., and Baulieu, E. E., 1985, Induction of labour with mifepristone after intrauterine fetal death, *Lancet* **2**:1019.

Calder, A. A., Embrey, M. P., and Tait, T., 1977, Ripening of the cervix with extra-amniotic prostaglandin E_2 in viscous gel before induction of labor, *Br. J. Obstet. Gynaecol.* **84**:264–268.

Caldeyro-Barcia, R., and Sereno, J., 1961, The response of the human uterus to oxytocin throughout pregnancy, in: *Oxytocin* (R. Caldeyro-Barcia and H. Heller, eds.), Pergamon Press, Oxford, pp. 177–202.

Caldwell, B. V., Tillson, S., Brock, W. A., and Speroff, L., 1972, The effects of exogenous progesterone and estradiol on prostaglandin F levels in ovariectomized ewes, *Prostaglandins* **1**:217–238.

Carsten, M. E., and Miller, J. D., 1985, Ca^{2+} release by inositol trisphosphate from Ca^{2+}-transporting microsomes derived from uterine sarcoplasmic reticulum, *Biochem. Biophys. Res. Commun.* **130**:1027–1031.

Casey, M. L., and MacDonald, P. C., 1984, Endocrinology of preterm birth, *Clin. Obstet. Gynecol.* **27**:562–571.

Casey, M. L., Cutrer, S. I., and Mitchell, M. D., 1983a, Origin of prostanoids in human amniotic fluid: The fetal kidney as a source of amniotic fluid prostanoids, *Am. J. Obstet. Gynecol.* **147**:547–551.

Casey, M. L., MacDonald, P. C., and Mitchell, M. D., 1983b, Stimulation of prostaglandin E_2 production in amnion cells in culture by a substance(s) in human fetal and adult urine, *Biochem. Biophys. Res. Commun.* **114**:1056–1063.

Casey, M. L., MacDonald, P. C., and Mitchell, M. D., 1984, Characterization of prostaglandin formation by human amnion cells in monolayer culture, *Prostaglandins* **27**:421–427.

Challis, J. R. G., and Vaughan, M., 1987, Steroid synthetic and prostaglandin metabolizing activity is present in different cell populations from human fetal membranes and decidua, *Am. J. Obstet. Gynecol.* **157**:1474–1481.

Chamley, W. A., Bagoyo, M. M., and Bryant-Greenwood, G. D., 1977, *In vitro* response of relaxin-treated rat uterus to prostaglandins and oxytocin, *Prostaglandins* **14**:763–769.

Chan, W. Y., 1977, Relationship between the uterotonic action of oxytocin and prostaglandins: Oxytocin action and release of PG-activity in isolated nonpregnant and pregnant rat uteri, *Biol. Reprod.* **17**:541–548.

Chan, W. Y., 1980, The separate uterotonic and prostaglandin-releasing actions of oxytocin. Evidence and comparison with angiotensin and methacholine in the isolated rat uterus, *J. Pharmacol. Exp. Ther.* **213**:575–579.

Chan, W. Y., 1987, Enhanced prostaglandin synthesis in the parturient rat uterus and its effects on myometrial oxytocin receptor concentrations, *Prostaglandins* **34**:889–902.

Chang, W.-C., Nakao, J., Murota, S.-I., and Tai, H.-H., 1983, Induction of fatty acid cyclooxygenase in rat aortic smooth muscle cells by estradiol, *Prostaglandins Leukotrienes Med.* **10**:33–37.

Cheah, S. H., and Sherwood, O. D., 1980, Target tissues for relaxin in the rat: Tissue distribution of injected ^{125}I-labeled relaxin and tissue changes in adenosine $3',5'$-monophosphate levels after *in vitro* relaxin incubation, *Endocrinology* **106**:1203–1209.

Chegini, N., and Rao, C. V., 1988, The presence of leukotriene C_4- and prostacyclin-binding sites in nonpregnant human uterine tissue, *J. Clin. Endocrinol. Metab.* **66**:76–87.

Chegini, N., Rao, C. V., Wakim, N., and Sanfilippo, J., 1986, Prostaglandin binding to different cell types of human uterus: Quantitative light microscope autoradiographic study, *Prostaglandins Leukotrienes Med.* **22**:129–138.

Chester, R., Dukes, M., Slater, S. R., and Walpole, A. L., 1972, Delay of parturition in the rat by anti-inflammatory agents which inhibit the biosynthesis of prostaglandins, *Nature* **240**:37–38.

Chew, C. S., and Rinard, G. A., 1979, Glycogen levels in the rat myometrium at the end of pregnancy and immediately postpartum, *Biol. Reprod.* **20**:1111–1114.

Clark, J. H., and Markaverich, B. M., 1984, The agonistic and antagonistic actions of estriol, *J. Steroid Biochem.* **20**:1005–1013.

Clark, J. H., Hsueh, A. J. W., and Peck, E. J., Jr., 1977, Regulation of estrogen receptor replenishment by progesterone, *Ann. N.Y. Acad. Sci.* **286**:161–179.

Clegg, P. C., Hall, W. J., and Pickles, V. R., 1966, The action of ketonic prostaglandins on the guinea pig myometrium, *J. Physiol. (Lond.)* **183**:123–146.

Cooke, R. G., and Homeida, A. M., 1985, Suppression of prostaglandin $F_{2\alpha}$ release and delay of luteolysis after active immunization against oxytocin in the goat, *J. Reprod. Fertil.* **75**:63–68.

Cornette, J. C., Harrison, K. L., and Kirton, K. T., 1974, Measurement of prostaglandin $F_{2\alpha}$ metabolites by radioimmunoassay, *Prostaglandins* **5**:155–164.

Crankshaw, D. J., 1987, The sensitivity of the longitudinal and circular muscle layers of the rat's myometrium to oxytocin *in vitro* during pregnancy, *Can. J. Physiol. Pharmacol.* **65**:773–777.

Crankshaw, D. J., Crankshaw, J., Branda, L. A., and Daniel, E. E., 1979, Receptors for E type prostaglandins in the plasma membrane of nonpregnant human myometrium, *Arch. Biochem. Biophys.* **198**:70–77.

Creange, J. E., Schane, H. P., Anzalone, A. J., and Potts, G. O., 1978, Interruption of pregnancy in rats by azastene, an inhibitor of ovarian and adrenal steroidogenesis, *Fertil. Steril.* **30**:86–90.

Csapo, A. I., 1956, Progesterone block, *Am. J. Anat.* **98**:273–291.

Csapo, A. I., 1975, The "seesaw" theory of the regulatory mechanism of pregnancy, *Am. J. Obstet. Gynecol.* **121**:578–581.

Csapo, A. I., and Resch, B. A., 1979, Induction of preterm labor in the rat by antiprogesterone, *Am. J. Obstet. Gynecol.* **134**:823–827.

Csapo, A. I., and Takeda, H., 1965, Effect of progesterone on the electrical activity and intra-uterine pressure of pregnant and parturient rabbits, *Am. J. Obstet. Gynecol.* **91**:221–231.

Csapo, A. I., and Wiest, W. G., 1969, An examination of the quantitative relationship between progesterone and maintenance of pregnancy, *Endocrinology* **85**:735–746.

Csapo, A. I., Puri, C. P., Tarro, S., and Henzl, M. R., 1982, Deactivation of the uterus during normal and premature labor by the calcium antagonist nicardipine, *Am. J. Obstet. Gynecol.* **142**:483–491.

Danforth, D. N., 1947, Fibrous nature of human cervix, and its relation to isthmic segment in gravid and nongravid uteri, *Am. J. Obstet. Gynecol.* **53**:541–560.

Danforth, D. N., Veis, A., Breen, M., Weinstein, H. G., Buckingham, J. C., and Manalo, P., 1974, The effect of pregnancy and labor on the human cervix: Changes in collagen, glycoproteins, and glycosaminoglycans, *Am. J. Obstet. Gynecol.* **120**:641–651.

Darne, J., McGarrigle, H. H. G., and Lachelin, G. C. L., 1987, Saliva oestriol, oestradiol, oestrone and progesterone levels in pregnancy: Spontaneous labour at term is preceded by a rise in the saliva oestriol:progesterone ratio, *Br. J. Obstet. Gynaecol.* **94**:227–235.

Dey, F. L., Fisher, C., and Ranson, S. W., 1941, Disturbances in pregnancy and labor in guinea pigs with hypothalamic lesions, *Am. J. Obstet. Gynecol.* **42**:459–466.

Diczfalusy, E., 1974, Endocrine functions of the human fetus and placenta, *Am. J. Obstet. Gynecol.* **119**:419–433.

Di Renzo, G. C., Johnston, J. M., Okazaki, T., Okita, J. R., MacDonald, P. C., and Bleasdale, J. E., 1981, Phosphatidylinositol-specific phospholipase C in fetal membranes and uterine decidua, *J. Clin. Invest.* **67**:847–856.

Di Renzo, G. C., Anceschi, M. M., and Bleasdale, J. E., 1984a, Beta-adrenergic stimulation of prostaglandin production by human amnion tissue, *Prostaglandins* **27**:37–49.

Di Renzo, G. C., Venincasa, M. D., and Bleasdale, J. E., 1984b, The identification and characterization of β-adrenergic receptors in human amnion tissue, *Am. J. Obstet. Gynecol.* **148**:398–405.

Divers, W. A., Jr., Wilkes, M. M., Babaknia, A., and Yen, S. S. C., 1981, An increase in catecholamines and metabolites in the amniotic fluid compartment from middle to late gestation, *Am. J. Obstet. Gynecol.* **139**:483–486.

Downing, S. J., and Sherwood, O. D., 1985a, The physiological role of relaxin in the pregnant rat. I. The influence of relaxin on parturition, *Endocrinology* **116**:1200–1205.

Downing, S. J., and Sherwood, O. D., 1985b, The physiological role of relaxin in the pregnant rat. II. The influence of relaxin on uterine contractile activity, *Endocrinology* **116**:1206–1214.

Downing, S. J., and Sherwood, O. D., 1985c, The physiological role of relaxin in the pregnant rat. III. The influence of relaxin on cervical extensibility, *Endocrinology* **116**:1215–1220.

Downing, S. J., Bradshaw, J. M. C., and Porter, D. G., 1980, Relaxin improves the coordination of rat myometrial activity *in vivo*, *Biol. Reprod.* **23**:899–903.

Dubin, N. H., Ghodgaonkar, R. B., and King, T. M., 1979, Role of prostaglandin production in spontaneous and oxytocin-induced uterine contractile activity in *in vitro* pregnant rat uteri, *Endocrinology* **105**:47–51.

Edman, K. A. P., and Schild, H. O., 1962, The need for the calcium in the contractile responses induced by acetylcholine and potassium in the rat uterus, *J. Physiol. (Lond.)* **161**:424–441.

Ekman, G., Forman, A., Marsál, K., and Ulmsten, U., 1983, Intravaginal versus intracervical application of prostaglandin E_2 in viscous gel for cervical priming and induction of labor at term in patients with an unfavorable cervical state, *Am. J. Obstet. Gynecol.* **147**:657–661.

Ekman, G., Malmström, A., Uldbjerg, N., and Ulmsten, U., 1986, Cervical collagen: An important regulator of cervical function in term labor, *Obstet. Gynecol.* **67**:633–636.

Ellendorff, F., Forsling, M., Parvizi, N., Williams, H., Taverne, M., and Smidt, D., 1979, Plasma oxytocin and vasopressin concentrations in response to prostaglandin injection into the pig, *J. Reprod. Fertil.* **56:**573–577.

Embrey, M. P., 1969, The effect of prostaglandins on human pregnant uterus, *J. Obstet. Gynaecol. Br. Commonw.* **76:**783–789.

Falck Larsen, J., Kern Hansen, M., Hesseldahl, H., Kristoffersen, K., Larsen, P. K., Osler, M., Weber, J., Eldon, K., and Lange, A., 1980, Ritodrine in the treatment of preterm labour. A clinical trial to compare a standard treatment with three regimens involving the use of ritodrine, *Br. J. Obstet. Gynaecol.* **87:**949–957.

Falck Larsen, J., Eldon, K., Lange, A. P., Leegaard, M., Osler, M. Sederberg Olsen, J., and Permin, M., 1986, Ritodrine in the treatment of preterm labor: Second Danish multicenter study, *Obstet. Gynecol.* **67:**607–613.

Ferguson, J. K. W., 1941, A study of the motility of the intact uterus at term, *Surg. Gynecol. Obstet.* **73:**359–366.

Fields, P. A., and Larkin, L. H., 1980, Enhancement of uterine cervix extensibility in oestrogen-primed mice following administration of relaxin, *J. Endocrinol.* **87:**147–152.

Fisher, C., Magoun, H. W., and Ranson, S. W., 1938, Dystocia in diabetes insipidus. The relation of pituitary oxytocin to parturition, *Am. J. Obstet. Gynecol.* **36:**1–9.

Fitzpatrick, F. A., Aguirre, R., Pike, J. E., and Lincoln, F. H., 1980, The stability of 13,14-dihydro-15 keto-PGE_2, *Prostaglandins* **19:**917–931.

Flint, A. P. F., and Sheldrick, E. L., 1982, Ovarian secretion of oxytocin is stimulated by prostaglandins, *Nature* **297:**587–588.

Flint, A. P. F., Leat, W. M. F., Sheldrick, E. L., and Stewart, H. J., 1986, Stimulation of phosphoinositide hydrolysis by oxytocin and the mechanism by which oxytocin controls prostaglandin synthesis in the ovine endometrium, *Biochem. J.* **237:**797–805.

Flower, R. J., and Blackwell, G. J., 1979, Anti-inflammatory steroids induce biosynthesis of a phospholipase A_2 inhibitor which prevents prostaglandin generation, *Nature* **278:**456–459.

Forman, A., Gandrup, P., Andersson, K.-E., and Ulmsten, U., 1982, Effects of nifedipine on oxytocin- and prostaglandin $F_{2\alpha}$-induced activity in the postpartum uterus, *Am. J. Obstet. Gynecol.* **144:**665–670.

Fox, A. W., Friedman, P. A., and Abel, P. W., 1987, Vasopressin receptor mediated contraction and [^{3}H]inositol metabolism in rat tail artery, *Eur. J. Pharmacol.* **135:**1–10.

Fuchs, A.-R., 1972, Prostaglandin effects on rat pregnancy. I. Failure of induction of labor, *Fertil. Steril.* **23:**410–416.

Fuchs, A.-R., 1985, Oxytocin in animal parturition, in: *Oxytocin. Clinical and Laboratory Studies* (J. A. Amico, and A. G. Robinson, eds.), Elsevier, Amsterdam, pp. 207–235.

Fuchs, A.-R., and Fuchs, F., 1984, Endocrinology of human parturition: A review, *Br. J. Obstet. Gynaecol.* **91:**948–967.

Fuchs, A.-R., and Poblete, V. R., Jr., 1970, Oxytocin and uterine function in pregnant and parturient rats, *Biol. Reprod* **2:**387–400.

Fuchs, A.-R., Mok, E., and Sundaram, K., 1974, Luteolytic effects of prostaglandins in rat pregnancy, and reversal by luteinizing hormone, *Acta Endocrinol. (Kbh).* **76:**583–596.

Fuchs, A.-R., Fuchs, F., Husslein, P., Soloff, M. S., and Fernstrom, M., 1982, Oxytocin receptors and human parturition: A dual role for oxytocin in the initiation of labor, *Science* **215:**1396–1398.

Fuchs, A.-R., Periyasamy, S., Alexandrova, M., and Soloff, M. S., 1983a, Correlation between oxytocin receptor concentration and responsiveness to oxytocin in pregnant rat myometrium. Effects of ovarian steroids, *Endocrinology* **113:**742–749.

Fuchs, A.-R., Goeschen, K., Husslein, P., Rasmussen, A. B., and Fuchs, F., 1983b, Oxytocin and the initiation of human parturition. III. Plasma concentrations of oxytocin and 13,14-dihydro-15-keto-prostaglandin $F_{2\alpha}$ in spontaneous and oxytocin-induced labor at term, *Am. J. Obstet. Gynecol.* **147:**497–502.

Fuchs, A.-R., Fuchs, F., Husslein, P., and Soloff, M. S., 1984, Oxytocin receptors in human uterus during pregnancy and parturition, *Am. J. Obstet. Gynecol.* **150:**734–741.

Fuchs, A.-R., Fuchs, F., and Soloff, M. S., 1985, Oxytocin receptors in nonpregnant human uterus, *J. Clin. Endocrinol. Metab.* **60:**37–41.

Fukai, H., Den, K., Sakamoto, H., Kodaira, H., Uchida, F., and Takagi, S., 1984, Study of oxytocin receptor: II. Oxytocin and prostaglandin $F_{2\alpha}$ receptors in human myometria and amnion–decidua complex during pregnancy and labor, *Endocrinol. Jpn.* **31:**565–570.

Furr, B. J. A., Valcaccia, B., and Challis, J. R. G., 1976, The effects of Nolvadex (tamoxifen citrate; ICI 46,474) on pregnancy in rabbits, *J. Reprod. Fertil.* **48:**367–369.

Garfield, R. E., Kannan, M. S., and Daniel, E. E., 1980, Gap junction formation in myometrium: Control by estrogens, progesterone, and prostaglandins, *Am. J. Physiol.* **238:**C81–C89.

Gennser, G., Ohrlander, S., and Eneroth, P., 1977, Fetal cortisol and the initiation of labour in the human, in: *The Fetus and Birth, Ciba Foundation Symposium,* Elsevier/Excerpta Medica/North-Holland, Amsterdam, pp. 401–426.

Gerzer, R., Brash, A. R., and Hardman, J. G., 1986, Activation of soluble guanylate cyclase by arachidonic acid and 15-lipoxygenase products, *Biochim. Biophys. Acta* **886:**383–389.

Giannopoulos, G., Goldberg, P., Shea, T. B., and Tulchinsky, D., 1980, Unoccupied and occupied estrogen receptors in myometrial cytosol and nuclei from nonpregnant and pregnant women, *J. Clin. Endocrinol. Metab.* **51:**702–710.

Gibb, W., Lavoie, J.-C., and Roux, J. F., 1978, 3β-Hydroxysteroid dehydrogenase activity in human fetal membranes, *Steroids* **32:**365–372.

Gietzen, K., Seiler, S., Fleischer, S., and Wolf, H. U., 1980, Reconstitution of the Ca^{2+}-transport system of human erythrocytes, *Biochem. J.* **188:**47–54.

Gillespie, A., 1972, Prostaglandin–oxytocin enhancement and potentiation and their clinical applications, *Br. Med. J.* **1:**150–152.

Gillespie, A., Brummer, H. C., and Chard, T., 1972, Oxytocin release by infused prostaglandin, *Br. Med. J.* **1:**543–544.

Glasser, S. R., Northcutt, R. C., Chytil, F., and Strott, C. A., 1972, The influence of an antisteroidogenic drug (aminoglutethimide phosphate) on pregnancy maintenance, *Endocrinology,* **90:**1363–1370.

Golichowski, A. M., 1986, Biochemical basis of cervical maturation, in: *The Physiology and Biochemistry of the Uterus in Pregnancy and Labor* (G. Huszar, ed.), CRC Press, Boca Raton, FL, pp. 261–280.

Golichowski, A. M., and Tzeng, D. Y., 1985, Binding of the calcium antagonist [^{3}H]nitrendipine to human myometrial plasmalemma, *Biol. Reprod.* **33:**1105–1112.

Gordon, A. J., and Calder, A. A., 1977, Oestradiol applied locally to ripen the unfavourable cervix, *Lancet* **2:**1319–1321.

Goren, H. J., Geonzon, R. M., Hollenberg, M. D., Lederis, K., and Morgan, D. O., 1980, Oxytocin action: Lack of correlation between receptor number and tissue responsiveness, *J. Supramol. Struct.* **14:**129–138.

Granström, E., Hamberg, M., Hansson, G., and Kindahl, H., 1980, Chemical instability of 15-keto-13,14-dihydro-PGE$_2$: The reason for low assay reliability, *Prostaglandins* **19:**933–957.

Gréen, K., Bygdeman, M., Toppozoda, M., and Wiqvist, N., 1974, The role of PGF$_{2\alpha}$ in human parturition. Endogenous plasma levels of 15-keto-13,14-dihydroprostaglandin F$_{2\alpha}$ during labor, *Am. J. Obstet. Gynecol.* **120:**25–31.

Grover, A. K., Kwan, C.-Y., Luchowski, E., Daniel, E. E., and Triggle, D. J., 1984, Subcellular distribution of [^{3}H]nitrendipine binding in smooth muscle, *J. Biol. Chem.* **259:**2223–2226.

Gutknecht, G. D., Duncan, G. W., and Wyngarden, L. J., 1972, Inhibition of prostaglandin F$_{2\alpha}$ or LH induced luteolysis in the pseudopregnant rabbit by 17β-estradiol, *Proc. Soc. Exp. Biol. Med.* **130:**406–413.

Habenicht, A. J. R., Goerig, M., Grulich, J., Rothe, D., Gronwald, R., Loth, U., Schettler, G., Kommerell, B., and Ross, R., 1985, Human platelet-derived growth factor stimulates prostaglandin synthesis by activation and by rapid *de novo* synthesis of cyclooxygenase, *J. Clin. Invest.***75:**1381–1387.

Haldar, J., Kupfer, L., and Sokol, H. W., 1982, Decreased sensitivity to oxytocin of uteri from homozygous Brattleboro rats, *Ann. N.Y. Acad. Sci.* **394:**46–49.

Harden, T. K., 1983, Agonist-induced desensitization of the β-adrenergic receptor-linked adenylate cyclase, *Pharmacol. Rev.* **35:**5–32.

Harris, B. A., Jr., Huddleston, J. F., Sutliff, G., and Perlis, H. W., 1983, The unfavorable cervix in prolonged pregnancy, *Obstet. Gynecol.* **62:**171–174.

Ham, E. A., Cirillo, V. J., Zanetti, M. E., and Kuehl, F. A., Jr., 1975, Estrogen-directed synthesis of specific prostaglandins in uterus, *Proc. Natl. Acad. Sci. U.S.A.* **72:**1420–1427.

Hertelendy, F., 1973, Block of oxytocin-induced parturition and oviposition by prostaglandin inhibitors, *Life Sci.* **13:**1581–1589.

Hilliard, J., 1973, Corpus luteum function in guinea pigs, hamsters, rats, mice and rabbits, *Biol. Reprod.* **8:**203–221.

Hirata, F., Matsuda, K., Notsu, Y., Hattori, T., and del Carmine, R., 1984, Phosphorylation at a tyrosine residue of lipomodulin in mitogen-stimulated murine thymocytes, *Proc. Natl. Acad. Sci. U.S.A.* **81:**4717–4721.

Hochman, J., Weiss, G., Steinetz, B. G., and O'Byrne, E. M., 1978, Serum relaxin concentrations in prostaglandin- and oxytocin-induced labor in women, *Am. J. Obstet. Gynecol.* **130:**473–474.

Hoffman, B. B., Lavin, T. N., Lefkowitz, R. J., and Ruffolo, R. R., Jr., 1981, Alpha adrenergic receptor subtypes in rabbit uterus: Mediation of myometrial contractions and regulation by estrogens, *J. Pharmacol. Exp. Ther.* **219:**290–295.

Hofmann, G. E., Rao, C. V., Barrows, G. H., and Sanfilippo, J. S., 1983, Topography of human uterine prostaglandin E and $F_{2\alpha}$ receptors and their profiles during pathological states, *J. Clin. Endocrinol. Metab.* **56:**360–366.

Hollingsworth, M., Gallimore, S., and Isherwood, C. N. M., 1980, Effects of prostaglandins $F_{2\alpha}$ and E_2 on cervical extensibility in the late pregnant rat, *J. Reprod. Fertil.* **58:**95–99.

Hong, S. L., and Deykin, D., 1981, The activation of phosphatidylinositol-hydrolyzing phospholipase A_2 during prostaglandin synthesis in transformed mouse BALB/3T3 cells, *J. Biol. Chem.* **256:**5215–5219.

Hooper, S. B., Watkins, W. B., and Thorburn, G. D., 1986, Oxytocin, oxytocin-associated neurophysin, and prostaglandin $F_{2\alpha}$ concentrations in the utero–ovarian vein of pregnant and nonpregnant sheep, *Endocrinology* **119:**2590–2597.

Horton, E. W., and Poyser, N. L., 1976, Uterine luteolytic hormone: A physiological role for prostaglandin $F_{2\alpha}$, *Physiol. Rev.* **56:**595–651.

Hsu, C. J., McCormack, S., and Sanborn, B. M., 1985, The effect of relaxin on cyclic adenosine 3′,5′-monophosphate concentrations in rat myometrial cells in culture, *Endocrinology* **116:**2029–2035.

Husslein, P., Fuchs, A.-R., and Fuchs, F., 1981, Oxytocin and the initiation of human parturition. I. Prostaglandin release during induction of labor by oxytocin, *Am. J. Obstet. Gynecol.* **141:**688–693.

Husslein, P., Kofler, E., Rasmussen, A. B., Sumulong, L., Fuchs. A.-R., and Fuchs, F., 1983, Oxytocin and the initiation of human parturition. IV. Plasma concentrations of oxytocin and 13,14-dihydro-15-keto-prostaglandin $F_{2\alpha}$ during induction of labor by artificial rupture of the membranes, *Am. J. Obstet. Gynecol.* **147:**503–507.

Huszar, G., 1986, Cellular regulation of myometrial contractility and essentials of tocolytic therapy, in: *The Physiology and Biochemistry of the Uterus in Pregnancy and Labor* (G. Huszar, ed.), CRC Press, Boca Raton, FL, pp. 107–126.

Huszar, G., Cabrol, D., and Naftolin, F., 1986, The relationship between myometrial contractility and cervical maturation in pregnancy and labor, in: *The Physiology and Biochemistry of the Uterus in Pregnancy and Labor* (G. Huszar, ed.), CRC Press, Boca Raton, FL, pp. 297–306.

Ichida, S., Tokunaga, H., Oda, Y., Fujita, N., Hirata, A., and Hata, T., 1983, Increase of serotonin receptors in rat uterus induced by estradiol, *J. Biol. Chem.* **258:**13438–13443.

Irvine, R. F., 1982, How is the level of free arachidonic acid controlled in mammalian cells? *Biochem. J.* **204:**3–16.

Janis, R. A., and Triggle, D. J., 1986, Effects of calcium channel antagonists on the myometrium, in: *The Physiology and Biochemistry of the Uterus in Pregnancy and Labor* (G. Huszar ed.), CRC Press, Boca Raton, FL, pp. 201–223.

Järvinen, P. A., Luukkainen, T., and Väistö, L., 1965, The effect of oestrogen treatment on myometrial activity in late pregnancy, *Acta Obstet. Gynecol. Scand.* **44:**258–264.

Johnson, M., Jessup, R., Jessup, S., and Ramwell, P. W., 1974, Correlation of prostaglandin E_1 receptor binding with evoked uterine contraction: Modification by disulfide reduction, *Prostaglandins* **6:**433–449.

Jones, S. A., and Summerlee, A. J. S., 1987, Effects of chronic infusion of porcine relaxin on oxytocin release in lactating rats, *J. Endocrinol.* **114:**241–246.

Joseph, M. K., Fernstrom, M. A., and Soloff, M. S., 1982, Switching of β- to α-tubulin phosphorylation in uterine smooth muscle of parturient rats, *J. Biol. Chem.* **257:**11728–11733.

Judson, D. G., Pay, S., and Bhoola, K. D., 1980, Modulation of cyclic AMP in isolated rat uterine tissue slices by porcine relaxin, *J. Endocrinol.* **87:**153–159.

Kamm, K. E., and Stull, J. T., 1985, The function of myosin and myosin light chain kinase phosphorylation in smooth muscle, *Annu. Rev. Pharmacol. Toxicol.* **25:**593–620.

Kao, C. Y., 1976, Electrophysiological properties of uterine smooth muscle, in: *Biology of the Uterus* (R. M. Wynn, ed.), Plenum Press, New York, pp. 423–496.

Karim, S., 1971, Action of prostaglandin in the pregnant woman, *Ann. N.Y. Acad. Sci.* **180:**483–498.

Karim, S. M. M., and Devlin, J., 1967, Prostaglandin content of amniotic fluid during pregnancy and labour, *J. Obstet. Gynaecol. Br. Commonw.* **74:**230–234.

Keirse, M. J. N. C., 1983, Prostaglandins during human parturition, in: *Initiation of Parturition: Prevention of Prematurity* (P. C. MacDonald and J. Porter, eds.), Ross Laboratories, Columbus, OH, pp. 137–144.

Keirse, M. J. N. C., and Turnbull, A. C., 1973, E Prostaglandins in amniotic fluid during late pregnancy and labour, *J. Obstet. Gynaecol. Br. Commonw.* **80:**970–973.

Keirse, M. J. N. C., and Turnbull, A. C., 1975, Metabolism of prostaglandins within the pregnant uterus, *Br. J. Obstet. Gynaecol.* **82:**887–893.

Keirse, M. J. N. C., Mitchell, M. D., and Turnbull, A. C., 1977, Changes in prostaglandin F and 13,14-dihydro-15-keto-prostaglandin F concentrations in amniotic fluid at the onset of and during labour, *Br. J. Obstet. Gynaecol.* **84:**743–746.

Kertiles, L. P., and Anderson, L. L., 1979, Effect of relaxin on cervical dilatation, parturition and lactation in the pig, *Biol. Reprod.* **21:**57–68.

Khan-Dawood, F. S., and Dawood, M. Y., 1984, Estrogen and progesterone receptor and hormone levels in human myometrium and placenta in term pregnancy, *Am. J. Obstet. Gynecol.* **150**:501–505.

Kinoshita, K., Satoh, K., and Sakamoto, S., 1977, Biosynthesis of prostaglandin in human decidua, amnion, chorion, and villi, *Endocrinol. Jpn.* **24**:343–350.

Klopper, A. I., and Dennis, L. K., 1962, Effect of oestrogens on myometrial contractions, *Br. Med. J.* **2**:1157–1159.

Kolesnick, R. N., Musacchio, I., Thaw, C., and Gershengorn, M. C., 1984, Arachidonic acid mobilizes calcium and stimulates prolactin secretion from GH_3 cells, *Am. J. Physiol.* **246**:E458–E462.

Krall, J. F., Mori, H., Tuck, M. L., LeShon, S. L., and Korenman, S. G., 1978, Demonstration of adrenergic catecholamine receptors in rat myometrium and their regulation by sex steroids, *Life Sci.* **23**:1073–1081.

Kroc, R. L., Steinetz, B. G., and Beach, V. L., 1959, The effects of estrogens, progestagens, and relaxin in pregnant and nonpregnant laboratory rodents, *Ann. N.Y. Acad. Sci.* **75**:942–980.

Kuriyama, H., and Suzuki, H., 1976, Effects of prostaglandin E_2 and oxytocin on the electrical activity of hormone-treated and pregnant rat myometria, *J. Physiol. (Lond.)* **260**:335–349.

Lackritz, R., Tulchinsky, D., Ryan, K. J., and Levine, L., 1978, Plasma prostaglandin metabolites in human labor, *Am. J. Obstet. Gynecol.* **131**:484–489.

Lange, A. P., Secher, N. J., Westergaard, J. G., and Skovgård, I. B., 1982, Prelabor evaluation of inducibility, *Obstet, Gynecol,* **60**:137–147.

Leake, R. D., Weitzman, R. E., Glatz, T. H., and Fisher, D. A., 1981, Plasma oxytocin concentrations in men, nonpregnant women, and pregnant women before and during spontaneous labor, *J. Clin. Endocrinol. Metab.* **53**:730–733.

Leaver, H. A., and Richmond, D. H., 1984, The effects of oxytocin, estrogen, calcium ionophore A23187 and hydrocortisone on prostaglandin $F_{2\alpha}$ and 6-oxo-prostaglandin $F_{1\alpha}$ production by cultured human endometrial and myometrial explants, *Prostaglandins Leukotrienes Med.* **13**:179–196.

Leaver, H. A., and Seawright, A., 1982, Controls of endometrial prostaglandin output *in vitro* during the estrous cycle of the guinea pig: influence of estradiol 17β, progesterone, oxytocin and calcium ionophore A23187, *Prostaglandins Leukotrienes Med.* **9**:657–668.

Levine, L., and Gutierrez-Cernosek, R. M. C., 1973, Levels of 13,14-dihydro-15-keto-$PGF_{2\alpha}$ in biological fluids as measured by radioimmunoassay, *Prostaglandins* **3**:785–804.

Lewis, R. B., and Schulman, J. D., 1973, Influence of acetylsalicylic acid, an inhibitor of prostaglandin synthesis, on the duration of human gestation and labour, *Lancet* **2**:1159–1161.

Liggins, G. C., Fairclough, R. J., Grieves, S. A., Kendall, J. Z., and Knox, B. S., 1973, The mechanism of initiation of parturition in the ewe, *Recent Prog. Horm. Res.* **29**:111–159.

Lopez Bernal, A., Hansell, D. J., Alexander, S., and Turnbull, A. C., 1987, Prostaglandin E production by amniotic cells in relation to term and preterm labour, *Br. J. Obstet. Gynaecol.* **94**:864–869.

Lumsden, M. A., and Baird, D. T., 1986, The effect of intrauterine administration of prostacyclin on the contractility of the non-pregnant uterus *in vivo*, *Prostaglandins* **31**:1011–1022.

Lye, S. J., and Challis, J. R. G., 1982, Inhibition by PGI_2 of myometrial activity *in vivo* in non-pregnant ovariectomized sheep, *J. Reprod. Fertil.* **66**:311–315.

Maathuis, J. B., and Kelly, R. W., 1978, Concentrations of prostaglandins $F_{2\alpha}$ and E_2 in the endometrium throughout the human menstrual cycle, after the administration of clomiphene or an oestrogen–progestogen pill and in early pregnancy, *J. Endocrinol.* **77**:361–371.

MacDonald, P. C., Schultz, F. M., Duenhoelter, J. H., Gant, N. F., Jimenez, J. M., Pritchard, J. A., Porter, J. C., and Johnston, J. M., 1974, Initiation of human parturition. I. Mechanism of action of arachidonic acid, *Obstet. Gynecol.* **44**:629–636.

MacKenzie, I. Z., and Embrey, M. P., 1977, Cervical ripening with intravaginal prostaglandin E_2 gel, *Br. Med. J.* **2**:1381–1384.

MacKenzie, I. Z., and Mitchell, M. D., 1981, Serial determinations of prostaglandin E in amniotic fluid following the vaginal administration of a prostaglandin E_2 gel, *Prostaglandins Med.* **7**:43–47.

MacLennan, A. H., Green, R. C., Bryant-Greenwood, G. D., Greenwood, F. C., and Seamark, R. F., 1980, Ripening of the human cervix and induction of labour with purified porcine relaxin, *Lancet* **1**:220–223.

Majerus, P. W., 1983, Arachidonate metabolism in vascular disorders, *J. Clin. Invest.* **72**:1521–1525.

Manzai, M., and Liggins, G. C., 1984, Inhibitory effects of dispersed human amnion cells on production of prostaglandin E and F by endometrial cells, *Prostaglandins* **28**:297–307.

Marc, S., Leiber, D., and Harbon, S., 1986, Carbachol and oxytocin stimulate the generation of inositol phosphates in the guinea pig myometrium, *FEBS Lett.* **201**:9–14.

Marshall, J. M., 1959, Effects of estrogen and progesterone on single uterine muscle fiber in the rat, *Am. J. Physiol.* **197**:935–942.

Marshall, J. M., 1974, Effects of neurohypophysial hormones on the myometrium, in: *The Pituitary Gland and its Neuroendocrine Control,* Part 1, *Handbook of Physiology,* Section 7: *Endocrinology,* Vol. IV (R. O.

Greep, E. B. Astwood, E. Knobil, W. H. Sawyer, and S. R. Geiger, eds.), American Physiological Society, Washington, pp. 469–492.

McCoshen, J. A., Johnson, K. A., Dubin, N. H., and Ghodgaonkar, R. B., 1987, Prostaglandin E_2 release on the fetal and maternal sides of the amnion and chorion–decidua before and after term labor, *Am. J. Obstet. Gynecol.* **156:**173–178.

McCracken, J. A., Carlson, J. C., Glew, M. E., Goding, J. R., Baird, D. T., Green, K., and Samuelsson, B., 1972, Prostaglandin $F_{2\alpha}$ identified as luteolytic hormone in sheep, *Nature (New Biol)* **238:**129–134.

McPhail, L. C., Clayton, C. C., and Snyderman, R., 1984, A potential second messenger role for unsaturated fatty acids: Activation of Ca^{2+}-dependent protein kinase, *Science* **224:**622–625.

Mercado-Simmen, R. C., Bryant-Greenwood, G. D., and Greenwood, F. C., 1980, Relaxin receptor in the rat myometrium: Regulation by estrogen and relaxin, *Endocrinology* **110:**220–226.

Mercado-Simmen, R. C., Goodwin, B., Ueno, M. S., Yamamoto, S. Y., and Bryant-Greenwood, G. D., 1982, Relaxin receptors in the myometrium and cervix of the pig, *Biol. Reprod.* **26:**120–128.

Metz, S. A., Draznin, B., Sussman, K. E., and Leitner, J. W., 1987, Unmasking of arachidonate-induced insulin release by removal of extracellular calcium, *Biochem. Biophys. Res. Commun.* **142:**251–258.

Milewich, L., Gant, N. F., Schwarz, B., Chen, G. T., and MacDonald, P. C., 1977, Initiation of human parturition. VIII. Metabolism of progesterone by fetal membranes of early and late human gestation, *Obstet. Gynecol.* **50:**45–48.

Miller, M. D., and Marshall, J. M., 1965, Uterine response to nerve stimulation; Relation to hormonal status and catecholamines, *Am. J. Physiol.* **209:**859–865.

Miller, W. C., and Moore, J. B., Jr., 1984, High affinity binding sites for [³H]-nitrendipine in rabbit uterine smooth muscle, *Life Sci.* **34:**1717–1724.

Mitchell, B., Cruickshank, B., McLean, D., and Challis, J., 1982, Local modulation of progesterone production in human fetal membranes, *J. Clin. Endocrinol. Metab.* **55:**1237–1239.

Mitchell, B. F., Challis, J. R. G., and Lukash, L., 1987, Progesterone synthesis by human amnion, chorion, and decidua at term, *Am. J. Obstet. Gynecol.* **157:**349–353.

Mitchell, M. D., Flint, A. P. F., and Turnbull, A. C., 1975a, Stimulation by oxytocin of prostaglandin F levels in uterine venous effluent in pregnant and puerperal sheep, *Prostaglandins* **9:**47–56.

Mitchell, M. D., Keirse, M. J. N. C., Anderson, A. B. M., and Turnbull, A. C., 1975b, Evidence for a local control of prostaglandins within the pregnant human uterus, *Br. J. Obstet. Gynaecol.* **84:**35–38.

Mitchell, M. D., Flint, A. P. F., and Turnbull, A. C., 1976a, Plasma concentrations of 13,14-dihydro-15-keto-prostaglandin F during pregnancy in sheep, *Prostaglandins* **11:**319–329.

Mitchell, M. D., Patrick, J. E., Robinson, J. S., Thorburn, G. D., and Challis, J. R. G., 1976b, Prostaglandins in the plasma and amniotic fluid of rhesus monkeys during pregnancy and after intra-uterine foetal death, *J. Endocrinol.* **71:**67–76.

Mitchell, M. D., Flint, A. P. F., Bibby, J., Brunt, J., Arnold, J. M., Anderson, A. B. M., and Turnbull, A. C., 1977, Rapid increases in plasma prostaglandin concentrations after vaginal examination and amniotomy, *Br. Med. J.* **2:**1183–1185.

Mitchell, M. D., Bibby, J., Hicks, B. R., and Turnbull, A. C., 1978, Specific production of prostaglandin E by human amnion *in vitro*, *Prostaglandins* **15:**377–382.

Mitchell, M. D., Strickland, D. M., Brennecke, S. P., and Saeed, S. A., 1983, New aspects of arachidonic acid metabolism in human parturition, in: *Initiation of Parturition: Prevention of Prematurity* (P. C. MacDonald and J. Porter, eds.), Ross Laboratories, Columbus, OH, pp. 145–150.

Mitchell, M. D., MacDonald, P. C., and Casey, M. L., 1984, Stimulation of prostaglandin E_2 synthesis in human amnion cells maintained in monolayer culture by a substance(s), in amniotic fluid, *Prostaglandins Leukotrienes Med.* **15:**399–407.

Montrucchio, G., Alloatti, G., Tetta, C., Roffinello, C., Emanuelli, G., and Camusi, G., 1986, *In vitro* contractile effect of platelet-activating factor on guinea pig myometrium, *Prostaglandins* **32:**539–554.

Mukku, V. R., and Stancel, G. M., 1985, Regulation of epidermal growth factor receptor by estrogen, *J. Biol. Chem.* **260:**9820–9824.

Murphy, B. E. P., 1982, Human fetal serum cortisol levels related to gestational age: evidence of mid-gestational fall and a steep late rise, independent of sex or mode of delivery, *Am. J. Obstet, Gynecol.* **144:**276–282.

Musah, A. I., Schwabe, C., Willham, R. L., and Anderson, L. L., 1986, Relaxin on induction of parturition in beef heifers, *Endocrinology* **118:**1476–1482.

Nagata, I., Sunaga, H., Furuya, K., Makimura, N., and Kato, K., 1987, Changes in the plasma prostaglandin $F_{2\alpha}$ metabolite before and during spontaneous labor and labor induced by amniotomy, oxytocin, and PGE_2, *Endocrinol. Jpn.* **34:**153–159.

Nakla, S., Skinner, K., Mitchell, B. F., and Challis, J. R. G., 1986, Changes in prostaglandin transfer across human fetal membranes obtained after spontaneous labor. *Am. J. Obstet. Gynecol.* **155:**1337–1341.

Nieder, J., and Augustin, W., 1983, Increase of prostaglandin E and F equivalents in amniotic fluid during late pregnancy and rapid PGF elevation after cervical dilatation, *Prostaglandins Leukotrienes Med.* **12:**289–297.

Niesert, S., Christopherson, W., Korte, K., Mitchell, M. D., MacDonald, P. C., and Casey, M. L., 1986, Prostaglandin E$_2$ 9-ketoreductase activity in human decidua vera tissue, *Am. J. Obstet. Gynecol.* **155:**1348–1352.

Nishihara, J., Ishibashi, T., Imai, Y., and Muramatsu, T., 1984, Mass spectrometric evidence for the presence of platelet-activating factor (1-O-alkyl-2-acetyl-*sn*-glycero-3-phosphocholine) in human amniotic fluid during labor, *Lipids* **19:**907–910.

Nishikori, K., Weisbrodt, N. W., Sherwood, O. D., and Sanborn, B. M., 1983, Effects of relaxin on rat uterine myosin light chain kinase activity and myosin light chain phosphorylation, *J. Biol. Chem.* **258:**2468–2474.

Northover, B. J., 1972, The effects of indomethacin on calcium, sodium, potassium and magnesium fluxes in various tissues of the guinea-pig, *Br. J. Pharmacol.* **45:**651–659.

Novy, M. J., 1983, Endocrine control of parturition in rhesus monkeys, in: *Initiation of Parturition: Prevention of Prematurity* (P. C. MacDonald and J. Porter, eds.), Ross Laboratories, Columbus, OH, pp. 62–71.

Novy, M. J., Cook, M. J., and Manaugh, L., 1974, Indomethacin block of normal onset of parturition in primates, *Am. J. Obstet. Gynecol.* **118:**412–416.

O'Grady, J. P., Caldwell, B. V., Auletta, F. J., and Speroff, L., 1972, The effects of an inhibitor of prostaglandin synthesis (indomethacin) on ovulation, pregnancy, and pseudopregnancy in the rabbit, *Prostaglandins* **1:**97–106.

Okazaki, T., Casey, M. L., Okita, J. R., MacDonald, P. C., and Johnston, J. M., 1981, Initiation of human parturition. XII. Biosynthesis and metabolism of prostaglandins in human fetal membranes and uterine decidua, *Am. J. Obstet. Gynecol.* **139:**373–381.

Olson, D. M., Skinner, K., and Challis, J. R. G., 1983a, Prostaglandin output in relation to parturition by cells dispersed from human intrauterine tissues, *J. Clin. Endocrinol. Metab.* **57:**694–699.

Olson, D. M., Opavsky, M. A., and Challis, J. R. G., 1983b, Prostaglandin synthesis by human amnion is dependent upon extracellular calcium, *Can. J. Physiol. Pharmacol.* **61:**1089–1092.

Omini, C., Folco, G. C., Pasargiklian, R., Fano, M., and Berti, F., 1979, Prostacyclin (PGI$_2$) in pregnant human uterus, *Prostaglandins* **17:**113–120.

Padayachi, T., Norman, R. J., Reddi, K., Schweni, M., Philpott, H., and Joubert, S. M., 1986, Changes in amniotic fluid prostaglandins with oxytocin-induced labor, *Obstet. Gynecol.* **68:**610–613.

Pavlik, E. J., and Coulson, P. B., 1976, Modulation of estrogen receptors in four different target tissues: Differential effects of estrogen vs. progesterone, *J. Steroid Biochem.* **7:**369–376.

Pearce, D. J., 1977, Pre-induction priming of the uterine cervix with oral prostaglandin E$_2$ and a placebo, *Prostaglandins* **14:**571–576.

Pearlmutter, A. F., and Soloff, M. S., 1979, Characterization of the metal ion requirement for oxytocin-receptor interaction in rat mammary gland membranes, *J. Biol. Chem.* **254:**3899–3906.

Perry, G., Siegal, B., and Held, B., 1977, Second trimester abortion: Single dose intra-amniotic injection of prostaglandin F$_{2\alpha}$ with intraveous oxytocin augmentation, *Prostaglandins* **13:**987–994.

Pharriss, B. B., and Wyngarden, L. J., 1969, The effect of prostaglandin F$_{2\alpha}$ on the progestogen content of ovaries from pseudopregnant rats, *Proc. Soc. Exp. Biol. Med.* **130:**92–94.

Pinto, R. M., Fisch, L., Schwarcz, R. L., and Montuori, E., 1964, Action of estradiol upon uterine contractility and the milk ejecting effect in pregnant women, *Am. J. Obstet. Gynecol.* **90:**99–107.

Pinto, R. M., Leon, C., Mazzocco, N., and Scasserra, V., 1967, Action of estradiol-17β at term and at onset of labor, *Am. J. Obstet. Gynecol.* **98:**540–546.

Piper, P., and Vane, J., 1971, The release of prostaglandins from lungs and other tissues, *Ann. N.Y. Acad. Sci.* **180:**363–385.

Porter, D. G., Downing, S. J., and Bradshaw, J. M. C., 1979, Relaxin inhibits spontaneous and prostaglandin-driven myometrial activity in anaesthetized rats, *J. Endocrinol.* **83:**183–192.

Porter, D. G., Downing, S. J., and Bradshaw, J. M. C., 1981, Inhibition of oxytocin- or prostaglandin F$_{2\alpha}$-driven myometrial activity by relaxin in the rat is oestrogen dependent, *J. Endocrinol.* **89:**399–404.

Poyser, N. L., Horton, E. W., Thompson, C. J., and Los, M., 1971, Identification of prostaglandin F$_{2\alpha}$ released by distention of guinea-pig uterus *in vitro, Nature* **230:**526–528.

Rath, W., Adelmann-Grill, B. C., Pieper, U., and Kuhn, W., 1987, The role of collagenases and proteases in prostaglandin-induced cervical ripening, *Prostaglandins* **34:**119–127.

Raziano, J., Ferin, M., and Vande Wiele, R. L., 1972, Effects of antibodies to estradiol-17β and to progesterone on nidation and pregnancy in rats, *Endocrinology* **90:**1133–1138.

Reddi, K., Kambaran, S. R., Norman, R. J., Joubert, S. M., and Philpott, H., 1984, Abnormal concentrations of prostaglandins in amniotic fluid during delayed labour in multigravid patients, *Br. J. Obstet. Gynaecol.* **91:**781–787.

Rehnström, J., Ishikawa, M., Fuchs, F., and Fuchs, A.-R., 1983, Stimulation of myometrial and decidual prostaglandin production by amniotic fluid from term, but not midterm pregnancies, *Prostaglandins* **26**:973–981.

Reynolds, S. R. M., Hellman, L. M., and Bruns, P., 1948, Patterns of uterine contractility in women during pregnancy, *Obstet. Gynecol. Surv.* **3**:629–646.

Riemer, R. K., Goldfien, A. C., Goldfien, A., and Roberts, J. M., 1986, Rabbit uterine oxytocin receptors and *in vitro* contractile response: Abrupt changes at term and the role of eicosanoids, *Endocrinology* **119**:699–709.

Riley, S. C., and Poyser, N. L., 1987, Prostaglandin production by the guinea-pig endometrium: Is calcium necessary? *J. Endocrinol.* **113**:463–471.

Roberts, J. M., Insel, P. A., and Goldfien, A., 1981, Regulation of myometrial adrenoreceptors and adrenergic response by sex steroids, *Mol. Pharmacol.* **20**:52–58.

Roberts, J. S., and McCracken, J. A., 1976, Does prostaglandin $F_{2\alpha}$ released from the uterus by oxytocin mediate the oxytocic action of oxytocin? *Biol. Reprod.* **15**:457–463.

Roberts, J. S., Barcikowski, B., Wilson, L., Skarnes, R. C., and McCracken, J. A., 1975, Hormonal and related factors affecting the release of prostaglandin $F_{2\alpha}$ from the uterus, *J. Steroid Biochem.* **6**:1091–1097.

Roberts, J. S., McCracken, J. A., Gavagan, J. E., and Soloff, M. S., 1976, Oxytocin-stimulated release of prostaglandin $F_{2\alpha}$ from ovine endometrium *in vitro*: Correlation with estrous cycle and oxytocin–receptor binding, *Endocrinology* **99**:1107–1114.

Robinson, J. S., Chapman, R. L. K., Challis, J. R. G., Mitchell, M. D., and Thorburn, G. D., 1978, Administration of extra-amniotic arachidonic acid and the suppression of uterine prostaglandin synthesis during pregnancy in the rhesus monkey, *J. Reprod. Fertil.* **54**:369–373.

Romero, R., Lafreniere, D., Hobbins, J. C., and Mitchell, M. D., 1987, A soluble product from human decidua inhibits prostaglandin production by human amnion, *Prostaglandins Leukotrienes Med.* **30**:29–35.

Saeed, S. A., and Mitchell, M. D., 1982, Stimulants of prostaglandin biosynthesis in human fetal membranes, uterine decidua vera and placenta, *Prostaglandins* **24**:475–484.

Saeed, S. A., McDonald-Gibson, W. J., Cuthbert, J., Copas, J. L., Schneider, C., Gardiner, P. J., Butt, N. M., and Collier, H. O. J., 1977, Endogenous inhibitor of prostaglandin synthetase, *Nature* **270**:32–36.

Saeed, S. A., Strickland, D. M., Young, D. C., Dang, A., and Mitchell, M. D., 1982, Inhibition of prostaglandin synthesis by human amniotic fluid: Acute reduction in inhibitory activity of amniotic fluid obtained during labor, *J. Clin. Endocrinol. Metab.* **55**:801–803.

Sakai, K., Yamaguchi, T., Morita, S., and Uchida, M., 1983, Agonist-induced contraction of rat myometrium in Ca-free solution containing Mn, *Gen. Pharmacol.* **14**:391–400.

Saldana, L. R., Schulman, H., Yang, W. H., Cunningham, M. A., and Randolf, G., 1974, Midtrimester abortion by prostaglandin impact, *Obstet. Gynecol.* **44**:579–585.

Salomy, M., Halbrecht, I., and London, R., 1975, Mid-trimester abortion with intra-amniotic prostaglandin $F_{2\alpha}$ and intravenous oxytocin infusion, *Prostaglandins* **9**:271–279.

Samuelsson, B., Granström, E., Gréen, K., Hamberg, M., and Hammarström, S., 1975, Prostaglandins, *Annu. Rev. Biochem.* **44**:669–695.

Samuelsson, B., Goldyne, M., Granström, E., Hamberg, M., Hammarström, S., and Malmsten, C., 1978, Prostaglandins and thromboxanes, *Annu. Rev. Biochem.* **47**:997–1029.

Sanborn, B. M., 1986, The role of relaxin in uterine function, in: *The Physiology and Biochemistry of the Uterus in Pregnancy and Labor* (G. Huszar, ed.), CRC Press, Boca Raton, FL, pp. 225–238.

Sanborn, B. M., Kuo, H. S., Weisbrodt, N. W., and Sherwood, O. D., 1980, The interaction of relaxin with the rat uterus. I. Effect on cyclic nucleotide levels and spontaneous contractile activity, *Endocrinology* **106**:1210–1215.

Sawyer, W. H., Frieden, E. H., and Martin, A. S., 1953, *In vitro* inhibition of spontaneous contractions of the rat uterus by relaxin-containing extracts of sow ovaries, *Am. J. Physiol.* **178**:547–552.

Schatz, F., Markiewicz, L., and Gurpide, E., 1984, Effects of estriol on $PGF_{2\alpha}$ output by cultures of human endometrium and endometrial cells, *J. Steroid Biochem.* **20**:999–1003.

Schatz, F., Markiewicz, L., and Gurpide, E., 1987, Differential effects of estradiol, arachidonic acid, and A23187 on prostaglandin $F_{2\alpha}$ output by epithelial and stromal cells of human endometrium, *Endocrinology* **120**:1465–1471.

Schillinger, E., and Prior, G., 1976, Characteristics of prostaglandin receptor sites in human uterine tissue, *Adv. Prostaglandin Thromboxane Res.* **1**:259–263.

Schirar, A., Capponi, A., and Catt, K. J., 1980, Regulation of uterine angiotensin II receptors by estrogen and progesterone, *Endocrinology* **106**:5–12.

Schofield, B. M., 1957, The hormonal control of myometrial function during pregnancy, *J. Physiol. (Lond.)* **138**:1–10.

Schofield, B. M., 1964, Myometrial activity in the pregnant guinea-pig, *J. Endocrinol.* **30**:347–354.

Schofield, B. M., 1968, Parturition, in: *Advances in Reproductive Physiology*, Vol. 3 (A. McLaren, ed.), Academic Press, New York, pp. 9–32.

Schrey, M. P., Read, A. M., and Steer, P. J., 1986, Oxytocin and vasopressin stimulate inositol phosphate production in human gestational myometrium and decidual cells, *Biosci. Rep.* **6**:613–619.

Schwabe, C., Steinetz, B., Weiss, G., Segaloff, A., McDonald, J. K., O'Byrne, E., Hochman, J., Carriere, B., and Goldsmith, L., 1978, Relaxin, *Recent Prog. Horm. Res.* **34**:123–211.

Schwalm, H., and Dubrauszky, V., 1966, The structure of the musculature of the human uterus–muscles and connective tissue, *Am. J. Obstet. Gynecol.* **94**:391–404.

Scott, R. S., and Rennie, P. I. C., 1970, Factors controlling the lifespan of the corpora lutea in the pseudopregnant rabbit, *J. Reprod. Fertil.* **23**:415–422.

Sellers, S. M., Hodgson, H. T., Mitchell, M. D., Anderson, A. B. M., and Turnbull, A. C., 1982, Raised prostaglandin levels in the third stage of labor, *Am. J. Obstet. Gynecol.* **144**:209–212.

Seppala, M., Kajanona, P., Widholm, O., and Vara, P., 1972, Prostaglandin–oxytocin abortion: A clinical trial on intra-amniotic prostaglandin $F_{2\alpha}$ in combination with intravenous oxytocin, *Prostaglandins* **2**:311–319.

Sharma, S. C., and Fitzpatrick, R. J., 1974, Effect of oestradiol-17β and oxytocin on prostaglandin F alpha release in the anoestrus ewe, *Prostaglandins* **6**:97–105.

Sheldrick, E. L., Mitchell, M. D., and Flint, A. P. F., 1980, Delayed luteal regression in ewes immunized against oxytocin, *J. Reprod. Fertil.* **59**:37–42.

Sherwood, O. D., Nara, B. S., Crnekovic, V. E., and First, N. L., 1969, Relaxin concentrations in pig plasma after the administration of indomethacin and prostaglandin $F_{2\alpha}$ during late pregnancy, *Endocrinology* **104**:1716–1721.

Skinner, K. A., and Challis, J. R. G., 1985, Changes in the synthesis and metabolism of prostaglandins by human fetal membranes and decidua at labor, *Am. J. Obstet. Gynecol.* **151**:519–523.

Skinner, S J. M., Liggins, G. C., Wilson, T., and Neale, G., 1984, Synthesis of prostaglandin F by cultured human endometrial cells, *Prostaglandins* **27**:821–838.

Soloff, M. S., and Alexandrova, M., 1981, Parturition, lactation and the regulation of oxytocin receptors, in: *Reproductive Processes and Contraception* (K. W. McKerns, ed.), Plenum Press, New York, pp. 281–303.

Soloff, M. S., and Grzonka, Z., 1986, Effects of manganese on relative affinities of receptors for oxytocin analogues. Binding studies with rat myometrial and mammary gland membranes, *Endocrinology* **119**:1564–1569.

Soloff, M. S., and Swartz, T. L., 1974, Characterization of a proposed oxytocin receptor in the uterus of the rat and sow, *J. Biol. Chem.* **249**:1376–1381.

Soloff, M. S., and Sweet, P., 1982, Oxytocin inhibition of $(Ca^{2+} + Mg^{2+})$ATPase activity in rat myometrial plasma membranes, *J. Biol. Chem.* **257**:10687–10693.

Soloff, M. S., Alexandrova, M., and Fernstrom, M. J., 1979, Oxytocin receptors: Triggers for parturition and lactation? *Science* **204**:1313–1315.

Soloff, M. S., Fernström, M. A., Periyasamy, S., Soloff, S., Baldwin, S., and Wieder, M., 1983, Regulation of oxytocin receptor concentration in rat uterine explants by estrogen and progesterone, *Can. J. Biochem. Cell Biol.* **61**:625–630.

Spellacy, W. N., Cruz, A. C., Birk, S. A., and Buhi, W. C., 1979, Treatment of premature labor with ritodrine: A randomized controlled study, *Obstet. Gynecol.* **54**:220–223.

Speroff, L., Caldwell, B. V., Brock, W. A., Anderson, G. G., and Hobbins, J. C., 1972, Hormone levels during prostaglandin $F_{2\alpha}$ infusions for therapeutic abortion, *J. Clin. Endocrinol. Metab.* **34**:531–536.

Strauss, J. F. III, and Stambaugh, R. L., 1974, Induction of 20α-hydroxysteroid dehydrogenase in rat corpora lutea of pregnancy by prostaglandin $F_{2\alpha}$ *Prostaglandins* **5**:73–85.

Strauss, J. F. III, Sokoloski, J., Caploe, P., Duffy, P., Mintz, G., and Stambaugh, R. L., 1975, On the role of prostaglandins in parturition in the rat, *Endocrinology* **96**:1040–1043.

Strickland, D. M., Saeed, S. A., Casey, M. L., and Mitchell, M. D., 1983, Stimulation of prostaglandin biosynthesis by urine of the human fetus may serve as a trigger for parturition, *Science* **220**:521–522.

Stys, S. J., 1986, Endocrine regulation of cervical functions during pregnancy, in: *The Physiology and Biochemistry of the Uterus in Pregnancy and Labor* (G. Huszar, ed.), CRC Press, Boca Raton, FL, pp. 281–295.

Summerlee, A. J. S., O'Byrne, K. T., Paisley, A. C., Breeze, M. F., and Porter, D. G., 1984, Relaxin affects the central control of oxytocin release, *Nature* **309**:372–374.

Szlachter, N., O'Byrne, E., Goldsmith, L., Steinetz, B. G., and Weiss, G., 1980, Myometrial inhibiting activity of relaxin-containing extracts of human corpora lutea of pregnancy, *Am. J. Obstet. Gynecol.* **136**:584–586.

Takahashi, K., Diamond, F., Bieniarz, J., Yen, H., and Burd, L., 1980, Uterine contractility and oxytocin sensitivity in preterm, term, and postterm pregnancy, *Am. J. Obstet. Gynecol.* **136**:774–779.

Tansey, T. R., and Padykula, H. A., 1978, Cellular responses to experimental inhibition of collagen degradation in the postpartum rat uterus, *Anat. Rec.* **191**:287–309.

Taylor, M. J., Webb, R., Mitchell, M. D., and Robinson, J. S., 1982, Effect of progesterone withdrawal in sheep during late pregnancy, *J. Endocrinol.* **92**:85–93.

Tetta, C., Montrucchio, G., Alloatti, G., Roffinello, C., Emanuelli, G., Benedetto, C., Camussi, G., and Massobrio, M., 1986, Platelet-activating factor contracts human myometrium *in vitro, Proc. Soc. Exp. Biol. Med.* **183**:376–381.

Theobald, G. W., 1959, The choice between death from postmaturity or prolapsed cord and life from induction of labour, *Lancet* **1**:59–65.

Theobald, P. W., Rath, W., Kühnle, H.,and Kuhn, W., 1982, Histologic and electron-microscopic examinations of collagenous connective tissue of the non-pregnant cervix, the pregnant cervix, and the pregnant prostaglandin-treated cervix, *Arch. Gynecol.* **231**:241–245.

Thorbert, G., 1978, Regional changes in structure and function of adrenergic nerves in guinea-pig uterus during pregnancy, *Acta Obstet. Gynecol. Scand. [Suppl.]* **79**:1–32.

Thorbert, G., Alm, P., Björklund, A. B., Owman, C., and Sjöberg, N.-O., 1979, Adrenergic innervation of the human uterus: Disappearance of the transmitter and transmitter-forming enzymes during pregnancy, *Am. J. Obstet. Gynecol.* **135**:223–226.

Thorburn, G. D., and Challis, J. R. G., 1979, Endocrine control of parturition, *Physiol. Rev.* **59**:863–918.

Thorburn, G. D., Challis, J. R. G., and Robinson, J. S., 1977, Endocrine control of parturition, in: *Biology of the Uterus* (R. M. Wynn, ed.), Plenum Press, New York, pp. 653–732.

Touqui, L., Rothhut, B., Shaw, A. M., Fradin, A., Vargaftig, B. B., and Russo-Marie, F., 1986, Platelet activation—a role for a 40K anti-phospholipase A_2 protein indistinguishable from lipocortin, *Nature* **321**:177–180.

Ulmsten, U., Andersson, K.-E., and Wingerup, L., 1980, Treatment of premature labor with the calcium antagonist nifedipine, *Arch. Gynecol.* **229**:1–5.

Valentine, B. H., 1977, Intravenous oxytocin and oral prostaglandin E_2 for ripening of the unfavourable cervix, *Br. J. Obstet. Gynecol.* **84**:846–854.

Vane, J. R., and Williams, K. I., 1972, Prostaglandin production contributes to the contractions of the rat isolated uterus, *Br. J. Pharmacol.* **45**:146P.

Vesin, M.-F., Khac, L. D., and Harbon, S., 1978, Modulation of intracellular adenosine cyclic $3',5'$-monophosphate and contractility of rat uterus by prostaglandins and polyunsaturated fatty acids, *Mol. Pharmacol.* **14**:24–37.

Vu Hai, M. T., Logeat, F., Warembourg, M., and Milgrom, E., 1977, Hormonal control of progesterone receptors, *Ann. N.Y. Acad. Sci.* **286**:199–209.

Wahl, L. M., Blandau, R. J., and Page, R. C., 1977, Effect of hormones on collagen metabolism and collagenase activity in the pubic symphysis ligament of the guinea pig, *Endocrinology* **100**:571–579.

Wallner, B. P., Mattaliano, R. J., Hession, C., Cate, R. L., Tizard, R., Sinclair, L. K., Foeller, C., Chow, E. P., Browning, J. L., Ramachandran, K. L., and Pepinsky, R. B., 1986, Cloning and expression of human lipocortin, a phospholipase A_2 inhibitor with potential anti-inflammatory activity, *Nature* **320**:77–81.

Walsh, S. W., Kittinger, G. W., and Novy, M. J., 1979a, Maternal peripheral concentrations of estradiol, estrone, cortisol, and progesterone during late pregnancy in rhesus monkeys (*Macaca mulatta*) and after experimental fetal anencephaly and fetal death, *Am. J. Obstet. Gynecol.* **135**:37–42.

Walsh, S. W., Norman, R. L., and Novy, M. J., 1979b, *In utero* regulation of rhesus monkey fetal adrenals: Effects of dexamethasone, adrenocorticotropin, thyrotropin-releasing hormone, prolactin, human chorionic gonadotropin, and α-melanocyte-stimulating hormone on fetal and maternal plasma steroids, *Endocrinology* **104**:1805–1813.

Walsh, S. W., Resko, J. A., Grumbach, M. M., and Novy, M. J., 1980 *In utero* evidence for a functional fetoplacental unit in rhesus monkeys, *Biol. Reprod.* **23**:264–270.

Waltman, R., Tricomi, V., and Palav, A., 1973, Aspirin and indomethacin: Effect on instillation/abortion time on mid-trimester hypertonic saline induced abortion, *Prostaglandins* **3**:47–58.

Warnock, D. H., and Csapo, A. I., 1975, Progesterone withdrawal induced by ICI 81008 in pregnant rats, *Prostaglandins* **10**:715–724.

Warrick, C., Skinner, K., Mitchell, B. F., and Challis, J. R. G., 1985, Relation between cyclic adenosine monophosphate and prostaglandin output by dispersed cells from human amnion and decidua, *Am. J. Obstet. Gynecol.* **153**:66–71.

Wiegerinck, M. A. H. M., Poortman, J., Donker, T. H., and Thijssen, J. H. H., 1983, *In vivo* uptake and subcellular distribution of tritium-labeled estrogens in human endometrium, myometrium, and vagina, *J. Clin. Endocrinol. Metab.* **56:**76–86.

Wiest, W. G., Kidwell, W. R., and Balogh, K., Jr., 1968, Progesterone catabolism in the rat ovary: A regulatory mechanism for progestational protency during pregnancy, *Endocrinology* **82:**844–859.

Wikland, M., Lindblom, B., Hammarström, S., and Wiqvist, N., 1983, The effect of prostaglandin I_2 on the contractility of the term pregnant human myometrium, *Prostaglandins* **26:**905–916.

Wilhelmsson, L., Wikland, M., and Wiqvist, N., 1981, PGH_2, TXA_2 and PGI_2 have potent and differentiated actions on human uterine contractility, *Prostaglandins* **21:**277–286.

Williams, K. I., Dembinska-Kiec, A., Zmuda, A., and Gryglewski, R. J., 1978, Prostacyclin formation by myometrial and decidual fractions of the pregnant rat uterus, *Prostaglandins* **15:**343–350.

Williams, K. I., El-Tahir, K. E. H., and Marcinkiewicz, E., 1979, Dual actions of prostacyclin (PGI_2) on the rat pregnant uterus, *Prostaglandins* **17:**667–672.

Williams, L. T., and Lefkowitz, R. J., 1977, Regulation of rabbit myometrial alpha adrenergic receptors by estrogen and progesterone, *J. Clin. Invest.* **60:**815–818.

Willman, E. A., and Collins, W. P., 1978, The metabolism of prostaglandin E_2 by tissues from the human uterus and foeto-placental unit, *Acta Endocrinol. (Kbh).* **87:**632–642.

Wiqvist, N., Lundström, V., and Gréen, K., 1985, Premature labor and indomethacin, *Prostaglandins* **10:**515–526.

Wlodawer, P., Kindahl, H., and Hamberg, M., 1976, Biosynthesis of prostaglandin $F_{2\alpha}$ from arachidonic acid and prostaglandin endoperoxides in the uterus, *Biochim. Biophys. Acta* **431:**603–614.

Wolf, B. A., Turk, J., Sherman, W. R., and McDaniel, M. L., 1986, Intracellular Ca^{2+} mobilization by arachidonic acid, *J. Biol. Chem.* **261:**3501–3511.

Zarrow, M. X., Anderson, N. C., and Callantine, M. R., 1963, Failure of progesterone to prolong pregnancy in the guinea pig, *Nature* **198:**690–692.

Zeitler, P., and Handwerger, S., 1985, Arachidonic acid stimulates phosphoinositol hydrolysis and human placental lactogen release in an enriched fraction of placental cells, *Mol. Pharmacol.* **28:**549–554.

Zuckerman, H., Reiss, U., and Rubinstein, I., 1974, Inhibition of human premature labor by indomethacin, *Obstet. Gynecol.* **44:**787–792.

Index